Coding for Pediatrics 2019

A Manual for Pediatric Documentation and Payment

For Use With AMA CPT® 2019

24th Edition

Author
Committee on Coding and Nomenclature (COCN)
American Academy of Pediatrics

Linda D. Parsi, MD, MBA, CPEDC, FAAP, Editor

Cindy Hughes, CPC, CFPC, Consulting Editor
Becky Dolan, MPH, CPC, CPEDC, Staff Editor

American Academy of Pediatrics

DEDICATED TO THE HEALTH OF ALL CHILDREN®

American Academy of Pediatrics Publishing Staff

Mary Lou White, *Chief Product and Services Officer/SVP, Membership, Marketing, and Publishing*

Mark Grimes, *Vice President, Department of Publishing*

Barrett Winston, *Senior Manager, Publishing Acquisitions and Business Development*

Mary Kelly, *Senior Editor, Professional/Clinical Publishing*

Leesa Levin-Doroba, *Production Manager, Practice Management*

Jason Crase, *Manager, Editorial Services*

Peg Mulcahy, *Manager, Art Direction and Production*

Mary Jo Reynolds, *Marketing Manager, Practice Publications*

Published by the American Academy of Pediatrics
345 Park Blvd
Itasca, IL 60143
Telephone: 630/626-6000
Facsimile: 847/434-8000
www.aap.org

The American Academy of Pediatrics is an organization of 67,000 primary care pediatricians, pediatric medical subspecialists, and pediatric surgical specialists dedicated to the health, safety, and well-being of infants, children, adolescents, and young adults.

While every effort has been made to ensure the accuracy of this publication, the American Academy of Pediatrics (AAP) does not guarantee that it is accurate, complete, or without error.

The recommendations in this publication do not indicate an exclusive course of treatment or serve as a standard of medical care. Variations, taking into account individual circumstances, may be appropriate. Vignettes are provided to illustrate correct coding applications and are not intended to offer advice on the practice of medicine.

Products and Web sites are included for informational purposes only. Inclusion in this publication does not imply endorsement. The American Academy of Pediatrics does not recommend any specific brand of products or services.

This publication has been developed by the American Academy of Pediatrics. The contributors are expert authorities in the field of pediatrics. No commercial involvement of any kind has been solicited or accepted in development of the content of this publication.

Special discounts are available for bulk purchases of this publication. E-mail Special Sales at aapsales@aap.org for more information.

CPT® copyright 2018 American Medical Association (AMA). All rights reserved.

Fee schedules, relative value units, conversion factors, and/or related components are not assigned by the AMA, are not part of *CPT*, and the AMA is not recommending their use. The AMA does not directly or indirectly practice medicine or dispense medical services. The AMA assumes no liability for data contained or not contained herein.

CPT® is a registered trademark of the AMA.

This publication has prior approval of the American Academy of Professional Coders (AAPC) for 4.0 continuing education units. Granting of this approval in no way constitutes endorsement by AAPC of the publication content or publication sponsor.

11-35M   1 2 3 4 5 6 7 8 9 10

MA0875
ISBN: 978-1-61002-203-3
eBook: 978-1-61002-204-0
ISSN: 1537-324X

Disclaimer

||||ı||ı||ı

Every effort has been made to include the new and revised 2019 *Current Procedural Terminology (CPT®)*; *International Classification of Diseases, 10th Revision, Clinical Modification (ICD-10-CM)*; and Healthcare Common Procedure Coding System (HCPCS) codes, their respective guidelines, and other revisions that might have been made. Due to our publishing deadlines and the publication date of the American Medical Association *CPT*, additional revisions and/or additional codes may have been published subsequent to the date of this printing. It is the responsibility of the reader to use this manual as a companion to the *CPT, ICD-10-CM,* and HCPCS publications. Vignettes are provided throughout this publication to illustrate correct coding applications. They are not intended to offer medical advice on the practice of medicine. Further, it is the reader's responsibility to access the American Academy of Pediatrics Web site (www.aap.org/cfp) routinely to find any corrections due to errata in the published version.

Copyright Acknowledgment

Current Procedural Terminology (*CPT*®) is a listing of descriptive terms and 5-digit numeric identifying codes and modifiers for reporting medical services and procedures performed by physicians. This presentation includes only the *CPT* descriptive terms, numeric identifying codes, and modifiers for reporting medical services and procedures that were selected by the American Academy of Pediatrics (AAP) for inclusion in this publication. The inclusion of a *CPT* service or procedure description and its code number in this publication does not restrict its use to a particular specialty group. Any procedure or service in this publication may be used to report the services provided by any qualified physician or, when appropriate, other qualified health care professional.

The American Medical Association (AMA) and the AAP assume no responsibility for the consequences attributable to or related to any use or interpretation of any information or views contained in or not contained in this publication.

Any 5-digit numeric *CPT* code, service descriptions, instructions, and/or guidelines are copyright 2018 (or such other date of publication of *CPT* as defined in the federal copyright laws) AMA. All rights reserved.

The most current *CPT* is available from the AMA.

No fee schedules, basic unit values, relative value guides, conversion factors or scales, or components thereof are included in *CPT*.

Contents

|||ᵢ|||||ᵢ|

Foreword

The American Academy of Pediatrics (AAP) is pleased to publish this, the 24th edition of *Coding for Pediatrics*—an instructional manual and reference tool for use by primary care pediatricians, pediatric subspecialists, and others involved in the provision of care to children. The purpose of this manual is to support the delivery of quality care to children by providing the pediatric practitioner with the knowledge to best support appropriate business practices. Many changes have been made to this edition, including updating the 2019 *Current Procedural Terminology* (*CPT®*) codes and update of *International Classification of Diseases, 10th Revision, Clinical Modification* (*ICD-10-CM*) codes with guidelines for their application. A quick reference to new procedure codes is provided to assist with updating of other coding references (eg, superbills) and to alert readers to changes that may be of most interest to their practice.

With a focus on creating ease of reference, *Coding for Pediatrics 2019* is divided into the following parts:

1. The Quick References include all new and revised *CPT* and *ICD-10-CM* codes applicable to pediatrics. They also identify codes that have deleted for 2019.
2. Coding Basics and Business Essentials includes information on code sets, compliance, and business topics such as billing and payment methodologies.
3. Primarily for the Office and Other Outpatient Settings includes information on coding and billing of services such as office visits, outpatient consultations, and preventive services.
4. Primarily for Hospital Settings includes information on coding for inpatient and observation services, including newborn care and surgical procedures.
5. Digital Medicine Services includes discussion of coding for telemedicine services, remote monitoring and interpretation, and other services provided via digital technology.
6. The American Academy of Professional Coders continuing education quiz gives readers the chance to earn 4.0 continuing education units.
7. The appendixes include worksheets for chronic and complex patient management and vaccine coding information.

As in previous years, the AAP is also pleased to continue to offer *Coding for Pediatrics 2019* as an eBook.

Any corrections that may be necessary subsequent to the publication of the manual will be available to readers of *Coding for Pediatrics 2019* by accessing www.aap.org/cfp. *Coding for Pediatrics 2019* does not replace *CPT, ICD-10-CM,* or the Healthcare Common Procedure Coding System; rather, it supplements those manuals. Every effort has been made to include the 2019 codes and their respective guidelines; however, revised codes and/or guidelines may have been published subsequent to the date of this printing. Updates to this manual will be posted as appropriate on the *Coding for Pediatrics* Web site (www.aap.org/cfp).

The AAP actively works with the American Medical Association (AMA) *CPT* Editorial Panel and the AMA/Specialty Society Relative Value Scale Update Committee (RUC) to develop pediatric specialty codes and assign them appropriate relative value units. Since 1995, the AAP has contributed to the process that evaluates and reviews changes to the Medicare Resource-Based Relative Value Scale (RBRVS). Pediatricians have been actively involved in the AMA RUC Practice Expense Review Committee to review direct practice expenses for all existing codes. As importantly, the AAP is represented on the AMA *CPT* Editorial Advisory Panel and on the *ICD-10-CM* Editorial Advisory Board. The AAP continues to be involved in all areas of payment. The AAP Committee on Coding and Nomenclature oversees all areas of coding as they relate to pediatrics, including *CPT* procedure coding, *ICD-10-CM* diagnosis coding, and the valuation of *CPT* services through the Medicare RBRVS.

The AAP will continue to request new code changes and attempt to expeditiously notify membership of changes through various means. *AAP Pediatric Coding Newsletter*™—a monthly newsletter available in print and online—provides members and their office personnel with up-to-date coding and payment information. The newsletter and other online resources can be accessed through the AAP newsletter Web site (http://coding.aap.org). Other resources include coding seminars presented at the AAP National Conference & Exhibition; webinars sponsored by the AAP (www.aap.org/webinars/coding); instructional materials in *AAP News,* including the

Coding Corner; *Pediatric ICD-10-CM: A Manual for Provider-Based Coding;* and various quick reference cards. The use of these resources should provide pediatricians with the skills needed to report their services appropriately. The AAP Health Care Financing Strategy staff at the AAP headquarters stands ready to assist with coding problems and questions not covered in this manual. The AAP Coding Hotline can be accessed through e-mail at aapcodinghotline@aap.org.

Acknowledgments

Coding for Pediatrics 2019, 24th Edition, is the product of the efforts of many dedicated individuals.

Our mission is to make coding easier to understand so that pediatric providers can continue to serve children well. We have strived to make this book easier to understand by categorizing areas and by using many examples (vignettes) of different coding situations. This knowledge is key to help all pediatric providers stay in compliance and correctly code with confidence. We hope you enjoy reading this book, and we will continue to strive to make this easier to serve you always with excellence.

This work has been made immeasurably easier and the final edition dramatically improved by the dedicated work of many collaborators. First and foremost, I must thank Cindy Hughes, CPC, CFPC, consulting editor, for her professional input. Additionally, I must thank the Committee on Coding and Nomenclature (COCN) support staff at the American Academy of Pediatrics (AAP), particularly Becky Dolan, MPH, CPC, CPEDC, staff editor, for her many excellent suggestions as well as for reviewing major portions of the project. Thank you also to Teri Salus, MPA, CPC, CPEDC, for her review of new *Current Procedural Terminology* (*CPT®*) codes and suggestions for changes to content. I would also like to thank the members of COCN and the AAP Coding Publications Editorial Advisory Board. The members of these committees have each contributed extensive time in reviewing and updating content of the manual. We want to especially thank the following reviewers:

Vita Boyar, MD, FAAP
David M. Kanter, MD, MBA, CPC, FAAP
Steven E. Krug, MD, FAAP
Edward A. Liechty, MD, FAAP
Jeffrey F. Linzer Sr, MD, FAAP
Jeanne Marconi, MD, FAAP
Richard A. Molteni, MD, FAAP
Renee F. Slade, MD, FAAP
Sanjeev Y. Tuli, MD, FAAP
Lynn Wegner, MD, FAAP

None of this work is possible without the support of the COCN members who work tirelessly to develop and value codes and fight for pediatrics "at the table." The committee strives to keep pediatrics at the forefront of coding and valuation. The excellent teams listed as follows are truly experts in these areas and are devoted to representing the AAP and its members:

CPT **Team**
Joel F. Bradley, MD, FAAP (*CPT* Advisor)
David M. Kanter, MD, MBA, CPC, FAAP (*CPT* Alternate Advisor)
Teri Salus, MPA, CPC, CPEDC (AAP Staff to *CPT*)

American Medical Association/Specialty Society Relative Value Scale Update Committee (RUC) Team
Steven E. Krug, MD, FAAP (RUC Advisor)
Margie C. Andreae, MD, FAAP (RUC Representative)
Eileen D. Brewer, MD, FAAP (RUC Alternate Representative)
Linda Walsh, MAB (AAP Staff to RUC)

International Classification of Diseases (*ICD*) **Team**
Jeffrey F. Linzer Sr, MD, FAAP (AAP Representative to *ICD*)
Edward A. Liechty, MD, FAAP (AAP Alternate Representative to *ICD*)
Becky Dolan, MPH, CPC, CPEDC (AAP Staff to *ICD*)

I am most grateful to the invaluable input of the following AAP committees and individuals: the Committee on Medical Liability and Risk Management, specifically James P. Scibilia, MD, FAAP, and AAP staff Julie Ake, senior health policy analyst; the Private Payer Advocacy Advisory Committee, specifically Sue Kressly, MD, FAAP, and AAP staff Lou Terranova, senior health policy analyst; the Section on Telehealth Care, specifically

Peter Dehnel, MD, FAAP; and the Section on Neonatal-Perinatal Medicine coding trainers. In addition, we reached out to other AAP members for their expertise on specific content areas. A special thank you to Mary Landrigan-Ossar, MD, FAAP, for her assistance with the anesthesia chapter and Suzanne Berman, MD, FAAP, for her assistance with the coding continuum.

This project would not have been completed were it not for the outstanding work of AAP staff. In Membership, Marketing, and Publishing, Barrett Winston, senior manager, publishing acquisitions and business development; Mary Kelly, senior editor, professional/clinical publishing; Jason Crase, manager, editorial services; Peg Mulcahy, manager, art direction and production; Leesa Levin-Doroba, production manager, practice management; and Mary Jo Reynolds, marketing manager, practice publications, deserve special recognition for their outstanding skill and dedication to this project. At the AAP, I am especially appreciative of the support and professional expertise of Linda Walsh, MAB, director, and AAP staff support to the AAP COCN, dedicated advocates for all of us who provide medical care to children. A special thank-you to our AAP Board of Directors reviewer, Richard Tuck, MD, FAAP. Dr Tuck is a former COCN member and is an expert on this topic. We are so grateful to have his leadership and review for this manual!

Finally, we all would like to give a big thank-you to all our readers, billers, coders, medical team, and dedicated pediatric providers who work tirelessly around the clock to provide the best care to all children. Your work inspires us to work very hard behind the scenes to provide you the latest and most accurate coding information. By all of us working together, we can accomplish the highest standards of care for our future.

Linda D. Parsi, MD, MBA, CPEDC, FAAP
Editor

Quick Reference to 2019 *ICD-10-CM* Pediatric Code Changes

We have made every effort to include those diagnosis code changes that are applicable to pediatric practices. However, revisions and/or additional codes may have been published subsequent to the date of this printing. This list does not include all changes made to *International Classification of Diseases, 10th Revision, Clinical Modification (ICD-10-CM)*. Refer to your 2019 *ICD-10-CM* coding reference (eg, manual, data files) for a complete listing of new and revised codes, complete descriptions, and instructions for reporting. Codes are valid October 1, 2018. Topics for update for 2019 include

Quick Reference to 2019 *ICD-10-CM* Pediatric Code Changes	
Topic	**2019 *ICD-10-CM* Codes**
Alkalosis of newborn	**P74.41** Alkalosis of newborn
Appendicitis	**K35.20** Acute appendicitis with generalized peritonitis, without abscess
	K35.21 Acute appendicitis with generalized peritonitis, with abscess
	K35.30 Acute appendicitis with localized peritonitis, without perforation or gangrene
	K35.31 Acute appendicitis with localized peritonitis and gangrene, without perforation
	K35.32 Acute appendicitis with perforation and localized peritonitis, without abscess
	K35.33 Acute appendicitis with perforation and localized peritonitis, with abscess
	K35.890 Other acute appendicitis without perforation or gangrene
	K35.891 Other acute appendicitis without perforation, with gangrene
Cannabis dependence	**F12.23** Cannabis dependence with withdrawal
	F12.93 Cannabis use, unspecified, with withdrawal
Congenital Zika virus disease	**P35.4** Congenital Zika virus disease
Ecstasy poisoning	**T43.641A** Poisoning by ecstasy, accidental (unintentional), initial encounter **T43.641D** Poisoning by ecstasy, accidental (unintentional), subsequent encounter **T43.641S** Poisoning by ecstasy, accidental (unintentional), sequela
	T43.642A Poisoning by ecstasy, intentional self-harm, initial encounter **T43.642D** Poisoning by ecstasy, intentional self-harm, subsequent encounter **T43.642S** Poisoning by ecstasy, intentional self-harm, sequela
	T43.643A Poisoning by ecstasy, assault, initial encounter **T43.643D** Poisoning by ecstasy, assault, subsequent encounter **T43.643S** Poisoning by ecstasy, assault, sequela
	T43.644A Poisoning by ecstasy, undetermined, initial encounter **T43.644D** Poisoning by ecstasy, undetermined, subsequent encounter **T43.644S** Poisoning by ecstasy, undetermined, sequela
Factitious disorder	**F68.A** Factitious disorder imposed on another **F68.10** Factitious disorder, imposed on self, unspecified **F68.11** Factitious disorder imposed on self, with predominantly psychological signs and symptoms **F68.12** Factitious disorder imposed on self, with predominantly physical signs and symptoms **F68.13** Factitious disorder imposed on self, with combined psychological and physical signs and symptoms

Quick Reference to 2019 *ICD-10-CM* Pediatric Code Changes (*continued*)	
Topic	**2019 *ICD-10-CM* Codes**
Family history of elevated lipoprotein(a)	**Z83.430** Family history of elevated lipoprotein(a) **Z83.438** Family history of other disorder of lipoprotein metabolism and other lipidemia
Fetal inflammatory response syndrome (newborn)	**P02.70** Newborn affected by fetal inflammatory response syndrome
Hyperchloremia of newborn	**P74.421** Hyperchloremia of newborn
Hyperkalemia of newborn	**P74.31** Hyperkalemia of newborn
Hyperlipidemia	**E78.41** Elevated lipoprotein(a) **E78.49** Other hyperlipidemia
Hypernatremia of newborn	**P74.21** Hypernatremia of newborn
Hypochloremia of newborn	**P74.422** Hypochloremia of newborn
Hypokalemia of newborn	**P74.32** Hypokalemia of newborn
Hyponatremia of newborn	**P74.22** Hyponatremia of newborn
Immunization not carried out due to unavailability of vaccine	**Z28.83** Immunization not carried out due to unavailability of vaccine
Infection following a procedure	**T81.40XA** Infection following a procedure, unspecified, initial encounter **T81.40XD** Infection following a procedure, unspecified, subsequent encounter **T81.40XS** Infection following a procedure, unspecified, sequela
	T81.41XA Infection following a procedure, superficial incisional surgical site, initial encounter **T81.41XD** Infection following a procedure, superficial incisional surgical site, subsequent encounter **T81.41XS** Infection following a procedure, superficial incisional surgical site, sequela
	T81.42XA Infection following a procedure, deep incisional surgical site, initial encounter **T81.42XD** Infection following a procedure, deep incisional surgical site, subsequent encounter **T81.42XS** Infection following a procedure, deep incisional surgical site, sequela
	T81.43XA Infection following a procedure, organ and space surgical site, initial encounter **T81.43XD** Infection following a procedure, organ and space surgical site, subsequent encounter **T81.43XS** Infection following a procedure, organ and space surgical site, sequela
	T81.44XA Sepsis following a procedure, initial encounter **T81.44XD** Sepsis following a procedure, subsequent encounter **T81.44XS** Sepsis following a procedure, sequela

Quick Reference to 2019 *ICD-10-CM* Pediatric Code Changes (*continued*)

Topic	2019 *ICD-10-CM* Codes
Infection following a procedure (*continued*)	**T81.49XA** Infection following a procedure, other surgical site, initial encounter **T81.49XD** Infection following a procedure, other surgical site, subsequent encounter **T81.49XS** Infection following a procedure, other surgical site, sequela
Lipoprotein	**E78.41** Elevated lipoprotein(a)
Muscular dystrophy	**G71.00** Muscular dystrophy, unspecified **G71.01** Duchenne or Becker muscular dystrophy **G71.02** Facioscapulohumeral muscular dystrophy **G71.09** Other specified muscular dystrophies
Newborn affected by fetal inflammatory response syndrome	**P02.70** Newborn affected by fetal inflammatory response syndrome
Newborn affected by maternal medication	**P04.11** Newborn affected by maternal antineoplastic chemotherapy **P04.12** Newborn affected by maternal cytotoxic drugs **P04.13** Newborn affected by maternal use of anticonvulsants **P04.14** Newborn affected by maternal use of opiates **P04.15** Newborn affected by maternal use of antidepressants **P04.16** Newborn affected by maternal use of amphetamines **P04.17** Newborn affected by maternal use of sedative-hypnotics **P04.18** Newborn affected by other maternal medication **P04.19** Newborn affected by maternal use of unspecified medication **P04.1A** Newborn affected by maternal use of anxiolytics
Newborn affected by maternal use of cannabis	**P04.81** Newborn affected by maternal use of cannabis
Newborn affected by maternal use of drugs of addiction	**P04.40** Newborn affected by maternal use of unspecified drugs of addiction **P04.42** Newborn affected by maternal use of hallucinogens
Plasminogen deficiency	**E88.02** Plasminogen deficiency
Postpartum depression (for use on mother)	**Z13.32** Encounter for screening for maternal depression
Screening for	**Z13.30** Encounter for screening examination for mental health and behavioral disorders, unspecified **Z13.31** Encounter for screening for depression **Z13.32** Encounter for screening for maternal depression (For use on maternal record only) **Z13.39** Encounter for screening examination for other mental health and behavioral disorders **Z13.40** Encounter for screening for unspecified developmental delays **Z13.41** Encounter for autism screening **Z13.42** Encounter for screening for global developmental delays (milestones)
Sulfatase deficiency	**E75.26** Sulfatase deficiency
Transitory electrolyte disturbance of newborn	**P74.49** Other transitory electrolyte disturbance of newborn

Quick Reference to 2019 *ICD-10-CM* Pediatric Code Changes (*continued*)	
Topic	**2019 *ICD-10-CM* Codes**
Williams syndrome	Q93.82 Williams syndrome
Zika exposure	Z20.821 Contact with and (suspected) exposure to Zika virus

Quick Reference to 2019 *CPT*® Pediatric Code Changes

We have made every effort to include those procedures and services that are applicable to pediatric practices. However, revisions and/or additional codes may have been published subsequent to the date of this printing. This list does not include all changes made to *Current Procedural Terminology* (*CPT*®) *2019*. Always refer to *CPT 2019* for a complete listing of new codes, complete descriptions, and revisions. Any errata to *CPT 2019* will be posted to the American Medial Association Web site, https://www.ama-assn.org/practice-management/errata-technical-corrections. These changes take effect January 1, 2019. Do not report the changes or codes prior to that.

Quick Reference to 2019 *CPT*® Pediatric Code Changes

Evaluation and Management

2018	2019
99487–99490 Physician time may be included to support reporting of chronic care management services, but these codes were valued based on time of clinical staff.	#●99491 Chronic care management services, provided personally by a physician or other qualified health care professional, at least 30 minutes of physician or other qualified health care professional time, per calendar month, with the following required elements: multiple (two or more) chronic conditions expected to last at least 12 months, or until the death of the patient, chronic conditions place the patient at significant risk of death, acute exacerbation/decompensation, or functional decline; comprehensive care plan established, implemented, revised, or monitored *(See Chapter 12, Managing Chronic and Complex Conditions.)*
*0188T Remote real-time interactive video-conferenced critical care, evaluation and management of the critically ill or critically injured patient; first 30–74 minutes *+0189T each additional 30 minutes	No codes *(See Chapter 18, Critical and Intensive Care, and Chapter 20, Digital Medicine Services: Technology-Enhanced Care Delivery.)*
99446 Interprofessional telephone/Internet/electronic health record assessment and management service provided by a consultative physician including a verbal and written report to the patient's treating/requesting physician/qualified health care professional; 5–10 minutes of medical consultative discussion and review 99447 11–20 minutes of medical consultative discussion and review 99448 21–30 minutes of medical consultative discussion and review 99449 31 minutes or more of medical consultative discussion and review	▲99446 Interprofessional telephone/Internet/electronic health record assessment and management service provided by a consultative physician including a verbal and written report to the patient's treating/requesting physician/qualified health care professional; 5–10 minutes of medical consultative discussion and review ▲99447 11–20 minutes of medical consultative discussion and review ▲99448 21–30 minutes of medical consultative discussion and review ▲99449 31 minutes or more of medical consultative discussion and review #●99451 Interprofessional telephone/Internet/electronic health record assessment and management service provided by a consultative physician including a written report to the patient's treating/requesting physician/qualified health care professional; 5 or more minutes of medical consultative time #●99452 Interprofessional telephone/Internet/electronic health record referral service(s) provided by a treating/requesting physician/qualified health care professional; 30 minutes *(See Chapter 20, Digital Medicine Services: Technology-Enhanced Care Delivery.)*

Refer to **Table 1-4** for full details. #, re-sequenced code; ●, new code; +, add-on code; ▲, revised code; ★, telemedicine code; *, deleted code for 2019.

Quick Reference to 2019 *CPT* Pediatric Code Changes (*continued*)

Evaluation and Management (continued)

2018	2019
Medicine **Special Services, Procedures and Reports** **Miscellaneous Services** **99090* Analysis of clinical data stored in computers (eg, ECGs, blood pressures, hematologic data) *Deleted from Medicine section and moved to Evaluation and Management section* **99091** Collection and interpretation of physiologic data (eg, ECG, blood pressure, glucose monitoring) digitally stored and/or transmitted by the patient and/or caregiver to the physician or other qualified health care professional, qualified by education, training, licensure/regulation (when applicable) requiring a minimum of 30 minutes of time	**Evaluation and Management** **Non–Face-to-Face Services** **Digitally Stored Data Services/Remote Physiologic Monitoring** #●99453 Remote monitoring of physiologic parameter(s) (eg, weight, blood pressure, pulse oximetry, respiratory flow rate), initial; set-up and patient education on use of equipment #●99454 device(s) supply with daily recording(s) or programmed alert(s) transmission, each 30 days #▲99091 Collection and interpretation of physiologic data (eg, ECG, blood pressure, glucose monitoring) digitally stored and/or transmitted by the patient and/or caregiver to the physician or other qualified health care professional, qualified by education, training, licensure/regulation (when applicable) requiring a minimum of 30 minutes of time, each 30 days **Remote Physiologic Monitoring Treatment Management Services** #●99457 Remote physiologic monitoring treatment management services, 20 minutes or more of clinical staff/physician/other qualified health care professional time in a calendar month requiring interactive communication with the patient/caregiver during the month *(See Chapter 12, Managing Chronic and Complex Conditions, and Chapter 20, Digital Medicine Services: Technology-Enhanced Care Delivery.)*

Musculoskeletal System

*20005 Incision and drainage of soft tissue abscess, subfascial (ie, involves the soft tissue below the deep fascia)	**20005** has been deleted. For incision and drainage of subfascial soft tissue abscess, see appropriate incision and drainage for specific anatomic sites (eg, 27603, incision and drainage, leg or ankle; deep abscess or hematoma).

Cardiovascular System

33411 Replacement, aortic valve; with aortic annulus enlargement, noncoronary sinus **33412** with transventricular aortic annulus enlargement (Konno procedure) **33413** by translocation of autologous pulmonary valve with allograft replacement of pulmonary valve (Ross procedure)	#●33440 Replacement, aortic valve; by translocation of autologous pulmonary valve and transventricular aortic annulus enlargement of the left ventricular outflow tract with valved conduit replacement of pulmonary valve (Ross-Konno procedure) ▲33411 with aortic annulus enlargement, noncoronary sinus ▲33412 with transventricular aortic annulus enlargement (Konno procedure) ▲33413 by translocation of autologous pulmonary valve with allograft replacement of pulmonary valve (Ross procedure) *(See Chapter 19, Common Surgical Procedures and Sedation in Facility Settings.)*

*Refer to **Table 1-4** for full details. #, re-sequenced code; ●, new code; +, add-on code; ▲, revised code; ★, telemedicine code; *, deleted code for 2019.*

Quick Reference to 2019 *CPT*® Pediatric Code Changes (*continued*)

Cardiovascular System (continued)

2018	2019
36568 Insertion of peripherally inserted central venous catheter (PICC), without subcutaneous port or pump; younger than 5 years of age 36569 age 5 years or older 36584 Replacement, complete, of a peripherally inserted central venous catheter (PICC), without subcutaneous port or pump, through same venous access	▲36568 Insertion of peripherally inserted central venous catheter (PICC), without subcutaneous port or pump, without imaging guidance; younger than 5 years of age ▲36569 age 5 years or older #●36572 Insertion of peripherally inserted central venous catheter (PICC), without subcutaneous port or pump, including all imaging guidance, image documentation, and all associated radiological supervision and interpretation required to perform the insertion; younger than 5 years of age #●36573 age 5 years or older ▲36584 Replacement, complete, of a peripherally inserted central venous catheter (PICC), without subcutaneous port or pump, through same venous access, including all imaging guidance, image documentation, and all associated radiological supervision and interpretation required to perform the replacement *(See Chapter 19, Common Surgical Procedures and Sedation in Facility Settings.)*

Digestive System

2018	2019
*43760 Change of gastrostomy tube, percutaneous, without imaging or endoscopic guidance	●43762 Replacement of gastrostomy tube, percutaneous, includes removal, when performed, without imaging or endoscopic guidance; not requiring revision of gastrostomy tract ●43763 requiring revision of gastrostomy tract *(See Chapter 19, Common Surgical Procedures and Sedation in Facility Settings.)*

Medicine Part 1

2018	2019
(Use 93568 in conjunction with 93451, 93453, 93456, 93457, 93460, 93461, 93530–93533)	(Use 93568 in conjunction with 93451, 93453, 93456, 93457, 93460, 93461, 93530–93533, 93582) The parenthetical for +93568 (injection procedure during cardiac catheterization including imaging supervision, interpretation, and report; for pulmonary angiography) is revised to include 93582 (percutaneous transcatheter closure of patent ductus arteriosus). *(See Chapter 19, Common Surgical Procedures and Sedation in Facility Settings.)*
94780 Car seat/bed testing for airway integrity, neonate, with continual nursing observation and continuous recording of pulse oximetry, heart rate and respiratory rate, with interpretation and report; 60 minutes +94781 each additional full 30 minutes	▲94780 Car seat/bed testing for airway integrity, for infants through 12 months of age, with continual clinical staff observation and continuous recording of pulse oximetry, heart rate and respiratory rate, with interpretation and report; 60 minutes +▲94781 each additional full 30 minutes *(See Chapter 18, Critical and Intensive Care.)*

*Refer to **Table 1-4** for full details. #, re-sequenced code; ●, new code; +, add-on code; ▲, revised code; ★, telemedicine code; *, deleted code for 2019.*

Quick Reference to 2019 *CPT*® Pediatric Code Changes (*continued*)

Medicine Part 2

2018	2019
*96111 Developmental testing (includes assessment of motor, language, social, adaptive, and/or cognitive functioning by standardized developmental instruments), with interpretation and report	●96112 Developmental test administration (including assessment of fine and/or gross motor, language, cognitive level, social, memory and/or executive functions by standardized developmental instruments when performed), by physician or other qualified health care professional, with interpretation and report; first hour +●96113 each additional 30 minutes (List separately in addition to code for primary procedure)
96125 Standardized cognitive performance testing (eg, Ross Information Processing Assessment) per hour of a qualified health care professional's time, both face-to-face time administering tests to the patient and time interpreting these test results and preparing the report	#96125 Standardized cognitive performance testing (eg, Ross Information Processing Assessment) per hour of a qualified health care professional's time, both face-to-face time administering tests to the patient and time interpreting these test results and preparing the report *(See Chapter 14, Mental and Behavioral Health Services.)*
96116 Neurobehavioral status exam (clinical assessment of thinking, reasoning and judgment, eg, acquired knowledge, attention, language, memory, planning and problem solving, and visual spatial abilities), per hour of the psychologist's or physician's time, both face-to-face time with the patient and time interpreting test results and preparing the report	★▲96116 Neurobehavioral status exam (clinical assessment of thinking, reasoning and judgment [eg, acquired knowledge, attention, language, memory, planning and problem solving, and visual spatial abilities]), by physician or other qualified health care professional, both face-to-face time with the patient and time interpreting test results and preparing the report; first hour +●96121 each additional hour *(See Chapter 14, Mental and Behavioral Health Services.)*
*96101 Psychological testing (includes psychodiagnostic assessment of emotionality, intellectual abilities, personality and psychopathology, eg, MMPI, Rorschach, WAIS), per hour of the psychologist's or physician's time, both face-to-face time administering tests to the patient and time interpreting these test results and preparing the report *96102 Psychological testing (includes psychodiagnostic assessment of emotionality, intellectual abilities, personality and psychopathology, eg, MMPI and WAIS), with qualified health care professional interpretation and report, administered by technician, per hour of technician time, face-to-face	●96130 Psychological testing evaluation services by physician or other qualified health care professional, including integration of patient data, interpretation of standardized test results and clinical data, clinical decision making, treatment planning and report, and interactive feedback to the patient, family member(s) or caregiver(s), when performed; first hour +●96131 each additional hour (List separately in addition to code for primary procedure) ●96132 Neuropsychological testing evaluation services by physician or other qualified health care professional, including integration of patient data, interpretation of standardized test results and clinical data, clinical decision making, treatment planning and report, and interactive feedback to the patient, family member(s) or caregiver(s), when performed; first hour +●96133 each additional hour ●96136 Psychological or neuropsychological test administration and scoring by physician or other qualified health care professional, two or more tests, any method, first 30 minutes

*Refer to **Table 1-4** for full details. #, re-sequenced code; ●, new code; +, add-on code; ▲, revised code; ★, telemedicine code; *, deleted code for 2019.*

Quick Reference to 2019 *CPT*® Pediatric Code Changes (*continued*)

Medicine Part 2 (continued)

2018	2019
*96103 Psychological testing (includes psychodiagnostic assessment of emotionality, intellectual abilities, personality and psychopathology, eg, MMPI), administered by a computer, with qualified health care professional interpretation and report *96118 Neuropsychological testing (eg, Halstead-Reitan Neuropsychological Battery, Wechsler Memory Scales and Wisconsin Card Sorting Test), per hour of the psychologist's or physician's time, both face-to-face time administering tests to the patient and time interpreting these test results and preparing the report *96119 Neuropsychological testing (eg, Halstead-Reitan Neuropsychological Battery, Wechsler Memory Scales and Wisconsin Card Sorting Test), with qualified health care professional interpretation and report, administered by technician, per hour of technician time, face-to-face *96120 Neuropsychological testing (eg, Wisconsin Card Sorting Test), administered by a computer, with qualified health care professional interpretation and report	+●96137 each additional 30 minutes after first 30 minutes (List separately in addition to code for primary procedure) ●96138 Psychological or neuropsychological test administration and scoring by technician, two or more tests, any method; first 30 minutes +●96139 each additional 30 minutes (List separately in addition to code for primary procedure) ●96146 Psychological or neuropsychological test administration, with single automated, standardized instrument via electronic platform, with automated result only *(See Chapter 14, Mental and Behavioral Health Services.)*

Medicine Part 3

2018	2019
*0359T Behavior identification assessment, by the physician or other qualified health care professional, face-to-face with patient and caregiver(s), includes administration of standardized and non-standardized tests, detailed behavioral history, patient observation and caregiver interview, interpretation of test results, discussion of findings and recommendations with the primary guardian(s)/caregiver(s), and preparation of report	#●97151 Behavior identification assessment, administered by a physician or other qualified health care professional, each 15 minutes of the physician's or other qualified health care professional's time face-to-face with patient and/or guardian(s)/caregiver(s) administering assessments and discussing findings and recommendations, and non-face-to-face analyzing past data, scoring/interpreting the assessment, and preparing the report/treatment plan #●97152 Behavior identification supporting assessment, administered by one technician under the direction of a physician or other qualified health care professional, face-to-face with the patient, each 15 minutes

*Refer to **Table 1-4** for full details. #, re-sequenced code; ●, new code; +, add-on code; ▲, revised code; ★, telemedicine code; *, deleted code for 2019.*

Quick Reference to 2019 *CPT*® Pediatric Code Changes (*continued*)

Medicine Part 3 (continued)

2018	2019
*0360T Observational behavioral follow-up assessment, includes physician or other qualified health care professional direction with interpretation and report, administered by one technician; first 30 minutes of technician time, face-to-face with the patient	▲**0362T** Behavior identification supporting assessment, each 15 minutes of technicians' time face-to-face with a patient, requiring the following components: ⚙ administration by the physician or other qualified health care professional who is on site; ⚙ with the assistance of two or more technicians; ⚙ for a patient who exhibits destructive behavior; ⚙ completion in an environment that is customized to the patient's behavior
*+0361T each additional 30 minutes of technician time, face-to-face with the patient	#●**97153** Adaptive behavior treatment by protocol, administered by technician under the direction of a physician or other qualified health care professional, face-to-face with one patient; each 15 minutes
0362T Exposure behavioral follow-up assessment, includes physician or other qualified health care professional direction with interpretation and report, administered by physician or other qualified health care professional with the assistance of one or more technicians; first 30 minutes of technician(s) time, face-to- face with the patient	#●**97154** Group adaptive behavior treatment by protocol, administered by technician under the direction of a physician or other qualified health care professional, face-to-face with two or more patients, each 15 minutes
*+0363T each additional 30 minutes of technician(s) time, face-to-face with the patient	#●**97155** Adaptive behavior treatment with protocol modification administered by physician or other qualified health care professional, which may include simultaneous direction of technician, face-to-face with one patient, each 15 minutes
*0364T Adaptive behavior treatment by protocol, administered by technician, face-to-face with one patient; first 30 minutes of technician time	#●**97158** Group adaptive behavior treatment with protocol modification, administered by physician or other qualified health care professional face-to-face with multiple patients, each 15 minutes
*+0365T each additional 30 minutes of technician time	▲**0373T** Adaptive behavior treatment with protocol modification, each 15 minutes of technicians' time face-to-face with a patient, requiring the following components: ⚙ administration by the physician or other qualified health care professional who is on site; ⚙ with the assistance of two or more technicians; ⚙ for a patient who exhibits destructive behavior; ⚙ completion in an environment that is customized to the patient's behavior.
*0366T Group adaptive behavior treatment by protocol, administered by technician, face-to-face with two or more patients; first 30 minutes of technician time	
*+0367T each additional 30 minutes of technician time	#●**97156** Family adaptive behavior treatment guidance, administered by physician or other qualified health care professional (with or without the patient present), face-to-face with guardian(s)/caregiver(s), each 15 minutes
*0368T Adaptive behavior treatment with protocol modification administered by physician or other qualified health care professional with one patient; first 30 minutes of patient face-to-face time	#●**97157** Multiple-family group adaptive behavior treatment guidance, administered by physician or other qualified health care professional (without the patient present), face-to-face with multiple sets of guardians/caregivers, each 15 minutes
*+0369T each additional 30 minutes of patient face-to-face time	

Refer to **Table 1-4** for full details. #, re-sequenced code; ●, new code; +, add-on code; ▲, revised code; ★, telemedicine code; *, deleted code for 2019.

Quick Reference to 2019 *CPT*® Pediatric Code Changes (*continued*)

Medicine Part 3 (continued)

2018	2019
*0370T Family adaptive behavior treatment guidance, administered by physician or other qualified health care professional (without the patient present) *0371T Multiple-family group adaptive behavior treatment guidance, administered by physician or other qualified health care professional (without the patient present) *0372T Adaptive behavior treatment social skills group, administered by physician or other qualified health care professional face-to-face with multiple patients 0373T Exposure adaptive behavior treatment with protocol modification requiring two or more technicians for severe maladaptive behavior(s); first 60 minutes of technicians' time, face-to-face with patient *+0374T each additional 30 minutes of technicians' time face-to-face with patient	

*Refer to **Table 1-4** for full details. #, re-sequenced code; ●, new code; +, add-on code; ▲, revised code; ★, telemedicine code; *, deleted code for 2019.*

Part 1:
Coding Basics and Business Essentials

Part 1: Coding Basics and Business Essentials

CHAPTER 1

||||||||

The Basics of Coding

||||||||

Contents

An Introduction to the Official Code Sets

In the United States, the Health Insurance Portability and Accountability Act of 1996 (HIPAA) requires the use of 5 specific code sets for purposes of health care transactions. The 4 code sets primarily used by physicians are listed in **Table 1-1**. The fifth designated code set, *Code on Dental Procedures and Nomenclature (CDT)*, is used to report dental procedures primarily to dental insurance plans.

By creating national standards for code sets, HIPAA sharply restricted the creation of codes by local or regional payers that created duplicative and complex reporting methodologies. Each code set, other than *CDT*, is used to facilitate communication of standardized health information for purposes such as prior authorization of medical care and submission of health care claims in pediatric practice. Understanding the purpose and constructs of the 4 code sets used by physicians is important to successful interactions with health plans and supports accurate health care statistics.

Table 1-1. Code Sets Required by Health Insurance Portability and Accountability Act of 1996

Code Set	Used to Report	Examples
International Classification of Diseases, 10th Revision, Clinical Modification (ICD-10-CM)	Diagnoses and other reasons for encounters	**Z38.00** Single liveborn infant, delivered vaginally **J00** Acute nasopharyngitis (common cold)
Current Procedural Terminology (CPT®)[a]	Most professional services, vaccine and immune globulin products, and tracking performance measurement	**99238** Hospital discharge day management; 30 minutes or less **90680** Rotavirus vaccine, pentavalent (RV5), 3 dose schedule, live, for oral use
Healthcare Common Procedure Coding System (HCPCS)[b]	Supplies, medications, and services (when a *CPT* code does not describe the service as covered by health plan benefits)	**S0630** Removal of sutures; by a physician other than the physician who originally closed the wound **J0698** Injection, cefotaxime sodium, per g
National Drug Code (NDC)	Specific prescription drug, vaccine, and insulin products and dosages	**00006-4047-20** RotaTeq 2-mL single-dose tube, package of 20 **60574-4114-01** Synagis 0.5-mL in 1 vial, single dose

[a] Also known as Level I of the HCPCS code set.
[b] Refers to Level II HCPCS codes assigned by the Centers for Medicare & Medicaid Services.

International Classification of Diseases, 10th Revision, Clinical Modification (ICD-10-CM)

The *International Classification of Diseases (ICD)* is published by the World Health Organization (WHO) for epidemiological tracking and collection of mortality statistical data worldwide. The *ICD* is currently in its 10th revision. The United States adopted a clinical modification of *ICD-10, International Classification of Diseases, 10th Revision, Clinical Modification (ICD-10-CM)*, on October 1, 2015.

Another code set, *ICD-10-Procedure Coding System (ICD-10-PCS)*, is only used to show hospital inpatient resource utilization and is not intended to show physician or other outpatient services. Physicians continue to report services and resources provided through use of *Current Procedural Terminology (CPT®)* and Healthcare Common Procedure Coding System (HCPCS) codes.

ICD-10-CM is the official system for reporting morbidity and mortality associated with health care data in the United States. The clinical modifications in the US version are generally proposed by specialty medical societies to improve injury and illness tracking and are reviewed by the *ICD-10* Coordination and Maintenance Committee. For diagnosis codes, this process is coordinated by the National Center for Health Statistics (NCHS) of the Centers for Disease Control and Prevention, which then publishes new and revised codes in the public domain after approval by the secretary of the US Department of Health and Human Services. Updates to *ICD-10-CM* are implemented each October 1 following publication by the NCHS and the Centers for Medicare & Medicaid Services (CMS) in early to midsummer.

Oversight and resolution of coding questions related to *ICD-10-CM* is performed by the American Hospital Association (AHA) Editorial Advisory Board for *Coding Clinic for ICD-10-CM and ICD-10-PCS* and the public-private "cooperating parties": CMS, NCHS, AHA, and American Health Information Management Association. The increased granularity and specificity in *ICD-10-CM* are also at the specific request of certain medical societies. No clinical diagnosis codes are added for payment purposes.

> **~ More From the AAP ~**
>
> The American Academy of Pediatrics provides timely information in advance of code set updates through its *AAP Pediatric Coding Newsletter*™.

The American Academy of Pediatrics (AAP) holds a seat on the editorial advisory board. Findings are published quarterly by the AHA in *Coding Clinic*. *ICD-10-CM* codes and accompanying guidelines and findings by the editorial advisory board are part of the standard transaction code sets under HIPAA and must be recognized by all payers. For *ICD-10-CM,* the hierarchy of official coding guidelines and instructions is as follows:

- *ICD-10-CM* alphabetic index and tabular list
- *Official Guidelines for Coding and Reporting*
- AHA *Coding Clinic* advice

The *ICD-10-CM* Coordination and Maintenance Committee typically meets in March and September of each year to consider proposals for new codes or revisions to existing codes or instructions. Annual updates of *ICD-10-CM* are implemented on October 1 each year.

Pediatricians with suggestions for new or changes to existing *ICD-10-CM* codes related to pediatric care are encouraged to forward their suggestions to coding staff at the AAP headquarters. The AAP staff and advisor who are involved in the process can be of great assistance. E-mail the coding staff at aapcodinghotline@aap.org.

ICD-10-CM *Code Structure*

In *ICD-10-CM*, a code is a complete set of alphanumeric characters for which there are no further subdivisions, 3 to 7 characters long, describing a condition or reason for an encounter or related factors, such as external causes. The first character of each code is a letter ranging from A to T or V to Z (the letter U is not used). The second through seventh characters may be letters or numbers. For codes that extend beyond 3 characters, the first 3 characters are found to the left of a decimal with the remaining characters to the right.

Pattern: XXX.XXXX

Although typically illustrated in capital letters, the alphabetic characters are not case sensitive. Each 3-character code category may then be further expanded with etiology, severity, site, manifestations, or intent within the fourth through sixth characters. When required, a seventh character is an extension to further define the episode of care, status of fracture healing, number of the fetus in obstetric conditions, or site of recording of the Glasgow Coma Scale. *ICD-10-CM* uses the letter X as a placeholder. When a subcategory of fewer than 6 characters requires 7 characters for a complete code, an X must be used as a placeholder to fill in for any undefined characters.

> **~ More From the AAP ~**
>
> For more information on *International Classification of Diseases, 10th Revision, Clinical Modification (ICD-10-CM)* guidelines, see the *AAP Pediatric Coding Newsletter*™ ICD-10-CM Collection at http://coding.aap.org (subscription required).

Examples of complete codes include

R05	Cough
J06.9	Acute upper respiratory infection
H65.04	Acute recurrent serous otitis media, right ear

Z00.129   Encounter for routine child health examination without abnormal findings
W07.XXXA   Fall from chair, initial encounter

Note the letter **X** is used as a placeholder in code **W07.XXXA**. The tabular listing for this code is **W07** with no further subcategories but with an instruction that the appropriate seventh character **A**, **D**, or **S** must be added to code **W07** to indicate the initial encounter, subsequent encounter, or encounter for a sequela of the fall from chair, respectively. The placeholder must be used to complete the code so the seventh character is in the appropriate position. If **W07.A** were submitted, the associated claim would likely be rejected because this is not a valid *ICD-10-CM* code. The letter **X** is also embedded in some codes to provide for future expansion of a code category (eg, **H60.8X1**, other otitis externa of the right ear).

ICD-10-CM *Guidelines*

The official conventions found in the *ICD-10-CM Official Guidelines for Coding and Reporting* are outlined in sections that include descriptions of symbols, abbreviations, and other instructional notes. The guidelines are organized into 4 sections. Only sections I and IV pertain to physicians reporting services. Sections II and III relate to hospital or facility technical services and are not discussed here. *ICD-10-CM* guidelines can be found in *ICD-10-CM* manuals or at www.cdc.gov/nchs/icd/icd10cm.htm.

The *ICD-10-CM* Guidelines box provides an overview of the information pertinent to pediatric care as provided in each section of the guidelines.

ICD-10-CM Guidelines (*continued*)
Section I—Conventions, General Coding Guidelines, and Chapter-Specific Guidelines (*continued*)
ICD-10-CM Guidelines
Section I—Conventions, General Coding Guidelines, and Chapter-Specific Guidelines

A. Conventions
Punctuation
[ ] In the alphabetic index, brackets identify manifestation codes. Brackets are used in the tabular list to enclose synonyms, alternative wording, or explanatory phrases.
( ) Parentheses are used in the alphabetic index and tabular list to enclose supplementary words (ie, nonessential modifiers) that may be included in the medical record but do not affect code selection. If a nonessential modifier is mutually exclusive to a sub-term of the main term, the sub-term is given priority.
- A dash (-) at the end of an alphabetic index entry indicates that additional characters are required for code completion. *A dash is also used throughout this publication to indicate incomplete codes.*

Notes
⊛ **Includes:** Further defines or gives examples of the content of a category.
⊛ **Excludes1:** Not coded here—used to indicate codes for conditions that would not occur in conjunction with the code category where the note is found. An exception to the *Excludes1* definition is the circumstance when the 2 conditions are unrelated to each other. If it is not clear whether the 2 conditions involving an *Excludes1* note are related, coders are instructed to query the provider.
⊛ **Excludes2:** Not included here—used to indicate codes for conditions not included in the code category where the note is found but that may be additionally reported when both conditions are present.
⊛ **Code first:** A sequencing rule in the tabular list to report first a code for an underlying cause or origin of a disease (etiology), if known.
⊛ **Code also:** An instruction that another code may be necessary to fully describe a condition. The sequence of the codes depends on the circumstances of the encounter.
⊛ **See:** In the alphabetic index, this instructs that another term should be referenced to find the appropriate code.
⊛ **See also:** In the alphabetic index, this instructs that another term may provide additional entries that may be useful.
⊛ **Use an additional code:** A sequencing rule often found at the listing of an etiology code, this instruction directs to also report a code for the manifestation.

ICD-10-CM Guidelines (*continued*)

Section I—Conventions, General Coding Guidelines, and Chapter-Specific Guidelines (*continued*)

Terminology

- **And:** Means and/or in *ICD-10-CM*.
- **Combination code:** A single code that represents multiple conditions or a single condition with an associated secondary process or complication.
- **First-listed diagnosis:** For reporting of professional services, the diagnosis, condition, problem, or other reason for the encounter or visit shown in the medical record to be chiefly responsible for the services provided is listed first and followed by other conditions that affected management or treatment.
- **NEC:** Not elsewhere classifiable. Indicates a code for other specified conditions that is reported when the medical record provides detail that is not captured in a specific code.
- **NOS:** Not otherwise specified. NOS indicates a code for an unspecified condition that is reported when the medical record does not provide sufficient detail for assignment of a more specific code.
- **Sequela:** A late effect of an illness or injury that is no longer in the acute phase. There is no time limit on when a sequela code can be used. The residual may be apparent early, such as in cerebral infarction, or it may occur months or years later, such as that due to a previous injury.
- **With and In:** The classification presumes a causal relationship between the 2 conditions linked by the terms *with* or *in* in the alphabetic index or tabular list. These conditions should be coded as related even in the absence of provider documentation explicitly linking them, unless the documentation clearly states that the conditions are unrelated or when another guideline exists that specifically requires a documented linkage between 2 conditions (eg, sepsis guideline for "acute organ dysfunction that is not clearly associated with the sepsis"). For conditions not specifically linked by these relational terms in the classification or when a guideline requires that a linkage between 2 conditions be explicitly documented, provider documentation must link the conditions to code them as related.

B. General Coding Guidelines

- First and foremost, begin by finding a term in the alphabetic index, and then turn to the tabular list to be sure you are selecting a complete code and follow code instructions for that chapter and code category.
- Assign a code for signs and symptoms when no definitive diagnosis has been reached at an encounter.
- Do not report additional codes for conditions that are integral or routinely associated with a disease process (eg, wheezing in asthma).
- When the same condition is documented as acute and chronic, codes for both conditions are reported if the alphabetic index lists the conditions at the same indentation level. The acute condition is sequenced first.
- When a combination code describes 2 diagnoses, or a diagnosis and its associated manifestation or complication, report only the combination code. If a manifestation or complication is not identified in a combination code, it may be separately reported.
- When reporting a sequela (late effect) of an injury or illness, report first the current condition and then the sequela code.
- If both sides are affected by a condition and the code category does not include a code for the bilateral condition, assign codes for right and left. When a patient has a bilateral condition and each side is treated during separate encounters, assign the bilateral code for each encounter where the condition exists on both sides. Do not assign a bilateral code if the condition no longer exists bilaterally.
- Coders generally may not assume a complication of care without documentation of the cause-and-effect relationship (eg, infection in a patient with a central venous line).
- Unspecified codes are appropriately selected when information to support a more specific code was not available at the time of the encounter (eg, type of pneumonia is not known). Unspecified codes are not appropriate when information to support a more specific code would generally be known (eg, laterality, type of attention-deficit/hyperactivity disorder). See the Appropriate Use of Unspecified Codes box later in this chapter for more information.

ICD-10-CM Guidelines (*continued*)

Section I–Conventions, General Coding Guidelines, and Chapter-Specific Guidelines (*continued*)

C. Chapter-Specific Guidelines
- See these guidelines for specific diagnoses and/or conditions found in each chapter.
- When selecting electronic coding applications, look for inclusion of chapter-specific guidelines when using the code search functionality.

Chapter 16, Certain Conditions Originating in the Perinatal Period (P00–P96)
- For conditions that originate in the perinatal or neonatal period, the provider selects diagnostic codes from Chapter 16 in *ICD-10-CM*, P00–P96. For coding and reporting purposes, the *perinatal period* is defined as before birth through the 28th day following birth. Should a condition originate in the perinatal period and continue to have health care implications throughout the life of the patient, the Chapter 16 code should continue to be used regardless of the patient's age. If the reason for a particular encounter is a perinatal or neonatal condition (ie, originated in the perinatal or neonatal period), the Chapter 16 code may be sequenced first (exception: the Z38 series type of delivery code ranks as primary for care by the attending physician during the admission that began with the neonate's birth). *ICD* coding guidelines allow for exclusive use of perinatal or neonatal period codes to characterize a patient's clinical condition on an encounter claim so long as the condition(s) originated in the perinatal or neonatal period and so long as the condition(s) continues to have clinical implications for the care of the patient. Typical scenarios that may require exclusive use of perinatal or neonatal codes beyond the perinatal period are often found in neonatal intensive care unit settings where early gestational ages and evolving maturation extend diagnostic effect, such as in drug withdrawal syndrome of infant of dependent mother (P96.1), chronic respiratory disease arising in the perinatal period (P27.-), necrotizing enterocolitis (P77.-), and prematurity (P07.-). (Note that these codes are not reported for conditions with onset after the patient is 28 days old. For example, necrotizing enterocolitis with onset after the neonatal period is reported with codes K55.30–K55.33.)

Chapter 19: Injury, Poisoning and Certain Other Consequences of External Causes (S00–T88)
- Most categories in Chapter 19 have a seventh character requirement for each applicable code. Most categories in this chapter have 3 seventh character values (with the exception of fractures): A, initial encounter; D, subsequent encounter; and S, sequela. Categories for traumatic fractures have additional seventh character values. While the patient may be seen by a new or different provider over the course of treatment for an injury, assignment of the seventh character is based on whether the patient is undergoing active treatment (services to establish a pattern of healing) and not whether the provider is seeing the patient for the first time. *Tip:* It may help to think of seventh character A as active treatment/management, D as during healing, and S as scars and other sequela.

Section IV–Diagnostic Coding and Reporting Guidelines for Outpatient Services

Selecting a code
- The coding conventions and guidelines of Section I take precedence over these outpatient guidelines.
- Never assign a code for a condition that is unconfirmed (eg, probable obstruction). Instead, assign codes for signs and symptoms.
- Use codes in categories Z00–Z99 when circumstances other than a disease or injury are recorded as the reason for encounter.

Sequencing of diagnosis codes
- Physicians and other providers of professional services should list first the condition, symptom, or other reason for encounter that is chiefly responsible for the services provided. List also any coexisting conditions. (Note: Some codes and chapters have specific guidelines with regard to sequencing.)

Reporting previously treated conditions
- Do not code conditions that have been previously treated but no longer exist. Personal history codes Z85–Z87 may be used to identify a patient's historical conditions. Codes for family history that affects current care are also reported (Z80–Z84).
- Report codes for chronic or recurring conditions as many times as the patient receives care for each condition.

ICD-10-CM Guidelines (*continued*)
Section IV–Diagnostic Coding and Reporting Guidelines for Outpatient Services (*continued*)

Reporting diagnoses for diagnostic examinations

- The condition, symptoms, or other reason for a diagnostic examination or test should be linked to the service. For laboratory or radiology testing in the absence of related conditions, signs, or symptoms, report code **Z01.89**, encounter for other specified special examinations.
- When diagnostic tests have been interpreted by a physician and the final report is available at the time of coding, code any confirmed or definitive diagnosis(es) documented in the interpretation. Do not code related signs and symptoms as additional diagnoses.

Reporting preoperative evaluations

- When the reason for an encounter is a preoperative evaluation, a code from subcategory **Z01.81-**, encounter for pre-procedural examinations, is reported first, followed by codes for the condition that is the reason for surgery and codes for any findings of the preoperative evaluation.

Reporting health examinations (preventive care)

- Codes for pediatric health examinations are found in subcategory **Z00.1-**. Encounters for routine child health examinations are reported based on findings—with or without new abnormal findings. Abnormal findings in the context of a routine examination are new (not previously diagnosed) or exacerbated conditions. When reporting an encounter with abnormal findings, report also codes to describe the findings. When a previously diagnosed condition is stable but managed at the same encounter as a routine child health examination, this is not reported as an abnormal finding of the routine child examination. Codes for conditions managed may be assigned in addition to the code for a routine child health examination without abnormal findings (**Z00.129**).

Application of the Guidelines and Conventions of ICD-10-CM

It is important to recognize and follow instructions found in the alphabetic index and tabular list. These are the prevailing instructions for reporting that are supplemented by the guidelines and guidance published in AHA *Coding Clinic for ICD-10-CM*. The indentation and instructions in the alphabetic index guide the user to the correct chapter and category of the tabular list. The alphabetic index may include many sub-terms for a single main entry. The indentation of each term directs to the appropriate listing.

To correctly select codes in *ICD-10-CM*, it is important to know how the alphabetic index and tabular list are used to locate the most specific code for documented diagnoses.

The Pathway to *ICD-10-CM* Code Selection

Alphabetic Index

Code selection in *ICD-10-CM* begins in the alphabetic index. The main portion of the alphabetic index consists of an alphabetic list of terms for diseases, injuries, and other reasons for encounters with their corresponding codes or code categories. The alphabetic index also includes an index to external causes of injuries, a table of neoplasms, and a table of drugs and chemicals.

In **Table 1-2**, the alphabetic index pathway to acute recurrent allergic nonsuppurative otitis media is illustrated. Note how the number of dashes (-) leads you from the sub-term through various levels of qualifiers to the most specific diagnosis code (less an additional character for laterality found in the tabular index).

Note how the index listings for otitis media start with an unspecified code category (**H66.90**, otitis media, unspecified, unspecified ear). This is the default entry that is reported only if no further specification is provided in the medical record. The dash following code numbers indicates that the tabular list will provide additional characters to complete the code with specific details such as laterality.

> ⅼⅼⅼⅼⅼⅼ **Coding Pearl** ⅼⅼⅼⅼⅼⅼ
>
> Look for instructional notes at each division within the tabular list (eg, block, category, or code), as these give important guidance to correct code selection.

Table 1-2. Alphabetic Index Layout	
Levels	**Examples**
Main term (bold type)	**Otitis** (acute) **H66.90**
Sub-term—essential qualifier of main term	- with effusion -*see also* Otitis, media, nonsuppurative - media (hemorrhagic) (staphylococcal) (streptococcal) **H66.9-**
2nd qualifier—modifier of the preceding sub-term	- - nonsuppurative **H65.9-**
3rd qualifier—modifier of the preceding 2nd qualifier	- - - acute or subacute NEC **H65.19-**
4th qualifier—modifier of the preceding 3rd qualifier	- - - - allergic **H65.11-**
5th qualifier—modifier of the preceding 4th qualifier	- - - - - recurrent **H65.11-**
Abbreviation: NEC, not elsewhere classifiable.	

A "see also" note is found at the sub-term "with effusion." The see also note here instructs that another term may provide additional entries that may be useful (e.g., otitis, - media, - - nonsuppurative). An additional qualifier under the sub-term "with effusion" is "- - purulent - see Otitis, media, suppurative." The "see" instruction directs the reader to another term that should be referenced to find the appropriate code (eg, otitis, - media, - - suppurative).

Tabular List

The tabular list is the end point for code selection. It is an alphanumeric list of *ICD-10-CM* codes structured as an indented list of 21 chapters with further divisions, including blocks, categories, subcategories, and codes. Chapters are based on condition, body system, consequences of external causes, external causes, and other factors influencing health status or contact with health services. Table 1-3 provides examples of notes found at each level of the tabular list (eg, chapter, block).

Diagnosis Coding Tips

- Specificity in coding is important to demonstrating the reason for a service or encounter, including the nature or severity of conditions managed. However, there are times when a diagnosis is established at a non-specific level (eg, pneumonia without specification of the causal organism). See further discussion of this important topic in the Appropriate Use of Unspecified Codes box.
- Physicians and other practitioners should become familiar with the documentation elements that are captured in *ICD-10-CM* code categories for conditions commonly seen in their practice. For example, when documenting care for otitis media, key documentation elements include whether the condition affects the right, the left, or both ears; is acute, acute recurrent, or chronic; is suppurative or nonsuppurative; and is with or without spontaneous rupture of the tympanic membrane. Exposure to or use of tobacco is also reported in conjunction with otitis media.
- Pay close attention to the terminology for nonspecific diagnoses. For example, the diagnosis "reactive airways disease" is to be coded as asthma per the guidelines. In children treated for an asthma-like condition who have not been diagnosed with asthma, it may be more appropriate to report the signs or symptoms as the primary diagnosis.
- When testing is performed to rule out or confirm a suspected diagnosis or condition on a patient with a sign(s) or symptom(s), it is considered a diagnostic examination and is not screening. Therefore, the code that explains the reason for the test (ie, sign or symptom) should be reported. Screening codes may be reported as the primary code if the reason for the visit is specifically for the screening examination or test.

Chapter 1: The Basics of Coding

Table 1-3. Tabular List Notes

Type of Note	Example
Chapter-level notes (apply to all codes in a chapter) 1. The first note advises that codes from Chapter 16 are never used on the maternal record. 2. The inclusion note further defines that codes in this chapter represent conditions that originate in the newborn period but may be reported even if morbidity occurs later. 3. The *Excludes2* note provides information on potentially coexisting conditions that may be separately reported but are not included in this chapter.	**Chapter 16** **Certain Conditions Originating in the Perinatal Period** (P00–P96) **Note:** Codes from this chapter are for use on newborn records only, never on maternal records. **Includes:** Conditions that have their origin in the fetal or perinatal period (before birth through the first 28 days after birth) even if morbidity occurs later **Excludes2:** congenital malformations, deformations, and chromosomal abnormalities (Q00–Q99) endocrine, nutritional, and metabolic diseases (E00–E88) injury, poisoning, and certain other consequences of external causes (S00–T88) neoplasms (C00–D49) tetanus neonatorum (A33)
Block-level notes (apply to all codes in the block [eg, P00–P04])	**Newborn affected by maternal factors and by complications of pregnancy, labor, and delivery** (P00–P04) **Note:** These codes are for use when the listed maternal conditions are specified as the cause of confirmed morbidity or potential morbidity which have their origin in the perinatal period (before birth through the first 28 days after birth).
Category-level notes (apply to all codes in the category [eg, H67.1–H67.9] unless otherwise specified) 1. The **"code first"** note is a sequencing rule. When an underlying condition is identified, the code for that condition is listed first. 2. The **"use additional code"** note is also a sequencing note instructing that codes for associated perforated tympanic membrane are reported secondary to the code for otitis media. 3. *Excludes1* is followed by a list of conditions that typically would not occur at the same encounter as the conditions in this code category or, as in this case, are represented by combination codes (eg, otitis media in influenza).	H67 Otitis media in diseases classified elsewhere Code first underlying disease, such as: viral disease NEC (B00–B34) Use additional code for any associated perforated tympanic membrane (H72.-) **Excludes1** otitis media in: influenza (J09.X9, J10.83, J11.83) measles (B05.3) scarlet fever (A38.0) tuberculosis (A18.6)
Subcategory-level notes (apply to all codes within the subcategory [eg, R06.00–R06.09])	R06.0 Dyspnea **Excludes1:** tachypnea NOS (R06.82) transient tachypnea of newborn (P22.1)
Code-level note (applies only to the code above the instruction)	R06.2 Wheezing **Excludes1:** asthma (J45.-)

Appropriate Use of Unspecified Codes

Unspecified codes are valid *ICD-10-CM* codes used to report conditions for which a more specific diagnosis has not yet been determined and/or testing to determine a more specific diagnosis would not be medically necessary. However, misuse of unspecified codes may result in claim denials and unnecessary delays in receiving prior authorizations for testing or procedures.

Do not report the default code (first code listed in the alphabetic index) when more detail about the patient's conditions should be documented to support another, more specific code. For example, do not report **J45.909** for unspecified asthma, uncomplicated, for reevaluation of asthma, which includes clinical classification of intermittent, mild-persistent, moderate-persistent, or severe-persistent asthma. The diagnosis code reported should reflect what is known at the end of the current encounter.

Examples of unspecified codes that should be acceptable, provided by Jeffrey F. Linzer Sr, MD, AAP representative to the Editorial Advisory Board for the AHA *Coding Clinic for ICD-10-CM and ICD-10-PCS,* are as follows:
- Viral intestinal infection, unspecified (**A08.4**)
- Infectious gastroenteritis and colitis, unspecified (**A09**)
- Hb-SS disease with crisis, unspecified (**D57.00**)
- Acute pharyngitis, unspecified (**J02.9**)
- Pneumonia, unspecified organism (**J18.9**)
- Sprain of unspecified site of right knee (**S83.91X-**)
- Sprain of unspecified ligament of right ankle (**S93.401-**)

Dr Linzer also provides the following examples of unspecified codes that indicate inappropriate coding due to failure to document information that would typically be known at the time of the encounter and/or inappropriate code selection:
- Acute suppurative otitis media without spontaneous rupture of eardrum, unspecified ear (**H66.009**)
- Otitis media, unspecified, unspecified ear (**H66.90**)
- Cutaneous abscess of limb, unspecified (**L02.419**)
- Extremely low birth weight newborn, unspecified weight (**P07.00**)
- Abrasion of unspecified finger (**S60.419-**)
- Sprain of unspecified ligament of unspecified ankle (**S93.409-**)

In short, unspecified codes are necessary and should be reported when appropriate. However, physicians must document in sufficient detail to capture what is known at the time of the encounter and codes selected must reflect the documented diagnosis(es). If, at the time of code selection, documentation does not appear to include information that would be known at the time of the encounter, it is appropriate for coders to query the physician for more information and/or request an addendum to the documentation to more fully describe the conditions addressed at the encounter.

- Codes for routine examinations that include "with abnormal findings" in the code descriptor are reported only when there are new abnormal findings at the time of the preventive encounter (ie, new problem or exacerbation of previously managed problem). If preexisting (ie, known) conditions are stable but addressed at the preventive encounter but there are no new abnormal findings, report first the code for routine examination without abnormal findings (eg, Z00.129) and then the code(s) appropriate for the conditions addressed.
- When routine vision, developmental, and/or hearing screening services are performed in conjunction with a preventive medicine visit, the diagnosis code for a routine infant or child health check should be linked to the appropriate screening service.
- Codes for reporting live-born neonates according to type of birth (*ICD-10-CM* codes Z38.0–Z38.8) are reported by the attending physician as the first-listed diagnosis for a newborn at the time of birth and for the duration of the birth admission as long as the baby is consuming health care (ie, crib or bassinet occupancy). This includes reporting for a neonate kept in the normal newborn nursery (eg, awaiting adoption) or mother's room (awaiting a mother's discharge) and those neonates who stay in the birth hospital for a prolonged period.

- Codes in Chapter 16, Certain Conditions Originating in the Perinatal Period (P00–P99), are used when the diagnosis is made on a fetus or a neonate who is 28 days or younger. WHO defines the day of birth as day of life 0 (zero). A baby reaches 28 days of life on day 29 of age. These codes are only to be reported when the condition originates in this time but can be reported beyond the perinatal period if the condition(s) causes morbidity or is the primary reason for or contributing to why the patient is receiving health care.

- If, after evaluation and study of a suspected condition, there is no diagnosis or signs or symptoms that are appropriate, report the codes for observation and evaluation for suspected conditions not found. Codes for observation and evaluation for suspected conditions not found in a neonate (ICD-10-CM codes Z05.0–Z05.9) are distinct from those for reporting suspected conditions not found in older children and adults (ICD-10-CM code Z03.89).

- Disorders of newborn related to slow fetal growth and fetal malnutrition are reported with codes in category P05. Codes in subcategory P05.0- are reported for newborn light for gestational age. WHO defines light for gestational age as usually referring to weight below but length above the 10th percentile for gestational age (may be referenced as *asymmetrical*). In contrast, codes in subcategory P05.1 are reported for newborn small for gestational age, including the newborn who is small and light for dates. This usually refers both to weight and length below the 10th percentile (often called *symmetrical*). Note that head circumference is *not* considered in choosing light versus small.

- Use aftercare codes (Z42–Z49, Z51) for patients who are receiving care to consolidate treatment or managing residual conditions.

- Conditions that were previously treated and no longer exist cannot be reported. Therefore, it is correct coding to report care following completed treatment with ICD-10-CM code Z09, encounter for follow-up examination after completed treatment for conditions other than malignant neoplasm. Personal history codes (Z86.-, Z87.-) may be used to provide additional information on follow-up care. If a payer does not accept follow-up care codes as primary and requires that the service be reported with the diagnosis code that reflects the condition that had been treated, report the follow-up care codes as secondary. However, get the payer's policy in writing and inquire why it is not following coding guidelines.

- Do not select a diagnosis code that is "closest to" the diagnosis or condition documented in the medical record. If a specific diagnosis code is not included on your encounter form, write it in. For example, do not report unspecified joint pain (M25.50) if the diagnosis is right knee pain (M25.561).

- Pay attention to age factors within certain code descriptors. For example, ICD-10-CM code R10.83 is used to report infantile colic. Colic in the child older than 12 months is reported with ICD-10-CM code R10.84.

- There is no limit to the number of diagnosis codes that can be reported. Although space is only allotted for up to 12 codes on the CMS-1500 claim form and each service line may be connected to 1 to 4 of the included codes, you may submit as many claim forms as necessary to report the diagnoses. Electronic claims in HIPAA version 5010 may also include up to 12 diagnosis codes.

- "Unspecified" codes can still be reported if, at the time of the encounter, more information cannot be obtained. However, it will be important to not report "unspecified" for conditions or information that should be documented, such as laterality.

- "Recurrent" is not defined by ICD. Therefore, to use a recurrent code, the documentation should reflect that a practitioner believes it to be a recurrence.

- "Confirmed" influenza or other conditions do not require a positive laboratory test result or other test. What is required is that the practitioner, through training and experience, believes the patient has the condition based on clinical assessment and documents the condition in the chart.

Resources

The AAP *Pediatric ICD-10-CM: A Manual for Provider-Based Coding* is a condensed version of the entire ICD-10-CM manual and provides only the guidelines and codes that are applicable and of importance to pediatric practitioners. The manual was designed for use in conjunction with the complete ICD-10-CM code set. The ICD-10-CM codes are found at www.cdc.gov/nchs/icd/icd10cm.htm.

AAP *Pediatric Coding Newsletter*™ provides articles on diagnosis coding for pediatric conditions.

Healthcare Common Procedure Coding System (HCPCS)

The HCPCS coding system includes Level I codes (*CPT*®) and Level II codes (CMS national codes). Level III codes (local codes assigned and used by Medicare and other carriers) were part of the HCPCS code set but were eliminated under HIPAA. HCPCS Level II codes are the standardized coding system for describing and identifying health care services, equipment, and supplies in health care transactions that are not identified by HCPCS Level I (*CPT*) codes. To differentiate discussion of *CPT* and HCPCS Level II codes, the term HCPCS typically is used in reference to Level II codes unless otherwise stated.

HCPCS codes begin with a single letter (A–V) followed by 4 numeric digits (eg, Q4011, cast supplies, short arm cast, pediatric [0-10 years], plaster). Commonly used categories of HCPCS include H codes for services such as alcohol/drug and behavioral services, J codes for drugs administered by other than oral method and chemotherapy drugs, Q codes that represent temporary codes (although many codes have been used for years) for certain tests and procedures and supplies such as cast supplies, S codes for screenings and examinations in alignment with certain payer policies (often Blue Cross Blue Shield plans), and T codes, used mainly by Medicaid agencies to describe specific services such as nursing and certain behavioral health services.

HCPCS codes may be reported when the narrative differs from the *CPT* code for the service. Payer policies, particularly Medicaid plan policies, often drive the decision between reporting with *CPT* versus HCPCS. For instance, *CPT* does not include a code for removal of sutures by a physician other than the physician who repaired the wound and instructs to report an evaluation and management (E/M) service for encounters for suture removal. HCPCS includes code S0630 (removal of sutures by a physician other than the physician who originally closed the wound). When allowed or required by a payer, code S0630 may be reported in lieu of an E/M service for suture removal.

HCPCS J codes (eg, J0696, injection, ceftriaxone sodium, per 250 mg) represent medications only and not the administration of the medication. The term *injection* is included in the descriptor to specify that the medication code is reported for the medication when provided via injection or infusion and not oral or topical applications. Separate procedure codes, typically *CPT* codes, are used to report medication administration by injection or infusion. HCPCS codes for drugs specify the unit of measure for each unit reported on the claim (eg, 250 mg of ceftriaxone sodium equals 1 unit on the claim line reporting provision of the medication). (See National Drug Code [NDC] section later in this chapter for information on reporting units of service in conjunction with NDC reporting.)

Modifiers are also included in the HCPCS code set. Modifiers indicate that a service or procedure has been altered by some specific circumstance but not changed in its basic code definition. HCPCS modifiers are more comprehensive than the modifiers included in *CPT*, offering modifiers that designate anatomical sites, provider types, and services payable under specific benefits or policies. Examples include

F4	Left hand, fifth digit
EP	Service provided as part of Medicaid early periodic screening diagnosis and treatment (EPSDT) program
AJ	Clinical social worker

Modifiers are further discussed in Chapter 2 and illustrated throughout this publication.

New permanent HCPCS codes are released by the CMS each November for implementation on January 1 of each year. However, temporary HCPCS codes may be implemented on a quarterly basis. Temporary codes are added to address the need for a reporting mechanism prior to the annual update (eg, to meet the requirements of a legislative mandate).

Current Procedural Terminology (CPT®)

CPT is published annually by the American Medical Association (AMA). *CPT* codes are known as Level I codes of HCPCS but are commonly treated as a separate code set. This is the primary procedural coding system for professional services by physicians and other qualified health care professionals (QHPs).

CPT includes 3 categories of codes.

☀ Category I codes represent procedures or services that have been determined consistent with current medical practice and are performed by many practitioners in clinical practice in multiple locations. Category I codes are 5-digit numeric codes, with exception of codes for proprietary laboratory analyses, which include 4 numeric digits followed by the letter U. Category I codes are divided into the following sections and code ranges:

Evaluation and management	**99201–99499**
Anesthesia	**01000–01999, 99100–99140**
Surgery	**10004–69990**
Radiology	**70010–79999**
Pathology and laboratory	**80047–89398, 0001U–0017U**
Medicine	**90281–99199, 99500–99607**

Each section of codes is preceded by guidelines specific to code selection and reporting of services included in that section.

CPT Category I codes are updated annually with release of new codes each fall to allow physicians and payers to prepare for implementation on January 1 of each year. Exceptions include the vaccine product codes, which are updated twice annually (January and July) and may be released earlier when specific criteria for rapid release are met. New vaccine codes released July 1 are implemented on January 1, and vice versa.

New codes effective with services provided on or after January 1, 2019, are listed in the Quick Reference to 2019 *ICD-10-CM* Pediatric Code Changes on page xiii and Quick Reference to 2019 *CPT*® Pediatric Code Changes on page xvii.

☀ Category II *CPT* codes are a set of supplemental tracking codes that can be used for performance measurement. Category II codes are 5-digit alphanumeric codes that include 4 numbers followed by the letter F. Category II code changes since the printing of the last *CPT* manual are posted to https://www.ama-assn.org/practice-management/category-ii-codes. A document available at that Web site, "CPT Category II Codes Alphabetical Clinical Topics Listing," includes the latest code changes with revision, implementation, and publication dates. See Chapter 3 for further discussion and illustration of Category II codes.

☀ Category III *CPT* codes are a set of temporary codes for emerging technology, services, procedures, and service paradigms. Category III codes allow data collection to substantiate the usage of new services/procedures. Assignment of a Category III code to a service is not a statement of support, or lack thereof, for the efficacy of, use of, or payment for the service.

  ❖ Category III codes are 5-character alphanumeric codes with 4 numbers followed by the letter T.
  ❖ Category III codes are not assigned relative value units (RVUs), and payment for these services is based strictly on payer policies. If you are performing any procedure or service identified with a Category III *CPT* code, work with your payers to determine their coverage and payment policies.
  ❖ Category III codes are released biannually with an implementation date 6 months following the release date. For instance, a code released on July 1, 2017, is implemented on January 1, 2018, and published in *CPT 2019*. The most recent Category III code listing is found at https://www.ama-assn.org/practice-management/category-iii-codes.
  ❖ In general, Category III codes must be replaced for reporting by Category I codes or approved for continued Category III status within 5 years following the Category III code assignment. Category III codes that are not renewed for continued utilization are archived and the codes are not reused.

CPT includes an index of procedures used to find codes and code ranges to help guide the user to the correct section(s) of codes. Codes should not be selected from the index without verification in the main text of the manual. Terms in the index include procedures and services, organs and anatomic sites, conditions, synonyms, eponyms, and abbreviations (eg, EEG).

Appendixes in *CPT* provide quick references to modifiers; a summary of new, revised, and deleted codes; clinical examples of E/M services; add-on and modifier-exempt codes; and other procedure code references. Based on changes to the coding manual, the appendixes may vary from year to year.

The AMA hosts a Web site devoted to *CPT*, https://www.ama-assn.org/practice-management/cpt-current-procedural-terminology, with information on code development and maintenance, summaries of recent *CPT* Editorial Panel actions, and newly released codes.

CPT *Conventions and Guidelines*

CPT is structured to save space in the listing of codes by use of indentations to identify variations of services that have a common base descriptor. For example

99381	Initial comprehensive preventive medicine evaluation and management of an individual including an age and gender appropriate history, examination, counseling/anticipatory guidance/risk factor reduction interventions, and the ordering of laboratory/diagnostic procedures, new patient; infant (age younger than 1 year)
99382	early childhood (age 1 through 4 years)
99383	late childhood (age 5 through 11 years)
99384	adolescent (age 12 through 17 years)
99385	18–39 years

The portion of the code descriptor for **99381** before the semicolon also applies to codes **99382–99385**. Increased indentation of codes that share a portion of the first code's descriptor helps to identify which codes share a common base procedure.

Symbols are used throughout *CPT* to indicate specific characteristics of codes and instructions. As shown in **Table 1-4**, symbols indicate new or revised codes, new instructions, and other important characteristics of a code (eg, vaccine pending US Food and Drug Administration approval).

Table 1-4. *Current Procedural Terminology*® Symbols

Symbols	Description
●	A bullet at the beginning of a code means the code is a new code for the current year. For example #●**99452** Interprofessional telephone/Internet/electronic health record referral service(s) provided by a treating/requesting physician or qualified health care professional, 30 minutes
▲	A triangle means the code descriptor has been revised. For example ▲**94780** Car seat/bed testing for airway integrity, for infants through 12 months of age, with continual clinical staff observation and continuous recording of pulse oximetry, heart rate and respiratory rate, with interpretation and report; 60 minutes
+	A plus sign means the code is an add-on code. For example +▲**94781** each additional full 30 minutes (List separately in addition to code for primary procedure)
∅	A null sign means the code is a "modifier **51** exempt" code and, therefore, does not require modifier **51** (multiple procedures) even when reported with other procedures. For example ∅**31500** Intubation, endotracheal, emergency procedure
⚡	The lightning bolt identifies codes for vaccines that are pending US Food and Drug Administration approval. For example ⚡**90587** Dengue vaccine, quadrivalent, live, 3 dose schedule, for subcutaneous use
#	The pound symbol is used to identify re-sequenced codes that are out of numerical sequence. This allows related codes to be placed in an appropriate location, making it easier to locate a procedure or service.
○	The **○** symbol precedes codes that are recycled or reinstated.
★	A star means the service represented by the code is included in Appendix P as a code to which modifier **95** may be appended to indicate the service was rendered via real-time telemedicine services.

CPT includes specific guidelines that are located at the beginning of each section and additional prefatory instructions for categories of codes throughout the *CPT* manual. Code-specific instructions often follow a code in parentheses (referred to as *parenthetical instructions*). While code selection is often incorporated in electronic health records (EHRs), knowledge of and access to these guidelines and instructions is important to correct coding. Correct coding is important to obtaining correct claims payment. Always read the applicable guidelines and instructions before selecting a code.

Additional guidance can be found in *CPT Assistant*, a monthly newsletter published by the AMA that provides additional information about the intended use of codes, the related guidelines, and parenthetical instructions. Although widely considered authoritative, *CPT* instruction and *CPT Assistant* are not part of the standard transaction code sets under HIPAA. All payers must accept *CPT* codes but are not required to adhere to the published guidelines and instructions. Where payer policy differs from *CPT*, payer contracts typically require adherence to payer policy.

Some key instructions are

- In the *CPT* code set, the term *procedure* is used to describe services, including diagnostic tests. The section of the book in which a code is placed is not indicative of whether the service is a surgery or not a surgery for insurance or other purposes.

- Select the code for the procedure or service that accurately identifies the service performed. Do not select a code that merely approximates the service provided. If no such specific code exists, report the service using the appropriate unlisted procedure code. Unlisted procedure codes are provided in each section of *CPT* (eg, 99429, unlisted preventive medicine service). In some cases, a modifier may be used to indicate a reduced, discontinued, or increased procedural service.

- *CPT* distinguishes a physician or other QHP from clinical staff.

  - A physician or QHP is an individual who is qualified by education, training, licensure, or regulation (when applicable), and facility privileging (when applicable), who performs a professional service within his or her scope of practice and independently reports that professional service.

  - A clinical staff member is a person who works under the supervision of a physician or other QHP and who is allowed by law, regulation, and facility policy to perform or assist in the performance of a specified professional service but who does not individually report that professional service.

- Many diagnostic services require a technical and a professional component. It is important to understand that the technical component (eg, obtaining an electrocardiogram) leads to results or findings. The interpretation and creation of a report of the results or findings is a professional service. Some services specifically require a professional's interpretation and report. Other services include only a technical component and require only documentation of the results or findings (eg, scoring of a developmental screening instrument). Codes and modifiers exist to report the technical or professional component when the complete service is not provided by the same individual or provider (eg, facility provides technical component and physician provides professional component).

- Add-on codes (marked with a + before the code) are always performed in addition to a primary procedure and are never reported as stand-alone services. Add-on codes describe additional intraservice work and are not valued to include pre- and post-service work like most other codes.

Example

99291	Critical care, evaluation and management of the critically ill or critically injured patient; first 30–74 minutes
99292	each additional 30 minutes (List separately in addition to code for primary service)

Code 99292 is never reported in the absence of code 99291 on the same date of service.

Use of Time in Procedure Coding

Most procedures and services in *CPT* are described by specific components of physician work (eg, 94011, measurement of spirometric forced expiratory flows in an infant or child through 2 years of age). However, time (especially intraservice time) is also used as a proxy for physician work. Many services are reported based solely on time of service or, as in the case of many E/M services, may be reported based on key components of work (history, examination, and medical decision-making [MDM]) *or* typical time when most of the time of service was spent in counseling and/or coordination of care.

Understanding the correct application of time in code selection is important to reporting the code that most accurately describes the service provided. *CPT* provides general and category/code-specific instructions for reporting services based on time. An understanding of these instructions is key to selecting codes that most accurately capture the services provided. This chapter will review the general guidelines for reporting time and guidelines specific to time-based reporting of E/M services. Service-specific instructions and examples are also provided throughout this manual to help illustrate time-based coding.

The Value of Documenting Time

Failure to document time of service may be costly even when it is possible to report a service without documenting time.

Example

➤ **Discharge summary: Continued on intravenous (IV) antibiotics until this morning, breastfeeding well, no further fevers.** Vital signs and general appearance and examination of the heart, lungs, abdomen, and skin are performed. Blood and urine cultures remain negative after 48 hours. Intravenous antibiotics discontinued. Final diagnosis: fever, likely viral infection. Patient discharged home with instructions for home care and follow-up. A total of 35 minutes was spent on the floor reviewing the hospital course, expected follow-up, and signs and symptoms of possible sepsis or infection with mother.

The physician documents that 35 minutes was spent in discharge management services. A summary of the activities is documented to support the time of service.	*CPT* 99239 (hospital discharge day management; more than 30 minutes)
Viral infection is not reported because diagnoses documented as uncertain (eg, likely) are not reported. Instead codes for signs and symptoms, such as fever, are reported.	*ICD-10-CM* R50.9 (fever)

Teaching Point: If time were not documented, lesser code 99238 (hospital discharge day management; 30 minutes or less) would be reported because time of greater than 30 minutes must be documented to support code 99239. Code 99238 has 2.07 total RVUs, while code 99239 is assigned 3.05 total RVUs. Persistent failure to document the time of discharge day management services may result in significant loss of otherwise earned revenue. For example, a payer contract allows $40 per RVU, so a practice is paid $82.80 ($40 × 2.07) for code 99238 and $122 ($40 × 3.05) for code 99239. Therefore, $39.20 of potential revenue is lost due to lack of documentation; for 10 services, $392 of potential revenue is lost.

Likewise, failure to document time eliminates the possibility of reporting prolonged services and may negatively affect the level of service reported when multiple episodes of care occur on the same date (eg, multiple hospital care services). Routinely noting the time spent face-to-face (outpatient) or on a patient's unit or floor (observation and inpatient) and those instances when more than 50% of that time is spent in counseling and/or coordination of care allows for recognition of occasions where reporting based on time is most advantageous.

General Guidelines

CPT provides overall instructions for time-based reporting in the "Instructions for Use of the CPT Codebook" found in the Introduction of the coding manual. These instructions are followed for reporting time-based services when there are no section guidelines, prefatory instructions, parenthetical instructions, or specified time requirements in code descriptors.

☼ If your EHR or other coding reference does not include the prefatory and parenthetical instructions provided in *CPT*, consider whether secondary code verification prior to billing is necessary. Alternatively, it may be possible to insert instructions in the form of notes or alerts in an EHR.

- Time is the physician or other reporting provider's face-to-face or unit/floor time with the patient, unless otherwise stated. Time spent by clinical staff is reported only when specified in *CPT* or allowed under incident-to policy established by a payer. (Learn more about incident-to services in Chapter 13, Allied Health and Clinical Staff Services.)

- A unit of time is met when the midpoint is *passed* (eg, an hour is attained when 31 minutes have passed), unless otherwise specified by *CPT* or payer policy. (Some payers may require that the typical time assigned to a service be met or exceeded rather than approximated as allowed by *CPT*.) The midpoint rule is not applied when *CPT* includes category- or code-specific instructions to the contrary. Examples of when the midpoint rule does and does not apply are included throughout this chapter.

- It is important to note that a code that is reported "per day" (eg, 99468, initial inpatient neonatal critical care, per day, for the E/M of a critically ill neonate, 28 days of age or younger) is not reported for all services in a 24-hour period but, rather, all services on a single date. Likewise, a code describing services "on the same date" (eg, 99463, initial hospital or birthing center care, per day, for E/M of normal newborn infant admitted and discharged on the same date) is reported only for services on a single date of service.

> ||||||| ***Coding Pearl*** |||||||
>
> Section and prefatory instructions, code descriptors, and parenthetical instructions override the general instruction for time-based reporting.

Documentation of Time

- Documentation of time spent providing services should be evident in the medical record for each service reported based on time (ie, start and stop times or total minutes of service).

- Documentation of time may be automated in an EHR, but physicians should be able to demonstrate that the EHR functionality captures the correct time for code selection as specified by *CPT*. For instance, only intra-service time is used to select codes for moderate sedation. Documentation should clearly reflect the start and stop times for this service.

- When multiple services are provided on the same date, the time spent in time-based services must be clearly distinguished from time spent providing other services.

- In addition to documentation of start and stop or total time of service, documentation should clearly support the service reported. For example, documentation of psychotherapy should include factors such as modalities and frequency, functional status, mental status examination, diagnosis, treatment plan, prognosis, and progress.

- All documentation must be signed or electronically authenticated with the name and credentials of the physician or other provider of care and date of service.

Time of Evaluation and Management (E/M) Services

There are very few E/M service codes for which typical time is never a factor in reporting the service. Other criteria are used for the selection of the specific codes (eg, defined components, services reported per day).

Certain E/M services are always reported based on time. However, many E/M services are described by either key components (ie, history, examination, MDM) or typical time. For these services, time may be the basis for code selection in lieu of key components when appropriate per *CPT* instruction.

E/M Services That Are Always Based on Time

Certain E/M services are never reported based on key components but, rather, are time-based services. These codes are often not subject to the general instructions for reporting based on time, as prefatory language and code descriptors provide reporting instructions.

Examples

➤ **A single code is reported for all hospital discharge day services based on time of 30 minutes or less (99238) or of more than 30 minutes (99239).** See The Value of Documenting Time section earlier in this chapter for more information on these codes.

99238	Hospital discharge day management; 30 minutes or less
99239	more than 30 minutes

➤ **The code descriptor for 99291 is critical care, E/M of the critically ill or critically injured patient; first 30 to 74 minutes.** Per prefatory instruction, code 99291 is not reported for critical care of less than 30 minutes (ie, the midpoint rule does not apply). Code 99291 is reported only once per date by the reporting individual, even if time spent providing critical care is not continuous, and only for time of at least 30 minutes.

99291   Critical care, evaluation and management of the critically ill or critically injured patient; first 30–74 minutes

+99292   each additional 30 minutes (List separately in addition to code for primary service)

Reporting Time in Lieu of Key Components

Key guidelines for using time as the controlling factor in the selection of an E/M service that may otherwise be reported based on key components include

- Time shall be used as the key component in the selection of an E/M code if there is an assigned typical time and counseling and/or coordination of care accounts for *more than 50%* of the physician face-to-face time (for outpatient) or floor or unit time (for inpatient) with the patient and/or family.

- When reporting based on time spent counseling and/or coordinating care, codes are selected based on typical times assigned to the E/M code in the category appropriate to the service rendered (eg, office or other outpatient visit). Typical times are included in the code descriptors of E/M services that may be reported by either key components or time.

- What makes up time differs in the facility/hospital setting from the office or other outpatient reporting (**Table 1-5**).

Example

99214   Office or other outpatient visit for the evaluation and management of an established patient, which requires at least 2 of these 3 key components:

       - A detailed history;
       - A detailed examination;
       - Medical decision making of moderate complexity.

       Counseling and/or coordination of care with other physicians, other qualified health care professionals, or agencies are provided consistent with the nature of the problem(s) and the patient's and/or family's needs. Usually, the presenting problem(s) are of moderate to high severity. Typically, 25 minutes are spent face-to-face with the patient and/or family.

- For typical times for E/M services in outpatient settings, see Chapter 7, Evaluation and Management Services in the Office and Outpatient Clinics, and Chapter 8, Evaluation and Management Services in Home or Nursing Facility Settings. For typical times for E/M services in inpatient or observation settings, see Chapter 16, Noncritical Hospital Evaluation and Management Services.

- The time spent in counseling and/or coordination of care may be with the patient, family, and/or those who may have assumed responsibility for the care of the patient (eg, foster parents, legal guardian, person acting in loco parentis).

- The term *counseling* is broadly defined by *CPT* as most activities that are not procedures and includes discussions about a condition and/or its management. Per *CPT*, counseling includes

     ❖ Diagnostic results, impressions, and/or recommended diagnostic studies
     ❖ Prognosis
     ❖ Risks and benefits of management (treatment) options
     ❖ Instructions for management (treatment) and/or follow-up
     ❖ Importance of compliance with chosen management (treatment) options
     ❖ Risk factor reduction
     ❖ Patient and family education

- Counseling about a condition emerging as part of the information gathering for the primary diagnosis may appropriately be included in total time of counseling (eg, discussing ways to increase caloric intake in a patient with anorectic effects of medication for attention-deficit/hyperactivity disorder).

☀ Time of an E/M service is categorized as face-to-face or unit or floor time.

　❖ Face-to-face time applies in non-facility settings for services such as office and other outpatient E/M visits and consultations. Only the time that a physician or other QHP spends face-to-face with a patient and/or caregiver(s) is used for determining the level of service provided.

　❖ Unit or floor time is used in a facility setting (including outpatient observation) and includes the physician's or QHP's time directed to care of a single patient, including face-to-face time and time spent on the unit or floor managing and coordinating that patient's care (eg, reviewing charts, communicating with clinical staff). Time spent off the unit or floor (eg, in radiology viewing images) is not included in the unit or floor time used in code selection.

Table 1-5. *CPT* Definition of Face-to-face Time	
Consultation or Visit in Office/Outpatient, Home, Domiciliary	**Inpatient Hospital, Observation Setting, Nursing Home, Hourly Critical Care**
Direct physician to patient and/or family member/other with responsibility for care of the patient	Floor/unit time dedicated to the one patient Includes the time spent at the patient's bedside, counseling the family/patient, and on the floor documenting and coordinating care with the patient's care team members

☀ Although codes are valued to include typical preservice and post-service time, only the typical time (face-to-face or unit/floor) is used in code selection.

Example

➤ **The typical time assigned to a level 3 established patient office or other outpatient E/M service (99213) is 15 minutes.** Code 99213 is valued to include 3 minutes of preservice time (eg, time reviewing history obtained by clinical staff) and 5 minutes of post-service time (eg, time documenting the service provided, care coordination, and communication with patient/caregivers between current and next encounter). Because services are valued to include preservice and post-service time, code selection is affected only when the time of service significantly exceeds the typical time (eg, prolonged service is reported only for 30 minutes or more beyond the 15-minute typical time of code 99213).

☀ Time spent on a particular calendar day does not have to be continuous. A physician may spend face-to-face time with a patient before and after clinical staff administer treatments or monitor the patient, but only the physician's total face-to-face time with the patient is considered in selecting a level of service unless otherwise specified.

☀ When service time is discontinuous, each episode of care should include documentation of time.

☀ Only physicians or QHPs with their own National Provider Identifier may report services using time as the key component. Incident-to policy, as developed by Medicare, generally allows for reporting of services by QHPs working under direct physician supervision as if the services were personally performed by the physician. However, most Medicare contractors will not allow reporting of incident-to services based on time of counseling and/or coordination of care. Please refer to the Medicare Incident-to Requirements: Supervision of Nonphysician Health Care Professionals section in Chapter 13, Allied Health and Clinical Staff Services. Keep in mind that the incident-to requirements are Medicare policy; *commercial payers may have their own policies.*

☀ When time is used as the controlling factor in the selection of an E/M code and the service is provided by a resident, the time reported is based on the face-to-face time (for outpatient) or floor or unit time (for inpatient) spent by the teaching physician with the patient or caregiver. Refer to the Guidelines for Reporting E/M Services Under Teaching Physician Guidelines section in Chapter 6, Evaluation and Management Documentation Guidelines.

☀ When a range of codes includes sequential times (eg, office or other outpatient E/M services) and the time of service is between the times assigned to codes, report the code with the typical time closest to the actual time of service. If the actual time of service falls exactly between the typical times of 2 codes, report the code with *the lower typical time* (ie, the midpoint must be passed to report the greater service).

- Time-based services are reported based only on time devoted to that particular service. When a separately reportable service is performed concurrently with a time-based service, the time associated with providing the concurrent service *is not* counted toward the time used in reporting the time-based service.
- When separately reportable services are rendered in the same encounter as time-based services, the time spent in the separately reportable service should be distinguishable from that of the time-based service (eg, start and stop times of procedural services are noted).

Documentation of Time Spent in Counseling and/or Coordination of Care

According to the guidelines as specified in the AMA publication, *Principles of CPT® Coding,* when selecting a code based on time, the medical record documentation must reflect

1. The amount of time and extent of counseling and/or coordination of care services provided
2. Distinguishing of that time from time spent performing key components by reporting time separately
3. The total time spent face-to-face (for outpatient) or floor or unit (for inpatient)
4. A summary of the discussion items and/or the coordination of care efforts

If the entire face-to-face encounter is spent in counseling only, the total time spent and a summary of the discussion items must be clearly documented.

In distinguishing the time and extent of counseling and/or coordination of care services for a service that includes time spent performing key components, physicians may document the estimated number of minutes or the percentage of the documented total face-to-face time that was spent in counseling and/or coordination of care.

The summary of discussion items and/or coordination of care efforts should be sufficient in detail to support the selection of a code based on time (eg, include options discussed, patient/caregiver concerns addressed, and summary of patient and family education).

Examples for Documenting Time

Counseling in the office might be documented as follows:
- Spoke with Ms Jones about _____, and
  - ❖ *40-minute visit with approximately 25 minutes spent in counseling, or*
  - ❖ T = # minutes*; C = # minutes; counseled, *or*
  - ❖ "I personally spent a total time of <_> minutes in the care of this patient; of that, <_> minutes was spent in counseling and coordinating care face-to-face."

*If you choose to use the second method for documentation of time, be sure to include a description of T (total time) and C (counseling and/or coordination of care time) in your office policy. Otherwise, the documentation should state "total time" or "counseling time."

Hospital/observation care progress notes might be documented as follows:
- ❖ 25 minutes spent on floor with patient, nursing staff, and physical therapy regarding Ms Jones, *or* document time in and time out.
- ❖ Timed chart entry in the progress notes or orders may be enough to support floor time. Caseworkers, physical therapists, etc, may document the time spent communicating with the physician. These documented entries may support total floor time.

If you use a template for your progress notes, include space for reporting face-to-face time, counseling time, and a summary of discussion items. If you are using an EHR, make software changes to accommodate the documentation requirements. Do not just use the "office time" as shown in your EHR because that does not reflect face-to-face time.

A summary of the patient/caregiver concerns and questions, your responses and recommendations, and plan of care must be documented to support the medical necessity of the time spent counseling and/or coordinating care.

Time of Clinical Staff

In recent years, there has been greater recognition of the need for payment to support activities such as care coordination that require clinical staff time performing services under physician supervision rather than direct delivery of care by the physician. Services such as chronic care management, psychiatric collaborative care management, and prolonged clinical staff service are now described by specific *CPT*® codes reported based on the time spent by clinical staff. However, as with time-based services provided by physicians and QHPs, documentation to support services based on clinical staff time requires specific elements. These include

- Documentation of an authenticated order for the service by the ordering or supervising physician.
- Documentation of the time and care activity performed for each episode of service rendered by clinical staff during the reporting period, including authentication (written or electronic signature with credentials and date of service).
- Documentation and authentication of physician time spent in care activities that might otherwise be performed by clinical staff and were not otherwise reportable during the reporting period, when applicable.
- Evidence of the supervising physician's ongoing involvement in the patient's care, such as review and/or revision of the patient care plan.
- Only the time of clinical staff whose services are a practice expense to the reporting physician are included in the time of service (ie, services by clinical staff of a facility are not reportable by a physician who has no contractual or employment relationship with the staff).
- When multiple clinical staff members meet about a patient, count the time only once.

> ||||||| *Coding Pearl* |||||||
>
> See the prefatory language in *Current Procedural Terminology*® when reporting sequential time-based services, such as critical care, prolonged service, and moderate (conscious) sedation, to find specific instructions and helpful tables illustrating code assignment by time of service.

Time-Based Reporting of Non-E/M Services

In addition to time-based reporting of E/M services, many other services are reported based on the time of service. Only include time spent in activities such as interpretation and report when the code descriptor indicates time spent in such activities is used in code selection.

See Chapter 10, Surgery, Infusion, and Sedation in the Outpatient Setting, and Chapter 19, Common Surgical Procedures and Sedation in Facility Settings, for other information on reporting anesthesia or therapeutic and surgical procedures.

Time-Based Coding Examples

➤ Moderate (conscious) sedation services are reported based on 15-minute time increments of intra-service time beginning with administration of a sedating agent(s) and ending after the procedure is completed and the physician or QHP providing the sedation is no longer in personal continuous face-to-face contact with the patient.

➤ Intra-arterial and IV infusions are reported based on time and whether the infusion is the initial infusion service or a subsequent infusion service.

➤ Care plan oversight services for ventilator management of a patient in a home or domiciliary setting are reported for 30 minutes or more per month.

Examples

➤ Code 96116 (neurobehavioral status exam [clinical assessment of thinking, reasoning and judgment, eg, acquired knowledge, attention, language, memory, planning and problem solving, and visual spatial abilities], by physician or other qualified health care professional, both face-to-face time with the patient and time interpreting test results and preparing the report; first hour) specifically states that *the physician's time of interpreting tests and preparing the report is counted toward the time of service.*

➤ **Code 94780** (car seat/bed testing for airway integrity, for infants through 12 months of age, with continual clinical staff observation and continuous recording of pulse oximetry, heart rate and respiratory rate, with interpretation and report; 60 minutes) is reported based on the time spent (typically by clinical staff) monitoring the infant during the testing period and not on time spent by the physician interpreting the outcome and preparing a report.

Teaching Point: The physician's time interpreting the testing and preparing a report is not used in code selection, but the service was valued to include the typical post-service time that a physician spends in interpreting and preparing a report.

Time-based services may overlap 2 dates of service (ie, beginning prior to midnight and continuing on the next date). If the service is continuous, report as if provided on the initial date of service. However, once the initial service has ended, any new service provided on the second date is reported as an initial service.

Examples

➤ **A physician provides remote intraoperative neurophysiology monitoring from 8:00 pm on one date to 1:00 am on the next date.** The service is reported as performed on the date the service began with code 95941 (continuous intraoperative neurophysiology monitoring, from outside the operating room [remote or nearby] or for monitoring of more than one case while in the operating room, per hour) times 5 units.

➤ **A facility may report 2 initial IV push services (96374) when provided from 11:30 to 11:40 pm and again from 1:30 to 1:40 am, as the service was not continuous.** However, an IV push started at 11:55 pm and ending at 12:05 am is reported as one continuous service on the date the service started.

Key Takeaways for Reporting Time

Examples of time-based reporting are included throughout this manual to further the understanding of time-based reporting. The examples emphasize some key tips for reporting based on time.

❂ Time must be documented to support coding of time-based services. Failure to document time may lead to lost revenue.
❂ Time is met when the midpoint is passed unless otherwise specified in *CPT*® instruction or code descriptors.
❂ Time is that of the physician or other individual reporting the service unless otherwise specified (eg, code descriptor specifies clinical staff time).
❂ Documentation should include the context of time spent in counseling and/or coordination of care, when applicable.

National Drug Code (NDC)

The NDCs are universal product identifiers for prescription drugs including vaccines and insulin products. Codes are 10-digit, 3-segment numbers that identify the product, labeler, and trade package size. Medicare, Medicaid, and other government payers (eg, Tricare), as well as some private payers, require the use of NDCs when reporting medication and vaccine product codes. The HIPAA standards for reporting NDCs do not align with the 10-digit format; they require an 11-digit code. Conversion to an 11-digit code in 5-4-2 format is required. Leading zeros are added to the appropriate segment to accomplish the 5-4-2 format as illustrated in **Table 1-6**.

Table 1-6. National Drug Code Format Examples

Product	10-digit NDC Formats	11-digit NDC Formats (Added 0 [zero] is underscored.)
RotaTeq 2-mL single-dose tube, package of 20	0006-4047-20 (4-4-2)	<u>0</u>0006-4047-20 (5-4-2)
Fluzone Quadrivalent 0.25-mL prefilled single-dose syringe, package of 10	49281-517-25 (5-3-2)	49281-<u>0</u>517-25 (5-4-2)
Synagis 0.5-mL in 1 vial, single dose	60574-4114-1 (5-4-1)	60574-4114-<u>0</u>1 (5-4-2)
Abbreviation: NDC, National Drug Code.		

It is important to verify each payer's requirements for NDC reporting. Some payers require reporting of the NDC that is provided on the outer packaging when a vaccine or other drug is supplied in bulk packages. However, other payers require reporting of the NDC from the vial that was administered. If a payer uses the Medicare NDC-to-HCPCS crosswalk with HCPCS (ie, matches NDC to HCPCS/*CPT*® codes), the required NDC for vaccine products is specified in the average wholesale price.

The correct number of NDC units must also be included on claims. The NDC units are often different from HCPCS/*CPT* units. For most payers, NDC units are reported as grams (GR), milligrams (ME), milliliters (ML), or units (UN). The qualifiers GR, ME, ML, and UN are reported before the number of NDC units on a claim to indicate the measure. For instance, a claim for supply of 0.5-mL, single-dose, prefilled syringe of pneumococcal 13-valent conjugate vaccine would include 1 unit of service on the claim line with *CPT* code **90670** and ML05 units on the NDC line for this service, as illustrated in the 1500 form example in **Table 4-1** on page 85.

If you are not currently reporting vaccines with NDCs, be sure to coordinate the requirements with your billing software company. For more information on NDCs, visit www.fda.gov/drugs/informationondrugs/ucm142438.htm or link through www.aap.org/cfp, access code AAPCFP24.

> **~ More From the AAP ~**
>
> For more information on reporting National Drug Codes, see "Reporting the National Drug Code: A Refresher" in the August 2014 *AAP Pediatric Coding Newsletter*™ at http://coding.aap.org (subscription required).

Beyond Code Sets

Who Assigns the Codes?

Diagnoses should be assigned by the clinician (pediatrician, pediatric nurse practitioner, or physician assistant) indicating a principal (primary) diagnosis that best explains the reason with the highest risk of morbidity or mortality for the patient encounter. All contributing (secondary) diagnoses that help explain the medical necessity for the episode of care should also be listed. However, only those conditions that specifically affect the patient's encounter should be listed. Code assignment may take place in conjunction with documentation or later, depending on the workflow processes of the practice. When codes are selected by physicians at the time of EHR documentation, it is advisable to have trained administrative staff verify that the codes are selected in compliance with *ICD-10-CM* guidelines and conventions. Electronic health records often fail to show complete code descriptors and/or *ICD-10-CM* instructions (eg, exclusion notes).

Assignment of the specific diagnosis code by a nonphysician provider or administrative staff should be done under the physician's or reporting provider's supervision. The first-listed code on the claim should be the principal diagnosis unless the tabular instructions direct to "code first" a

> **||||||| *Coding Pearl* |||||||**
>
> Documentation of diagnoses, signs and symptoms, or other reasons for a service is not accomplished through code assignment. Per official guidance from *Coding Clinic*, selection of a code cannot replace a written diagnostic statement. Multiple clinical conditions may be represented by a single diagnosis code, and more than one code may be required to fully describe a condition. Codes should be assigned to the documented diagnostic statement.

specific condition (eg, code first cystic fibrosis [**E84.-**] in a patient with secondary diabetes [**E08.-**] due to cystic fibrosis).

Procedure codes may be selected at the time of documentation or later by administrative staff working under the supervision of the reporting provider. Verification of the levels of service, need for modifiers, and compliance with *CPT* and payer policies is advised prior to billing.

For those practices using a printed encounter form, including 50 to 100 of the most commonly used diagnoses *and* their respective codes on the outpatient encounter form allows the physician or health care professional to mark the appropriate code(s), indicating which is primary. If a specific diagnosis code is not included on the form, write it in! Do not select a diagnosis code that is "closest to" the diagnosis. The AAP has developed an encounter form including *ICD-10-CM* codes. For a copy, go to www.aap.org/cfp (access code AAPCFP24). Refer to Chapter 4, The Business of Medicine: Working With Current and Emerging Payment Systems, for tips on designing an encounter form.

Telling the Encounter Story

After learning to appropriately select codes for diagnoses, services, supplies, and medications, it is important to understand how these are relayed to health plans for payment. In the end, a claim tells a story of what happened during a patient encounter. Because physicians do not submit full documentation, use the various code sets and other supportive information to tell payers what happened and what should be paid (**Figure 1-1**).

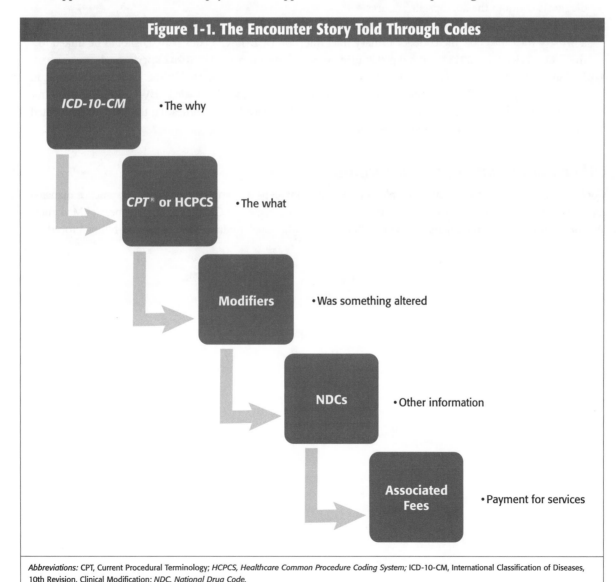

Figure 1-1. The Encounter Story Told Through Codes

- *ICD-10-CM* — • The why
- *CPT*® or HCPCS — • The what
- Modifiers — • Was something altered
- NDCs — • Other information
- Associated Fees — • Payment for services

Abbreviations: CPT, Current Procedural Terminology; *HCPCS, Healthcare Common Procedure Coding System;* ICD-10-CM, International Classification of Diseases, 10th Revision, Clinical Modification; *NDC, National Drug Code.*

Reporting Codes for Payment

In addition to establishing standard code sets, HIPAA also established standardized electronic transaction standards for patient benefit inquiries and submission of health claims and related reports. Claims for professional services are typically submitted electronically in a format referenced as 837P (professional claim) as currently configured in version 5010A1. Paper claim form submissions using the National Uniform Claim Committee 1500 claim form, version 02/12 (1500 form), are allowed for providers who meet an exception to the HIPAA requirements for electronic claim submission (eg, provider with <10 full-time employees). However, paper claims submission increases the length of time between submission and payment and increases the chance of error in either completion of the form or claims processing. Because of this, few physicians routinely submit paper claims. The 1500 form, however, contains the same information as an electronic claim and is valuable for demonstrating how codes and other information necessary for claims processing must be relayed to payers. An example of a completed 1500 form is found on page 85.

Linking the Diagnosis to the Service

* Every claim line for a physician service must be linked to the appropriate *ICD-10-CM* code that represents the reason for the service.
* When using an EHR, physicians should list the primary diagnosis in the EHR first and make certain the software knows that it should be reported as the first listed. In addition, the EHR should be able to link diagnosis codes to the appropriate services.
* The diagnosis code may be the same for each service performed. For example, if a child is diagnosed with a urinary tract infection, the code for urinary tract infection (*ICD-10-CM* code **N39.0**) should be linked to the E/M service (eg, **99213**) and a dipstick urinalysis without microscopy (**81002**) performed.
* Linking of the *ICD-10-CM* code to the service on the billing form is illustrated in the 1500 form example in Table 4-1 on page 85. Each *ICD-10-CM* code is placed in a diagnosis field labeled 21A–L. A diagnosis pointer in field 24E indicates which diagnosis code relates to each service line by indicating the letter of the related diagnosis field. More than one diagnosis field may be linked to a service.

Other Coding and Billing Information

Correct code assignment and claims completion are important steps in compliant and effective practice management. However, many other processes and policies are required. Please see Chapter 4, The Business of Medicine: Working With Current and Emerging Payment Systems, for additional guidance on coding and billing procedures.

Modifiers and Coding Edits

Contents

Chapter 2: Modifiers and Coding Edits

Chapter 2: Modifiers and Coding Edits

Current Procedural Terminology® Modifiers

Current Procedural Terminology (*CPT*®) defines a *modifier* as a means to indicate that a service or procedure has been altered by some specific circumstance but not changed in its basic code definition. Because a modifier is used to report a service or procedure that was altered, medical record documentation must always support the use of the modifier.

In addition to *CPT* modifiers, the Centers for Medicare & Medicaid Services (CMS) maintains a list of modifiers for use with Healthcare Common Procedure Coding System (HCPCS) and *CPT* codes. Most state Medicaid programs and many commercial payers follow CMS guidelines and may recognize HCPCS modifiers as well.

When are modifiers needed? In brief, a modifier or combination of modifiers is appended to a procedure code when it is necessary to add context of how or when the service was provided. Context often affects payment, such as when a procedure for which the code does not indicate unilateral or bilateral is performed bilaterally. By appending modifier **50** (bilateral procedure), the claim for services provides context allowing claims adjudication systems to process for payment at a higher rate (typically 150% of the allowable amount for the unilateral service). Examples of information provided by modifiers include

- A service provided on the same date or within the global period of a previous service is unrelated, more extensive, performed on a different body area, or performed at separate encounters.
- A face-to-face service was provided via telemedicine using real-time, interactive communication technology.
- The same service was repeated on the same date.
- An evaluation and management (E/M) service that might otherwise be considered part of another service is significantly beyond the typical preservice and/or post-service components of the other service.
- The units of services provided were medically necessary but exceed the payer's unit of service edits.
- A service that may be provided for diagnostic or preventive purposes was provided for preventive purposes.

Some modifiers are used exclusively with E/M services, and others are reported only with surgical or other procedures. Refer to **Table 2-1** to review modifiers used with E/M service codes and those used only for other services. Multiple modifiers can be appended to a single *CPT* or HCPCS code.

Payers use coding edits (paired codes and/or unit of service limitations) to aid in automated claims adjudication. Modifiers play an important role in this process. When a modifier is appropriately applied to one code in a pair or to a code for services that exceed the units of service typically allowed by payer edits, the payer may allow charges that would otherwise be denied as bundled or non-covered. Further illustration of the use of modifiers in relation to payer edits is discussed in the Coding Edits section later in this chapter.

The Health Insurance Portability and Accountability Act of 1996 requires recognition of all *CPT* modifiers, but payers may have their own payment and billing policies for the use of modifiers that can vary from *CPT* guidelines. Know and understand their policies. When payment is denied inappropriately because of nonrecognition or the incorrect application of a modifier, appeal the denied services. For more information, contact the American Academy of Pediatrics (AAP) Coding Hotline (aapcodinghotline@aap.org).

Table 2-1. Modifiers and Evaluation and Management Services	
24, 25, 57	E/M-only modifiers
22, 26, 47, 50, 51, 52, 53, 54, 55, 56, 58, 59, 62, 63, 66, 76, 77, 78, 79, 80, 81, 82, 91	Procedure-only (non-E/M service) modifiers
32, 33, 92, 95, 96, 97, 99	Either E/M or procedures
Abbreviation: E/M, evaluation and management.	

22–Increased Procedural Services

- Modifier **22** is used to report procedures when the work required to provide a service is substantially greater than typically required.
- Modifier **22** is only appended to anesthesia, surgery, radiology, laboratory, pathology, and medicine codes.

❖ Documentation must support the substantial additional work and the reason for the additional work (eg, increased intensity, time, technical difficulty of procedure, severity of patient's condition, physical and mental effort required). Reporting of additional diagnosis codes to support the increased work is also helpful.

❖ Most payers will require that a copy of the medical record documentation be sent with the claim when modifier **22** is reported. Make certain the procedure or progress note clearly reflects the complexity of the procedure and/or the increased time that was required. Report additional diagnoses that contributed to the increased work.

❖ For an electronic claim, indicate "additional documentation available on request" in the claim level loop (2300 NTE) or in the line level loop (2400 NTE) segment. If the payer allows electronic claim attachments, follow the payer's instructions to submit the procedure note and, if necessary, a physician statement about the increased difficulty of the procedure.

Examples—Modifier 22

➤ The physician required 45 minutes to perform a simple repair of a 1-cm laceration on a 2-year-old because the child was combative and several stops and starts were necessary.

    12011 22 (simple repair superficial wound of face; ≤2.5 cm)

➤ An appendectomy is performed on a morbidly obese 12-year-old. The surgery is complicated and requires additional time because of the obesity.

    44950 22 (appendectomy)

24—Unrelated E/M Service by the Same Physician or Other Qualified Health Care Professional During a Postoperative Period

❖ Modifier **24** is appended to an E/M code when the physician or other qualified health care professional (QHP) who performed a procedure provides an unrelated E/M service during the postoperative period.

❖ The CMS has its own system for definition of global periods, and some payers will follow those guidelines or assign a specific number of follow-up days for surgical procedures. (See Chapter 10, Surgery, Infusion, and Sedation in the Outpatient Setting, and Chapter 19, Common Surgical Procedures and Sedation in Facility Settings, for information on global surgery guidelines.)

Link the appropriate *International Classification of Diseases, 10th Revision, Clinical Modification* (ICD-10-CM) code to the E/M visit to support that the service was unrelated to the surgical procedure. Do not report the surgical diagnosis code if it was not the reason for the encounter.

Example—Modifier 24

➤ The physician sees a 6-year-old established patient for swimmer's ear (right ear) and performs a problem-focused history and physical examination. Eight days prior to this visit, the physician had performed a removal of a subcutaneous foreign body (by incision) not involving the fascia from the foot. The CMS has assigned a 10-day global postoperative period to code **10120** (removal foreign body subcutaneous tissues, simple), indicating that payment for all follow-up visits within that period related to that surgical service are included under the code. Many payers will follow the CMS global period.

ICD-10-CM	CPT®
H60.331 (acute swimmer's ear, right ear)	**99212 24** (established office/outpatient E/M)

25—Significant, Separately Identifiable E/M Service by the Same Physician or Other Qualified Health Care Professional on the Same Day of the Procedure or Other Service

~ More From the AAP ~

For more information on reporting evaluation and management or procedural services in the global period of another service, see "The Surgical Package and Related Services" in the May 2018 *AAP Pediatric Coding Newsletter*™ at http://coding.aap.org (subscription required).

- Modifier 25 is used when a procedure or service identified by a *CPT* code is performed by the same physician or other QHP, or physician or other health care professional of the same specialty and group, and the patient's condition requires a significant, separately identifiable E/M service (99201–99499) above and beyond the other service provided or beyond the usual preoperative and postoperative care associated with the procedure that was performed.

- Different diagnoses are not required for reporting of the E/M service on the same date.

- Separate documentation is required for the E/M service and the procedure or other service. Documentation for both services may be on one progress note. The performed and documented E/M components must support the level of service reported and be separately identifiable from the procedure or other service documentation.

- *CPT* procedure codes include evaluative elements routinely performed prior to the procedure and the routine postoperative care. An assessment of the problem with an explanation of the procedure to be performed is considered inherent to the procedure and should not be reported separately with an E/M service code. (See Chapter 10, Surgery, Infusion, and Sedation in the Outpatient Setting, and Chapter 19, Common Surgical Procedures and Sedation in Facility Settings, for information on global surgery guidelines.)

~ More From the AAP ~

For more information on reporting modifier 25, see "Revisiting Modifier 25: Still Confused After All These Years" in the February 2016 *AAP Pediatric Coding Newsletter*™ at http://coding.aap.org (subscription required).

- When appropriate, modifier 25 may be reported on more than one E/M service for a single encounter. An example would be if a physician performed and reported a preventive medicine service (eg, 99393 25) along with a problem-oriented service (eg, 99212 25) in addition to giving the patient vaccines with counseling (eg, 90460).

- **DO *NOT* USE MODIFIER 25 WHEN**
  - ❖ The medical record does not support both services.
  - ❖ A problem encountered during a preventive medicine visit is insignificant or incidental (eg, minor diaper rash, renewal of prescription medications, minor cold, stable chronic problem) or did not require additional work to perform the key components (history, physical examination, medical decision-making [MDM], or time) of the E/M service.
  - ❖ The E/M service is a routine part of the usual preoperative and postoperative care.
  - ❖ Modifier 57 (decision for surgery) is more appropriate. The ultimate decision on whether to use modifier 25 or 57 requires knowledge of payer policies. (See modifier 57 later in this chapter.)

Examples—Modifier 25

➤ **A 2-year-old established patient is seen in the office for a preventive medicine visit.** The mother reports that he has had vomiting and diarrhea since last evening. An expanded-level history and physical examination are performed and the patient is treated for acute gastroenteritis. The work performed for the illness (history, physical examination, and MDM) is documented in addition to the preventive medicine service.

ICD-10-CM	CPT
Z00.121 (routine child health examination with abnormal findings)	99392 (preventive medicine visit, established patient, 1–4 years of age)
K52.9 (unspecified noninfective gastroenteritis and colitis)	99213 25 (established office/outpatient E/M)

Teaching Point: See Chapter 9, Preventive Services, for additional examples and guidelines for reporting a preventive medicine visit and a problem-oriented visit on the same day of service. Be aware of certain circumstances in which there is no patient co-payment for preventive medicine visits, yet there is for office visits. Non-preventive services are often subject to coinsurance or co-payment and deductible amounts even when provided on the same date as a preventive service.

➤ **A patient is scheduled for an office encounter for excision of ingrown toenail.** The physician takes a problem-focused history from the patient, who has no other complaints; examines the affected nail; and agrees with excision, explaining the procedure, risks, and benefits. The ingrown nail is corrected by wedge excision of the nail fold.

ICD-10-CM	CPT®
L60.0 (ingrowing nail)	**11765** (wedge excision of skin of nail fold)

Teaching Point: An E/M service with modifier **25** is *not* reported. A separate charge for an E/M service is reported only when the E/M service is significant and separately identifiable from the preservice work of a procedure reported on the same date.

➤ **An established patient is seen for evaluation after falling from a tree in her backyard.** An expanded history and physical examination are performed to evaluate the extent of injuries. She has a 1-cm laceration (repaired) on the left forearm and abrasions on her right elbow and right hand.

ICD-10-CM	CPT
S50.311A (abrasion right elbow, initial encounter) **S60.511A** (abrasion right hand, initial encounter) **S51.812A** (laceration without foreign body, left forearm, initial encounter) **W14.XXXA** (fall from tree, initial encounter) **Y92.017** (injury occurred in the yard of a private residence) **Y93.39** (injury occurred while climbing)	**99213 25** (established patient office visit) **12001** (simple repair superficial wound of forearm; ≤2.5 cm)

Teaching Point: Because the patient required E/M significantly beyond the typical preservice work of a minor laceration repair (eg, evaluation of all apparent and potential injuries), a separate E/M service is reported. Place of occurrence (category **Y92**) and activity (category **Y93**) codes are used only once, at the initial encounter for treatment. These codes do not require seventh characters.

➤ **An E/M service is performed on a 6-year-old established patient.** He is given 600,000 units of Bicillin (penicillin G benzathine) by intramuscular injection for strep throat.

ICD-10-CM	CPT
J02.0 (streptococcal pharyngitis)	**99212–99215 25** (established patient E/M visit, office) **J0561** × 6 units (injection penicillin G benzathine, 100,000 units) **96372** (administration therapeutic injection)

Teaching Point: *CPT* requires that modifier **25** be appended to a significant and separately identifiable E/M service when also reporting the administration of a therapeutic injection.

➤ **A 12-year-old established patient is seen for his preventive medicine visit.** The patient complains of an increasingly severe itchy rash on his hands, arms, and legs for 3 days. A problem-focused history related to the complaint is performed. He is diagnosed and treated for a moderately severe case of poison ivy, requiring a prescription for a topical steroid. He has not yet received his tetanus, diphtheria, and acellular pertussis (Tdap) or meningococcal (MenACWY, intramuscular) vaccines. The physician counsels the parents on the risks and protection from each of the diseases. The Centers for Disease Control and Prevention (CDC) Vaccine Information Statements are given to the parents and the nurse administers the vaccines.

ICD-10-CM	CPT
Z00.121 (well-child check with abnormal findings) **Z23** (encounter for immunization)	**99394 25** (preventive medicine visit, established patient, age 12 through 17 years) **90715** (Tdap, 7 years or older, intramuscular) **90734** (MenACWY) **90460** × 2 units **90461** × 2 units
L23.7 (allergic contact dermatitis due to plants, except food)	**99212 25** (office/outpatient E/M, established patient)

Teaching Point: Medical record documentation supports that a significant, separately identifiable E/M service was provided and is reported in addition to the preventive medicine service. Modifier **25** is appended to code **99212** to signify it is significant and separately identifiable from the preventive medicine service. Modifier **25** is also appended to code **99394** to signify it is significant and separately identifiable from immunization administration (required by payers that have adopted Medicare and Medicaid bundling edits).

> ## CMS Versus *CPT* Guidelines: Reporting a Significant, Separately Identifiable E/M Service and Minor Procedures
>
> The CMS allows modifier **25** to be used when a significant, separately identifiable E/M service is provided by the same physician or other QHP on the same day as a minor procedure (eg, suturing, removal of foreign bodies, endoscopy) but not with a major procedure. (See modifier **57**.) The CMS defines a *minor procedure* as one with a 0- to 10-day Medicare global period.
>
> *CPT* does not define global periods, but most commercial payers will assign their own definition of a global service period for minor procedures. Medical record documentation must clearly support the care as distinct or over and above the usual preoperative care associated with the procedure.

26–Professional Component

⬦ Certain procedures (eg, electrocardiograms [ECGs], radiographs, surgical diagnostic tests, laboratory tests) include a professional and technical component. The professional component includes the physician work (eg, interpretation of the test, written report). Modifier **26** is used to indicate that only the physician or other QHP component (supervision and interpretation) is being reported on a procedure that includes technical and professional (physician) components.

⬦ When reporting the professional component of diagnostic tests, interpretation should be documented in a report similar to that which is typical for the physicians who predominantly provide the service and should include indication(s) for testing, description of test, findings, limitations (when applicable), and impression or conclusion.

⬦ If the report of a physician's interpretation is included in the documentation of another service (eg, office visit), it is important that the report is distinct and complete.

⬦ The professional component is not reported when a physician reviews a test and notes agreement with the interpreting physician or when only a quick read without formal interpretation is provided.

- Some codes were developed to distinguish between technical and professional components (eg, routine ECG codes **93000–93010**). Modifier **26** is not appropriate when reporting codes that distinguish professional and technical components.

Examples–Modifier 26

> A physician interprets a radiograph of the foot that was taken at the outpatient department of the hospital and creates a report of the findings.
>
> **73620 26** (x-ray foot, 2 views)
>
> The physician reports modifier **26**, indicating professional component only, because the hospital provided the technical component.

> A physician reviews a radiograph of the foot that was taken at the outpatient department of the hospital and interpreted by a radiologist at that facility. The physician notes agreement with the interpretation.
>
> The review of the radiograph is not separately reported. The physician did not perform the medically necessary interpretation and report that constitutes the professional component of the foot radiograph. However, the physician's review of the image increases the level of MDM in a related E/M service.

> A surgeon reprograms a cerebrospinal fluid shunt in the radiology department of the hospital.
>
> The surgeon would report code **62252 26** (reprogramming of programmable cerebrospinal shunt) and the hospital would report code **62252 TC**.

Reporting Procedures With Modifier TC

CPT® does not have a modifier for reporting only the technical component. However, most payers recognize HCPCS modifier **TC** (technical component only). If a service includes a professional and technical component and the physician owns the equipment, employs the staff to perform the service, and interprets the test, the procedure is reported without a modifier. The physician who does not own the equipment but performs the written interpretation and report should report the service with modifier **26** appended to the appropriate *CPT* code. The facility or provider who owns the equipment and is responsible for the overhead and associated costs would report the same procedure code with modifier **TC** appended.

32–Mandated Services

- Modifier **32** is appended to services (eg, second opinion) that are mandated by a third-party payer or governmental, legislative, or regulatory requirements.
- The modifier is not limited to E/M services.
- Modifier **32** would be used when, for example, radiologic services are requested from a worker's compensation carrier, laboratory testing (eg, drug tests) is requested by a court system, or a physical therapy assessment is requested by an insurer.

Example–Modifier 32

> A developmental pediatrician is asked by a managed care organization (MCO) to provide a second opinion on a family physician's patient for selected treatment services for autism spectrum disorder (ASD). A comprehensive history and physical examination with high MDM are performed and documented and a report with recommendations is sent back to the MCO.

ICD-10-CM	*CPT*
F84.0 (autistic disorder)	**99245 32** (office/outpatient consultation)

33—Preventive Services

CPT modifier **33** is used to communicate to payers that a preventive medicine service (defined by the Patient Protection and Affordable Care Act [PPACA] provisions listed as follows) was performed on a patient enrolled in a health care plan subject to the preventive service coverage requirements of PPACA and, therefore, should not be subject to cost sharing.

- The appropriate use of modifier **33** will reduce claim adjustments related to preventive services and corresponding payments to members.
- Modifier **33** should only be appended to codes represented in one or more of the following 4 categories:
  - ❖ Services rated A or B by the US Preventive Services Task Force
  - ❖ Immunizations for routine use in children, adolescents, and adults as recommended by the Advisory Committee on Immunization Practices of the CDC
  - ❖ Preventive care and screenings for children as recommended by Bright Futures (AAP) and newborn testing (American College of Medical Genetics and Genomics)
  - ❖ Preventive care and screenings provided for women supported by the Health Resources and Services Administration
- **DO *NOT* USE MODIFIER 33**
  - ❖ **When the *CPT* code(s) is identified as inherently preventive (eg, preventive medicine counseling)**
  - ❖ **When the service(s) is not indicated in the categories noted previously**
  - ❖ **With an insurance plan that continues to implement the cost-sharing policy on preventive medicine services**
- Check with your payers before reporting modifier **33** to verify any variations in reporting requirements.

Example—Modifier 33

➤ **A 17-year-old established patient is seen for an office visit on Monday for missed period and suspected pregnancy.** The physician provides an E/M service with a problem-focused history and physical examination and straightforward MDM. The physician determines the patient is not pregnant and does not want to become pregnant but has been sexually active with multiple partners. The physician then spends approximately 10 minutes discussing contraception and risks of sexually transmitted infection (STI) with the patient. Point-of-care HIV-1 and HIV-2 testing is conducted with negative results. Specimen is collected for chlamydia and gonorrhea screening by an outside laboratory. The patient chooses to adopt barrier contraception methods and acknowledges understanding of risks and benefits.

ICD-10-CM	CPT
Z32.02 (encounter for pregnancy test, result negative)	Problem-oriented **99212 25** (office visit) **81025** (urine pregnancy test)
Z30.09 (encounter for other general counseling and advice on contraception) **Z11.4** (encounter for screening for HIV) **Z11.3** (encounter for screening for STI)	Preventive **99401** (preventive counseling, approximately 15 minutes) **86703 33 92** (antibody; HIV-1 and HIV-2; single assay)

Teaching Point: Append modifier **33** to code **86703** to indicate the test was performed as a preventive service because, although recommended as a preventive service, the test is also used for diagnostic purposes. Modifier **92** is reported to indicate use of the HIV test kit (not all payers recognize modifier **92**). Code **99401** is reported for 8 to 23 minutes of service based on the midpoint rule for billing based on time.

47—Anesthesia by Surgeon

- Modifier **47** is used only when a physician performing a procedure *also personally performs* the regional and/or general anesthesia. The physician performing the procedure may not report codes **00100–01999** for anesthesia services. Instead modifier **47** is appended to the code for the procedure performed.
- When performed, a code for regional anesthesia (nerve block) may be reported to indicate the site of the block.
- Modifier **47** is considered informational by many payers and does not affect payment.
    - ❖ Medicaid considers all anesthesia (other than moderate conscious sedation) provided by the same physician performing a procedure to be included in the procedure.
    - ❖ Other payers may restrict use of modifier **47** to specific procedure codes and provide specific reporting instructions. Be sure to verify payer policy prior to reporting.
- **DO *NOT* USE MODIFIER 47 WHEN**
    - ❖ **Administering local anesthesia because that is considered inherent to the procedure**
    - ❖ **Performing moderate (conscious) sedation** (See Chapter 10, Surgery, Infusion, and Sedation in the Outpatient Setting, and Chapter 19, Common Surgical Procedures and Sedation in Facility Settings, for information on moderate sedation.)

Example—Modifier 47

➤ The surgeon performs a nerve block on the brachial plexus (**64415**) and removal of a ganglion cyst on the wrist (**25111**).

   25111 47 and **64415**

   The regional anesthesia is separate from the procedure.

50—Bilateral Procedure

- Modifier **50** is used to identify bilateral procedures that are performed at the same session.
- It is used only when the services and/or procedures are performed on identical anatomical sites, aspects, or organs.
- Modifier **50** is not appended to any code with a descriptor that indicates the procedure includes "one or both" or "unilateral or bilateral."
- The Medicare Physician Fee Schedule (Resource-Based Relative Value Scale [RBRVS]) includes a column (Column Z, BILAT SURG) that identifies codes that may be reported with modifier **50**. Procedures with a 1 indicator can be reported with modifier **50**. Many private payers also publish lists of codes that may be reported as bilateral procedures.
- When the *CPT®* code descriptor indicates a bilateral procedure and only a unilateral procedure is performed, modifier **52** (reduced services) should be appended to the procedure code.
- For Medicaid claims that require use of modifier **50**, only report 1 unit of service on the line item for the bilateral procedure.

Examples—Modifier 50

➤ A physician performs an incision and drainage of abscesses on both legs.

   10060 50 (incision and drainage of abscess; simple or single)

   Report based on payer guidelines. (See Coding Conundrum: Modifier **50** box.)

➤ A physician performs bilateral computerized corneal topography.

   Modifier **50** would not be appended to code **92025** (computerized corneal topography, unilateral or bilateral, with interpretation and report) because the code descriptor indicates a unilateral or bilateral procedure. (Modifier **52** is also not required for reporting a unilateral service when the code descriptor includes unilateral or bilateral.)

Coding Conundrum: Modifier 50

CPT® guidelines and Medicaid National Correct Coding Initiative (NCCI) edits require that bilateral procedures be reported with modifier **50** and 1 unit of service. Some payers may require that the procedure be reported with modifier **50** appended to the second code. Other payers may require that HCPCS modifiers **RT** (right) and **LT** (left) be appended to the code.

    For example: Foreign bodies are removed from both ears.

    Report with code **69200 50** with 1 unit, *or*

    69200 50 with 2 units, *or*

    69200 and **69200 50**, *or*

    69200 RT and **69200 LT**

Know payer guidelines and report services accordingly.

51–Multiple Procedures

- Modifier **51** is appended to additional procedures(s) or service(s) when multiple procedures are performed at the same session by the same individual or individuals in the same group practice. The primary procedure or service is reported first without a modifier.

- When multiple procedures or services are reported, payers usually reduce the payment for the second code by 50% because there is some resource cost duplication when both are done at the same visit or session. Medicare and some state Medicaid programs follow this policy.

  - The Medicare Physician Fee Schedule (RBRVS) includes a column (Column S, MULT PROC) that identifies codes that are subject to multiple procedure payment adjustment. The numerical indicators for multiple procedures are

    — 0 Procedure is not subject to multiple procedure payment adjustment.

    — 2 Procedure is subject to standard multiple procedure payment adjustment if reported on the same date as other procedures with indicators of 2 or 3.

    — 3 Procedure is subject to special rules for endoscopy when reported on the same date as another procedure in the same endoscopy family.

    — 4 Procedure is subject to special rules for diagnostic imaging when reported on the same date as another procedure in the same diagnostic imaging family (affects technical component only).

    — 5 The practice expense component for certain therapy services is subject to 50% reduction.

    — 6 The technical component of a diagnostic cardiovascular service is subject to 25% reduction.

    — 7 The technical component of a diagnostic ophthalmology service is subject to 25% reduction.

    — 9 Concept does not apply.

  For more information on multiple surgery indicators and adjustments, see Chapter 12, Section 40.6, of the *Medicare Claims Processing Manual* at www.cms.gov/Regulations-and-Guidance/Guidance/Manuals/Downloads/clm104c12.pdf.

- **DO *NOT* USE MODIFIER 51 WHEN**

  - Reporting add-on procedures (codes identified with the + symbol are exempt from the need to report this modifier because the services are performed in addition to a primary procedure or service).

  - Reporting *CPT* codes identified with the symbol Ø (exempt from modifier 51) because they have no associated or work relative value units (RVUs) and are already reduced (see Appendix E in *CPT* for a list of these codes).

  - Different providers perform the procedures.

  - Two or more physicians perform different and unrelated procedures (eg, multiple trauma) on the same patient on the same day (unless one of the physicians performs multiple procedures).

  - Reporting E/M services, physical medicine and rehabilitation services, or provision of supplies (eg, vaccines).

- Most payers identify those procedures that are eligible for modifier **51** and, therefore, are subject to multiple procedure or service payment reductions. Although many claims adjudication systems now automatically identify the primary procedure, it is advisable that the first-reported service is that with the highest relative value, followed by additional services appended with modifier **51**, when applicable.
- Some payers, including some Medicare administrative contractors, have advised against reporting this modifier because their systems automatically assign multiple service reductions to the appropriate services. In these cases, the system ignores modifier **51**. Check payer policies prior to reporting services with this modifier.

Examples—Modifier 51

➤ A simple repair of a 1.5-cm laceration on the left forearm and an intermediate repair of a 2.0-cm laceration on the head are performed on a child who has fallen while in-line skating at the local park.

ICD-10-CM	CPT
S01.01XA (laceration without foreign body of scalp, initial encounter) **S51.812A** (laceration without foreign body of left forearm, initial encounter) **V00.111A** (fall from in-line roller skates, initial encounter) **Y93.51** (injury occurred while in-line skating) **Y92.830** (place of occurrence, public park)	**12031** (layer closure of wound of scalp; ≤2.5 cm) **12001 51** (simple repair of superficial wound of extremity; ≤2.5 cm)

Teaching Point: Code **12031** is reported without the modifier because it carries the highest relative value (6.74 non-facility total RVUs vs 2.54 for code **12001**).

➤ Incision and removal of a foreign body of the left foot in the fascia and cryotherapy wart removal for common warts were performed at an office visit.

ICD-10-CM	CPT
S90.852A (superficial foreign body, left foot, initial encounter) **B07.8** (other viral warts)	**28190** (removal foreign body, foot, subcutaneous) **17110 51** (destruction of benign lesions other than skin tags or cutaneous vascular proliferative lesions; up to 14 lesions)

Teaching Point: Code **28190** is reported without the modifier because it carries the highest relative value (7.42 non-facility total RVUs vs 3.14 for code **17110**).

52—Reduced Services

- Modifier **52** is used when a service or procedure is partially reduced or eliminated (ie, procedure started but discontinued) at the discretion of the physician or other QHP.
- Modifier **52** is not used when a procedure is canceled prior to the induction of anesthesia and/or surgical preparation in the operating room.
- A payer may require that a letter of explanation and/or copy of the procedure or operative report be submitted with the claim.
- The diagnosis code linked to the procedure reported with modifier **52** should reflect why the procedure was reduced.
- When reporting a reduced service or a procedure code with modifier **52**, do not reduce your normal fee. Let the payer reduce the payment based on its policy and review of the submitted progress note.

Examples—Modifier 52

➤ Evoked otoacoustic emissions; limited test is performed on one ear due to a congenital deformity.

ICD-10-CM	CPT
Q16.9 (congenital malformation of ear causing impairment of hearing, unspecified)	92587 52 (distortion product evoked otoacoustic emissions; limited)

Teaching Point: Code 92587 includes testing of both ears. Therefore, modifier 52 would be appended for the unilateral service.

➤ Polysomnography with sleep staging and 4 or more additional parameters of sleep, with attendance by a sleep technologist, is performed on a 7-year-old patient. The study is discontinued after 4 hours of recording.

ICD-10-CM	CPT
R06.83 (snoring)	95810 52 (polysomnography; age 6 or older, sleep staging with 4 or more additional parameters of sleep, attended by a technologist)

Teaching Point: Instructions for reporting polysomnography include appending of modifier 52 when there is less than 6 hours of recording for code 95800, 95801, 95806, 95807, 95810, or 95811.

Coding Conundrum: Modifier 52 or 53?

The main distinction between modifiers **52** (reduced services—service was started but the physician elected to reduce the scope or even eliminate the procedure or service) and **53** (discontinued procedure—reason for terminating the procedure is due to extenuating circumstances or because complications arise that place the patient at risk) is the basis for the decision to alter the procedure. Modifier **52** is often used when the physician plans to reduce the scope or extent of the procedure as noted, whereas modifier **53** is used for situations such as unexpected events that occur in the course of the procedure (eg, cardiac arrest, profuse bleeding, arrhythmia). The following examples demonstrate the appropriate application of these modifiers when a physician performs a routine circumcision:

52: A physician begins a circumcision (**54150**) on a 3-day-old boy. The physician elects to perform the circumcision without a dorsal penile or ring block. In this circumstance, modifier **52** would be reported with code **54150** to indicate the service was reduced from its full descriptor based on the physician's discretion.

53: A physician begins a circumcision (**54150**) on a 3-day-old boy. During the procedure, the physician notices the neonate is showing signs of respiratory distress. The physician determines that the procedure needs to be discontinued to assess the neonate. Due to the severity of the situation, the physician decides not to continue with the procedure. In this circumstance, the physician would append modifier **53** to code **54150**, linking it to *ICD-10-CM* codes **Z41.2** (encounter for routine and ritual male circumcision) and **P22.9** (respiratory distress, newborn) to indicate why the procedure was discontinued. When reporting a procedure with modifier **53**, it is important to indicate why the procedure was discontinued.

53—Discontinued Procedure

◈ Modifier 53 signifies that a procedure was terminated (ie, started but discontinued) due to extenuating circumstances or circumstances in which the well-being of the patient was threatened (eg, patient is at risk or has unexpected, serious complications, such as excessive bleeding, hypotension) during a procedure.

◈ It is not used to report the elective cancellation of a procedure prior to the patient's anesthesia induction and/or surgical preparation in the operating suite.

◈ The diagnosis code should reflect the reason for the termination of the procedure.

◈ Most payers will require that operative or procedure reports be submitted with the claim.

Examples—Modifier 53

➤ **An unsuccessful attempt is made to place a central line in the right subclavian vein.** The line is successfully placed in the left subclavian vein.

> **36555 53 RT** (insertion non-tunneled centrally inserted central venous catheter; younger than 5 years)
> **36555 LT**
>
> *Note:* Some payers do not recognize modifiers **RT** and **LT**. See the descriptions and use of these modifiers in the Healthcare Common Procedure Coding System Modifiers section later in this chapter.

➤ **During catheterization of the right side of the heart, the child experiences ventricular arrhythmia and the procedure is discontinued.**

> **93451 53** (right heart catheterization)

54—Surgical Care Only

❖ Modifier **54** is appended to the surgery procedure code when the physician does the procedure but another physician or other QHP (not of the same group practice) accepts a transfer of care and provides preoperative and/or postoperative management.

55—Postoperative Management Only

❖ Modifier **55** is appended to the surgical code to report that only postoperative care is performed because another physician or other QHP of another group practice has performed the surgical procedure and transferred the patient for postoperative care.

56—Preoperative Management Only

❖ Modifier **56** is appended to the surgical code when only the preoperative care and evaluation are performed because another physician or other QHP of another group practice has performed the surgical procedure.

Examples—Modifiers 54, 55, and 56

➤ **An infant undergoes a repair of tetralogy of Fallot.** The patient's pediatric cardiologist provides the postoperative management.

> The surgeon reports code **33692** (complete repair tetralogy of Fallot without pulmonary atresia) with modifier **54** appended, and the cardiologist reports code **33692 55** for postoperative care services.
>
> These split care arrangements will usually require a manual review by payers, with some variable amount of the global fee being carved out for the 2 physicians. Check with your payers for their payment policy if this is typical for your practice.

➤ **A child is admitted to the hospital by the pediatrician for intravenous antibiotics for a deep abscess on the right leg.** On the second day of the hospital stay, a surgeon is called in and performs an incision and drainage of the abscess. The child is discharged on day 3 and seen in follow-up by the pediatrician.

> Surgeon reports

ICD-10-CM	CPT®
L02.415 (cutaneous abscess of right lower limb)	**27603 54** (incision and drainage with surgical care only)

Pediatrician reports

ICD-10-CM	CPT
L02.415	27603 55 (incision and drainage with postoperative management only)

Coding Conundrum: Modifiers 54, 55, and 56

Modifiers **54**, **55**, and **56** typically are used to report surgical procedures that have a global period of 10 to 90 days. They are not reported with procedures that have 0-day global periods. It is important to learn which guidelines are followed by your major payers. When reporting these modifiers, coordination and communication between the physicians and their billing staff is imperative.

57–Decision for Surgery

* Modifier **57** is appended to an E/M service that resulted in the initial decision to perform the surgery or procedure.

* Appending modifier **57** to the E/M service indicates to the payer that the E/M service is not part of the global period. The global period for surgical procedures is assigned by the CMS, private payers, or state Medicaid and not by the American Medical Association.

* Many payers will follow the CMS Medicare payment policy that allows reporting of modifier **57** only when the visit on the day before or day of surgery results in a decision to perform a surgical procedure that has a 90-day global period (major procedure). Know commercial and state Medicaid policies, maintain a written copy of the policy, and adhere to the policy. (See Chapter 10, Surgery, Infusion, and Sedation in the Outpatient Setting, and Chapter 19, Common Surgical Procedures and Sedation in Facility Settings, for information on global surgery guidelines.)

Examples–Modifier 57

➤ **A 10-year-old is seen by the pediatrician for the evaluation of pain in her foot.** Radiograph reveals a metatarsal fracture, and the decision is made to treat the closed fracture.

The appropriate E/M code (**99201–99215 57**), based on the medical necessity and performance and documentation of the required key components, would be reported in addition to code **28470** (closed treatment, metatarsal fracture; without manipulation). Code **28470** has an assigned global surgery period of 90 days. An E/M code with modifier **57** is reported only by the physician or a physician of the same specialty and group practice of the physician who performs the procedure. Other physicians providing E/M services on the day before or day of a procedure would not append modifier **57**.

➤ **A circumcision is performed on the day of discharge on a 2-day-old born in the hospital, delivered vaginally.**

ICD-10-CM	CPT
Z38.00 (single liveborn infant, delivered vaginally) Z41.2 (encounter for routine male circumcision)	99238 25 (hospital discharge management) 54150 (circumcision using clamp/device with dorsal penile or ring block)

Teaching Point: The procedure has a 0-day global period. Per CMS guidelines, modifier **25** would be appended to the E/M service instead of modifier **57**.

Chapter 2: Modifiers and Coding Edits

58—Staged or Related Procedure or Service by the Same Physician or Other Qualified Health Care Professional During the Postoperative Period

- Modifier **58** is used to indicate that a procedure or service performed during the postoperative period was planned or anticipated (ie, staged), was more extensive than the original procedure, or was for therapy following a surgical procedure.
- Modifier **58** is a recognized modifier under the NCCI. (See the Appropriate NCCI Modifiers section later in the chapter for more on NCCI edits.) Refer to the Medicaid NCCI Web site, https://www.medicaid.gov/medicaid/program-integrity/ncci/index.html, for more details on the proper use of modifier **58** to override an edit.
- Typically, payers recognize modifier **58** only when there is a global surgical period associated with the procedure code.
- **DO *NOT* REPORT MODIFIER 58 WHEN**
  - ❖ Treatment of a problem requires a return to the operating/procedure room (eg, unanticipated clinical condition) (see modifier **78**).
  - ❖ Reporting procedures that include as part of their *CPT®* descriptor "one or more visits" or "one or more sessions."

Examples—Modifier 58

➤ An excision of a malignant lesion (1 cm) on the leg is performed. The pathology report indicates that the margins were not adequate, and a re-excision is performed 1 week later. The excised diameter is less than 2 cm.

   11602 58 (excision, malignant lesion including margins, leg; excised diameter 1.1–2.0 cm) for the second excision

   Note: The first excision would be reported using code **11601** (margin diameter 0.6–1.0 cm).

➤ Closure of a perineal urethrostomy, 5 weeks post-hypospadias repair, is performed as planned.

   53520 58 (closure of urethrostomy)

59—Distinct Procedural Service

- Modifier **59** is never appended to the code for an E/M service.
- Report modifier **59** only when no other modifier better describes the reason for separately reporting a service that might otherwise be bundled with another procedural service on the same date. Never append modifier **59** to bypass payer edits without clinical justification.
- See HCPCS modifiers **XE, XP, XS,** and **XU** for potential alternatives to modifier **59**.
- Per *CPT*, modifier **59** represents one of the following conditions of a procedure:
  - ❖ The procedure was provided at a different session from another procedure.
  - ❖ The procedure was a different procedure or surgery.
  - ❖ The procedure involved a different site or organ system.
  - ❖ The procedure required a separate incision or excision.
  - ❖ The procedure was performed on a separate lesion or injury (or area of injury in extensive injuries).

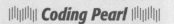
||||||| **Coding Pearl** |||||||

Never use modifier **59** in place of modifier **25** or on an evaluation and management service.

Examples—Modifier 59

➤ **The mother, teacher, and nanny each complete the Parents' Evaluation of Developmental Status.** The screenings are scored and interpreted.

96110 × 2 units and 96110 59 × 1 unit (developmental screen)

Medicaid Medically Unlikely Edits (MUEs) place a per-claim line limit on the units of service for 96110 at 2 units. When more than 2 units are clinically appropriate, the edit may be bypassed by reporting 2 units of service on one claim line and appending modifier 59 to additional claim lines. Remember that payers may have different reporting requirements for these services and, in addition, may have different upper limits on the number of units allowed.

➤ **Influenza A and B tests (87804) were performed. In this case, the rapid influenza test provides the physician with 2 distinct results.**

87804 (infectious agent antigen detection by immunoassay with direct optical observation; influenza)
87804 59

Modifier 59 would be appended to the second test to reflect that 2 distinct tests were performed.

Coding Conundrum: Modifier 51 (Multiple Procedures) or 59 (Distinct Procedural Service)?

Modifier **51** is most often used on surgical procedures that are performed during the same session and through the same incision. This modifier identifies potentially overlapping or duplicative RVUs related to the global surgical package or the technical component of certain services (eg, radiology services). Not all payers recognize or require modifier **51**.

Modifier **59** is used to identify distinct and independent procedures that are not normally reported together but are appropriate to the clinical circumstances. They are typically unrelated procedures or services performed on the same patient by the same provider on the same day on different anatomical sites or at different encounters. This is a modifier of last resort. When another modifier, such as **51**, is more appropriate, it should be reported in lieu of modifier **59**.

62—Two Surgeons

- Modifier 62 is used when 2 surgeons work together as primary surgeons performing a distinct part(s) of a procedure.
- Each surgeon should report his or her distinct operative work by adding modifier 62 to the procedure code and any associated add-on code(s) for that procedure as long as both surgeons continue to work together as primary surgeons.
- Each surgeon should report the co-surgery once using the same procedure code.
- If an additional procedure(s) (including an add-on procedure[s]) is performed during the same surgical session, a separate code(s) may also be reported without modifier 62 added.
- Column AB (CO SURG) of the Medicare Physician Fee Schedule (RBRVS) identifies procedures that may or may not be performed by co-surgeons. Indicator 1 is assigned to those procedures for which co-surgery is allowed under the Medicare program. See https://www.cms.gov/Medicare/Medicare-Fee-For-Service-Payment/PhysicianFeeSched/Index.html.

Example—Modifier 62

➤ **A neurosurgeon and general surgeon work together to place a ventriculoperitoneal shunt.**

Both physicians would report code 62223 62 with the same diagnosis code. The operative note must include the name of each surgeon, specific role of each surgeon, and necessity for 2 surgeons. Each surgeon should dictate his or her own operative report. Most payers will require authorization prior to the procedure.

63—Procedure Performed on Infants Less Than 4 kg

- Modifier **63** is used to report procedures performed on neonates and infants up to a present body weight of 4 kg that involve significantly increased complexity and physician work commonly associated with these patients.
- Unless otherwise designated, this modifier may only be appended to procedures or services listed in the **20100–69999** code series.
- Use of modifier **63** may require submission of an operative note with the claim. The operative note should include the patient's weight. It is also beneficial to report the patient's weight on the claim.
- **DO *NOT* REPORT MODIFIER 63**
  - ❖ When the code descriptor indicates the procedure is performed on young infants or neonates because the relative value for those procedures reflects the additional work (eg, code **49491** for repair initial inguinal hernia on preterm infant)
  - ❖ With any *CPT*® code listed in Appendix F of the *CPT* manual

Examples—Modifier 63

➤ A preterm neonate weighing 2.1 kg requires a physician's skill for central venous access.

    36568 63 (insertion of peripherally inserted central venous catheter without subcutaneous port or pump without imaging guidance; <5 years of age)

➤ A repair of patent ductus arteriosus by ligation is performed on an infant weighing less than 4 kg.

    33820 63 (repair of patent ductus arteriosus; by ligation)

66—Surgical Team

- Modifier **66** is appended to the basic procedure code when highly complex procedures (requiring the concomitant services of several physicians or other QHPs, often of different specialties, plus other highly skilled, specially trained personnel and various types of complex equipment) are carried out under the surgical team concept.
- Each surgeon reports modifier **66**.
- Each surgeon should dictate his or her own operative report and it should reflect the medical necessity for team surgery.
- Column AC (TEAM SURG) of the Medicare Physician Fee Schedule (RBRVS) identifies procedures that may or may not be performed by a team of surgeons. Indicator 1 is assigned to those procedures for which team surgery is allowed under the Medicare program.
- The operative notes are usually required by the payer.
- If a surgeon is assisting another surgeon, modifier **80, 81**, or **82** would be more applicable.

Example—Modifier 66

➤ Multiple surgeons perform different portions of an organ transplant.

    Each physician would report his or her services with modifier **66** appended to the procedure code.

76—Repeat Procedure or Service by Same Physician or Other Qualified Health Care Professional

- Modifier **76** is used when a procedure or service is repeated by the same physician or other QHP subsequent to the original procedure or service. Use of this modifier may prevent denial as a duplicate service line.
- The repeat procedure may be performed on different days. (Payer guidance may vary.)

- This modifier is appended to non-E/M procedure codes only and is not reported when the code definition indicates a repeat procedure.
- The use of this modifier advises the payer that this is not a duplicate service. (See modifier **91** for repeat clinical diagnostic laboratory test.)
- The CMS only recognizes this modifier on ECGs and radiographs or when a procedure is performed in an operating room or other location equipped to perform procedures. State Medicaid programs or other commercial payers may follow this guideline. Check with payers to determine their policy on use of the modifier.

Examples—Modifier 76

➤ **You see a patient in your office with severe asthma and give 3 nebulized albuterol treatments and steroids over the course of the visit.**

Report **94640** three times with modifier **76** appended to the second and third codes, or, if required by payers, report **94640 76** with 3 units.

(The Medicare and Medicaid NCCI manuals contradict *CPT* instruction for code **94640**, stating that *CPT* code **94640** should only be reported once during a single patient encounter regardless of the number of separate inhalation treatments that are administered.)

➤ **A physician performs incision and drainage of a cutaneous abscess of the right thigh (10060).** Within the 10-day global period of the procedure, the physician performs a repeat incision and drainage (**10060**) of the right thigh.

First date of service: **10060**
Second date of service: **10060 76**

77—Repeat Procedure or Service by Another Physician or Other Qualified Health Care Professional

- Modifier **77** is used when a procedure or service is repeated by another physician or health care professional subsequent to the original procedure or service.
- Payers may require documentation to support the medical necessity of performing the same service or procedure on the same day or during the global surgical period (if applicable).

Examples—Modifier 77

➤ **A simple repair of a 3-cm laceration of the knee is performed by the pediatrician.** Later that day, the child falls on the knee and opens the wound. A physician at the urgent care center performs another simple repair.

The second physician should report the service with code **12002 77**.

Remember that the diagnosis code selected must provide the medical necessity for the duplicate procedure. Payers may require a copy of the medical record.

78—Unplanned Return to the Operating/Procedure Room by the Same Physician or Other Qualified Health Care Professional Following Initial Procedure for a Related Procedure During the Postoperative Period

- Modifier **78** is used when another procedure is unplanned and related to the initial procedure, requires a return to the operating or procedure room, and is performed during the postoperative period of the initial procedure by the same physician.

- The related procedure might be performed on the same day or anytime during the postoperative period. (For repeat procedures, see modifier 76.)
- Link the appropriate diagnosis code(s) that best explains the reason for the unplanned procedure.

Examples—Modifier 78

➤ A pediatric surgeon returns to the operating room to stop bleeding from an abdominal procedure performed earlier in the day.

35840 78 (exploration for postoperative hemorrhage, thrombosis, or infection; abdomen)

The second procedure will usually be paid only for the intraoperative service, not the preoperative or postoperative care already paid in the original procedure.

➤ An incision and drainage of a deep abscess in the pelvis area 6 days following excision of a lipoma is performed.

26990 78 (incision and drainage, pelvis area; deep abscess)

79—Unrelated Procedure or Service by the Same Physician or Other Qualified Health Care Professional During the Postoperative Period

- The physician may need to indicate that the performance of a procedure or service during the postoperative period was unrelated to the original procedure. This circumstance may be reported by using modifier 79.
- The diagnosis must identify the reason for the new procedure within the global period. (For repeat procedures by the same physician on the same day, see modifier 76.)

Example—Modifier 79

➤ A patient had closed treatment of a shoulder dislocation with manipulation and 2 months later requires open treatment of a humeral shaft fracture.

24515 79 (open treatment of humeral shaft fracture with plate/screws, with or without cerclage)

80—Assistant Surgeon

- Modifier 80 is used when the assistant surgeon assists the surgeon during the entire operation.
- The primary surgeon reports the appropriate *CPT*® code for the procedure and the assistant surgeon reports the same code with modifier 80 appended.
- Payers vary on payment rules. The CMS establishes guidelines for payment of assistant surgery for each procedure code. Most payers, including the CMS, will not pay for nonphysician surgery technicians in this role.
- Many payers require documentation to support the necessity of an assistant surgeon.

81—Minimum Assistant Surgeon

- Modifier 81 is used when an assistant surgeon is required for a short time and minimal assistance is provided.
- The assistant surgeon reports the same procedure code as the surgeon with modifier 81 appended.
- Many payers require documentation to support the use of an assistant surgeon for only a portion of a procedure.

82—Assistant Surgeon (When Qualified Resident Surgeon Not Available)

- Modifier 82 is used in teaching hospitals when a resident surgeon is not available to assist the primary surgeon.

- The unavailability of a qualified resident surgeon is a prerequisite for the use of modifier 82 appended to the usual procedure code number(s).

Modifiers 80, 81, and 82

- The Medicare Physician Fee Schedule includes in column AA (ASST SURG) indicators identifying procedures that may or may not be billed by an assistant surgeon. Indicator 1 is assigned to those procedures for which an assistant surgeon is allowed to bill under the Medicare program. Note that a payer may require use of HCPCS modifier AS (physician assistant, nurse practitioner, or clinical nurse specialist services for assistant-at-surgery) for surgical assistance performed by a nonphysician QHP.

91—Repeat Clinical Diagnostic Laboratory Test

- Modifier 91 is used to indicate it is necessary to repeat the same laboratory test on the same day to obtain subsequent test results.
- Modifier 91 is only reported when the laboratory test is performed more than once on the same patient on the same day.
- Modifier 91 cannot be reported when repeat tests are performed to confirm initial results, because of testing problems with the specimen or equipment, or for any reason when a normal one-time, reportable result is all that is required.

Example—Modifier 91

➤ **In the course of treatment for hyperkalemia, a patient had 3 serum potassium determinations (84132) done on the same day in the same office.** The patient had severe diarrhea and dehydration and initial potassium was borderline high. An ECG demonstrated peaked T waves indicating need to recheck potassium values. The second potassium test came back as 6.0, and 10% calcium gluconate (10–15 mL/kg) was given to bring down potassium. A third potassium test was performed to see results.

    84132 91 × 3 units of service

92—Alternative Laboratory Platform Testing

Modifier 92 is used to indicate that laboratory testing was performed using a kit or transportable instrument that wholly or in part consists of a single-use, disposable analytical chamber.

- This modifier is not required or acknowledged by all payers.
- CPT® instructs to report this modifier with HIV test codes 86701–86703 and 87389.

Example—Modifier 92

➤ **A 17-year-old established patient is seen for a preventive medicine service.** The physician provides an age- and a gender-appropriate E/M service including discussion of contraception and risks of STI. Point-of-care HIV-1 and HIV-2 screening is conducted with negative results. Specimen is collected for chlamydia and gonorrhea screening by an outside laboratory. The patient chooses to adopt barrier contraception methods and acknowledges understanding of risks and benefits.

ICD-10-CM	CPT
Z00.129 (encounter for routine child health examination without abnormal findings)	99394 (preventive E/M service)
Z30.09 (encounter for other general counseling and advice on contraception) Z11.4 (encounter for screening for HIV) Z11.3 (encounter for screening for STI)	86703 33 92 (antibody; HIV-1 and HIV-2; single assay)

Teaching Point: Append modifier **33** to code **86703** to indicate the test was performed as a preventive service because, although recommended as a preventive service, the test is also used for diagnostic purposes. Modifier **92** is reported to indicate use of the HIV test kit (not all payers recognize modifier **92**).

95—Synchronous Telemedicine Service Rendered via a Real-time Interactive Audio and Video Telecommunications System

Modifier **95** is used to indicate a service was rendered via real-time (synchronous) interactive audio and video telecommunications system. This modifier is not applied if the communication is not real-time interactive audio and video. Codes to which modifier **95** may be applied are found in Appendix P of *CPT® 2019* and are preceded by a star symbol in the *CPT* manual.

Appendix P codes that may be of particular interest to pediatricians include

* New and established patient office or other outpatient E/M services (**99201–99205, 99212–99215**)
* Subsequent hospital care (**99231–99233**)
* Inpatient and outpatient consultations (**99241–99245, 99251–99255**)
* Subsequent nursing facility care (**99307–99310**)
* Prolonged services in the office or outpatient setting (**99354, 99355**)
* Individual behavior change interventions (**99406–99409**)
* Transitional care management services (**99495, 99496**)

Appendix P also includes codes for services such as psychotherapy, health and behavior assessment and intervention, medical nutrition therapy, and education and training for patient self-management, allowing for telemedicine services provided by certain qualified nonphysician health care professionals in addition to subspecialty physicians. For more information on reporting synchronous telemedicine services, see Chapter 20, Digital Medicine Services: Technology-Enhanced Care Delivery.

For a full listing of codes that may be reported for telemedicine services, see Appendix P in your *CPT* reference.

96—Habilitative Services

When a health plan is subject to the PPACA provision for equal benefits for habilitative and rehabilitative services, it may be necessary to append a modifier to identify those services that are habilitative (ie, intended to help the patient learn and retain new skills and functioning). As equal but separate benefit limitations for habilitative and rehabilitative services may apply, use of modifiers to distinguish services may allow for appropriate claims processing and support the patient's access to the full benefits for each type of service. Not all health plans are subject to the PPACA provision for habilitative and rehabilitative benefits, and covered services may vary. Be sure to verify benefits under each individual patient's plan prior to provision of services. When necessary, append modifier **96** (habilitative services) to the procedure code to indicate that the procedure provided was a habilitative service (eg, speech therapy for a child who is a late talker) versus rehabilitative (eg, speech therapy to assist a child with regaining speech following illness or injury). Some health plans have required HCPCS modifier **SZ** for designation of habilitative services and may or may not adopt modifier **96**. (See modifier **97** for reporting rehabilitative services. When both habilitative and rehabilitative services are rendered on the same date, append the appropriate modifier to the code for each service.)

Example—Modifier 96

➤ **A physician provides 30 minutes of adaptive behavior treatment with protocol modification for a child with ASD.** The patient's health plan requires a modifier to distinguish this habilitative service from rehabilitative services.

97155 96 (adaptive behavior treatment with protocol modification administered by physician or other qualified health care professional, which may include simultaneous direction of technician, face-to-face with one patient, each 15 minutes)

97–Rehabilitative Services

Modifier **97** is appended when it is necessary to designate that a service was rehabilitative in nature rather than for habilitative purposes. Under the PPACA, certain health plans must distinguish services that are rehabilitative (eg, services to help a patient walk following an accident that caused impairment) versus habilitative (eg, services to help a child with developmental delays learn to walk for the first time). As equal but separate benefit limitations for habilitative and rehabilitative services may apply, use of modifiers to distinguish services may allow for appropriate claims processing and support the patient's access to the full benefits for each type of service. Not all health plans are subject to the PPACA provision for habilitative and rehabilitative benefits. Be sure to verify benefits under each patient's plan prior to provision of services.

> **~ More From the AAP ~**
>
> For more information on reporting modifiers, see "When Are Modifiers Necessary?" in the November 2016 *AAP Pediatric Coding Newsletter*™ at http://coding.aap.org (subscription required).

Example–Modifier 97

➤ A physician provides 15 minutes of adaptive behavior treatment with protocol modification for a child with ASD.

    97155 97

Healthcare Common Procedure Coding System Modifiers

The HCPCS modifiers are used to report specific information not conveyed in code descriptors or by *CPT*® modifiers, such as procedural services performed at separate encounters on the same date (**XE**), performance of tests waived by Clinical Laboratory Improvement Amendments (CLIA) (**QW**), technical component only (**TC**), and anatomical sites, such as **RT** (right side) and **E1** (upper left eyelid). Medicaid programs often use a variety of HCPCS modifiers for state-defined purposes. See your state Medicaid provider manual for information on HCPCS modifiers and definitions assigned in your state (eg, modifier **SY** [persons who are in close contact with member of high-risk population] may be used with codes for certain immunizations). Be sure to review the list of HCPCS modifiers in your 2019 HCPCS reference.

Anatomical Modifiers

An anatomical modifier may be reported to identify specific sites, such as right foot, fifth digit (**T9**). The anatomical-specific modifiers are designated as appropriate modifiers under NCCI edits and are listed in the Modifiers That Can Be Used to Override NCCI Edits box later in this chapter. The Medicaid NCCI manual indicates that procedures performed on fingers should be reported with modifiers **FA** and **F1–F9**, and procedures performed on toes should be reported with modifiers **TA** and **T1–T9**. Medically Unlikely Edit values for many finger and toe procedures are 1 (one) based on use of these modifiers for clinical scenarios in which the same procedure is performed on more than one finger or toe. (See the Medically Unlikely Edits section later in this chapter for more information.)

Example–Anatomical Modifiers

➤ A physician must amputate the fourth and fifth phalanges of the left foot.
    28820 T3 (amputation, toe; metatarsophalangeal joint)
    28820 T4 (amputation, toe; metatarsophalangeal joint)
    Note: Some payers may require that modifier **59** (distinct procedural service) or **XS** (separate structure) be reported. Verify coding edits and payer policy before reporting.

X {E, P, S, U} Modifiers

Modifiers XE, XP, XS, and XU were implemented by Medicare and other payers to more specifically identify reasons for separate reporting of procedures or services that may previously have been identified by *CPT* modifier 59. However, instructions for correct use of these modifiers are still limited and may vary by payer. As the XE, XP, XS, and XU modifiers are more specific, payers may require reporting in lieu of modifier 59. Modifiers XE, XP, XS, and XU should not be appended to an E/M code. Do not append modifier 59 and the XE, XP, XS, and XU modifiers to the same service line of a claim (ie, single code). As payer adoption and guidance on use of these modifiers may vary, it is important to verify individual payer policy before reporting.

XE	Separate encounter (different operative session)
XP	Separate practitioner
XS	Separate structure (site/organ)
XU	Unusual nonoverlapping service

While accepted by most payers, few resources are available to describe appropriate reporting of these modifiers. National Correct Coding Initiative edits are not yet updated to require modifiers XE, XP, XS, and XU in lieu of modifier 59 for specific code pairs. *AAP Pediatric Coding Newsletter*™ will include articles featuring more information on these modifiers as it becomes available.

EP—Service Provided as Part of Medicaid Early and Periodic Screening, Diagnosis, and Treatment (EPSDT) Program

Some Medicaid and private payers require the use of modifier EP to denote services that are provided to covered patients as part of the Early and Periodic Screening, Diagnosis, and Treatment (EPSDT) program services required in the state.

❋ Can be appended to the preventive medicine service (eg, 99392) or screening services, such as developmental screening (96110)

Example—Modifier EP

➤ A 9-month-old established patient presents for her routine preventive medicine service. As part of her state EPSDT services, she receives an age-appropriate history and physical examination, preventive counseling, and anticipatory guidance. The patient's father also receives a standardized developmental screening, which is required of EPSDT services.

   99391 EP (preventive medicine service, established patient <1 year)
   96110 EP (developmental screening)

GA—Waiver of Liability Statement Issued as Required by Payer Policy, Individual Case

GU—Waiver of Liability Statement Issued as Required by Payer Policy, Routine Notice

GX—Notice of Liability Issued, Voluntary Under Payer Policy

❋ Modifiers GA, GU, and GX may or may not be recognized by Medicaid and private payers when reporting services that are not covered under the patient's benefit plan. Follow individual payer policies regarding provision and reporting of advance notice of noncoverage to patients/responsible parties.

GC—This Service Has Been Performed in Part by a Resident Under the Direction of a Teaching Physician

- When modifier **GC** is included on a claim, a teaching physician is certifying that the service was rendered in compliance with the CMS requirements for services reported by teaching physicians.
- Requirements for reporting modifier **GC** may vary among commercial health plans. This modifier is typically informational, meaning it does not affect the amount paid for a service.
- If the service was provided solely by the teaching physician, the claim should not be billed with the **GC** modifier.
- See further discussion of modifier **GC** in Chapter 6, Evaluation and Management Documentation Guidelines, and Chapter 19, Common Surgical Procedures and Sedation in Facility Settings.

JW—Drug Amount Discarded/Not Administered to Any Patient

- May be used as a tool to internally track wasted drugs and vaccines.
- This modifier is reported on claims only when required by certain payers. As of January 1, 2017, Medicare required use of modifier **JW** on codes for the unused portion of a drug or biological from a single-dose vial or package when the billing unit assigned to the drug in the HCPCS code descriptor has been exceeded. Medicaid plans may also require reporting of modifier **JW**.
- When required by payer policy, report only when the full amount of a single-dose vial is not used due to patient indications. Report only when the amount of drug wasted is equal to at least 1 billing unit (ie, do not report wastage when 7 mg of a 10-mg vial is administered and the billing unit is 10 mg, as the remaining 3 mg is already accounted for in the billing unit).
- Never report for discarded amounts from a multidose vial.
- Never report modifier **JW** for overfill wastage (ie, an excess amount placed in the single-dose vial by the manufacturer to ensure that an adequate amount can be drawn into the syringe for use).
- Modifier **JW** is not applicable for reporting the following circumstances. However, some practices use the modifier for internal tracking of drug waste.
  - ❖ A parent decides to forego an immunization after the vaccine had been drawn up.
  - ❖ The vial is dropped and the medication must be discarded.
  - ❖ A vaccine is discarded due to temperature out of range during storage.

> ### ~ More From the AAP ~
>
> The AAP Private Payer Advocacy Advisory Committee developed a paper, "The Business Case for Pricing Vaccines," to share with payers to address fair payment for vaccines above and beyond purchase price. Calculated in that rate is loss due to wastage. Given that many payers will not pay for a vaccine product not given, if payment rates are appropriate, there is compensation overall. See the paper at www.aap.org/cfp; use access code AAPCFP24.

QW—CLIA-Waived Tests

- The CLIA-waived tests are those commonly done in a laboratory or an office that are considered simple and low risk.
- One common test in the *CPT®* **80000** series that is CLIA waived is the rapid strep test (**87880**).
- Laboratories and physician offices performing waived tests may need to append modifier **QW** to the *CPT* code for CLIA-waived procedures. The use of modifier **QW** is payer specific.
- Some of the CLIA-waived tests are exempt from the use of modifier **QW** (eg, **81002**, **82272**). To review the list of CLIA-waived procedures, go to https://www.cms.gov/clia.

RT, LT—Right and Left Side

- Modifiers **RT** and **LT** are used for information only and do not affect payment of a procedure unless otherwise specified by a payer.
- Used to identify procedures performed on the left or right side of the body.
- Modifiers **RT** and **LT** are not used in place of modifier **50** but may be used in association with modifier **50**.

Some payers may require that modifier **59** (distinct procedural service) be reported in addition to or in lieu of the laterality modifiers.

Example—Modifiers RT and LT

➤ **The physician removes a subcutaneous foreign body that extended into the fascia from the left elbow and a subfascial foreign body from the right elbow.**

  24200 LT (removal of a subcutaneous foreign body from the elbow)

  24201 RT (removal of a deep foreign body from the elbow)

X1–X5 Patient Relationship Modifiers

- Modifiers **X1–X5** were introduced for voluntary reporting of the reporting physician or practitioner's relationship to a patient during an episode of care.

X1	Continuous/broad services
X2	Continuous/focused services
X3	Episodic/broad services
X4	Episodic/focused services
X5	Only as ordered by another clinician

- At this time, there is no requirement to report modifiers **X1–X5**, and there is no effect on payment when these modifiers are used or not used.
- In the future, the patient relationship modifiers are intended for use in value-based payment methodologies where the cost of care and outcomes may be attributed to specific physicians and other providers of care. (For more information on value-based payment methodologies, see Chapter 3, Coding to Demonstrate Quality and Value.)

Coding Edits

National Correct Coding Initiative (NCCI) Edits

The NCCI edits were developed for use by the CMS in adjudicating Medicare claims, but they are also used by many private payers, and all Medicaid programs use a Medicaid-specific version of the NCCI edits. The NCCI edits frequently form the basis for proprietary claims software.

The NCCI edits

- Have been developed based on *CPT* code descriptors and instructions, coding guidelines developed by national medical societies (eg, AAP), Medicare billing history, local and national Medicare carrier policies and edits, and analysis of standard medical and surgical practice.
- Are used by payers to translate payment policies into the claims processing system for physician services as well as to promote correct coding.
- Include 2 types of edits: procedure-to-procedure (PTP) and MUEs.

The Medicaid NCCI manual includes the following guidance: "Physicians should not inconvenience beneficiaries nor increase risks to beneficiaries by performing services on different dates of service to avoid MUE or NCCI PTP edits." This is likely in response to practice policies adopted by some physicians that are focused on achieving maximum payment. Delaying patient care to avoid code edits could be seen as an abusive billing practice and policies or practices to the effect should be avoided.

Procedure-to-Procedure Edits

- ❋ Identify code pairs that normally should not be billed by the same physician for the same patient on the same date of service.
- ❋ Include edits based on services that are mutually exclusive based on code descriptor or anatomical considerations, services that are considered to be inherent to each other, and edits based on coding instructions.
  - ❖ If 2 codes of an edit are billed by the same provider for the same patient for the same date of service without an appropriate modifier, the column 1 code is paid.
  - ❖ If clinical circumstances justify appending the appropriate modifier to the column 2 code, payment of both codes may be allowed.

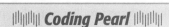

> **Coding Pearl**
>
> Medicaid NCCI files are published separately from Medicare files at https://www.medicaid.gov/medicaid/program-integrity/ncci/index.html.

Appropriate NCCI Modifiers

Modifier indicators are assigned to every code pair identified in the NCCI. They dictate whether modifiers are needed or will be accepted to override the edit. These indicators are

0   Under no circumstance may a modifier be used to override the edit.

1   An appropriate modifier may be used to override the edit.

9   This edit was deleted prior to its effective date or there is, essentially, no edit.

Modifiers That Can Be Used to Override NCCI Edits

24 Unrelated E/M service by the same physician or other qualified health care professional during a postoperative period	**FA** Left hand, thumb
	F1 Left hand, second digit
	F2 Left hand, third digit
25 Significant, separately identifiable E/M service by the same physician or other qualified health care professional on the same day of the procedure or other service	**F3** Left hand, fourth digit
	F4 Left hand, fifth digit
	F5 Right hand, thumb
	F6 Right hand, second digit
	F7 Right hand, third digit
57 Decision for surgery	**F8** Right hand, fourth digit
58 Staged or related procedure or service by the same physician or other qualified health care professional during the postoperative period	**F9** Right hand, fifth digit
	LC Left circumflex, coronary artery
	LD Left anterior descending coronary artery
59 Distinct procedural service	**LM** Left main coronary artery
78 Unplanned return to the operating/procedure room by the same physician or other qualified health care professional following initial procedure for a related procedure during the postoperative period	**LT** Left side
	RC Right coronary artery
	RI Ramus intermedius coronary artery
	RT Right side
	TA Left foot, great toe
79 Unrelated procedure or service by the same physician or other qualified health care professional during the postoperative period	**T1** Left foot, second digit
	T2 Left foot, third digit
	T3 Left foot, fourth digit
91 Repeat clinical diagnostic laboratory test	**T4** Left foot, fifth digit
E1 Upper left, eyelid	**T5** Right foot, great toe
E2 Lower left, eyelid	**T6** Right foot, second digit
E3 Upper right, eyelid	**T7** Right foot, third digit
E4 Lower right, eyelid	**T8** Right foot, fourth digit
	T9 Right foot, fifth digit
	XE Separate encounter (different operative session)
	XP Separate practitioner
	XS Separate structure (site/organ)
	XU Unusual nonoverlapping service

Only certain modifiers can be used to override edits when the service or procedure is clinically justified, and they may be used only on the code pairs that are assigned the 1 indicator. For overrides of mutually exclusive edits or correct coding edits, the appropriate modifier is always appended to the code that appears in column 2 because that is considered the bundled procedure. To append the appropriate modifier and override an edit, it is imperative that the conditions of that modifier are met.

Modifiers **22** (increased procedural services), **76** (repeat procedure or service by same physician or other QHP), and **77** (repeat procedure or service by another physician or other QHP) are not Medicaid NCCI-associated modifiers. Use of any of these modifiers does not bypass an NCCI PTP edit.

Examples of Medicaid NCCI Edits

Column 1	Column 2	Modifier Indicator	Effective Date
99460 Initial hospital or birthing center care, per day, for evaluation and management of normal newborn infant	**99462** Subsequent hospital care, per day, for evaluation and management of normal newborn	0	10/1/2010
The NCCI edits preclude any payment for the component code because they are mutually exclusive. Each code represents all normal newborn care on a single date of service by one physician or physicians of the same specialty and group practice.			
94640 Pressurized/non-pressurized inhalation treatment	**94664** Demonstration and/or evaluation patient use of nebulizer	1	10/1/2010
The comprehensive code (**94640**) would be paid and the component code (**94664**) would be denied unless a modifier indicating a distinct procedural service (eg, **59**) is appended to the component code (**94664**). Please note that under current CMS payment policy, both services are reported only if the nebulizer treatment and demonstration utilize different devices (eg, treatment with small volume nebulizer and demonstration of handheld inhaler with spacer) or occurred at separate encounters. Please refer to the CMS NCCI edit site for more information (https://www.medicaid.gov/medicaid/program-integrity/ncci/index.html).			
94060 Bronchodilation responsiveness, spirometry as in **94010**, pre- and post-bronchodilator administration	**94010** Spirometry	0	10/1/2010
The NCCI edits preclude any payment for the component code (ie, column 2 code **94010**).			
90460 Immunization administration through 18 years of age, first or only component, with counseling by physician	**99392** Preventive medicine service, established patient age 1–4	1	1/1/2013
The comprehensive code (**90460**) would be paid and the component code (**99392**) would be denied unless modifier **25** (significant, separately identifiable E/M service) is appended to the component code (**99392**). Be aware that the higher valued service may be listed as the component code and would be denied without the application of the correct modifier. Medicaid NCCI edits place routine child health examination codes (eg, **99392**) as component codes to immunization administration codes, although the counseling included in the routine child health examination is distinct from immunization counseling.			

Medically Unlikely Edits

The *National Correct Coding Initiative Policy Manual for Medicaid Services* describes MUEs as unit of service edits that were established by the CMS to prevent payment for an inappropriate number/quantity of the same service. An MUE for a HCPCS/*CPT*® code is the maximum number of units of service, under most circumstances, allowable by the same provider for the same beneficiary on the same date of service.

Medicaid MUEs

- Are applied separately to each line of a claim. If the unit of service on a line exceeds the MUE value, the entire line is denied.
- Are coding edits rather than medical necessity edits. State Medicaid agencies may apply payment policy that is more restrictive than the MUEs.
- May be established based on claims data. Claims data are also used in considering appeals of charges denied based on MUEs.
- May limit units of service based on anatomical structures.
- May limit the number of units of service based on *CPT®* code descriptors/*CPT* coding instructions.
- Are published on the CMS Medicaid NCCI Web site at https://www.medicaid.gov/medicaid/program-integrity/ncci/index.html.
- Are published with an "Edit Rationale" for each HCPCS/*CPT* code.
  - ❖ The MUE value assigned for code **96110** (developmental screening, per instrument) is 3 based on CMS NCCI policy. (No further explanation of this rationale is provided in the current Medicaid or Medicare NCCI manuals.)
  - ❖ The MUE value assigned to code **96127** (brief emotional/behavior assessment, per instrument) is 2 based on the nature of the service or procedure (typically determined by the amount of time required to perform a procedure/service or clinical application of a procedure/service).
- Are applied separately to each claim line for a service when modifiers (eg, **59**, **76**, **77**, anatomical) cause the same HCPCS/*CPT* code to appear on separate lines of a claim.

It is important to recognize the use of modifiers to override the MUE must be justified based on correct selection of the procedure code, correct application of the number of units reported, medical necessity and reasonableness of the number of services, and, if applicable, reason the physician's practice pattern differs from national patterns.

Keeping Up-to-date With NCCI

Medicaid and Medicare NCCI edits are updated quarterly. Each Medicare NCCI version ends with .0 (point zero), .1, .2, or .3 indicating its effective dates.

- Versions ending in .0 (point zero) are effective from January 1 through March 31 of that year.
- Versions ending in .1 are effective from April 1 through June 30 of that year.
- Versions ending in .2 are effective from July 1 through September 30 of that year.
- Versions ending in .3 are effective from October 1 through December 31 of that year.

The CMS releases the Medicare NCCI edits free of charge on its Web site (www.cms.gov/NationalCorrectCodInitEd/NCCIEP/list.asp). Medicaid NCCI files are published separately free of charge at https://www.medicaid.gov/medicaid/program-integrity/ncci/index.html. Although many of the Medicaid edits mirror Medicare edits, this is not always the case. The CMS has instructed that use of the appropriate NCCI file is important to correct coding. Online NCCI edits are posted in spreadsheet form, which allows users to sort by procedure code and effective date. Furthermore, there is a "Find" tool that allows users to look for a specific code. The edit files are indexed by procedure code ranges for simplified navigation. Policy manuals that explain the rationale for edits and correct use of NCCI-associated modifiers are published to the Web pages listed previously. Updated manuals for the year ahead are published annually in late fall. Changes in the manual are shown in red font for easy identification. Be sure to update your NCCI edit files quarterly and review changes to the NCCI manual each year.

Practice management and electronic health record software may also contain tools for identifying codes affected by NCCI edits.

Reviewing and Using These Edits

1. Be aware of all coding edits that are applicable to your specialty; as each update replaces the former edits, it is important to review them quarterly. Always look for new or deleted edits. Updated files can be found at www.aap.org/coding under the "Coding Resources, National Correct Coding Initiative (NCCI) Edits" tab.

2. Pay close attention to the modifier indicator because it may have changed from the last quarterly update. For example, a code set that initially would not allow override with a modifier may now subsequently allow one, or vice versa.

3. Pay attention to the effective date and deletion date of each code set. The edits are applicable only if they are effective. The effective date is based on the date of service, and not the date the claim was submitted. Sometimes a pair is retroactively terminated. If so, you may resubmit claims for payment if the date of service is within the filing time frame of the payer.

4. Use modifiers as appropriate. Modifiers should be used only when applicable based on coding standards, when medically justified or necessary, and when supported by medical record documentation (progress notes, operative notes, procedure notes, diagrams, or pictures), or, as previously mentioned, when dictated by payers. Refer to the CMS written guidelines (because they are very explicit about billing surgical procedures) or to your payer's provider manual.

5. When billing surgical procedures, you may need to look at several different codes for possible edits. Be sure to always use the code that is reflective of the total service performed.

6. If you are denied payment for services for which there is no edit, for which a reported modifier should have allowed payment, and/or for which the edit is inconsistent with *CPT* guidelines, you need to appeal the denial. Having knowledge of how this system works is to your benefit when appealing the denial.

7. Some payers have developed or adopted coding edit programs that are different from and often more comprehensive than the NCCI. If a payer policy differs from the CMS NCCI policy and is not clearly defined in its provider manual, refer to the payer's Web site. Make sure you get policies in writing for the services you commonly perform.

8. Report the services provided correctly based on *CPT* code guidelines (unless a payer has clearly stated otherwise). Remember that these edits are based on Medicare and Medicaid guidelines, and not all private payers follow all these edits.

> ### ~ More From the AAP ~
>
> For more information on NCCI edits, see "Back to Basics: The National Correct Coding Initiative" in the March 2015 *AAP Pediatric Coding Newsletter* at http://coding.aap.org (subscription required).

Chapter 2: Modifiers and Coding Edits

Coding to Demonstrate Quality and Value

Contents

Quality and performance measurement are important aspects of the pediatric medical home and the movement from payment by fee for service alone to value-based payment. Physicians who have successfully participated in quality measurement may see incentive payments, such as per-member/per-month payments, annual incentives, or a percentage of savings.

Physicians, payers, and accreditation organizations may use codes or claims data as a first line of quality measurement. When diagnosis or procedure codes provide necessary information for reviewing quality performance data, more time-consuming and costly medical record review may be avoided. In January 2017, the American Academy of Pediatrics (AAP) published a policy statement, "A New Era in Quality Measurement: The Development and Application of Quality Measures" (http://pediatrics.aappublications.org/content/139/1/e20163442). This policy statement includes a recommendation to national policy makers as follows:

"Quality measures, as much as possible, should be reportable by either *International Classification of Diseases, 10th Revision, Clinical Modification*, or *Current Procedural Terminology®* category II codes to reduce burden on pediatric health care providers. However, the inclusion of measures that also capture patient-centered perspectives on care is essential."

Clinical registries and other electronic data may also be used in quality measurement. This chapter discusses 2 ways that correct coding may support performance measurement: codes that may support Healthcare Effectiveness Data and Information Set (HEDIS) quality measurement and *Current Procedural Terminology (CPT®)* Category II codes.

For more information on value-based payment and other emerging payment models, see Chapter 4, The Business of Medicine: Working With Current and Emerging Payment Systems.

Healthcare Effectiveness Data and Information Set (HEDIS)

The National Committee for Quality Assurance (NCQA) describes HEDIS as a tool used by more than 90% of American health plans to measure performance on important dimensions of care and service. It is intended to allow purchasers and consumers to compare quality among health plans. The HEDIS measures are often incorporated in physician quality initiatives. Altogether, HEDIS consists of 94 measures across 7 domains of care (effectiveness of care, access/availability of care, experience of care, health plan stability, utilization, cost of care, and health plan descriptive information). To insure HEDIS stays current, the NCQA has established a process to update the measurement set annually.

The HEDIS measures address a broad range of important health issues. Among them are
- Asthma Medication Use
- Antidepressant Medication Management
- Childhood and Adolescent Immunization Status
- Childhood Weight/Body Mass Index (BMI) Assessment

Each health plan reviews a select set of measures each year. Because so many plans collect HEDIS data and the measures are so specifically defined, it is important to become familiar with the HEDIS system as it relates to quality measures and pay for performance (P4P).

Why HEDIS Matters to Pediatricians

The Centers for Medicare & Medicaid Services (CMS) has directly linked payment for health care services to patient outcomes. Consequently, health plans and providers, including physicians, are being asked to close gaps in care and improve overall quality. This focus on quality outcomes can help patients and members get the most from their benefits, which ultimately means better use of limited resources.

There are large sums of money at stake for health plans. For example, for a health plan with just 100,000 members being evaluated by HEDIS, each quality measure could mean millions in payments from federal or state agencies. When you consider that there are 20 to 25 measures directly tied

> ‖|‖| **Coding Pearl** ‖|‖|
>
> When a measure is met during an inpatient or observation stay (eg, newborn immunization during the birth admission), supporting documentation may be required in the record of the primary care physician even if the immunization was provided under supervision of a hospitalist or other physician or qualified health care professional.

to payment (depending on the health plan and population served), these are significant amounts of money! Now consider what that might look like for larger managed care organizations that have 1 million or more members enrolled. This is what keeps health care plans running. However, they cannot do it without physicians, and this is the fundamental concept behind P4P quality initiatives. The plans will pay the physicians to help them attain these funds from the CMS.

What Is a Pediatrician's Role in HEDIS?

You and your office staff can help facilitate the HEDIS process improvement by

- Providing the appropriate care within the designated time frames.
- Not all patients will be included in a physician's patient count for HEDIS purposes, as continuous enrollment in the health plan without a gap of more than 45 days may be required for inclusion. However, attention to the time frames for providing recommended screenings and services across the patient population is important. For instance, practices should have a reminder system to track immunizations for children younger than 24 months to avoid failure to provide the recommended immunizations prior to 25 months of age. If patients reach 25 months of age without receiving the recommended vaccines, this negatively affects the HEDIS score for the physician until the child turns 3 years old (ie, is no longer included in the patient count for the measure).
- Documenting all care in the patient's medical record.
- Accurately coding all claims. Providing information accurately on a claim may reduce the number of records requested.
- Responding to a health plan's requests for medical records in a timely fashion (typically within a week).

  The time frames are set each year.

- January to May 15: Medical record requests will come in from the plans. All data must be gathered by the plan by May 15, with no exceptions.
- June: The plans must report their results to the NCQA.
- July to October: The NCQA releases the new Quality Compass nationwide—commercial plans in July; Medicaid and Medicare in September and October.

Medical Record Requests

Some information cannot be captured through claims data, so requests for medical records related to health plan HEDIS surveys are necessary. The Health Insurance Portability and Accountability Act of 1996 allows disclosure of protected health information to a health plan for the plan's HEDIS purposes, so long as the period for which information is needed overlaps with the **period** for which the patient is or was enrolled in the health plan. Health plans may contract with outside vendors to conduct HEDIS record reviews.

- Providers are notified of record requests (often by fax but may vary by plan).
- The request will include a member list, the measure that is being evaluated, and the minimum necessary chart information needed.
- Data collection may vary by plan but may include fax, mail, on-site visits for large requests, remote electronic health record (EHR) access, and electronic data interchange via a secure Web portal.

HEDIS Measures and Codes

In **Table 3-1**, some of the pediatric HEDIS measures for 2018 are listed, including the codes that may be used in HEDIS review (HEDIS 2019 measures were not finalized at time of publication). These include *International Classification of Diseases, 10th Revision, Clinical Modification* (ICD-10-CM);

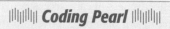

> ### |||||||| *Coding Pearl* ||||||||
>
> Previously, *International Classification of Diseases, 10th Revision, Clinical Modification (ICD-10-CM)* codes for pediatric body mass index (BMI) percentiles (**Z68.51–Z68.54**) were reported in conjunction with codes for counseling on nutrition and physical activity. However, the American Hospital Association *Coding Clinic* has advised that codes for BMI are only reported in conjunction with physician documentation of a related condition (eg, overweight, obesity). See **Table 3-1** for an illustration of reporting BMI measurement in compliance with *ICD-10-CM* guidelines through the use of *Current Procedural Terminology®* Category II code **3008F** (BMI, documented).

Healthcare Common Procedure Coding System; and *CPT®* codes. **Table 3-1** does not contain all measures applicable to the pediatric population. Note that each measure includes a defined patient population (eg, children who turn 2 years of age during the measurement year).

Physicians and group practices may also report HEDIS measures as part of a pediatric medical home or other quality improvement initiative using data pulled from internal administrative data (eg, number of preventive medicine service *CPT* codes reported for population of patients 3–6 years old). Pediatric medical home and quality improvement initiatives vary by state or region and may include a combination of HEDIS and other nationally recognized quality measures.

Table 3-1. Healthcare Effectiveness Data and Information Set Pediatric Performance Measure Codes

Measure/Description	Codes
Weight Assessment and Counseling for Nutrition and Physical Activity for Children and Adolescents (WCC) Description: Percentage of members 3–17 years of age who had an outpatient visit with a PCP or an OB/GYN that included evidence of BMI documentation with corresponding height and weight, counseling for nutrition, and/or counseling for physical activity	**Diagnosis** *(ICD-10-CM)* Counseling: nutrition **Z71.3** Counseling for physical activity **Z71.82** **Procedure** Nutrition counseling—*CPT®:* **97802–97804** HCPCS: **S9470, S9452, S9449, G0270, G0271,** or **G0447** Physical activity counseling—HCPCS: **S9451** *or* **G0447** BMI, documented—*CPT:* **3008F**
Immunizations for Adolescents (IMA) Description: Percentage of adolescents 13 years of age (during the year) with appropriate immunizations	**Procedure** (vaccine products) Meningococcal—*CPT:* **90734** Tdap—*CPT:* **90715** Td—*CPT:* **90714** or **90718** Tetanus—*CPT:* **90703** Diphtheria—*CPT:* **90719** Human papillomavirus (complete series)—*CPT:* **90649–90651**
Follow-up Care for Children Prescribed ADHD Medications Percentage of children newly prescribed ADHD medication who had at least 3 follow-up care visits within a 10-month period, one of which was within 30 days of when the first ADHD medication was dispensed. Two rates are reported. 1. Initiation phase: The percentage of members 6–12 years of age as of the IPSD with an ambulatory prescription dispensed for ADHD medication, who had one follow-up visit with practitioner with prescribing authority during the 30-day initiation phase. 2. Continuation and maintenance phase: The percentage of members 6–12 years of age as of the IPSD with an ambulatory prescription dispensed for ADHD medication, who remained on the medication for at least 210 days and who, in addition to the visit in the initiation phase, had at least 2 follow-up visits with a practitioner within 270 days (9 months) after the initiation phase ended. One of the 2 visits (during days 31–300) may be a telephone visit with any practitioner.	**Procedure** *CPT* Stand-alone visits: **90804–90815, 96150–96154, 98960–98962, 99078, 99201–99205, 99211–99215, 99217–99220, 99241–99245, 99341–99345, 99347–99350, 99381–99384, 99391–99394, 99401–99404, 99411, 99412, 99510** Telephone visits: **98966–98968, 99441–99443** HCPCS: **G0155, G0176, G0177, G0409–G0411, G0463, H0002, H0004, H0031, H0034–H0037, H0039, H0040, H2000, H2001, H2010–H2020, M0064, S0201, S9480, S9484, S9485, T1015** **Follow-up visits identified by the following *CPT* codes must be with a mental health practitioner:** *CPT* in most outpatient and partial hospitalization settings: **90791, 90792, 90801, 90802, 90816–90819, 90821–90824, 90826–90829, 90832–90834, 90836–90840, 90845, 90847, 90849, 90853, 90857, 90862, 90875, 90876** *CPT* in partial hospitalization or community mental health centers only: **99221–99223, 99231–99233, 99238, 99239, 99251–99255**

Abbreviations: ADHD, attention-deficit/hyperactivity disorder; BMI, body mass index; CPT, Current Procedural Terminology; HCPCS, Healthcare Common Procedure Coding System; ICD-10-CM, International Classification of Diseases, 10th Revision, Clinical Modification; IPSD, Index Prescription Start Date; OB/GYN, obstetrician/gynecologist; PCP, primary care physician; Td, tetanus, diphtheria; Tdap, tetanus, diphtheria toxoid, and acellular pertussis.

Chapter 3: Coding to Demonstrate Quality and Value

Chapter 3: Coding to Demonstrate Quality and Value

Examples

➤ **A physician sees a 12-year-old girl for a new patient office visit with a chief complaint of acne.** The physician identifies that the girl is not up-to-date with immunizations and has not received preventive care in the last year. The physician recommends and provides a preventive medicine service. Patient has a health supervision examination with normal BMI and mild acne on face only noted on examination. Over-the-counter products for acne are recommended. CRAFFT (*car, relax, alone, forget, friends, trouble*) and Patient Health Questionnaire-9 (PHQ-9) were given and the results were normal. The encounter includes documentation of the services recommended by the AAP *Bright Futures: Guidelines for Health Supervision of Infants, Children, and Adolescents,* 4th Edition, and counseling and administration of age-appropriate immunizations of preservative-free flu vaccine, human papillomavirus (HPV) vaccine, meningitis (MenACWY [Menactra]), and tetanus, diphtheria, and acellular pertussis (Tdap). Documentation does not support a separately identifiable evaluation and management (E/M) service but includes a diagnosis of mild acne vulgaris.

ICD-10-CM	CPT®
Z00.121 (encounter for routine child health examination with abnormal findings) **L70.0** (acne vulgaris) **Z71.3** (dietary counseling and surveillance) **Z68.52** (BMI pediatric, 5th percentile to <85th percentile for age) **Z71.82** (exercise counseling)	**99384** (initial comprehensive preventive medicine E/M, new patient; age 12–17 years old)
Z00.121 (encounter for routine child health examination with abnormal findings) **Z23** (encounter for immunization)	**90460** × 4 units (immunization administration, each initial component) **90461** × 2 units (immunization administration, each additional component) **90686** (IIV4 [influenza] vaccine) **90651** (9-valent human papillomavirus [9vHPV]) **90734** (MenACWY) **90715** (Tdap)
Z13.89 (encounter for screening for other disorder [alcohol or drug use, depression]) **Z13.31** (encounter for screening for depression)	**96160** (administration and interpretation of health risk assessment instrument [alcohol and drug assessment]) **96127** (brief emotional/behavioral assessment, with scoring and documentation, per standardized instrument [depression screening])

The physician in this scenario has proactively provided preventive care that is recommended for this patient and, in doing so, is able to report diagnosis and procedure codes demonstrating that quality measures have been met. For instance, HEDIS includes measurements for immunization for meningococcus; tetanus, diphtheria, and pertussis; and HPV for all adolescents prior to their 13th birthday, in addition to measures for adolescent well-care (health supervision) visits, BMI measurement, and counseling on nutrition and physical activity.

➤ **A physician sees an established patient for complaints associated with upper respiratory infection (URI).** The caregiver requests an antibiotic but is instructed that the condition is viral and to use over-the-counter medicine as necessary for the child's comfort. No antibiotic is ordered.

ICD-10-CM	CPT
J06.9 (acute URI, unspecified)	99213 (office or other outpatient visit for the E/M of an established patient, which requires at least 2 of these 3 key components: An expanded problem focused history; An expanded problem focused examination; Medical decision-making of low complexity.) (Counseling and coordination of care with other physicians, other qualified health care professionals, or agencies are provided consistent with the nature of the problem(s) and the patient's and/or family's needs. Usually, the presenting problem(s) are of low to moderate severity. Typically, 15 minutes are spent face-to-face with the patient and/or family.)

Because no antibiotic was ordered at this encounter, the HEDIS measure for appropriate treatment of children 3 months to 18 years old with URIs was met. The diagnosis of URI indicates this measure may apply. The health plan may measure this through comparison of medical claims data with prescription drug plan claims data. Similar measures may apply for antibiotics appropriately prescribed for diagnosis of streptococcal pharyngitis following positive laboratory test for group A streptococcal infection.

Category II *Current Procedural Terminology*® Codes: Pay for Performance Measures

Category II codes were developed and are used by physicians and hospitals to report performance measures and certain aspects of care not yet included in performance measures. The performance measures are developed by national organizations, including the NCQA and the American Medical Association (AMA) Physician Consortium for Performance Improvement (PCPI), and based on quality indicators currently accepted and used in the health care industry. As a member of the AMA PCPI, the AAP is involved with the development of performance measures for pediatric diseases or conditions. The AAP policy statement, "A New Era in Quality Measurement: The Development and Application of Quality Measures" (http://pediatrics.aappublications.org/content/139/1/e20163442) includes recommendations to physicians and policy makers on adoption and use of quality measures. Any updated information on quality improvement can be found at www2.aap.org/visit/qualityimppublic.htm.

Reporting Category II codes allows internal monitoring of performance, patient compliance, and outcomes.

Performance Measure Codes

Performance measure codes
- Are intended for reporting purposes only.
- Describe clinical conditions (including complete performance measurements sets) and screening measures.
- Have no relative values on the Medicare Physician Fee Schedule (Resource-Based Relative Value Scale).
- Are reported on a voluntary basis.
- Are reported in addition to, *not in place of,* Category I *CPT* codes.
- Describe the performance of a clinical service typically included in an E/M code or the result that is part of a laboratory procedure/test.

Category II code development and maintenance take place on an as-needed basis. Category II code changes since the printing of the last *CPT* manual are posted to https://www.ama-assn.org/practice-management/cpt-category-ii-codes. The online document, "CPT Category II Codes Alphabetical Clinical Topics Listing," includes the latest code changes with revision, implementation, and publication dates.

Codes are grouped within categories based on established clinical documentation methods (ie, history, physical findings, assessment, and plan). Each code identifies the specific clinical condition and performance measured.

Categories are defined in **Table** 3-2.

Table 3-2. Performance Measure Codes	
Category of Codes	**Examples**
Composite Measures—0000F Series Codes in the **0000F** range comprise several measures that are grouped to facilitate reporting of a clinical condition when all included components are performed.	Code **0012F** is reported when the assessment on an 18-year-old with community-acquired bacterial pneumonia includes all the following components: **1026F** Comorbid conditions assessed **2010F** Vital signs recorded **2014F** Mental status assessed **2018F** Hydration status assessed
Patient Management—0500F Series Codes in the **0500F** range are used to describe utilization measures or measures of patient care provided for specific clinical purposes (eg, prenatal care, presurgical and postsurgical care, referrals).	Code **0545F** is used to report that a plan for follow-up care was documented on a 15-year-old with a diagnosis of major depressive disorder.
Patient History—1000F Series Codes in the **1000F** range are used to describe measures for aspects of patient history and review of systems.	Code **1031F** is used to report that the smoking status and exposure to secondhand smoke in the home were assessed in patients with asthma. Code **1050F** is used to report a patient history of new or changing moles.
Physical Examination—2000F Series Codes in the **2000F** range describe aspects of the physical examination or clinical assessment.	Code **2030F** is reported when the hydration status is documented as normally hydrated on a 2-month-old with acute gastroenteritis.
Diagnostic/Screening Processes or Results—3006F Codes in the **3006F** range are used to report results of clinical laboratory tests and radiologic or other procedural examinations.	When the most recent hemoglobin A_{1c} level is less than 7.0% on an 18-year-old with diabetes mellitus, code **3044F** is reported.
Therapeutic, Preventive, or Other Interventions—4000F Codes in the **4000F** range are used to report pharmacologic, procedural, or behavioral therapies, including preventive services such as patient education and counseling.	Code **4058F** is reported when gastroenteritis education is provided to the mother of a 6-month-old with acute gastroenteritis and documented in the medical record.
Follow-up or Other Outcomes—5005F Codes in the **5005F** range are used to describe the review and communication of test results to patients, patient satisfaction and experience with care, patient functional status, and patient morbidity and mortality.	Code **5050F** is reported when a treatment plan is communicated to the provider(s) managing continuing care within 1 month of the diagnosis of melanoma.
Patient Safety—6005F Codes in the **6005F** range are used to describe patient safety practices.	Code **6005F** is used to report the rationale (eg, severity of illness and safety) for the recommended level of care (eg, home, hospital) for a patient with community-acquired bacterial pneumonia.
Structural Measures—7010F Codes in the **7010F** range are used to identify measures that address the setting or system of the delivered care and address aspects of the capabilities of the organization or health care professionals providing the care.	Code **7010F** is reported when patient information is entered into a recall system that includes a specified target date for the next examination of a patient with melanoma and a process to follow up with patients about missed or unscheduled appointments.
Non-measure Claims-Based Reporting—9001F Codes in the **9001F** range are used to identify certain aspects of care not currently represented by recognized performance measures but which may later be associated with measures approved by an appropriate quality improvement organization.	Code **9001F** is reported to identify the size of an abdominal aortic aneurysm less than 5.0 cm maximum diameter on centerline-formatted computed tomography (CT) or minor diameter on axial-formatted CT.

Category II Modifiers

Category II modifiers (1P, 2P, 3P, and 8P) are used to report services that were considered but not provided because of a medical reason(s), patient choice, or system reason. Modifier 8P is equivalent to "action not performed, reason not otherwise specified." Table 3-3 contains modifiers and examples.

Table 3-3. Category II Modifiers	
Category II Modifier	**Examples**
Modifier 1P (performance measure exclusion modifier due to medical reasons) Used to report that one of the performance measures was not performed because it was not indicated (eg, already performed) or was contraindicated (eg, due to a patient's allergy)	Modifier 1P is appended to code 6070F (documentation that patient was queried and counseled about antiepileptic drug [AED] side effects) because the patient is not receiving an AED.
Modifier 2P (performance measure exclusion modifier due to patient choice) Used to report that the performance measure was not performed due to a patient's religious, social, or economic reasons; the patient declined (eg, noncompliance with treatment); or other specific reasons	Modifier 2P is appended to code 3210F (group A streptococcus test performed) when a physician considered the testing for streptococcus but the parent refused testing.
Modifier 3P (performance measure exclusion modifier due to system reasons) Used to report that the performance measure was not performed because the payer does not cover the service, the resources to perform the service are not available, or other reasons attributable to the health care delivery system Keep in mind that in the emergency department setting, appropriate medical screening and stabilization must be provided regardless of any consideration of payment. Providers are prohibited by federal statute from making treatment decisions in these circumstances based on payer coverage.	Modifier 3P is appended to code 4062F (patient referral for psychotherapy documented) when a 15-year-old with a diagnosis of major depressive disorder is not referred for psychotherapy because it is not available.
Modifier 8P (performance measure reporting modifier—action not performed, not otherwise specified) Used to allow the reporting of circumstances when an action described in a measure's numerator is not performed and the reason is not otherwise specified	Modifier 8P would be appended to code 2001F (weight recorded) when a 2-year-old with acute gastroenteritis is not weighed and, therefore, does not meet the performance measurement requirement.

Category II modifiers
- Are used only when allowed based on the specific reporting instructions for each performance measure.
- Are appended only to Category II *CPT* codes.
- Serve as a denominator exclusion from a performance measure (when measure allows).

The medical record should include written documentation of the reason that the service was ultimately not provided. Category II modifiers are only appended to Category II codes.

Reporting Performance Measures Applicable to Pediatrics

Many performance measures apply to the pediatric population. In addition, pediatric practices caring for patients 18 years or older may report Category II codes for conditions such as hypertension, diabetes mellitus, chronic kidney disease, gastroesophageal reflux disease, and community-acquired bacterial pneumonia and screening codes for tobacco use and cessation. Refer to the Alphabetical Clinical Topics Listing (ACTL) at https://www.ama-assn.org/practice-management/category-ii-codes for updated measures and reporting instructions.
The ACTL should be used in coordination with the Category II section in *CPT*.

Alphabetical Clinical Topics Listing

◈ Includes an alphabetic index of performance measures by clinical condition or topic

◈ Includes the measure developer (eg, PCPI), the performance measure, a description of the measure, and the associated Category II code

◈ Directs the reader to the measure developer's Web site to access the complete description of the measure (eg, specifications and requirements for reporting performance measures for asthma are located at www.aaaai.org/practice-resources/practice-tools/quality-measures)

Access the measure developer's Web site for the specification documents (ie, clinical measurement set, measurement set numerators and denominators, measure specifications, specifications for paper and EHRs, an algorithm for measure calculation, data abstraction definitions, a medication table, and a retrospective data abstraction tool) of the performance measure.

The following Web sites provide information and resources:

◈ www.ncqa.org

◈ https://www.ama-assn.org/practice-management/category-ii-codes

◈ www.thepcpi.org

Each performance measure includes a symptom or activity assessment, numerator, denominator, percentage, and reporting instructions. A patient must meet the criteria specified in the denominator (diagnosis code) to be included in the numerator (Category II code) for a particular performance measure.

Reporting measures to a payer (electronically or with a CMS-1500 claim form) is done the same way as reporting any *CPT®* code. Report the appropriate E/M code (eg, **99201–99215, 99241–99245**) based on the level of service performed and documented with all the appropriate *diagnosis* codes that were addressed during the course of the visit. Report the Category II *CPT* code that relates to the performance measure with any applicable Category II modifier. Only the diagnosis code for the condition or disease will be linked to Category II *CPT* codes. Examples for some measures are included following the measures.

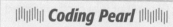

> ||ı|||ı|| **Coding Pearl** |||ı|||
>
> A patient must meet the criteria specified in the denominator (diagnosis code) to be included in the numerator (Category II code) for a particular performance measure. Only the diagnosis code for the condition or disease will be linked to Category II *Current Procedural Terminology®* codes.

Acute Otitis Externa

These codes apply to patients aged 2 years and older with a diagnosis of acute otitis externa (AOE). Clinical components are reported to denote if pain was assessed, if topical therapy was prescribed, and if systemic antimicrobial therapy was avoided.

Category II Codes: Acute Otitis Externa	Guidelines
1116F Auricular or periauricular pain assessed	Report at each encounter. Append modifier **1P** when the appropriate performance exclusion exists.
4130F Topical preparations (including over the counter) prescribed for acute otitis externa	If topical preparations are not prescribed, medical record documentation must indicate the medical and/or patient reasons, and modifier **1P** or **2P** would be appended to code **4130F** or drug allergy or other adverse effects would be indicated by diagnosis codes.
4131F Systemic antimicrobial therapy prescribed **4132F** Systemic antimicrobial therapy not prescribed	Report code **4132F** when systemic antimicrobial therapy is not prescribed. Report code **4131F** with modifier **1P** when there is a valid medical reason for prescribing systemic antimicrobial therapy. Exclusion modifiers cannot be reported with code **4132F**.

Example

➤ A 4-year-old presents with acute onset of right ear pain. An expanded-level history and physical examination are performed. The patient has been taking swimming lessons for the last 2 weeks. The diagnosis is AOE. The patient is sent home on topical antimicrobial and anti-inflammatory medication. All the criteria in the AOE measurement set as specified by the developer of the performance measurement are met. The applicable codes identified under the Category II *CPT* code section are reviewed and the ACTL is consulted for current measure criteria.

ICD-10-CM	CPT
H60.331 (swimmer's ear, right ear)	99213 (established patient; expanded history and physical examination with low-complexity medical decision-making) 1116F (auricular or periauricular pain assessed) 4130F (topical preparations [including over the counter] prescribed for AOE) 4132F (systemic antimicrobial therapy not prescribed)

Acute Otitis Media With Effusion

These codes apply to patients aged 2 months through 12 years with a diagnosis of acute otitis media with effusion. Clinical components reported as part of this measure signify that an assessment of tympanic membrane mobility was performed using pneumatic otoscopy or tympanometry, that hearing testing was performed within 6 months prior to a tympanostomy tube insertion, and whether or not antihistamines, decongestants, or systemic steroids were avoided.

Category II Codes: Acute Otitis Media With Effusion	Guidelines
2035F Tympanic membrane mobility assessed with pneumatic otoscopy or tympanometry	Reported at each encounter. Modifier 1P or 2P is appended when appropriate.
3230F Documentation that hearing test was performed within 6 months prior to a tympanostomy tube insertion	Reported at the time the tympanostomy tube insertion is performed. Medical record documentation must reflect the performance and results of the test or, if the test is performed by another physician or provider, should include a copy of the test results. Modifiers 1P or 3P may be appended to code 3230F as appropriate.
4131F Systemic antimicrobial therapy prescribed 4132F Systemic antimicrobial therapy not prescribed 4133F Antihistamines or decongestants prescribed or recommended 4134F Antihistamines or decongestants neither prescribed nor recommended 4135F Systemic corticosteroids prescribed 4136F Systemic corticosteroids not prescribed	Used to report the absence or overuse of medications for each patient. Modifier 1P is used with codes 4131F, 4133F, and 4135F when appropriate. Modifiers 1P, 2P, and 3P may not be reported with codes 4132F, 4134F, or 4136F.

Chapter 3: Coding to Demonstrate Quality and Value

Example

➤ **A 15-year-old new patient is seen with complaints of sleep disturbance and depressed mood.** The adolescent has not been eating well and has been increasingly irritable. A comprehensive history and detailed physical examination are performed. Behavioral health assessment instruments (PHQ-9, Mood and Feelings Questionnaire, and Screen for Child Anxiety Related Disorders) are completed and scored. The patient meets the *Diagnostic and Statistical Manual of Mental Disorders,* 5th Edition (*DSM-5*) criteria for moderate major depressive disorder (MDD). Treatment options, including psychotherapy and antidepressant medications, are discussed. The patient chooses to pursue psychotherapy but refuses medication, and a referral is provided. The patient is scheduled for follow-up by phone call from nurse in 1 week and appointment in 6 weeks.

ICD-10-CM	CPT
F32.1 (MDD single episode, moderate)	99203 (new patient; comprehensive history, detailed physical examination with moderate-complexity medical decision-making) 96127 x 3 (brief emotional/behavioral assessment (eg, depression inventory, attention-deficit/hyperactivity disorder [ADHD] scale), with scoring and documentation, per standardized instrument) 2060F (patient interviewed directly by evaluating clinician on or before date of diagnosis of MDD) 1040F (criteria for MDD documented at the initial evaluation) 3085F (suicide risk assessed) 4062F (patient referral for psychotherapy documented) 4063F (antidepressant pharmacotherapy considered and not prescribed) 0545F (plan for follow-up care documented)

Asthma

This measure is applicable to all patients 5 to 50 years of age with a diagnosis of asthma.

Category II Codes: Asthma	Guidelines
2015F Asthma impairment assessed 2016F Asthma risk assessed	Used for each patient who was evaluated at least once for asthma control. Evaluation of asthma impairment and asthma risk must occur during the same medical encounter. There are no exclusions to the measures. Code 2016F is also reported independently for each emergency department encounter or inpatient admission (with a diagnosis of acute asthma exacerbation). There are no performance exclusions for this measure.
1031F Smoking status and exposure to secondhand smoke in the home assessed	Report for each patient whose smoking status and exposure to secondhand smoke in the home was assessed. There are no performance exclusions.
1032F Current tobacco smoker OR currently exposed to secondhand smoke 1033F Current tobacco nonsmoker AND not currently exposed to secondhand smoke 4000F Tobacco use cessation intervention, counseling 4001F Tobacco use cessation intervention, pharmacologic therapy	Report code 1032F or 1033F to indicate tobacco use status. If reporting code 1032F, report 4000F OR 4001F to indicate type of tobacco use cessation intervention. There are no performance exclusions for this measure. Tobacco cessation interventions may be reported when provided to the patient's primary caregiver even if the caregiver is not the source of secondhand smoke in the home.

Category II Codes: Asthma (*continued*)	Guidelines
1038F Persistent asthma, mild, moderate, or severe **1039F** Intermittent asthma **4140F** Inhaled corticosteroids prescribed **4144F** Alternative long-term control medication prescribed	Report code **1038F** or **1039F** to indicate asthma severity. For patients with persistent asthma (**1038F**), report code **4140F**, **4144F**, or both. For patients with appropriate exclusion criteria, report code **4140F** or **4144F** with modifier **1P** or **2P**.
5250F Asthma discharge plan provided to patient	Report for each emergency department encounter or inpatient admission (with a diagnosis of acute asthma exacerbation) when an asthma discharge plan is provided to patient at time of discharge. There are no performance exclusions for this measure.

Example

➤ **A 10-year-old is seen with exacerbation of asthma.** His last exacerbation was 3 months ago. An expanded history and detailed physical examination are performed. Asthma control test is atypical at 19. Spirometry is performed and atypical for forced vital capacity (FVC), forced expiratory volume 1 (FEV_1), and FEV_1/FVC ratio. A nebulizer treatment with albuterol is administered. Examination following treatment shows decreased wheezing. Patient is sent home on albuterol and steroids administered by metered-dose inhaler with plan to follow up as necessary. Assessment of asthma status is documented as mild persistent. Category II codes for evaluation of asthma symptoms, persistent asthma, assessment of asthma status, and prescription of inhaled corticosteroids are reported. If documentation supports asthma risk (**2016F**), smoking status and exposure to secondhand smoke in the home (**1031F–1033F**), or tobacco use cessation intervention (**4000F, 4001F**), these may be additionally reported.

ICD-10-CM	CPT®
J45.31 (mild persistent asthma with exacerbation)	**99214 25** (established patient; expanded history, detailed physical examination with moderate-complexity medical decision-making) **94640** (aerosol treatment) **J7611** (albuterol, inhalation solution, US Food and Drug Administration–approved final product, non-compounded, administered through durable medical equipment concentrated form, 1 mg) **96160** (administration of patient-focused health risk assessment instrument [eg, health hazard appraisal] with scoring and documentation, per standardized instrument) **1005F** (asthma symptoms evaluated) **1038F** (persistent asthma, mild, moderate, or severe) **2015F** (assessment of asthma status) **4140F** (inhaled corticosteroids prescribed)

➤ If a payer follows Medicare and/or Medicaid National Correct Coding Initiative edits, spirometry (**94010**) is not separately reported during an encounter at which spirometry is performed. Check payer guidelines for coverage of administration of a patient-focused health risk instrument (**96160**).

Chapter 3: Coding to Demonstrate Quality and Value

Pediatric Acute Gastroenteritis

The pediatric acute gastroenteritis measure applies to patients aged 1 month through 5 years with a diagnosis of acute gastroenteritis.

Category II Codes: Pediatric Acute Gastroenteritis	Guidelines
4056F Appropriate oral rehydration solution recommended **4058F** Pediatric gastroenteritis education provided to caregiver	Used to report that the patient's caregiver was given a recommendation on an appropriate oral rehydration solution, diet education was performed, and the patient's caregiver was advised when to contact the physician. There are no performance exclusions.
2030F Hydration status documented, normally hydrated **2031F** Hydration status documented, dehydrated	Report when hydration status is documented in the medical record. When the patient is dehydrated and appropriate oral rehydration solution is recommended, report codes **4056F** and **2031F**. There are no performance exclusions.
2001F Weight recorded	Report when weight measurement is documented in the medical record. Modifiers **1P**, **2P**, and **3P** may not be reported. Modifier **8P** may be reported.

Pediatric Pharyngitis and Upper Respiratory Infection

The pediatric pharyngitis measure applies to patients 2 through 18 years of age (inclusive) with a diagnosis of pharyngitis who were dispensed or prescribed antibiotic treatment and/or received a group A streptococcus test.

The URI measure applies to patients 3 months through 18 years of age (inclusive) who were seen with a diagnosis of only URI and were appropriately not prescribed or dispensed an antibiotic.

Category II Codes: Pediatric Pharyngitis and Upper Respiratory Infection	Guidelines
3210F Group A streptococcus test performed	Report when a patient is diagnosed with pharyngitis, is dispensed or prescribed an antibiotic, and received a group A streptococcus test. Modifier **1P** for medical exclusions or **2P** for patient exclusions may be used.
4120F Antibiotic prescribed or dispensed **4124F** Antibiotic neither prescribed nor dispensed	Report as appropriate for both performance measures (pediatric pharyngitis and URI). Modifier **1P**, **2P**, or **3P** may not be reported with code **4120F** or **4124F** for pharyngitis. Modifier **1P** is reported with code **4124F** when appropriate for URI. If a patient was dispensed or prescribed an antibiotic and received the group A streptococcus test, codes **3210F** and **4120F** would be reported.

Pediatric End-stage Renal Disease

This measure applies to patients aged 17 years and younger with a diagnosis of end-stage renal disease receiving hemodialysis, having clearance of urea/volume (Kt/V) measurements as per the criteria listed in the codes, having received an influenza vaccine, and having a plan of care documented. This measure is reported during each calendar month that the patient is receiving hemodialysis.

Category II Codes: End-stage Renal Disease	Guidelines
0505F Hemodialysis plan of care documented	Report when the hemodialysis plan of care is documented in the medical record on a patient aged 17 years or younger.
3082F Clearance of urea/volume (Kt/V) less than 1.2 **3083F** Kt/V greater than or equal to 1.2 and less than 1.7 **3084F** Kt/V greater than or equal to 1.7	Report code applicable to the corresponding Kt/V measurement. If the Kt/V is <1.2 (**3082F**) and the patient has a plan of care for inadequate hemodialysis, also report code **0505F**. There are no performance exclusions for this measure.
4274F Influenza immunization administered or previously received	Report when a patient aged 6 months through 17 years (with a diagnosis of end-stage renal disease and receiving dialysis) is seen between November 1 and February 15 and receives the influenza immunization or has received the influenza immunization from another provider. The medical record must support that the vaccine was administered. Modifier **1P**, **2P**, or **3P** may be used when appropriate.

Epilepsy

This measure will be reported by the physician providing care to children and adults with a diagnosis of epilepsy.

Category II Codes: Epilepsy	Guidelines
1200F Seizure type(s) and current seizure frequency(ies) documented **1205F** Etiology of epilepsy or epilepsy syndrome(s) reviewed and documented	Report when the seizure type(s) and current seizure frequency for each seizure type are documented in the medical record. Modifier **1P** or **2P** may be reported if appropriate. When the medical record documentation includes the etiology of epilepsy or the epilepsy syndrome(s) is reviewed and documented (if known) or documented as unknown or cryptogenic, code **1205F** is reported. There are no performance exclusions for code **1205F**.
3650F Electroencephalogram (EEG) ordered, reviewed, or requested **1119F** Initial evaluation for condition **1121F** Subsequent evaluation for condition	Code **3650F** is used to report whether or not the patient with a diagnosis of epilepsy seen for an initial evaluation had at least one EEG ordered or, if an EEG was performed previously, results were reviewed or requested. If code **3650F** is reported on the same day as a new patient E/M service (**99201–99205**), neither code **1119F** nor **1121F** is reported. If code **3650F** is reported on the same day as an established patient E/M visit (**99211–99215**) or office or outpatient consultation (**99241–99245**), code **1119F** is also reported to denote an initial evaluation for the condition or code **1121F** is reported to denote a subsequent evaluation. Modifier **1P**, **2P**, or **3P** may be reported with code **3650F** when appropriate.
3324F Magnetic resonance imaging (MRI) or computed tomography (CT) scan ordered, reviewed, or requested **1119F** Initial evaluation for condition **1121F** Subsequent evaluation for condition	When a patient with the diagnosis of epilepsy has MRI (preferred imaging) or CT ordered or if results are reviewed or requested of an MRI or a CT previously obtained, code **3324F** is reported. If code **3324F** is reported on the same day as a new patient E/M service (**99201–99205**), neither code **1119F** nor **1121F** is reported. If code **3324F** is reported on the same day as an established patient E/M visit (**99211–99215**) or office or outpatient consultation (**99241–99245**), code **1119F** is also reported to denote an initial evaluation for the condition or code **1121F** is reported to denote a subsequent evaluation. Modifier **1P**, **2P**, or **3P** may be reported with code **3324F**.

Chapter 3: Coding to Demonstrate Quality and Value

Category II Codes: Epilepsy (*continued*)	Guidelines
6070F Patient queried and counseled about antiepileptic drug (AED) side effects	Report when the patient is queried and counseled about AED side effects and the counseling is documented in the medical record. Modifier **1P** may be reported. This includes patients who are not taking an AED.
5200F Consideration of referral for a neurologic evaluation of appropriateness for surgical therapy for intractable epilepsy within the past 3 years	Report when a patient with a diagnosis of intractable epilepsy was considered for referral for a neurologic evaluation of appropriateness for surgical therapy within the past 3 years. There are no performance exclusions applicable.
4330F Counseling about epilepsy-specific safety issues provided to patient (or caregiver[s])	Report when counseling is provided to a patient and/or their caregiver(s) about context-specific safety issues, appropriate to the patient's age, seizure type(s) and frequency(ies), and occupation and leisure activities (eg, injury prevention, burns, appropriate driving restrictions, bathing), at least once a year and is documented in the medical record. Modifier **3P** may be reported when appropriate.
4340F Counseling for women of childbearing potential with epilepsy	Report whether or not a female of childbearing potential (12–44 years old) was counseled about how epilepsy and its treatment may affect contraception and pregnancy and the counseling is documented in the medical record. Modifier **1P** may be reported.

Major Depressive Disorder—Child and Adolescent

This measure is applicable for reporting care to all patients aged 6 through 17 years with a diagnosis of MDD.

Category II Codes: Major Depressive Disorder	Guidelines
2060F Patient interviewed directly by evaluating clinician on or before date of diagnosis of MDD **1040F** *DSM-5* criteria for MDD documented at the initial evaluation **3085F** Suicide risk assessed	Report code **2060F** when a patient is interviewed directly by the evaluating clinician on or before the date of diagnosis. Report code **1040F** when there is documented evidence that the patient met the *DSM-5* criteria—at least 5 elements with symptom duration of 2 weeks or longer, including depressed mood (can be irritable mood in children and adolescents) or loss of interest or pleasure—during the visit in which the new diagnosis or recurrent episode was identified. Code **3085F** is reported when an assessment for suicide risk is performed and documented. Modifiers **1P**, **2P**, **3P**, and **8P** may not be reported.
4060F Psychotherapy services provided **4062F** Patient referral for psychotherapy documented	Report code **4060F** when a patient receives psychotherapy during an episode of MDD and the service is documented in the medical record. Report code **4062F** when a patient is referred for psychotherapy and the referral is documented in the medical record. Modifier **1P**, **2P**, or **3P** may be reported.
4063F Antidepressant pharmacotherapy considered and not prescribed **4064F** Antidepressant pharmacotherapy prescribed	Used to report whether the patient was considered or prescribed an antidepressant medication during an episode of MDD. Modifier **1P**, **2P**, or **3P** may not be reported.
0545F Plan for follow-up care for MDD, documented	Report when a plan for follow-up care is documented in the medical record. There are no performance exclusions for this measure.

HIV/AIDS

This measure is reported by the physician providing ongoing HIV care to children and adults. There are 29 Category II codes used in this measure. Each measure has a different denominator that is specific to the patient's age. Measures include reporting cell counts, use of antiretroviral therapy, screening for opportunistic infections and high-risk behaviors, administration of vaccines, and use of *Pneumocystis jiroveci* pneumonia prophylaxis. Refer to the ACTL at https://www.ama-assn.org/practice-management/category-ii-codes for details on the requirements for reporting these codes.

Chapter 3: Coding to Demonstrate Quality and Value

The Business of Medicine: Working With Current and Emerging Payment Systems

Contents

Chapter 4: The Business of Medicine: Working With Current and Emerging Payment Systems

To maintain a viable practice, physicians and their staff must continually refine their practice management skills as they respond to changing payment systems. The first section of this chapter provides an overview of how services are currently valued and how assigned values may be used to guide practice management. The second section reviews guidelines and tools that may be used to monitor and manage charge accumulation, claims filing, review of payments, the appeals process, contract negotiations, and the use of audits to protect against lost revenue and incorrect billing practices. The third section introduces emerging payment methodologies and how these may affect traditional and newer practice models, such as accountable care organizations (ACOs).

Connecting Codes to Payment and Budget

Before a claim is generated, a physician practice must establish fees for services that are greater than the cost of providing the service. A simple fee schedule methodology involves use of the Medicare Resource-Based Relative Value Scale (RBRVS). In 2019, most pediatric services are still valued and paid by Medicaid, Tricare, and commercial payers using a fee-for-service methodology based on the RBRVS. An understanding of how values are assigned to the codes for services, how the values relate to payment, and how this information contributes to a practice's finances is critical for the practice's financial viability and success.

The 3 components of the RBRVS are as follows:

1. *Physician work:* Physician work represents approximately 50% of the total relative value units (RVUs) assigned to most services. *Work* is described as time required to perform the service, mental effort and judgment, technical skill, physical effort, and psychological stress associated with concern about iatrogenic risk to the patient. Work is further broken down to preservice, intraservice, and post-service components. Understanding these components of work is important to code correctly, as preservice and post-service components should not be separately reported.

    ◈ *Preservice work:* For nonsurgical services, this preparatory non–face-to-face work includes typical review of records and communicating with other professionals. (Prolonged preservice work, such as extensive record review, may be separately reportable.) For surgical services, this includes physician work from the day before the service to the procedure but excludes the encounter that resulted in the decision for surgery or unrelated evaluation and management (E/M) services. (For more on the global period for surgery, see Chapter 10, Surgery, Infusion, and Sedation in the Outpatient Setting, and Chapter 19, Common Surgical Procedures and Sedation in Facility Settings.)

    ◈ *Intraservice work:* For nonsurgical services, this includes time spent by the physician or other qualified health care professional in direct patient care activities, such as obtaining history, examining the patient, and counseling the patient and/or caregivers. Surgical intraservice work begins with incision or introduction of instruments (eg, needle, scope) and ends with closure of the incision or removal of instruments.

    ◈ *Post-service work:* For nonsurgical services, post-service work includes arranging for further services, reviewing and communicating test results, preparing written reports, and/or communicating by telephone or secure electronic means. Separately reportable services, such as chronic care management or care plan oversight, are not included in post-service work. For surgical services, post-service work includes typical work in the procedure or operating room after the procedure has ended, stabilization of the patient in the recovery area, communications with family or other health care professionals, and visits on the day of surgery. Surgical services are also valued to include typical follow-up care for the presenting problem during a defined global period (eg, 10 or 90 days after the service).

2. *Practice expense:* This component is an estimate of preservice, intraservice, and post-service clinical staff time; medical supplies; and procedure-specific and overhead equipment. Practice expense makes up about 44% of the total RVUs for most services. Practice expense varies by site of service (facility vs non-facility). See the Place of Service Codes section later in this chapter for more information about how place of service affects payment.

3. *Professional liability:* This smallest component (about 4% of the total RVUs) is based on medical malpractice premium data.

   Figure 4-1 illustrates the percent of total RVU for each component.

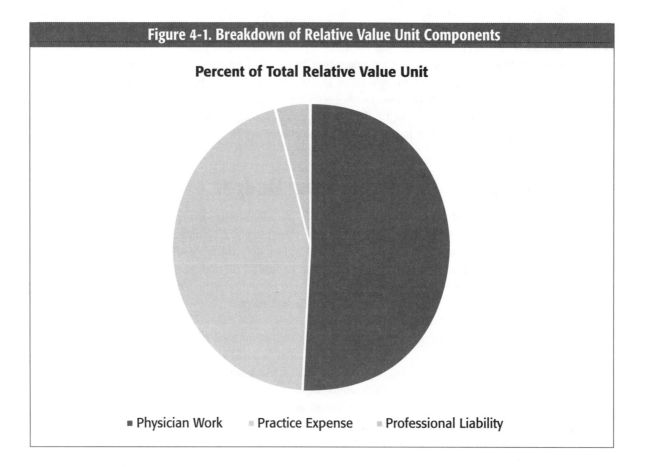

Figure 4-1. Breakdown of Relative Value Unit Components

Percent of Total Relative Value Unit

■ Physician Work   ■ Practice Expense   ■ Professional Liability

Each RVU component may be independently adjusted slightly upward or downward as a function of geographic area. The Centers for Medicare & Medicaid Services (CMS) calculates Medicare payment for a procedure code by multiplying total RVUs by a dollar conversion factor (CF) that is set annually.

Example

➤ **A payer uses the Medicare Physician Fee Schedule (MPFS) as a basis for physician payment with a CF or contracted fee schedule amount of $38 per RVU.** A physician submits established patient office visit code **99214** to the payer. The total Medicare non-facility RVUs (3.04) assigned to code **99214** are multiplied by the $38 CF to determine the allowed amount for the service.

(Total Medicare RVUs) × (Payer CF) = Allowed amount

(3.04) × ($38) = $115.52

Actual payment may vary based on the patient's out-of-pocket obligation. The total non-facility RVUs are a combination of RVUs for physician work (1.50), non-facility practice expense (1.44), and professional liability (0.10).

Medicaid fee schedules vary by state and, though often based on RVUs or the MPFS, state regulations may also designate amounts paid for specific services. Commercial payments for many procedure codes are often linked to a percentage of Medicare payment. Alternatively, payers may offer their own fee schedule for a practice's most used procedure codes. It is important to obtain the payer's fee schedule for all codes used or likely to be used by a practice and compare these with the MPFS and other published fee schedules. Although Medicare assigns a status of N (non-covered) to *Current Procedural Terminology* (*CPT*®) codes **99381–99385** and **99391–99395** in the MPFS, they do have component RVUs that allow calculation of Medicare equivalent payments. Medicaid and proposed commercial payments for pediatric preventive care can be evaluated in light of the Medicare equivalent payments. *Tip:* When reviewing a payer's fee schedule, make sure the payer also fully discloses its policies for paying for services that it considers to be *bundled* (ie, payment for 2 or more codes during the same encounter may be less than the sum of the individual payments). If a contract links payment to the MPFS, it is important to be specific about which fee schedule is used, as these change annually. Resetting payment based on the MPFS for the year of service may result in lower payments.

The RBRVS payment methodology may be used with practice- and physician-specific data generated from a practice's accounting and practice management systems to estimate an approximate cost of providing each service. The result should be a list of services each assigned a share of the practice's overhead cost as well as the margin and actual cost of providing the service. From the accounting system, an administrator may calculate the total practice expenses for a period, subtracting billable services that are not paid based on RVUs such as vaccines and medications. From the practice management system, reports may be generated to provide a total of the number of procedures billed by code, RVUs for each service, and total RVUs billed by the practice for the same period. By dividing total practice expenses by total RVUs, an administrator can calculate the practice cost per RVU. Additional calculations may be used to compare payment per RVU or per service among contracted payers. (Calculations should be viewed in context of other factors, such as history of timely and correct payment.)

Such calculations can be used to inform decisions on acceptance of contractual fee schedules, number of services necessary to break even or profit from provision of services, and return on investment potential for new equipment or services. The practice cost for providing a service may also be of significant value when approached by an ACO to participate in a financial agreement in which certain services are paid with a single lump payment that is then distributed among providers of service. A physician will need to know the cost of providing the service to negotiate a fair portion of the lump payment. (See the Accountable Care Organizations [ACOs] section later in this chapter.) More accurate estimates of cost may be determined on an actual cost basis. However, RVU calculations are straightforward and typically provide a reasonably reliable result.

Pediatric physicians can also play a role in recommending values for services to the CMS by participation in American Academy of Pediatrics (AAP) surveys conducted through the American Medical Association/Specialty Society Relative Value Scale Update Committee (RUC). These surveys are conducted to estimate the time and complexity of performing a service in comparison with another service. American Academy of Pediatrics staff sends out requests for participation to AAP section members to allow completion by physicians who most typically perform the service being surveyed. To learn more about participation in RUC surveys, see the "Understanding the RUC Survey Instrument" videos at https://www.youtube.com/watch?v=nu5unDX8VIs, and for information on code valuation, RBRVS, and payment, see https://www.aap.org/en-us/professional-resources/practice-transformation/getting-paid/Coding-at-the-AAP/Pages/Code-Valuation-and-PaymentRBRVS.aspx.

> **~ More From the AAP ~**
>
> For more information on relative value units, see the American Academy of Pediatrics policy statement, "Application of the Resource-Based Relative Value Scale System to Pediatrics," at http://pediatrics.aappublications.org/content/133/6/1158.full.pdf.

Clean Claims to Correct Payment

An effective charge accumulation system, accurate billing of procedure codes, and an efficient claims filing system are necessary but not sufficient to achieve clean claim submissions. Although the physician is ultimately responsible for the accuracy of codes selected and claims submitted, it typically takes a team effort to create and maintain an effective accounts receivable system, including

- Development and use of management tools.
  - Incorporation of claims processing tools for analysis of your claims processing procedures. A self-assessment tool for improving claims processing and payment can be found at https://www.aap.org/en-us/Documents/ImprovingClaimsProcessing.pdf.
  - Electronic health record (EHR) and/or billing systems may include automated tools to help identify errors prior to billing, alert to payments that do not align with contracted fees, and provide data for monitoring the time lapse from provision of service to payment.

- Continuing provider and staff education with constant oversight and communication with staff, payers, and patients.
  - ❖ Policies and procedures that support continuous monitoring of payer communications and disseminate information on benefit policy changes that affect coding and payment.
  - ❖ Assurance that staff assigned with responsibilities related to correct coding and billing have access to authoritative resources on coding and documentation (eg, current Medicaid National Correct Coding Initiative [NCCI] edits and manual). See Chapter 2, Modifiers and Coding Edits, and Chapter 5, Preventing Fraud and Abuse: Compliance, Audits, and Paybacks, for more information on code edits and compliant coding and billing.
- Performance of regular audits to identify potential corrective actions required to be compliant with billing standards, coding guidelines, and federal rules and regulations (eg, Health Insurance Portability and Accountability Act of 1996, Anti-Kickback Statute, False Claims Act). Audits benefit the practice by identifying
  - ❖ The number of timely and correctly submitted claims, resulting in faster and more appropriate payments
  - ❖ The need for physician and staff education on coding and documentation
  - ❖ Inappropriate carrier denials and reductions requiring appeals, thus decreasing practice costs
  - ❖ Issues for payer contract negotiations
  - ❖ Incorrect coding and related potential risk for charges of fraud or abuse
  - ❖ Areas in need of written office policies and procedures (eg, pre-authorizations and referrals processes, claims follow-up processes, control systems)
- Procedures for efficient review of payments. Timely identification of payment errors is necessary to obtain redress because contracts often specify a time limit on appeals.
- Guidance for write-offs and initiation of appeals processes.

The Encounter Form

Designing and Reviewing the Encounter Form

The encounter form, whether computer generated or printed, should be reviewed periodically and updated at the time of the *CPT*®; *International Classification of Diseases, 10th Revision, Clinical Modification* (ICD-10-CM); and Healthcare Common Procedure Coding System (HCPCS) updates (ie, January, April, July, and October) to be certain it includes most, if not all, of the services and procedures commonly performed in the practice and the codes are accurate.

See the Capturing Charges in the Electronic Health Record section later in this chapter for information on code maintenance and charge capture in an EHR.

Practices Generating Charges From a Printed Encounter Form (Superbill)

When developing the encounter form
- Include all levels of service for each category of E/M services (eg, **99201–99205, 99221–99223**) and ensure time is listed for coding based on time.
- List procedures (eg, laboratory) in alphabetic order within the category of service. For example, group vaccine administration codes and vaccine product codes together to maximize efficiency and workflow.
- Allow space on the printed encounter form to write in specific details of a procedure when required. For example

  Code **120**_____ Laceration repair; loc*_____; size_____ (*location)
- Include the most commonly reported diagnosis codes. Consider grouping diagnosis codes by organ system, and then alphabetically within the system.
- Leave space on the printed form to allow the reporting of the specific diagnosis and full *ICD-10-CM* code. For example
  ICD-10-CM: **M25.0**_____Joint pain; loc _____
- Include the most frequently used modifiers.

- Include add-on codes for prolonged and special services. For example

  99354   Prolonged service in the office or outpatient setting, first hour

  99058   Services provided on an emergency basis in the office, disrupting other scheduled services
- Develop a separate encounter form for hospital and outpatient hospital services. Make sure it includes all the services most commonly performed in the hospital setting.
- Leave space on the printed form to write in any services or diagnoses that are not included.
- When quality initiatives are dependent on codes reported (eg, codes supporting Healthcare Effectiveness Data and Information Set [HEDIS] measures), be sure that these codes are clearly indicated on the encounter form.

> **~ More From the AAP ~**
>
> The American Academy of Pediatrics Pediatric Office Superbill may be purchased from shopAAP at https://shop.aap.org/pediatric-office-superbill-2019.

Completing the Printed Encounter Form

Every practice should develop a written policy of the requirements needed to complete the form. Some points that should be part of the policy include

- The encounter form is *not* part of the medical record. Information such as the need for follow-up care, diagnostic tests, or referrals must always be documented in the medical record even if written on the encounter form.
- Services must be clearly identified (eg, circle procedure, use check mark).
- The person providing the service (eg, physician, laboratory technologist, medical assistant) should document that service on the encounter form to ensure only the procedures performed are reported. For example, it is common for a physician to mark a urinalysis on the encounter form when he or she orders the test. However, if a specimen could not be obtained, the procedure would have been billed inappropriately. If the nurse (under supervision of the physician) had been responsible for reporting the service when performed, it would not have been reported because the urine was not obtained.
- The physician is ultimately responsible for the services reported and billed.
- The physician should identify the diagnosis as, for example, primary or secondary.
- Diagnoses and services or procedures must be numbered and linked to each other. For example, an E/M service and removal of impacted cerumen from the right ear (69210) is performed. The physician reports the primary diagnosis (H66.001, acute suppurative otitis media without spontaneous rupture of eardrum, right ear) (1) and the secondary diagnosis (H61.21, impacted cerumen, right ear) (2). *ICD-10-CM* diagnosis code H66.001 is linked to the office visit and the secondary diagnosis code is linked to the procedure.

  99213 25 (1) H66.001 (1)

  69210 (2)   H61.21 (2)
- On a paper claim form, the linking of diagnoses to procedures would look like Table 4-1.

Table 4-1. Diagnosis Indicator on CMS-1500 Form

21. Diagnosis or nature of illness or injury (Relate A–L to service line below 24E)				ICD Ind. 0					
A. H66.001	B. H61.21	C.	D.						
E.	F.	G.	H.						
I.	J.	K.	L.						
24. A. Dates of service	B. Place of service	C. EMG	D. Procedures, services or supplies CPT/HCPCS	Modifier	E. Diagnosis Pointer	F. Charges	G. Days or units	H. EPSDT	I. ID Qual	J. Rendering Provider #
1/1/2019–1/1/2019	11		99213 (E/M)	25	A	$$$	1		NPI	1234567890
1/1/2019–1/1/2019	11		69210 (cerumen removal)		B	$$$	1		NPI	1234567890

Abbreviations: CPT, Current Procedural Terminology; E/M, evaluation and management; EMG, emergency; EPSDT, Early and Periodic Screening, Diagnosis, and Treatment; HCPCS, Healthcare Common Procedure Coding System; ICD, International Classification of Diseases; NPI, National Provider Identifier.

- Procedures or diagnoses must be written, if not preprinted, on the form.
- A billing manager or clerk should only add or change a service or diagnosis with the agreement of the provider of service.
- A system should be instituted to monitor and ensure capture of all the day's patient encounter forms (eg, cross-reference to the patient sign-in records).

Reviewing the Encounter Form

A staff member who understands correct coding and reporting guidelines should always review the completed encounter form before charges are posted and the claim submitted to ensure that all procedures and services are captured and accurate.

For example, the reviewer should look to see that

- An administration code is reported with vaccines and/or injections.
- A venipuncture or finger stick is reported with a laboratory test.
- A handling fee is reported when the specimen is prepared and sent to an outside laboratory.
- A modifier is appended when appropriate (eg, modifier **76** for repeat procedures or services).
- The office visit is reported using the correct new or established patient category of service. (See Chapter 6, Evaluation and Management Documentation Guidelines, for more information on new and established patient code selection.)
- The diagnoses reported as primary and secondary are appropriate and are linked to the appropriate services or procedures.
- The documentation to support each service has been completed with required dates and signatures.

Capturing Charges in the Electronic Health Record

Many physicians now capture encounter and billing information in the EHR. Compliant documentation and code selection is discussed in Chapter 5, Preventing Fraud and Abuse: Compliance, Audits, and Paybacks. The basics of charge capture in the EHR are accurate listing of diagnoses, selection of complete codes, and procedure code selection based on work performed and documented. While integrating charge capture into the encounter documentation should provide efficiency, there are pitfalls to be avoided.

When using an EHR, make sure that codes in the system are accurate and updated in accordance with code set updates. It is important to verify with your electronic system vendors how code updates are incorporated into the system. This may be via scheduled upgrades that may or may not require system downtime or may occur via automated upgrades during night or weekend hours. Code updates should be based on the effective date of changes (eg, deleted codes may be entered for charges with a date of service prior to the effective date of deletion even after the update has been made). Practice and billing managers must maintain contact with the system vendor's upgrade and support staff and verify what, if any, manual steps are required on the part of the practice in relation to code changes.

It is also important that code descriptors displayed in code selection are adequate for accurate code selection. Truncated descriptors may omit key information that differentiates one code from another (eg, hypertrophy of tonsils should provide options for hypertrophy of tonsils alone or hypertrophy of tonsils and adenoid and prompt reporting of a code for tonsillitis when both tonsillitis and hypertrophy are diagnosed).

Documentation of the diagnoses has been problematic in some EHR systems. As with the paper record, the physician must have the ability to fully describe patient diagnoses (eg, 1, attention-deficit/hyperactivity disorder [ADHD] predominately inattentive type on parent and teacher scales with a positive family history of ADHD; 2, underachievement in school with grades dropping this semester; 3, disruption of family by separation and divorce, which is causing behavioral issues at home and school) for each encounter.

- Systems should not use diagnosis codes for populating the physician's diagnostic statement or assessment. Code descriptors may provide only generalized information and would not capture the physician's differential diagnoses (eg, delayed milestone in childhood—late talker at 3 years old and in speech therapy with possible autism spectrum disorder because does not give much eye contact and likes to play alone).
- The EHR should not reorder diagnoses entered by the physician. Physicians should list first the diagnosis and code most responsible for the encounter, followed by additional diagnoses. An EHR that reorders documented diagnoses (eg, alphabetically) results in noncompliance with diagnosis coding guidelines.

- The patient problem list should not be pulled forward as the diagnoses for each encounter. Only those conditions addressed or that affected management or treatment of conditions addressed should be reported for each encounter. (Follow payer guidelines for reporting diagnosis codes for chronic conditions that may be reported annually [often at preventive service visits] for purposes of risk stratification. See Chapter 3, Coding to Demonstrate Quality and Value, for additional information.)

Automated code selection is also problematic. An EHR may be designed to determine the level of E/M service provided based on information documented. However, physicians must make the code determination based on the medically necessary key components or time spent counselling and/or coordinating care. Automatic population of records may result in documentation that overstates the level of work and intensity of the service provided. (See more on compliant EHR documentation in Chapter 5, Preventing Fraud and Abuse: Compliance, Audits, and Paybacks.) Therefore, when EHR functionality includes automated E/M code determinations, physicians must view the EHR code as a suggestion that must be confirmed or rejected based on documentation and medical necessity. Failure to override suggested codes when appropriate may be considered an abusive practice.

When encounter data is utilized to show performance of quality metrics, it is essential that the data are configured to correctly populate reports of the patients to whom the measure applies and whether there is documentation of the outcome or process of care specified in the measure (eg, all patients aged 3–17 years and the percentage of those patients who received counseling for diet and exercise).

Submitting Clean Claims

Many states have enacted laws that require prompt payment of "clean claims." In general, clean claims are those that contain sufficient and correct information for processing without further investigation or development by the payer (definitions may vary by state). Submitted claims must be accurate and in accordance with the process as outlined in the executed carrier or health plan agreement. Knowing a payer's claim requirements will decrease chances of denied claims. Make sure the practice understands payer rules, for example, for billing for nonphysician services and incident-to billing. (See Chapter 6, Evaluation and Management Documentation Guidelines, and Chapter 13, Allied Health and Clinical Staff Services, for more information on billing for nonphysician services.) Be aware of any updates issued by the carrier that affect billing and claims submission. Generally, a clean claim should have the following information:

- Practice information (name, address, phone, National Provider Identifier [NPI], group tax ID number)
- Patient information (patient name, birth date, policyholder, policy number, patient ID number, address)
- Codes (*CPT*®, *ICD-10-CM*, HCPCS, place of service), modifiers, and service dates
- Carrier information
- Secondary insurance information
- Referring physician name and NPI, if applicable
- Facility name and address, as appropriate

If additional information is necessary to support a service or explain an unusual circumstance (eg, unlisted procedure code, unusual procedure, complicated procedure)

- Use the attachments feature of your claims system, clearinghouse, or other electronic claim attachment procedure as directed by the payer (eg, submission of attachments by fax) or send a hard-copy claim with a cover letter and a narrative report or copy of the appropriate part of the medical record (eg, progress note, procedure note) to facilitate claim processing.
- Any documentation (eg, coordination of benefits information, letter of medical necessity, clinical reports) should include the patient's name, service date, and policy number on each page in case the papers become separated. Documentation submitted electronically may require inclusion of the payer's internal control number for the associated claim. The internal control number is found on the claim acknowledgment report generated after claim submission.
- Keep a copy of the claim and supporting information for follow-up of payment.
- When filing claims for patients with coordination of benefits, make certain all required information (ie, primary and secondary insurance information) has been obtained from the patient and claims are filed with the supporting information (eg, explanation of benefits [EOB] or electronic remittance advice information), according to plan requirements.

Claims should be submitted for payment as soon as possible and before the deadline specified in the agreement. The optimum time for filing outpatient claims is on the day of or the day following the service but no more than 2 to 3 days from the date of service. Inpatient encounter forms for patients with prolonged hospitalizations may allow codes to be documented for 7 consecutive days; in this case, claims should be filed within 2 to 3 days of the end of the service week. It is not necessary to withhold claims until the patient is discharged. Policy should be adopted requiring completion of medical record documentation within a specified period to support prompt billing of services. Physicians must understand that timely completion of documentation is required for appropriate code selection, claim filing, and, ultimately, prompt payment.

> ||ı|ı|| **Coding Pearl** ||ı|ı||
>
> Practices should monitor lag time between completion of each service and submission of a claim for the service to identify and correct any cause of delayed submission. Timely finalization of documentation is necessary to make sure that codes are supported by the documentation before claims are submitted. Many practices adopt policies for timely completion of documentation.

Place of Service Codes

The place of service is indicated on each claim by a *place of service code* (often integrated into billing systems without need for manual entry with each charge). The place of service may appear evident when reporting codes for services such as inpatient hospital care, but this is not always the case. When providing services in a facility such as a hospital outpatient clinic, it is important to report the correct place of service because differences in practice expense in a facility versus a non-facility setting affect physician payment. For instance, a procedure performed in a surgical center would be paid at a lower fee schedule amount than the same procedure performed in a physician's clinic (not hospital-based) because the fee schedule takes into account the overhead or practice expense of providing, for example, the procedure room, supplies, and clinical staff. If services provided in a facility setting are reported as if provided in a physician's clinic, an overpayment may occur.

Physicians in provider-based practices (ie, those practices owned and operated as a part of a hospital) should be aware that the place of service code is especially important in this setting. Because the physician and practice expense portions of the patient's charges are often billed separately, the same services provided in a provider-based practice are often costlier than those provided in an independent (physician-owned) practice. Facility fees charged by the provider are often significantly higher than the non-facility fees charged in independent practices. The increased number of high-deductible health plans has raised awareness of the greater costs to patients when services are rendered in provider-based facilities and have prompted Medicare and some states to take action to reduce the added costs. Practices should be aware of any such restrictions that apply to billing in their locality and under payer contracts.

Place of service codes that may be reported for pediatric services include

02	Telehealth
03	School
04	Homeless shelter
11	Office
12	Home
13	Assisted living facility
14	Group home
16	Temporary lodging
19	Off campus—outpatient hospital
20	Urgent care facility
21	Inpatient hospital
22	On campus—outpatient hospital
23	Emergency room—hospital
24	Ambulatory surgical center
25	Birthing center
26	Military treatment facility
33	Custodial care facility

| 71 | Public health clinic |
| 72 | Rural health clinic |

Place of service codes are further discussed for certain E/M services in chapters dedicated to those sites of service. See a full list of place of service codes at www.cms.gov/Medicare/Coding/place-of-service-codes/Place_of_Service_Code_Set.html.

Special Consideration for Medicare Claims

Many health plans receive Medicare claims automatically when they are the secondary payer. In this case, the explanation of Medicare benefits will indicate that the claim has been automatically crossed over for secondary consideration. Physicians and providers should look for this indication on their EOBs and should not submit a paper claim to the secondary payer.

> ### ~ More From the AAP ~
>
> For more information about place of service codes, see "Place of Service: Not Always Office" in the April 2015 *AAP Pediatric Coding Newsletter*™ at http://coding.aap.org (subscription required).

Monitoring Claim Status

An important aspect of billing operations is prompt and routine claim monitoring. A defined process for verifying that submitted claims were received and accepted by claim clearinghouses and/or payers should be included in the practice's or billing service's written billing procedures. Steps may include (see the last bullet if billing is outsourced or centralized outside the practice)

- Identify each type of report and/or dashboard feature of the practice's billing system for use in verifying claim submission and acceptance for processing, assigning follow-up activities for unpaid claims, and tracking average time from date of service or submission to receipt of payment.
- Assign responsibilities for verifying that electronic claim submissions were received and accepted for processing as soon after transmission as possible.
  - ❖ Most clearinghouses will send a report indicating acceptance or rejection of a batch of claims within minutes of transmission and a report with individual claim-level detail within 24 hours of submission.
  - ❖ It is also often necessary to log in to a payer's Web site or system to verify receipt of claims and monitor acceptance or rejection.
- Electronic claim submission reports must be promptly reviewed for rejections or denials. All rejected or denied claims must be investigated to determine what corrections or payer contact is necessary to resubmit or return the claim for re-adjudication (eg, when a payer system error is corrected).
- Claims should not be resubmitted without investigation, as resubmission of a claim containing errors is unlikely to result in payment. Resubmission of the claim with errors may reset the aging of the claim in the billing system and result in late follow-up or denial for lack of timely filing.
- Identify staff responsible for claims follow-up and establish standards for timely follow-up on unpaid claims. System-generated reports are useful in identifying the age of claims.
- Policies and procedures should address communication with patients and responsible parties when a payer requests additional information prior to claims processing (eg, many payers will request information on other coverage and/or details of where and how an injury was sustained). Failure to respond to payer requests for information in a timely manner can result in delayed or denied claims payment.
- If centralized billing or an outsourced billing service is used, maintain oversight of performance by reviewing reports that show any lag time between completion of documentation and submission of claims, aging reports that show the average number of days since claim submission for unpaid claims, and reports of amounts adjusted or written off. (Even salaried physicians are affected by lost revenue and should have interest in the effectiveness of the practice's billing processes.)

Monitoring Payments

Develop a process to monitor the timeliness of all payments. Tips for monitoring payments include

- Identify payers who do not pay clean claims within the time frame agreed on in your contract and follow up on all late payments with the payer. Check the provisions of your state prompt pay law and know the provisions for clean claims, timely filing, and penalties. Report the payer's practice of late or delinquent payments to the proper agency because your practice may be entitled to payment plus interest.

- Review each EOB and/or remittance advice (electronic or paper) carefully to determine if the payment is correct. Familiarity with standard claim adjustment reason codes and remittance advice remark codes is essential to identifying denial reasons, such as a non-covered service, bundled payment, or provision of service not typical for physician specialty (not relevant for taxonomy code), and any patient responsibility for denied charges.
- Compare the EOBs and/or remittance advice to a spreadsheet listing your top 40 codes and their allowable payments by carrier to monitor contract compliance. Practice management software may also include the ability to add contractual allowances by payer. Make certain that the payment is consistent with the fee schedule, write-offs, and discounts agreed to by the practice and payer. Follow up with the payer on any discrepancies.
- Identify any discrepancies, such as changes to codes, reduced payment, or denials.
- Review all payer explanations, particularly reasons for denials or down-coding. If the service provided is not a benefit covered by the plan, the patient should be billed directly (may need a signed waiver form).
- Make certain that any denials or reductions in payment are not due to practice billing errors (eg, incorrect modifiers, obsolete codes) or are incorrect applications of an NCCI edit that does not pertain to pediatrics. If so, correct the errors immediately and educate staff members as appropriate to ensure correct future claim submissions.

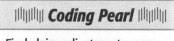

> |||||||| **Coding Pearl** ||||||||
>
> Find claim adjustment reason code and remittance advice remark code descriptions online at www.wpc-edi.com/reference.

- One efficiency of many electronic systems is automatic application of payments and adjustments. However, systems may apply incorrect adjustments based on payer remark codes. Staff should monitor all denials and reduced payments as appropriate and appeal incorrect adjustments when applicable.
- Maintain a log of all denials or payment reductions. This can be used as a basis for future negotiations or education of the payer. (Identify one individual who has billing and coding expertise to monitor as well as accept or reject denials.)
- Review your fee schedule to see if your practice is paid at 100% of the billed charges because this is an indication that your fees are below the maximum amount established by the carrier.
- Review your fees annually and understand the Medicare RBRVS, using it to value the services you provide. (For details on using the RBRVS, see "2019 RBRVS: What Is It and How Does It Affect Pediatrics?" at www.aap.org/coding, access code AAPCFP24.)
- Review your payment to make sure it exceeds your cost of providing that service.
- When contracting with payers, be aware of payment options that may be specified (eg, paper checks, electronic fund transfers, virtual credit card payment). It is important to understand the pros and cons of each (eg, credit card processing fees typically apply to card-based payment).
- Health plans must provide payment in compliance with electronic fund transfer standards of the Health Insurance Portability and Accountability Act rather than virtual card or wire transfer when requested by a physician. Agreements to accept electronic fund transfers should not allow health plans to debit an account without notification and consent. Banks may offer additional protections against unauthorized withdrawals.

Filing Appeals

Do not assume that the carrier's denials or audits are accurate. Be prepared to challenge the carrier. If you are coding correctly and in compliance with coding conventions, you should appeal all inappropriately denied claims and carrier misapplication of *CPT®* coding principles. Develop a system to monitor payer updates and any changes to the provider agreement so you are aware of the current payment policies and coding edits used by the payer.

- By accepting inappropriate claim denials, a practice may be setting itself up to charges of billing fraud.
- If a practice recodes claims as a result of inappropriate carrier denials, the resubmitted claim may not actually reflect the treatment the patient received.

Here is a summary of basic guidelines and tips for appealing payments.

- When in contact with the payer, always document the date, name, and title of the payer representative with whom you have talked and a summary of the details of the conversation. If a payer requests you submit a claim using codes or modifiers that are not consistent with clean coding standards, ask for documentation of the direction in writing.
  - Address issues with the person who has the authority to make decisions to overturn denials or reductions in payment.
  - Keep an updated file with names and contact information of the appropriate personnel with each of your contracted payers.
  - Request an e-mail or letter verifying the information provided and archive written correspondence containing payer representative advice and payer policies. If the carrier does not provide written documentation, prepare a summary and send it to your contact, stating that this will constitute the documentation of the discussion.
- Submit all appeals in writing.
  - Understand the payer's appeal process and appeal within its timeliness guidelines.
  - Format the letter to include the name of the patient, policy number, claim control number, and date of service(s) in question on each page of the letter.
  - The body of the letter should state the reason for the appeal and why you are in disagreement with the payer's adjudication of the claim.
  - Specify a date by which you expect the carrier to respond.
  - Support your case by providing medical justification and referencing *CPT®* coding guidelines. If necessary, consult with the AAP Coding Hotline for clarification of correct coding. It may be helpful to hire a certified coding expert with knowledge in pediatric coding to review your claims. (If hiring a full-time certified coding expert is not practical for a small practice, part-time employment or periodic consultation may be options for access to coding and compliance expertise.)
  - Consider sending correspondence to the carrier by certified mail to verify receipt. Document and retain copies of all communications with the carrier about the appeal.
- Maintain an appeals-pending file.
  - If there is no response from the payer within 4 weeks of the date of the letter, send a copy of the appeal letter stamped "Second Request."
  - If there is no response within 2 weeks, or if the matter continues to remain unresolved, contact the state department of insurance (or other appropriate agency in your state) to file a complaint or engage its assistance.
  - Contact your AAP chapter and pediatric council, if your chapter has one, to make them aware of the situation with the payer. American Academy of Pediatrics chapter pediatric councils meet with health plans to discuss carrier policies and practices affecting pediatrics and pediatricians.

The AAP has developed several sample appeal letters that may be used as templates in appealing payer decisions. The appeal letter templates can be found at https://www.aap.org/en-us/professional-resources/practice-transformation/getting-paid/Pages/Private-Payer-Advocacy-Templates-for-Appeal-Letters.aspx. Template topics include

- Bundling of services
- Immunization administration services (90460, 90461; 90471–90474)
- Inappropriate linking of *CPT* and diagnosis (*ICD-10-CM*) codes
- Modifier 25
- Well-child care (99381–99395) and sick visit (99201–99215) reported on the same calendar day

In addition, the AAP has posted a narrative that explains the appropriateness of reporting certain circumstances based on NCCI edits.

When the AAP recognizes systemic issues with payer policies, it sends letters to payers on specific issues that need resolution or for information. These letters and carrier responses are posted on the Practice Transformation/Getting Paid/Public and Private Payer Advocacy page (https://www.aap.org/en-us/professional-resources/practice-transformation/getting-paid/Pages/Private-Payer-Advocacy-Letters-to-Carriers.aspx).

Knowing when to appeal a payer denial is just as important as knowing how to properly appeal. Writing an effective appeal letter to payers requires knowledge of *CPT*® guidelines, CMS policy, and payer policy. The AAP Private Payer Advocacy Advisory Committee has developed resources to effectively respond to inappropriate claim denials and handling requests for refunds, managing private payer contracts and denials, and how to respond to payer audits. (See https://www.aap.org/en-us/professional-resources/practice-transformation/getting-paid/pages/Oops-We-Overpaid-You-How-to-Respond-to-Payer-Audits.aspx.)

> ### ~ More From the AAP ~
>
> For more information about resubmissions and appeals, see "Denials to Dollars: Resubmissions and Appeals" in the August 2016 *AAP Pediatric Coding Newsletter*™ at http://coding.aap.org (subscription required).

Negotiating With Payers

Payers need to be made aware and held accountable when their payment policies negatively affect the physician–carrier contractual arrangement. Previous class-action lawsuits against national carriers in response to payers' inappropriate down-coding and bundling of services have strengthened the position of physicians appropriately following *CPT* guidelines.

The following suggestions can facilitate negotiations:

- Know a health plan's policies and procedures and their effect on pediatric services. Develop a system to monitor all updates and changes to the physician contract. Be aware of updates that are provided with periodic e-mail bulletins or information posted on a payer Web site that practices have been instructed to review periodically. Practices must be aware that these alternative ways of disseminating payment information are often considered legal and binding.
- When adding new physicians to your practice, be aware of each payer's fee schedule policies. Do not assume that the same fee schedule will be applied across all physicians in the practice (eg, a payer may assign a reduced fee schedule to new physicians or carry forward a physician's contract from a previous practice).
- Be aware of any accountability (eg, penalties or other effect on shared savings) that a plan attributes to the practice when patients receive care outside their plan's network without referral by physicians within the practice.
- Know *CPT* codes, modifiers, and guidelines for their use.
- Understand how the NCCI adopted by some payers (including Medicaid) may relate to your practice.
- Understand and be able to describe the scope of services provided and the time requirements for the service.
- Be prepared to demonstrate cost savings that may be recognized by the plan as well as the value the practice brings to the plan in terms of savings, quality of care data, and/or patient satisfaction. This is your leverage. Negotiating payment with payers can be more successful if a practice is also prepared to provide quality of care data according to standard quality measures.
- Monitor and know the use (distribution) of codes by each physician and, if in a group practice, for the practice as a whole.
- Identify your payer mix. Know how many patients you have in each plan and what percentage of your total patients that represents. In addition, know what percentage of RVUs each payer pays for your most frequently used codes and how they compare in payment with each other. Accurate information on payer mix and potential value/loss to the practice is essential in making participation decisions.
- Know and understand the payment basis and process.
- Have specific codes or issues to discuss, not generalities (agreement with general ideas may not address specific issues).
- Try to negotiate for coverage and payment of services or, if payers refuse to cover services, get your contract amended to state that you can bill the service as non-covered. If the plan will allow for billing the patient for non-covered services, you must then advise your patients of this policy.
- If the plan does agree to provide coverage for a particular service, make certain you understand how the carrier will cover and pay for the service and if there will be any restrictions or limitations.
- Keep notes during the discussion and be certain you understand answers to any of your questions. Any specific agreements should be in writing and signed by both parties.

⚙ Engage parents or employers to work in partnership to help you negotiate with a plan. Encourage parents to work through their human resources department to communicate and appeal with payers. Petition from them can be very effective.

Many AAP chapters have developed pediatric councils, which meet with payers to address pediatric issues. Advise your chapter pediatric council of specific issues you have experienced and see how it can work with the plan. If your chapter does not have a pediatric council, this may be the right time to work with your chapter to begin developing one. To see if your state has a pediatric council or for more information, visit https://www.aap.org/en-us/professional-resources/practice-transformation/getting-paid/Pages/aap-pediatric-councils.aspx (AAP members only).

⚙ If the insurance company is not addressing your concerns satisfactorily, you should be willing to withdraw from its plan. Inform the payer (a formal notification process may be outlined in your contract), patients' families, and even the state insurance commission why continued participation is impossible. Some reasons for withdrawal might be slow payment, excessive documentation requirements, and substandard payment compared with other plans. Many times, negotiation begins when you walk away from the table.

Documentation and Coding Audits

Medicare, state Medicaid programs, and commercial payers will audit claims as well as monitor E/M coding profiles. Physician practices should also adopt standards for conducting internal audits or reviews. Internal audits provide important information to inform practice policy and procedures, detect missed revenue, protect against erroneous billing, and avoid issues with payers and outside auditors. Some key benefits of internal auditing are

⚙ Identification of negative billing and revenue trends, including

❖ Increased lag time between encounter and billing (eg, delays in finalization of documentation, delayed coding or billing functions, technology issues)

❖ Denial or underpayment of new services or new or revised procedure codes

❖ Significant unexpected increase or decrease in revenue

❖ Inappropriate adjustments or write-offs of unpaid or underpaid claims that should be appealed

⚙ Charge verification (eg, number of charges is equal to or greater than number of encounters, with exception of visits included in a global period)

⚙ Identification of incorrect billing and coding practices

⚙ Identification of payment that does not align with payer contract

⚙ Identification of electronic system or workflow issues

⚙ Identification of areas where new or additional training is necessary

See Chapter 5, Preventing Fraud and Abuse: Compliance, Audits, and Paybacks, for more detailed information on conducting internal audits.

Tools for the Pediatric Practice

Working with third-party payers on coding and payment issues can be a difficult task because there is little uniformity between carriers and, frequently, great inconsistencies within the same umbrella organization of carriers. The AAP Private Payer Advocacy Advisory Committee is charged with enhancing systems for members and chapters to identify and respond to issues with private carriers.

To assist the pediatric practice, the AAP has several available resources to consider.

⚙ American Academy of Pediatrics staff is available to provide clarification on coding issues. The AAP Coding Hotline can be accessed by e-mail at aapcodinghotline@aap.org.

⚙ Claim processing tools, a collection of template letters practices can use in appealing inappropriate carrier claim denials, and other claims processing tools are available through the AAP Resources for Payment site at https://www.aap.org/en-us/professional-resources/practice-transformation/getting-paid/Pages/resources-for-payment.aspx (AAP members only). Also, the AAP Coding Calculator allows physician practices to compare their actual E/M code use distribution to statistical norms and assess the potential effect on payment. It can be accessed at https://www.aap.org/en-us/professional-resources/practice-transformation/getting-paid/Coding-at-the-AAP/Pages/Coding-Calculator.aspx.

- Many AAP state chapters have developed pediatric councils to meet regularly with carriers to discuss pediatric issues related to access, coverage, and quality. Pediatric councils have the potential to facilitate better working relationships between pediatricians and carriers by identifying, informing, and educating payers on issues affecting pediatrics and pediatricians. The AAP chapter pediatric councils are not forums for contract negotiation, setting fees, or discussing payments. For information on pediatric councils, go to https://www.aap.org/en-us/professional-resources/practice-transformation/getting-paid/Pages/aap-pediatric-councils.aspx (AAP members only).

- The AAP has created tools to assist practices with managed care contracting. These resources are available at https://www.aap.org/en-us/professional-resources/practice-transformation/getting-paid/Pages/resources-for-payment.aspx.

- Members of the AAP are encouraged to access the AAP Hassle Factor Form online to report health plan issues. The information submitted is used to assist the AAP and chapters in identifying issues and facilitating public and private payer advocacy related to health plans, including discussion topics with national carriers and at chapter pediatric council meetings with regional carriers. The Hassle Factor Form can be accessed at https://www.aap.org/en-us/professional-resources/practice-transformation/getting-paid/Pages/Hassle-Factor-Form-Concerns-with-Payers.aspx (AAP members only) and can be submitted electronically.

- American Academy of Pediatrics members and their staff are encouraged to attend AAP Pediatric Coding Webinars, presented by pediatric coding experts. To obtain a list of scheduled webinars and to register, visit www.aap.org/webinars/coding.

- The *AAP Pediatric Coding Newsletter*™ provides articles on coding and documentation of specific services and supplies (eg, vaccines) with updates on new codes and emerging issues affecting coding and billing practices. Subscribers can access current and archived issues and coding resources at http://coding.aap.org.

Emerging Payment Methodologies

Many payers are in the process of transitioning from volume-based payments, such as fee for service, to value-based payment models that offer incentive payments to providers based on the quality of care, outcomes, and cost containment attributable to their practice. The intent is to promote patient value and efficiency, but one consequence is that some risk is shifted to physician practices. Under these emerging payment models, practice viability will depend on how well quality, cost, and efficiency are managed. Examples of some of these newer payment models include bundled payments, shared savings, and pay for performance. Physician payments may be based on a combination of fee for service and newer payment methodologies. Emerging forms of health care financing and delivery models include ACOs and integrated delivery systems.

- *Bundled payments:* These are a type of prospective payment in which health care providers (hospitals, physicians, and other health care professionals) share one payment for a specified range of services as opposed to paying each provider individually. The intent of bundled payment is to foster collaboration among multiple providers to coordinate services and control costs, thereby reducing unnecessary utilization.

- *Shared savings:* Under a shared savings arrangement, providers and payers seek to deliver care at a cost that is below current budgeted amounts, and the resulting savings are shared between the payer(s) and providers. The contractual arrangement between the payer(s) and providers will specify how the savings are calculated and distributed. Shared savings models may include upside reward exclusively or upside reward and downside risk. In an upside-reward–only arrangement, the provider only shares in any savings and is not at risk for a loss. Under reward-and-risk arrangements, the practice shares a reward if costs are less than budgeted but also would share the loss should actual total costs exceed budgeted costs. Shared savings should include an up-front agreement to continue additional payments for ongoing support of infrastructure for future years when the payer may want to cut back on the shared savings margin or reduce as those savings plateau. Quality metrics are typically tied to payment of shared savings, with physicians not meeting established quality benchmarks not receiving a portion of savings. See Chapter 3, Coding to Demonstrate Quality and Value, for more information on coding to support quality and performance measurement. For more information on shared savings, see https://www.aap.org/en-us/Documents/practicet_gainsharing_and_shared_savings.pdf or visit www.aap.org/cfp and enter password AAPCFP24

⬥ *Pay for performance:* In this arrangement, physician payments are based on a prospectively determined comparison of the provider's performance against acknowledged benchmarks. If the provider meets or exceeds those benchmarks, an enhanced payment or bonus is provided. Benchmarks are often similar to the National Committee for Quality Assurance HEDIS quality metrics (discussed in Chapter 3, Coding to Demonstrate Quality and Value). As examples, some of the most common metrics for pediatrics include rates of immunizations; rates of patient adherence to Early and Periodic Screening, Diagnosis, and Treatment visits; and rates of appropriate prescription of asthma medications. Pay for performance arrangements often include the following 4 types of measures:

   ❖ *Structure:* Measures use of staff capabilities, policies and procedures, and systems such as EHR and computerized physician order entry
   ❖ *Process:* Determines the extent to which providers consistently give patients specific services that are consistent with recommended guidelines for care
   ❖ *Outcome:* Measures the effects that one or more clinical interventions have had on patients' health, health status, and function
   ❖ *Patient experience:* Measures patient-reported experience of care

Each type of measure may include additional subtypes, and payers may use composite measures (ie, 2 or more measures that result in a single score).

In considering whether to participate in one of these newer payment models, a practice needs to determine expected costs and utilization and assess whether it can deliver services under the projected budget. Using *CPT*® codes and their RVUs will aid in this assessment. Projections can be made using RVUs of the services currently provided and projected to be provided. With these types of data, the practice can assess the effect of new payment methodologies to its bottom line.

⬥ In some parts of the country, practices can earn additional incentives if the total cost of care for their patients compares favorably to geographically and specialty matched peers. In addition, some payers are incentivizing around "care efficiency measures." Both of these are often risk adjusted based on claims data about the overall patient population of the practice.

Other considerations for pediatricians include

⬥ Depending on how the payment model is set up, managing a healthy population of patients may not result in significant cost savings.

⬥ Ability to access and monitor patient population and performance metric data is important to successful participation in new payment methodologies. Physicians must be aware of not only the patients they are seeing but those who are not receiving preventive and/or follow-up care.

⬥ Physicians need to understand the links between new payment methodologies and data collection to support quality metrics (eg, failure to report codes for screening services performed may result in negative performance measurement and lost opportunity for enhanced payment).

⬥ Physicians should understand how health plans attribute patients to individual physicians and/or groups for purposes of performance measurement and cost of care. Factors such as time of continuous enrollment with the health plan and number of visits to a provider may affect how patients are attributed. The CMS has initiated voluntary reporting of modifiers that identify the provider to patient relationship for an episode of care. However, these modifiers were created for Medicare, and because reporting is not required, adoption by other payers and physicians may be slow. (See HCPCS modifiers **X1–X5** in Chapter 2, Modifiers and Coding Edits, for more information on these relationship modifiers.)

⬥ In states where the Children's Health Insurance Program (CHIP) operates independent of a state Medicaid program, children covered by CHIP may or may not be included in new payment methodologies and/or performance measurement.

See the *AAP News* article, "PPAAC: Chapter pediatric councils work with payers on medical home programs," at www.aappublications.org/news/2016/03/18/PPAAC031816 for examples of how AAP chapters and their pediatric councils advocate for developing adequate financing for pediatric medical homes under value-based payment methodologies.

> ### ~ More From the AAP ~
>
> For more on value-based payment, alternative payment models, and accountable care organizations, go to https://www.aap.org/en-us/professional-resources/practice-transformation/getting-paid/Pages/value-based-payment.aspx.

Accountable Care Organizations (ACOs)

Most of the content about ACOs is adapted with permission from the January 2011 *AAP News* (accessed at http://www.aappublications.org/content/32/1/1.6). The information provided herein has been updated since publication of that article.

As defined by the CMS, an ACO is an organization of health care professionals that agrees to be accountable for the quality, cost, and overall care of beneficiaries. In return, the ACO will receive incentive payments based on quality and cost containment instead of volume and intensity. Eligible providers are likely to be individual and group practices, hospitals, integrated delivery systems, and others who create a legal entity with a management structure able to deliver and report on evidence-based and informed care to a defined population, effectively engage patients, and receive and distribute shared savings.

The Patient Protection and Affordable Care Act of 2010 included a number of provisions that establish ACOs in Medicare, Medicaid, and CHIP. In October 2011, the CMS issued final regulations to assist physicians, hospitals, and other health care professionals in coordinating care through ACOs.

Interest in ACOs is accelerating, and the market continues to witness a growth in their numbers. As of 2017, the CMS has documented 480 Medicare Shared Savings Program (MSSP) ACOs. In addition, there were currently 35 ACOs participating in the Advanced Payment ACO Model, which is designed for physician-based and rural providers who have come together voluntarily to provide coordinated care to the Medicare patients they serve. Participants in this model receive up-front and monthly payments, which they can use to make critical investments in their care coordination infrastructure. These approaches will evaluate the effectiveness of various payment models and how their approach can provide better care, work in conjunction with private payers, and reduce Medicare cost growth.

Beyond the federal government's push toward ACOs, commercial health insurers are also actively exploring the development of ACOs. One of the special features of commercially driven ACOs is their flexibility in implementing accountable care contracts. Many private ACOs emulate the CMS MSSP approach; however, the flexibility provided by market-driven ACOs permits them to undertake more creative approaches in modeling payment methodologies. Leavitt Partners, LLC, a national health intelligence firm, reported in 2017 that there are more than 900 public and private ACOs covering 32 million lives across every state in the United States.

Pediatricians must be in a position to assess the ACO transition locally. More importantly, pediatricians need to be actively engaged in this transition to a new care model to ensure it best serves the needs of children and families and the pediatric health care delivery system.

The growing interest in ACOs as a principal driver in the reconfiguration of the US health care delivery system aligns with the Triple Aim espoused by former CMS administrator Don Berwick, MD. In the aggregate, the Triple Aim is designed to improve the individual experience of care, improve the health of populations, and reduce per capita costs of care for populations.

The Pediatric ACO Demonstration Project, legislated as part of the Patient Protection and Affordable Care Act but unfunded, calls for participating state Medicaid programs to allow pediatric medical professionals to form ACOs and receive incentive payments. The US Department of Health and Human Services will develop quality guidelines that must be met. The applicant state and ACO must meet a certain level of savings or slow the rate of growth in health care costs to receive an incentive payment. However, if funded, it is anticipated the CMS will derive many of the ACO requirements on the basis of its MSSP.

> ### ~ More From the AAP ~
>
> Learn more from webinars on preparing your practice; go to https://www.aap.org/en-us/professional-resources/practice-transformation/getting-paid/Pages/alternative-payment-models.aspx and scroll down to "AAP Webinar Series on Alternative Payment Models."

AAP Resources for More Information on ACOs

In response to growing interest in the development of ACOs, in 2011, the AAP ACO Workgroup produced guidance for members on factors to consider in evaluating an opportunity to participate in an ACO (https://www.aap.org/en-us/professional-resources/practice-transformation/getting-paid/Pages/Accountable-Care-Organizations-and-Pediatricians-Evaluation-and-Engagement.aspx). The guidance was reevaluated in 2013 by a group of pediatrician experts in financing and economics and deemed to still be timely.

The AAP has since collaborated with Leavitt Partners to carry out a study of pediatric ACOs, including a series of 5 case studies of diverse pediatric models, a scan of Medicaid ACOs, and a summit of leaders in pediatric ACO development. These collaborative activities identified several issues in ACO formation and sustainability in pediatric settings and outlined a number of opportunities for the pediatric community in areas of organization, model change, and market dynamics; payment, financing, and contracting; quality and value; and use of new technologies. More information is available in the January 2017 *Pediatrics* article, "Pediatric Accountable Care Organizations: Insight From Early Adopters" (http://pediatrics.aappublications.org/content/early/2017/01/29/peds.2016-1840).

In addition, the CMS has published fact sheets that provide general information about ACOs and their operational and financial characteristics. They can be accessed at http://innovations.cms.gov/initiatives/ACO/index.html.

Preparing for New Payment Models

The new payment models discussed previously are already in place in some areas and will soon be adopted in others. Whether your practice provides primary or specialty care, there are steps that you should take to prepare for success. When payment is based on the costs of care and patient experience, practices must take responsibility for keeping costs low and quality of care and patient experience high. This includes such activities as

- Learn more about value-based payment options.
- Generate and use reports of your costs, quality measurement, etc.
- Learn who your active patients are and stay up-to-date through routine data analysis.
- Obtain lists of patients attributed to your practice by payers and reconcile to your active patient list.
- Identify and agree on a methodology by which any disputes over attributed patient panels will be reconciled.
- Embrace automation and alternatives to paper handling and traditional office-based care.
- Seek to remove inefficiencies by reviewing routine tasks and patient flow. Provide staff with incentives and an expectation to create consistency and efficiency.
- Learn about the communities of your patients—school and community resources, school schedules, average income and education of caregivers, urgent and emergency care utilization patterns—and use the information in providing care.
- Know the costs of the care you provide and order for your patients. Recognize that every provider within and outside of your practice must contribute to reducing the cost of care to reduce the practice's risk under new payment models.
  - ❖ Collaborate with subspecialists to ensure patients receive evidence-based and cost-effective care, including consideration of formulary and total cost of coordinated care.
- Consider options for adding nonphysician health care professionals, such as care coordinators, patient educators, and emotional/behavioral health specialists, to your practice.
- Embed clinical guidelines into care delivery through protocols and reminders.
- Configure and use your EHR and other automated systems to promote efficiency (eg, display generic drugs first when brand name is entered).
- When considering an alternative payment model contract, seek expert consultation to help identify and, as necessary, negotiate points of concern within the contract.

CHAPTER 5

Preventing Fraud and Abuse:
Compliance, Audits, and Paybacks

This chapter was contributed by the American Academy of Pediatrics Committee on Medical Liability and Risk Management.

Contents

Although most physicians work ethically, provide high-quality care, and submit appropriate claims for payment, unfortunately, there are some providers who exploit the health care system for personal gain. These few have necessitated an array of laws to combat fraud and abuse and protect the integrity of the health care payment system. Just as patients put enormous trust in physicians, so do payers. Medicare, Medicaid, other federal health care programs, and private payers rely on physicians' medical judgment to treat patients with appropriate services. They depend on physicians to submit accurate and truthful claims for the services provided to their enrollees. And most physicians intend to do just that. However, the process is made more difficult by the complex and dynamic nature of payer coding and billing procedures, which, despite efforts to standardize variations, persist from carrier to carrier, policy to policy, state to state, and month to month.

This chapter outlines the importance of safeguarding the health care system from fraud and abuse, describes how compliance programs can protect medical practices from unintentional billing errors, and provides general considerations on how to respond to overpayment notices and inquiries from auditors.

Defining Medical Fraud and Abuse

The federal government has more than a dozen laws in its anti-fraud and anti-abuse arsenal. The 5 most important laws that apply to physicians are the False Claims Act, Anti-Kickback Statute, Physician Self-Referral Law (Stark), Exclusion Authorities, and Civil Monetary Penalties Law. Abiding by these laws is not only the right thing to do; violating them, even (for some) unwittingly, could result in criminal penalties, civil fines, exclusion from federal health care programs, or loss of medical license from a state medical board. It all begins with understanding the definition of *fraud and abuse* in health care.

Fraud

Fraud is obtaining something of value through intentional misrepresentation or concealment of material facts. Examples of fraud in the physician's office may include

- Requiring that a patient return for a procedure that could have been performed on the same day
- Billing Medicare or Medicaid for services not provided, including no-shows
- Billing one member for services provided to another (non-covered) member
- Billing more than one party for the same service
- Billing services under a different National Provider Identifier (NPI) (except as allowed by payer guidance)
- Taking a kickback in money, in-kind, or other valuable compensation for referrals
- Completing a certificate of medical necessity for a patient who does not need the service or who is not professionally known by the provider

Abuse

Abuse includes any practice that is not consistent with the goals of providing patients with services that

- Are medically necessary
- Meet professionally recognized standards
- Are fairly priced

  Some examples of actions that will likely be considered to be abuse are
- Charging in excess for services or supplies
- Billing Medicare or Medicaid based on a higher fee schedule than for other patients
- Providing medically unnecessary services
- Submitting bills to Medicare or Medicaid that are the responsibility of another insurance plan
- Waiving co-payments or deductibles (except as permitted for financial hardship)
- Advertising for free services
- Coding all visits at the same level
- Unbundling claims—ie, billing separately for services that are correctly billed under one code
- Billing claims under the wrong NPI

Kickbacks, Inducements, and Self-referrals

Business arrangements in which physician practices refer business to an outside entity (eg, hospitals, hospices, nursing facilities, home health agencies, durable medical equipment suppliers, vendors) should be on a fair market value basis. Whenever a physician practice intends to enter into a business arrangement that involves making referrals, legal counsel familiar with anti-kickback and physician self-referral laws should review the arrangement.

Risk areas that may need to be addressed in policies and procedures include

- Offering inappropriate inducements to patients (eg, waiving coinsurance or deductible amounts without a good-faith determination that the patient is in financial need, failing to make reasonable efforts to collect the cost-sharing amount)
- Financial arrangements with outside entities to which the practice may refer federal health care program business
- Joint ventures with entities supplying goods or services to the physician practice or its patients
- Participation in an accountable care organization and/or compliance in the context of participation in a Medicaid Shared Savings Program
- Consulting contracts or medical directorships
- Laboratory payments based on volume of referred services
- Payments for services already covered by a federal health insurer (double-dipping)
- Office and equipment leases with entities to which the physician refers business
- Soliciting, accepting, or offering any gift or gratuity of more than nominal value to or from those who may benefit from a physician practice referral of federal health care program business

When considering whether to engage in a particular billing practice, enter into a particular business venture, or pursue an employment, consulting, or other personal services relationship, it is prudent to evaluate the arrangement for potential compliance problems. Use experienced health care lawyers to analyze the issues and provide a legal evaluation and risk analysis of the proposed venture, relationship, or arrangement. The state bar association may have a directory of local attorneys who practice in the health care field. The American Health Lawyers Association is another resource (www.healthlawyers.org).

> |ı|ı|ı|ı| **Coding Pearl** |ı|ı|ı|ı|
>
> Use experienced health care lawyers. To locate one, contact your state bar association or the American Health Lawyers Association (www.healthlawyers.org).

Anti-fraud and Anti-abuse Activities

The battle against health care fraud and abuse is being waged on many fronts—federal and state governments as well as private payers. More and more, these groups are sharing information, so that a provider under investigation by one government health care program will likely be contacted by another and possibly by private payers. The US Department of Health and Human Services (HHS) Office of Inspector General (OIG) has several anti-fraud campaigns underway. In addition to federal anti-fraud and anti-abuse laws, many states have enacted anti-fraud and anti-abuse legislation, and state Medicaid programs have established Medicaid fraud control units. That means physician practices are subject to several levels of scrutiny for possible fraudulent activity. The Patient Protection and Affordable Care Act (PPACA) introduced new Medicaid program integrity provisions, such as increased fraud detection methods, terminating providers previously terminated from other government health care programs, suspending future payments based on credible allegations of fraud, and adopting the National Correct Coding Initiative edits (see Chapter 2, Modifiers and Coding Edits, for more information on edits). All this means that the momentum and resources for rooting out fraud and abuse at the federal and state level have intensified.

In addition, Medicaid auditors have a financial incentive to find fraud. The Medicaid Recovery Audit Contractors (RAC) program allows states to hire private contractors to audit Medicaid payments and keep a percentage of what they collect. Contingency fees for these contractors vary by state and range from 5.25% to 17%, with most between 9% and 13%. Under some circumstances, there can be bonuses paid that increase these fees to greater than 20%. Because it is Medicaid, pediatricians may be included in RAC audits. The RAC program was established in provisions of the PPACA and modeled on a similar successful Medicare program. So far, the

Medicare and Medicaid RAC programs have gone after larger organizations, but it is not inconceivable that they will eventually turn their attention to physician practices. It's always better to be prepared. Information on the status of state Medicaid RAC programs is available through the Centers for Medicare & Medicaid Services (CMS) Medicaid site, www.medicaid.gov. This site includes the name and contact information for each state's RAC and medical directors and look-back period for audits.

Areas of Specific Concern

The Department of Health and Human Services and the Department of Justice Health Care Fraud and Abuse Control Program Annual Report for Fiscal Year 2017, published in April 2018, highlights some of the newer initiatives and findings of the Health Care Fraud and Abuse Program coordinated through the OIG. Many findings and initiatives put physician practices under high scrutiny for miscoded services, failure to adequately document services, and operating in a manner that conflicts with anti-kickback and self-referral laws. Examples of audit and evaluation findings in fiscal year (FY) 2017 include

* The FY 2017 national Medicaid improper payment rate is 10.1%, representing $36.7 billion in gross improper payments, compared with the FY 2016 improper payment rate of 10.48% or $36.1 billion in improper payments. The FY 2017 national Children's Health Insurance Program (CHIP) improper payment rate is 8.64%, representing $1.2 billion in gross improper payments, compared with a FY 2016 national CHIP improper payment rate of 7.99%, representing $0.7 billion in gross improper payments. As these error rates are well above targets set by the OIG, expect continued aggressive efforts to discover and reduce improper payments.
* Specific areas of concern that affect physicians include billing for a higher level of service than was provided, billing for services by clinical staff that do not meet incident-to provisions, and physician self-referral violations.
* Several cases in 2016–2017 involved inappropriate payments or other incentives to physicians for using particular medical devices or medications.
* The OIG has found that the CMS has incorrectly paid incentives for use of certified electronic health records (EHRs) to providers who could not substantiate their successful participation. The OIG expressed concerns about overpayments in relation to new and planned payment methodologies (eg, value-based purchasing) in the Medicare and Medicaid programs.
* Analysis of claims data is increasingly combined across payers and care settings to identify physicians and other providers who are outliers in their billing and referral patterns to identify potential fraud and abuse. The fraud and abuse control units of HHS and the US Department of Justice also continue to cross-reference enrollment information for the same physicians and providers when there is history of enrollment in multiple states and/or programs. By cross-referencing enrollment data, conflicting information and/or evidence of prior revocation of eligibility to participate in federal programs may be discovered.

Compliance Programs

Does your practice have a fraud and abuse prevention compliance program? For many years, compliance programs for small practices were voluntary. This is no longer the case; they are now required, even for small practices, but they can be scalable.

What is a compliance program? A compliance program establishes strategies to prevent, detect, and resolve conduct that does not conform to

* Federal and state law
* Federal, state, and private payer health care program requirements
* The practice's own ethical and business policies

Pediatric practices benefit from having compliance initiatives because they tighten billing and coding operations and documentation. Practices with written compliance programs report having better control on internal procedures, improved medical record documentation, and streamlined practice operations.

Section 6401(a) of the PPACA requires physicians and other providers and suppliers who enroll in Medicare, Medicaid, or CHIP to establish a compliance program with certain "core elements."

The 7 Elements of the Office of Inspector General Compliance Program

Although the OIG has yet to publish the official guidance for required compliance programs, it is helpful to look at the 7 core elements described in the OIG guidance on voluntary compliance program for small physician practices published in 2000.

- Conduct internal monitoring and auditing.
- Implement written compliance and practice standards.
- Designate a compliance officer, contact, or committee.
- Conduct appropriate training and education.
- Respond appropriately to detected offenses and develop corrective action.
- Develop open lines of communication.
- Enforce disciplinary standards through well-publicized guidelines.

It's also useful to consult the *United States Sentencing Commission Guidelines Manual,* which makes it clear that an organization under investigation may be given more sympathetic treatment if a good compliance program is in place. Compliance programs not only help to prevent fraudulent or erroneous claims, but they also show that the physician practice is making a good-faith effort to submit claims appropriately. However, that would require the program to be integrated into the daily operations of the practice. It cannot be a set of policies and procedures merely kept in a binder or on a computer unrelated to actual business operations.

Here are some reasons the *United States Sentencing Commission Guidelines Manual* identifies to implement an effective compliance program.

- It may save the practice money if it prevents costly civil suits and criminal investigations.
- It sends an unambiguous message to employees: Fraud and abuse will not be tolerated.
- It decreases the risk of employees bringing suit against the practice under the False Claims Act because employees will have an internal communication system for reporting questionable activities and resolving problems.
- It helps if an investigation occurs. Investigators may be more inclined to resolve the problem as a civil rather than a criminal matter, or it may lead to an administrative resolution rather than a formal false claim action.
- It may help reduce the range used for imposing fines under federal sentencing guidelines.
- It may influence an OIG decision whether to exclude a provider from participation in federal health care programs.
- It frequently results in improved medical record documentation.
- It improves coding accuracy, reduces denials, and makes claims and payment processes more effective.
- It educates physicians and employees on their responsibilities for preventing, detecting, and reporting fraud and abuse.
- It should meet governmental requirements for practices to have a formal compliance plan.

Steps to Developing a Compliance Program

The CMS has described the steps to create an effective compliance and ethics program. A key aspect is that the organization exercises due diligence to prevent and detect criminal conduct and promotes a culture that encourages ethical conduct and a commitment to compliance with the law.

The CMS specifies that in creating the compliance program, the practice

1. Develop and distribute written policies, procedures, and standards of conduct to prevent and detect inappropriate behavior.
2. Designate a chief compliance officer and other appropriate bodies (eg, a corporate compliance committee) charged with the responsibility of operating and monitoring the compliance program and who report directly to high-level personnel and the governing body.
3. Use reasonable efforts not to include any individual in the substantial authority personnel whom the organization knew, or should have known, has engaged in illegal activities or other conduct inconsistent with an effective compliance and ethics program.
4. Develop and implement regular, effective education and training programs for the governing body; all employees, including high-level personnel; and, as appropriate, the organization's agents.

5. Maintain a process, such as a hotline, to receive complaints and the adoption of procedures to protect the anonymity of complainants and protect whistle-blowers from retaliation. (In a small practice, a hotline could be replaced with an "anonymous fraud report box.")
6. Develop a system to respond to allegations of improper conduct and the enforcement of appropriate disciplinary action against employees who have violated internal compliance policies, applicable statutes, regulations, or federal health care program requirements.
7. Use audits and/or other evaluation techniques to monitor compliance and assist in the reduction of identified problem areas.
8. Investigate and remediate identified systemic problems, including making any necessary modifications to the organization's compliance and ethics program.

Written Policies and Procedures

A compliance program should have written compliance standards and procedures that the practice follows. They should specifically describe the lines of responsibility for implementing the compliance program. Those standards and procedures should reduce the likelihood of fraudulent activity while also helping to identify any incorrect billing practices. Policies and procedures should be updated periodically to address newly identified areas of risk, new regulations, or process changes in the practice. All staff should receive periodic education on policies and procedures to maintain up-to-date knowledge.

Coding and Billing

The following billing risk areas have been frequent areas of investigations and audits by the OIG and should be addressed in a good compliance program:

- Billing for items or services not provided or not provided as claimed
- Submitting claims for equipment, medical supplies, and services that are not reasonable and necessary
- Double billing
- Billing for non-covered services as if covered
- Known misuse of NPIs, which results in improper billing
- Billing separately for bundled services
- Misuse of modifiers
- Consistently under-coding or over-coding services
- Using only one evaluation and management (E/M) service code within a category of service

  Other areas that may trigger an audit include
- Profile of services reported differs from payer profiles of physicians of your specialty.
- Repeated use of unspecified diagnosis codes or use of codes that are not consistent with the service or your specialty.
- Surgical services not consistent with claims submitted by a facility.
- Number of procedures or services reported exceed the hours in a day.
- High numbers of denials.

> |||||||| **Coding Pearl** ||||||||
>
> Place of service errors are a targeted area of review for the Office of Inspector General. See Chapter 4, The Business of Medicine: Working With Current and Emerging Payment Systems, for more information on reporting correct place of service codes.

Medical Record Documentation

One of the most important physician practice compliance issues is the appropriate documentation of diagnosis and treatment. Patients and other providers must be able to trust that information within shared records is accurate and actionable for the care of the patient. With most pediatricians now using EHRs to document office-based services, compliant documentation must now encompass not only what should be documented but also what must be safeguarded from inaccuracies and potential noncompliant access to or disclosure of information.

The CMS has published guidance for physicians on detecting and responding to fraud, waste, and abuse associated with the use of EHRs (https://www.cms.gov/Medicare-Medicaid-Coordination/Fraud-Prevention/Medicaid-Integrity-Education/documentation-matters.html). The CMS instructs that physicians should apply the compliance program components previously discussed to take preventive action to deter the inappropriate use of EHR system features or inappropriate access to patient information. This includes a written compliance plan. The written compliance plan should specify that medical record documentation should comply with the following documentation principles and guidelines:

* The medical record should be complete (and legible, when handwritten) and individualized for each patient encounter. Do not allow cut-and-paste functionality in the EHR. Any use of copy and paste, copy forward, macros, or auto-population should be regulated by office policies that address maintenance of record integrity and supplementation via free text, where indicated. (Guidance from the CMS includes a decision table for ensuring proper use of EHR features and capabilities.)

* Retain all signatures when there are multiple authors or contributors to a document, so that each individual's contribution is unambiguously identified.

* All staff should receive initial and periodic education on compliant medical record documentation, including, as applicable, use of EHR functionality, use of individual sign-on, and appropriate access to records.

* Documentation should be completed at the time of service or as soon as possible afterward.

* The documentation of each patient encounter should include the reason for the encounter; any relevant history; physical examination findings; prior diagnostic test results, when pertinent; assessment, clinical impression, or diagnosis; plan of care; and date and legible identity of the observer.

* If not documented, the rationale for ordering diagnostic and other ancillary services should be easily inferred by an independent reviewer or third party. Past and present diagnoses and history should be accessible to the treating and/or consulting physician.

* Appropriate health risk factors should be identified. The patient's progress, patient's response to and any changes in treatment, and any revision in diagnosis should be documented.

* All pages in the medical record should include the patient name and an identifying number or birth date.

* Prescription drug management should include the name of the medication, dosage, and instructions.

* Clinically important telephone calls should be documented, including date, time, instructions, and follow-up.

* Anticipatory guidance, patient education, and counseling are best documented when performed.

* Any addenda should be identifiable with the author's signature and labeled with the date the addendum was made. The compliance plan should address what circumstances justify making changes to the EHR record and identify who can make changes, requirements for amendments and corrections to an EHR, and what information cannot be changed (ie, author, date, and time of original note).

* Consent forms should be dated, the procedure documented, and the form signed by the patient or his or her legal representative. Documentation should include a summary of the discussion of the procedure and risks.

* All abbreviations used should be explicit.

* Patient noncompliance, including immunization refusal, should be documented as well as discussion of the risks and adverse consequences of noncompliance.

* Allergies and adverse reactions should be prominently displayed.

* Immunization and growth charts must be maintained and current.

* Problem and medication lists should be completed and current, including over-the-counter medications.

* The EHR audit log should be enabled at all times so it creates an accurate chronological history of changes to the EHR. Practice procedures should describe any exceptions, including who can disable the log and under what circumstances this may be appropriate.

See the Coding Conundrum: Pitfalls of Electronic Health Record Coding box later in this chapter for other considerations specific to EHR documentation.

> ~ **More From the AAP** ~
>
> See also "What Does Your EHR Documentation Say?" in the March 2017 *AAP Pediatric Coding Newsletter* at http://coding.aap.org (subscription required).

Retention of Records

Policies and procedures should be written to include the creation, distribution, retention, and destruction of documents. In designing a record-retention system, privacy concerns and federal and state regulatory requirements should be taken into consideration. In addition to maintaining appropriate and thorough medical records on each patient, the OIG recommends that the system include the following types of documents:

- All records and documentation (eg, billing and claims documentation) required for participation in federal, state, and private-payer health care programs
- All records necessary to demonstrate the integrity of the physician practice's compliance process and to confirm the effectiveness of the program

    The following record-retention guidelines should be used:

- The length of time that a physician's medical record documentation is to be retained should be specified. Federal and state statutes should be consulted for specific time frames.
- Consulting with an attorney or risk management department of a medical liability insurer is prudent to determine the appropriate retention period. At a minimum, pediatricians may want to retain records until patients obtain the age of majority plus the statute of limitations in their jurisdiction. Longer retention periods may be prudent, depending on the circumstances.
- Medical records, including electronic correspondence, should be secured against loss, destruction, unauthorized access, unauthorized reproduction, corruption, and damage.
- Policies and procedures should stipulate the disposition of medical records in the event the practice is sold or closed.

    The American Academy of Pediatrics (AAP) provides free Health Insurance Portability and Accountability Act of 1996 (HIPAA) privacy and security manuals with downloadable templates, policies, and procedures at https://www.aap.org/en-us/professional-resources/practice-transformation/managing-practice/Pages/HIPAA-Privacy-and-Security-Compliance-Manuals.aspx.

Document Advice From Payers

A physician practice should document its efforts to comply with applicable federal, state, and private health care program requirements. For example

- When requesting advice from a government agency charged with administering a federal or state health care program or from a private payer, document and retain a record of the request and of all written or oral responses.
- Maintain a log of oral inquiries between the practice and third parties.
- Keep copies of all provider manuals, provider bulletins, and communications from payers about coding and submission of claims.

Designate a Compliance Officer

To administer the compliance program, the practice should designate an individual responsible for overseeing the program. More than one employee may be designated with the responsibility of compliance monitoring, or a practice may outsource all or part of the functions of a compliance officer to a third party. Attributes and qualifications of a compliance officer include

- Independent position to protect against any conflicts of interest from "regular" position responsibilities and compliance officer duties
- Attention to detail
- Experience in billing and coding
- Effective communication skills (oral and written) with employees, physicians, and carriers

    The primary responsibilities of a compliance officer include

- Overseeing and monitoring the implementation of the compliance program.
- Establishing methods, such as periodic audits, to improve the practice's efficiency and quality of services and reduce the practice's vulnerability to fraud and abuse.

Coding Conundrum: Pitfalls of Electronic Health Record Coding

One of the advantages of using electronic health records (EHRs) is enhanced documentation of services. Documentation of an evaluation and management (E/M) service may be easier because of the use of templates or drop-down options, and legibility is not an issue. However, there are disadvantages to EHRs when it comes to documentation. When completing an audit, be aware of

- The use of templates may not accurately describe pertinent patient history or abnormal findings on examination. Some EHRs do not allow free texting, thereby prohibiting more detailed, appropriate documentation. If a system does not allow free texting, work with the vendor to add this capability, or add any and all abnormal findings that might be pertinent in the template so documentation can be complete and accurate.

- Avoid templates and documentation tools that feature predefined text that may include information that is not relevant to the patient presentation and/or services rendered. Review and edit all defaulted data to ensure only patient-specific data is recorded for that visit, while removing all other irrelevant data pulled in by the default template.

- Users should be familiar with the manner in which the EHR constructs a note from the data entered into each field and how the system may be customized to enhance the final note.

- Only the history and physical examination that are pertinent to the problem or condition should be used in selection of an E/M code. Therefore, physicians should code each E/M service and override the EHR-assigned E/M code when appropriate.

- The physician must document history of present illness (HPI). The EHR will usually capture all documentation, whether performed by ancillary staff or the provider. Make certain it is clear who documented each portion of the service. For example, if HPI is documented by a nurse or medical assistant, the physician *must* document his or her HPI. (Electronic health record systems include audit trails that may be used to prove who entered specific elements of documentation. It is important to understand how the practice's EHR system creates and produces an audit trail.)

- The use of a scribe to enter information relayed by a physician or provider must be clearly entered in each record, when applicable. Most payers require identification of the scribe that includes a statement such as "acting as a scribe for Dr X." The physician or provider must review the note for accuracy and cosign indicating his or her words and actions were accurately recorded.

- If an EHR system automatically transfers the documented review of systems (ROS) and past, family, and social history from one encounter to the next or lists every medication that has been prescribed in the past, make certain the physician reviews the information to verify it is still accurate and documents his or her review of the pertinent copied information to support the level of history that was necessary and performed.

- The same information may be documented in the HPI and ROS (eg, HPI, "fever of 102°F"; ROS, "fever"). The repeated comment should only be used as HPI or ROS, not both, based on the context for which it was obtained (eg, description of problem, question to better define problem). The EHR system may not differentiate and will count the redundant information twice (or more), leading to a higher level of history.

- Most EHR systems have integrated an E/M coding system using the Centers for Medicare & Medicaid Services 1995 or 1997 *Documentation Guidelines for Evaluation and Management Services.* Systems measure or count the elements of each of the required key components (ie, history, physical examination, and medical decision-making) without regard to the nature of the presenting problem, severity of illness, or medical necessity. Therefore, if a physician elects to perform a detailed or comprehensive-level history and physical examination on every established patient, the reported E/M code will always be a potentially inappropriate higher-level E/M service.

- If previous diagnoses are carried over from one encounter to the next, make sure only those that are pertinent to the current visit are considered when determining the complexity of the service provided.

- List the primary diagnosis first because the EHR may report the diagnoses in the order in which they are documented.

- To support management options, it may be necessary to document the diagnoses being considered. These suspected or ruled-out diagnoses should not be reported by the EHR system in the outpatient setting.

- Make certain that any separately reportable procedure or service has documentation to support that it was performed.

- Don't depend on the software vendor to add *Current Procedural Terminology®*; *International Classification of Diseases, 10th Revision, Clinical Modification*; or Healthcare Common Procedure Coding System codes to the system. Review all new, deleted, and revised codes each year. Notify the vendor if codes have not been revised and educate physicians and billing staff on their appropriate use.

- Revising the compliance program in response to changes in the needs of the practice or changes in the law and in the policies and procedures of government and private payer health plans.
- Developing, coordinating, and participating in a training program that focuses on the elements of the compliance program and seeks to ensure that training materials are appropriate.
- Checking the HHS OIG List of Excluded Individuals and Entities and the federal System for Award Management to ascertain whether any potential new hires, current employees, medical staff, or independent contractors are listed; advising management of findings; and seeing that appropriate action is taken as described in the compliance program.
- Informing employees and physicians of pertinent federal and state statutes, regulations, and standards and monitoring their compliance.
- Investigating any report or allegation concerning suspected unethical or improper business practices and monitoring subsequent corrective action, compliance, or both.
- Assessing the practice's situation and determining what best suits the practice in terms of compliance oversight.
- Maintaining records of compliance-related activities, including meetings, educational activities, and internal audits. Particular attention should be given to documenting violations found by the compliance program and documenting the remedial actions.

The Audit/Review Process

1. Obtain and review a productivity report from your billing system.
2. Calculate the percentage distribution of E/M codes within each category of service (new and established office or outpatient visits, initial observation or inpatient services, use of modifier **25**) for each physician in the practice. (Most billing software provides these calculations.) You might also use the AAP Coding Calculator, found at https://www.aap.org/en-us/professional-resources/practice-transformation/getting-paid/Coding-at-the-AAP/Pages/Coding-Calculator.aspx, to help you profile your E/M code use and distribution.
3. Use data from a 12-month period because they include seasonal trends and are more reflective of practice patterns.
4. Perform a comparative analysis of the distribution with each physician in the practice. Remember that data only reflect the billing patterns, and not if one is more correct than another. More frequent oversight and monitoring is necessary for services provided by physicians who are new to the practice and may use documentation or coding guidance that conflicts with practice policy.
5. Review the report to ensure that all procedures performed are being captured and reported appropriately. For example, are discharge visits (**99238** and **99239**) being billed and is the number proportionate to the number of newborn and other hospital admissions performed?
6. Review the practice encounter form or code selection application to ensure that *Current Procedural Terminology* (*CPT®*) and *International Classification of Diseases, 10th Revision, Clinical Modification* (*ICD-10-CM*) codes are correct and match the corresponding description.
7. Review the actual encounter and claim form with the medical record to ensure the claim is submitted with the appropriate codes and/or modifiers. (See the Documentation and Coding Audits section later in this chapter.)
8. Review medical records to ensure they are compliant with national standards and office policies. Standards for maintenance of medical records can be found on the National Committee for Quality Assurance Web site (www.ncqa.org).
9. Review each medical record and encounter form (as applicable) with these questions in mind.
   - Are the patient's name, identification number, and/or date of birth on every page in the medical record?
   - Does the medical record contain updated demographic information?
   - Are allergies noted and prominently displayed?
   - Is the date of service documented?
   - Was the service medically necessary?
   - Does the documentation support the level of E/M service based on the required key components and/or type of service (eg, consultation, preventive medicine service)?

- Are all the services and/or procedures documented/captured on the encounter form?
- Does the documentation for the preventive medicine visit meet the requirements of the Medicaid Early and Periodic Screening, Diagnosis, and Treatment program when applicable?
- Does the documentation support the procedure billed (eg, administration of injection, catheterization, impacted cerumen removal)?
- Does the documentation support the diagnosis code(s) billed?
- If using an EHR, does the documentation support physician review and personal documentation? For example, if the EHR always brings up the patient's history, is there a notation that the physician reviewed it? If not, it should not be counted as part of the service.
- Is there a completed growth chart and immunization record?
- Is the documentation legible?
- Does any order for medication include the specific dosage and use?
- Is there documentation of a follow-up plan?
- Are diagnostic reports (eg, laboratory tests, radiograph) signed and dated to reflect review?
- Does documentation include the name and credentials of each contributing author in a manner that reflects each author's individual contributions?
- Was an appropriate modifier reported with sufficient documentation?
- Is the documentation in compliance with Physicians at Teaching Hospitals guidelines and/or incident-to provisions as appropriate?

Documentation and Coding Audits

Medicare, state Medicaid programs, and commercial payers will audit claims as well as monitor E/M coding profiles. While the specialty-specific E/M profiles published by the CMS provide helpful information, keep in mind that these distributions only reflect code use and not code accuracy. An atypical distribution of codes may be the result of care for a more complex patient population than average, including patients with chronic diseases or with social and economic challenges. Correct coding appropriately identifies the risk stratification for your patients and may directly affect your payments.

Also, just because you got paid does not mean that payers will not retrospectively audit and demand repayment or withhold future payments, particularly if claims were processed incorrectly or in error according to your contract. Practices are advised to become familiar with state laws addressing retrospective audits and repayments and with payer procedures for repayment. Your AAP chapter or state medical society may be able to help you understand your state-specific laws.

Preparing for the Audit

Before using documentation and coding audits to reduce the practice's vulnerability to fraud and abuse, it is important to consider how your practice can best conduct and use findings of an internal audit. Individual practices must consider how to conduct audits in a manner that offers the most benefit and least disruption to the practice. **Figure 5-1** offers steps to consider when developing a chart audit process.

Performing the Audit

Make certain that the reviewer has all appropriate and necessary tools, which may include

- The CMS *Documentation Guidelines for Evaluation and Management Services* (1995 and/or 1997) that are used by the practice or physician.
- Current *CPT®, ICD-10-CM,* and Healthcare Common Procedure Coding System manuals.
- Access to or copies of all payer newsletters or information bulletins that outline coding and/or payment policies.

> ### ~ More From the AAP ~
>
> The *Pediatric Evaluation and Management Coding Card* is an audit tool for verifying evaluation and management levels. The card is available for purchase at http://shop.aap.org/pediatric-evaluation-and-management-coding-card-2019.

- An audit worksheet. This may be one designed by your practice, or one of many published templates may be used. Note that the CMS has never endorsed any specific audit form or coding template. Make certain the audit form used includes appropriate requirements for selection of an E/M service.
- A log to document findings for each provider (**Table 5-1**). This log should include a summary detail of findings for each encounter reviewed. The log and E/M audit worksheets can be used as teaching tools at the conclusion of the audit.

Table 5-1. Sample Audit Log[a]					
Physician:		**Date:**		**Auditor:**	
Patient Name	**Patient ID/ DOB**	**Date of Service**	**Reported Code**	**Audited Code**	**Comments**
Jane	5/1/09	6/3/13	99214	99213	Total and counseling time not documented; key components = 99213; plan for return not documented
			J45.31; R06.2	J45.31	Wheezing is inherent to asthma (J45.31).
Zach	2/4/10	6/4/13	69210	0	Cerumen not documented as impacted
Gracie	11/12/08	6/4/13	99213	99214	Key components = 99214

Abbreviations: DOB, date of birth; ID, identification.

[a] Also available at www.aap.org/cfp; use access code AAPCFP24.

Following the Audit

- Discuss audit findings with each provider.
- Educate providers and staff as necessary.
- If a problem is encountered (eg, inappropriate use of modifiers, miscoding), a more focused retrospective review should be conducted to determine how long the error has been occurring and its effect. This is especially important when reviewing claims for physicians new to the practice or when a particular coding guideline or code has changed.
- If overpayments have occurred due to miscoding or billing errors, the errors should be corrected and education of appropriate staff performed. The errors may need to be disclosed and incorrect payments refunded. Always refer to payer contracts and agreements to understand their requirements and policies for overpayments and disclosure. Always seek advice from the practice's attorney prior to disclosure or repayment.
- Schedule follow-up audits, if indicated, to determine if problems have been resolved (eg, improved documentation, capturing procedures, correct use of modifiers).
- Determine if audits need to be performed on a quarterly or annual basis and follow through with audits on a routine basis.
- If changes need to be made to the EHR system, contact the vendor and discuss how these might be accomplished. Educate physicians and providers on the changes made or need for additional physician documentation.
- Establish or update written policies and procedures.
- Maintain records of your compliance efforts and training.

Figure 5-1. Preparing and Planning Medical Chart Audits

Focus
- Focus audits on documentation and coding of the most commonly performed services, adherence to medical record standards, appropriate reporting of diagnosis codes, use of modifiers, and adherence to coding and federal guidelines (eg, Physicians at Teaching Hospitals guidelines, physician self-referral laws).

Agree
- Make certain all physicians in the practice are in agreement with how any audit will be conducted and how results will be used.

Auditor
- The auditor (eg, physician, physician extender, coder or other administrative employee, outside consultant, a combination thereof) must be proficient at coding, understand payer guidelines and requirements, and know medical terminology. Consider a team approach (eg, nurse and coder). If a physician is not actually performing record reviews, one should be available to assist as necessary.

Legal
- Determine if audits should be performed under the direction of a health care attorney who may offer assistance with developing an audit process and provide guidance on any internal compliance concerns discovered in the process.
- Attorney–client privilege may apply when audits are directed by an attorney.

Timing
- Determine if your audit will be retrospective (ie, performed on paid claims and services) or prospective (ie, performed on services and claims that have not yet been billed).
- Prospective reviews are recommended because any necessary corrections can be made before a claim is filed. Although a prospective review will delay claims submission and introduce additional practice expense, this practice may have a net positive financial effect.

Services
- Select the types of services to be included in the audit. For example, if the review will include only office or outpatient services, include services most frequently reported (eg, a sampling of new and established patient problem-oriented and preventive medicine visits, documentation of nebulizer treatments).
- Include newborn care, critical care, initial and subsequent observation, and inpatient services when performing an audit of inpatient services.

Number
- Determine how many records or encounters will be included in the audit. Most coding consultants recommend at least 10 records per physician or provider per baseline or subsequent review. If a more focused review is required, the sample size may need to be increased. Medical records should be randomly selected for each evaluation and management level of service and from different dates of service.

Schedule
- Determine the frequency of audits. Large practices might consider conducting audits on a rotating schedule of one physician or provider per week or one physician or provider per month throughout the year.

Don't Get Caught Without a Plan

Most practices will never have to deal with demands for paybacks or fraud audits. Nevertheless, all practices should have a plan just in case they occur. Because time is of the essence in responding to these communications, it would be a calamity to have a letter sit on someone's desk while precious days tick away. Often, a response must be received within 30 days of the date of the request, and the paperwork demanded is not insignificant.

The first communication may be a request for repayment based on payer software analysis of claims history to detect claims paid in conflict with payment policies. It is important for all staff to be trained to recognize these requests and know to get them to the compliance officer immediately. Then, qualified staff tasked with receiving all requests for paybacks can determine the veracity of the request and, if inaccurate, act in accordance with the payer's rebuttal and appeal processes in a timely manner. Likewise, requests for records must be handled carefully and expeditiously.

Responding to Repayment Demands

In an effort to control costs and stamp out fraud, carrier claims processing and special investigative units use sophisticated software programs to identify providers with atypical coding patterns that could indicate erroneous coding and potential overpayments. For example, some carriers may flag providers considered outliers in frequently reporting high-level E/M codes or frequent use of modifiers. They then extrapolate the alleged overpayments over several years and demand across-the-board repayments. Worse, carriers will reduce payments on future claims to correct alleged overpayments on past claims. These requests require a swift and skilled response. Usually, several thousand dollars are involved. Given the compressed timeline and dollars at stake, seeking legal advice is invaluable in these situations.

Here is some general guidance for your consideration.

- If it is truly due to a billing error by the practice, take action to correct the problem and demonstrate to the carrier how it has or will be corrected and the measures implemented to avoid the problem in the future.
- Reply in writing to inform the carrier you are willing to work with it, and ask that it identify each of the claims in question as well as the specific criteria or standards it is applying to the audit.
- Make sure the practice and the carrier consistently apply current *CPT®* guidelines. Reference *CPT* coding guidelines and have appropriate documentation for support. The AAP Coding Hotline can be a resource to you as well; inquiries can be made to aapcodinghotline@aap.org.
- Review your carrier contract's clauses on audits and dispute resolution as well as applicable state laws on audits and repayments with your attorney.
- Focus any overpayment recovery efforts on a case-by-case basis. Avoid unilateral take-backs by not allowing the carrier to extrapolate repayments on any or all future claims.
- Have the carrier provide documentation as proof of overpayment for each contested claim.
- Obtain and secure written documentation of all contacts with the carrier on this issue. Should a carrier payment policy require reporting that varies from *CPT* guidelines, obtain written, dated documentation from the carrier to verify that is the case. Keep this documentation permanently.
- Use legal counsel skilled in carrier contracting when negotiating contracts and confronted with repayment demands.

The AAP Private Payer Advocacy Advisory Committee has a resource for AAP members on responding to retrospective audit and carrier take-back. To access it, go to www.aap.org/cfp (use access code AAPCFP24).

What if Your Practice Is Audited?

- Contact legal counsel as soon as possible. Make sure the attorney or legal practice has experience with audits. If it is a Medicaid audit, it is preferable to have an attorney with Medicaid audit experience. An audit is a complex legal process with significant consequences. It is unwise to attempt to maneuver through this process without sound legal advice.

- Designate one physician or staff member to serve as the primary contact with the attorney and auditors. However, keep in mind that all physicians and staff members may need to work with auditors to some extent.
- Request that the auditor provide you with an opening and closing conference. At the initial meeting, ask for the individual's credentials and job title and ask him or her to summarize the purpose of the review or audit.
- Know how far back auditors may conduct reviews, the number of records a contractor may request, the amount of time allowed to respond to each request, any rebuttal process in place, and steps necessary to appeal adverse findings.
- If the time requirements for producing copies or gathering medical records are unmanageable, contact the auditing entity and request an extension in writing. Provide a clear justification for the extension request.
- Keep copies of all written communication (eg, letters, directives, memos, e-mails). Keep the postmarked envelopes of all letters, including the original notice.
- Fully document all verbal communication, including time, date, persons involved, substance of the discussion, and conclusions and agreements.
- In response to requests for information, provide only the information requested and maintain copies of what you provide auditors. Before providing files, remove any information unrelated to the audit. For example, in a Medicaid audit, you could exclude information related to services provided when the patient was covered under a commercial plan or was uninsured.
- Do not alter any documents or medical records.
- Respond only to questions from the auditors; do not try to engage them in any conversations. If the auditors are conducting the review in your office, try to place them in a separate office away from patients, staff, and business operations.
- Be prepared to respond promptly to each request received. Keep a log of requests received by date, response due date, requesting party, any communication with the requestor, date of response, and outcome.
- Know HIPAA privacy regulations, documentation principles, coding guidelines, and payment policies, and verify that all supporting documentation is included in each response.
- If legibility of the record is questionable, include a transcribed copy with attestation by the author of the original document stating that the transcription is accurate and provided to ensure legibility. Any unsigned entry should also be accompanied by a separate attestation by its author.
- Copied or scanned medical records should be carefully reviewed to be sure that all pages were legibly copied (front and back, if applicable) and are straight and within the margins on the page.
- Any questions about the sufficiency of medical record documentation should be addressed with the physician or provider who ordered or documented the service prior to responding to the request for records. Any corrections to an entry should be performed in a manner that maintains legibility of the original content (eg, single-line strike-through) and should be signed and dated. A summary of the service provided may be included to provide more information but should be distinctly labeled as such and not as part of the original record.
- Include any policy or correspondence from the payer that was used to guide your billing and coding practices related to the service. (Archived payer manuals supportive of claims from previous years may be available on state Medicaid Web sites.) Clinical practice guidelines, policy statements, textbooks, and manuals may also be supportive of medical necessity.
- Send records in a manner that allows for confirmation of receipt.
- Secure a copy of auditors' contact information in case you need to follow up.
- Obtain, in writing, the expected date of a written summary of findings.

Can This Really Happen?

Conventional wisdom says that auditors will probably go after big organizations when it comes to investigating fraud and abuse, but the OIG has said repeatedly that it has zero tolerance for fraud, so, technically, everyone is at risk. Because most of the software programs used to detect unusual coding and billing patterns are based on adult services, pediatricians may be identified as outliers because their coding does not conform to adult-based parameters. Unfortunately, valid pediatric coding may be tagged as improper and honest providers may have to respond to inappropriate recoupment requests or audits. The AAP works hard to minimize these problems and help chapters respond when state Medicaid programs target pediatric coding as inappropriate. This is an ongoing challenge.

Sadly, there are instances of fraud involving pediatricians. A review of past OIG reports to Congress revealed the following cases:

- In August 2017, a New Jersey pediatrician was found guilty of 48 counts of health care claims fraud and one count of Medicaid fraud for billing for more than 24 hours of services per day on 48 days despite her office being open only 3 days per week for 8 hours per day. The pediatrician was sentenced to 3 years in prison.

- In November 2017, 4 people were convicted of fraud involving fraudulent billing of mental and behavioral health services under the stolen identities of a psychologist and licensed clinical social workers. The conviction indicates that the stolen identities of children who were eligible for Medicaid in several states were used to bill the Medicaid programs for more than $3.7 million.

- In August 2015, in Newark, NJ, 3 physicians were sentenced to a combined 7 years and 2 months in jail and ordered to pay a combined $434,300 in restitution after pleading guilty to charges related to a test-referral kickback scheme. As part of the kickback scheme, a laboratory entered into sham consulting agreements and sham rental and service agreements and offered cash and other inducements, such as third-party businesses, credit card payments, and valuable items (cars and electronics). The laboratory used the patient blood specimens to submit more than $100 million in claims to Medicare and private insurers. In April and May 2015, the physicians admitted to accepting approximately $1,500 or more per month in return for referring patient blood specimens. The laboratory's owner pleaded guilty to conspiracy to commit bribery and money laundering and is awaiting sentencing.

- Operation Free Shot focuses on health care providers who bill Medicaid and other insurance programs for childhood vaccines the providers received free of charge from the Vaccines for Children (VFC) program, a joint federal and state program that provides childhood immunizations. Under the VFC program, doctors and other health care providers receive free vaccines distributed by HHS and agree not to bill Medicaid or any other third party for the cost of the vaccines. The provider may recover a minimal fee for administrative costs associated with inoculating a child. Fraudulent claims have led to civil and criminal convictions with millions of dollars recovered and civil settlements as high as $430,000 against one practice.

- A pediatrician who operated an immunization program utilizing federal VFC program funds agreed to pay the government $65,000. The pediatrician allegedly administered 3,851 vaccine doses to children who were not eligible to receive the free immunizations. He also allegedly administered expired vaccines to children in at least 2 cases.

Explore the Need for Additional Insurance

Many medical liability insurers and insurance brokers offer products to provide additional coverage for the consequences of billing errors and omissions. Pediatric practices may want to contact their insurers to see whether their current medical liability policies cover any of the following problems. If they don't, it might be worthwhile to explore insurance options for obtaining that additional protection.

- Defense coverage for a Medicaid audit
- Qui tam action (False Claims Act)
- Unintentional billing errors and omissions
- Physician Self-Referral Law (Stark) violations
- Unintentional release of medical or financial data
- Breach of computers or network security
- Data recovery
- Health Insurance Portability and Accountability Act fines or investigation costs

Summary

These are interesting times for pediatric practices that require thoughtful preparation and ongoing concern. Learn about the fraud and abuse enforcement climate in your state. Implement an effective compliance program and follow it. Be sure your staff knows what a demand for repayment or audit notice looks like and what they need to do with it just on the off chance that something should happen. Have a response plan in place should an auditor knock on your door or a recoupment letter come in the mail. Consult with an attorney when needed. Think about the need for insurance for billing errors and omissions. Keep current with coding and billing updates.

CHAPTER 6

Evaluation and Management
Documentation Guidelines

Contents

Evaluation and Management (E/M) Documentation and Coding Guidelines

Three versions of evaluation and management (E/M) guidelines exist, including Current Procedural Terminology (CPT®) and the 1995 and 1997 guidelines published by the Centers for Medicare & Medicaid Services (CMS). Most Medicaid and private payers allow use of either the 1995 or 1997 CMS guidelines in E/M code selection but include elements of the CPT guidelines for E/M services (eg, guidelines for distinguishing between new and established patients).

Current Procedural Terminology *Guidelines*

- The vaguest of all versions; defines the components of E/M services and provides general guidance on selecting levels of history, examination, and medical decision-making (MDM).
- Includes specialty-specific clinical examples in Appendix C of the American Medical Association (AMA) *CPT 2019.*
- Provides expanded guidelines for topics such as distinguishing new patients from established patients, use of time in E/M code selection, and distinguishing between physicians and other qualified health care professionals (QHPs) and clinical staff.

  The AMA clinical examples are only examples and should not be used as a basis for coding patient encounters with the same diagnosis because the selection of a code must be based on the medically necessary services performed and documented and may include clinical variations.

Centers for Medicare & Medicaid Services Documentation Guidelines for Evaluation and Management Services

- Two sets of guidelines, 1995 and 1997 (see in this chapter or online at www.aap.org/cfp, access code AAPCFP24).
- Followed by the Medicare program, most private payers, and state Medicaid programs.
- Go beyond the *CPT* definitions and guidance for selecting levels of service providing specific documentation guidance. For example,
  - The chief complaint (CC), review of systems (ROS), and past, family, and social history (PFSH) may be listed as separate elements of history, or they may be included in the description of history of present illness (HPI).
  - Specific abnormal and relevant negative findings of the examination of the affected or symptomatic body area(s) or organ system(s) should be documented. A notation of "abnormal" without elaboration is insufficient.
- The CMS documentation guidelines were based on the adult population because few children are covered under the Medicare program. However, the 1995 and 1997 guidelines state that a history and/or examination performed on a pediatric patient may vary from the adult standard and yet be appropriate when considering the selection of an E/M code. As noted in the 1997 guidelines, under Section III, Documentation of E/M Services, paragraph 5:

  "These Documentation Guidelines for E/M services reflect the needs of the typical adult population. For certain groups of patients, the recorded information may vary slightly from that described here. Specifically, the medical records of infants, children, adolescents, and pregnant women may have additional or modified information recorded in each history and examination area.

  "As an example, newborn records may include under history of the present illness (HPI) the details of mother's pregnancy, and the infant's status at birth; social history will focus on family structure; family history will focus on congenital anomalies and hereditary disorders in the family. In addition, the content of a pediatric examination will vary with the age and development of the child. Although not specifically defined in these documentation guidelines, these patient group variations on history and examination are appropriate."

AAP commentary is indicated by green tint and italic sans serif body type.

* The key difference between the 1995 and 1997 E/M guidelines is the examination component. The 1997 guideline includes specific examination elements for a general multisystem examination and for single-system examinations (eg, cardiovascular, respiratory, skin). See more in the 1995 Guidelines for Documentation of Examination and 1997 Guidelines for Documentation of Examination sections later in this chapter.

Pediatric clinical vignettes are presented throughout this manual. These, too, are only examples, and the associated CPT codes should not be used for every patient with the same diagnosis.

Coding E/M Services From a Clinical Perspective

The definitions of the levels of service and requirements for each key component (ie, history, physical examination, and MDM) are ambiguous, and the steps defined in the requirements for selection of the code are not consistent with a physician's approach to addressing and treating an illness or problem. A physician does not enter a room and perform first a history, and then a physical examination, and finally MDM. Rather, the key components of an E/M service are performed in conjunction with one another. The MDM typically supports the level of history and/or physical examination medically necessary and is derived from the following obtained information:

* The documented CC helps to formulate the presenting problem or nature of the patient presentation.
* The level of history obtained and documented is based on the nature of the patient presentation. Concurrently, the physician is forming his or her impression of the problem's severity, possible diagnoses, other factors that require consideration in patient management, and a potential plan of care.
* The level of the performed physical examination is based on the presenting problem(s) and history. From the moment the physician observes the patient and while obtaining the history, the physician simultaneously is starting his or her physical assessment and examination (eg, general appearance). Additional history may be obtained concurrently with the examination. While performing the examination, the physician again is determining the severity or risk, need for diagnostic testing, differential diagnosis(es), and treatment plan.
* The documentation of the history, physical examination, ordered and performed diagnostic studies, assessment, and plan infer and support the complexity of MDM.

> **~ More From the AAP ~**
>
> Get a quick reference to inpatient and outpatient evaluation and management codes and key components with the American Academy of Pediatrics *Pediatric Evaluation and Management (E/M) Coding Card* (https://shop.aap.org/pediatric-evaluation-and-management-em-coding-card-2019).

Categories of E/M Codes

There are 26 categories of E/M codes (eg, office or outpatient services, consultations, prolonged physician services, newborn care). Specific guidelines for reporting codes within these categories are described in detail in chapters of this manual devoted to E/M services provided in specific settings (eg, office, emergency department) and type of service (eg, critical care). Many E/M codes require the performance and documentation of key components. Table 6-1 outlines those components. Those E/M services that do not require the key components as the basis for code selection include those services that are

* Bundled as a daily care code (eg, pediatric and neonatal critical care)
* Bundled as a period of care (eg, transitional care management)
* Based on specific guidelines (eg, normal newborn care, preventive medicine visits)
* Based on time (eg, hourly critical care, discharge services, prolonged service)

AAP commentary is indicated by green tint and italic sans serif body type.

E/M Code Components

Table 6-1. *Seven* Components Are Considered When Selecting the Level of Evaluation and Management Service Code		
Components	**Overarching Component**	**Description**
1. History	Key components	Used to select a level of E/M service, using all 3 or 2 of 3
2. Examination		
3. Medical decision-making		
4. Counseling	Contributory factors	May contribute to but are not required for the selection of a code. However, usually affect the extent of the key components that are performed.
5. Coordination of care		
6. Nature of presenting problem		
7. Time	Explicit component	Used to select a level of E/M service when time becomes the controlling factor

Abbreviation: E/M, evaluation and management.

Key Components

Most E/M services require performance and documentation of the key components (ie, history, physical examination, and MDM).

Contributory Factors

CPT® defines a presenting problem as "a disease, condition, illness, injury, symptom, sign, finding, complaint or other reason for encounter, with or without a diagnosis being established at the time of the encounter." This may be better described as patient presentation and may include psychosocial issues or ethical considerations determined by the physician or other QHP to require consideration in patient management. The nature of the patient presentation may be more extensive or different from the patient's CC (eg, adolescent girl states her reason for visit is headaches but also presents with anxiety about possible unwanted pregnancy). It is the nature of the presenting problem that generally determines the level of history and physical examination performed and documented and supports MDM.

For example, an infant with high fever and wheezing warrants a more comprehensive history and/or examination to determine the diagnosis or condition than an infant presenting with a diaper rash. This does not mean that all elements of examination, for example, require individual justification.

> |||||||| **Coding Pearl** ||||||||
>
> The nature of the presenting problem is defined by severity, risk, and probability of functional impairment.

Levels of presenting problems are defined in the CMS Table of Risk (see pages 146–147).

Explicit Component: Time

Time shall be used as the key or controlling factor in the selection of some E/M services (those that are assigned a typical time) when more than 50% of the physician face-to-face patient and/or family encounter is spent in counseling and/or coordination of care. (See Chapter 1, The Basics of Coding, for more on time-based billing.)

AAP commentary is indicated by green tint and italic sans serif body type.

Chapter 6: Evaluation and Management Documentation Guidelines

1995 and 1997 Documentation Guidelines for Evaluation and Management Services

It is important to note that history, MDM, and time do not vary between 1995 and 1997 guidelines. The examination element is the only difference.

I. Introduction

What is documentation and why is it important?

Medical record documentation is required to record pertinent facts, findings, and observations about an individual's health history including past and present illnesses, examinations, tests, treatments, and outcomes. The medical record chronologically documents the care of the patient and is an important element contributing to high-quality care. The medical record facilitates

- The ability of the physician and other health care professionals to evaluate and plan the patient's immediate treatment, and to monitor his/her health care over time
- Communication and continuity of care among physicians and other health care professionals involved in the patient's care
- Accurate and timely claims review and payment
- Appropriate utilization review and quality of care evaluations
- Collection of data that may be useful for research and education

An appropriately documented medical record can reduce many of the "hassles" associated with claims processing and may serve as a legal document to verify the care provided, if necessary.

What do payers want and why?

Because payers have a contractual obligation to enrollees, they may require reasonable documentation that services are consistent with the insurance coverage provided. They may request information to validate

- The site of service
- The medical necessity and appropriateness of the diagnostic and/or therapeutic services provided
- That services provided have been accurately reported

II. General Principles of Medical Record Documentation

The principles of documentation listed below are applicable to all types of medical and surgical services in all settings. For E/M services, the nature and amount of physician work and documentation varies by type of service, place of service, and the patient's status. The general principles listed below may be modified to account for these variable circumstances in providing E/M services.

1. The medical record should be complete and legible.
2. The documentation of each patient encounter should include
   - Reason for the encounter and relevant history, physical examination findings, and prior diagnostic test results
   - Assessment, clinical impression, or diagnosis
   - Plan for care
   - Date and legible identity of the observer
3. If not documented, the rationale for ordering diagnostic and other ancillary services should be easily inferred.
4. Past and present diagnoses should be accessible to the treating and/or consulting physician.
5. Appropriate health risk factors should be identified.
6. The patient's progress, response to and changes in treatment, and revision of diagnosis should be documented.

AAP commentary is indicated by green tint and italic sans serif body type.

7. The *CPT* and *ICD-10-CM* codes reported on the health insurance claim form or billing statement should be supported by the documentation in the medical record.

III. *Documentation of E/M Services*

This publication provides definitions and documentation guidelines for the three key components of E/M services and for visits that consist predominantly of counseling or coordination of care. The three key components—history, examination, and medical decision making—appear in the descriptors for office and other outpatient services, hospital observation services, hospital inpatient services, consultations, emergency department services, nursing facility services, domiciliary care services, and home services. While some of the text of *CPT* has been repeated in this publication, the reader should refer to *CPT* for the complete descriptors for E/M services and instructions for selecting a level of service. **Documentation guidelines are identified by the symbol •*DG.***

The descriptors for the levels of E/M services recognize seven components that are used in defining the levels of E/M services. These components are

- History
- Examination
- Medical decision making
- Counseling
- Coordination of care
- Nature of presenting problem
- Time

The first three of these components (ie, history, examination, and medical decision making) are the **key** components in selecting the level of E/M services. An exception to this rule is the case of visits that consist predominantly of counseling or coordination of care; for these services time is the key or controlling factor to qualify for a particular level of E/M service.

For certain groups of patients, the recorded information may vary slightly from that described here. Specifically, the medical records of infants, children, adolescents, and pregnant women may have additional or modified information recorded in each history and examination area.

As an example, newborn records may include under history of the present illness (HPI) the details of mother's pregnancy and the infant's status at birth; social history will focus on family structure; family history will focus on congenital anomalies and hereditary disorders in the family. In addition, information on growth and development and/or nutrition will be recorded. Although not specifically defined in these documentation guidelines, these patient group variations on history and examination are appropriate.

A. 1995/1997 Documentation of History

While the history requirements for both sets of documentation guidelines are nearly identical, there is one change to note in the History of Present Illness (HPI) section later in this chapter.

The levels of E/M services are based on four types of history (problem focused, expanded problem focused, detailed, and comprehensive.) Each type of history includes some or all of the following elements:

- Chief complaint (CC)
- History of present illness (HPI)
- Review of systems (ROS)
- Past, family, and/or social history (PFSH)

The extent of history of present illness; review of systems; and past, family, and/or social history that is obtained and documented is dependent upon clinical judgment and the nature of the presenting problem(s).

AAP commentary is indicated by green tint and italic sans serif body type.

Chapter 6: Evaluation and Management Documentation Guidelines

Table 6-2 shows the progression of the elements required for each type of history. To qualify for a given type of history, **all three elements in the table must be met**. (A chief complaint is indicated at all levels.)

History of Present Illness (HPI)	Review of Systems (ROS)	Past, Family, and/or Social History (PFSH)	Type of History
Brief	N/A	N/A	Problem focused
Brief	Problem pertinent	N/A	Expanded problem focused
Extended	Extended	Pertinent	Detailed
Extended	Complete	Complete	Comprehensive

Table 6-2. Progression of Elements Required for Each Type of History

•**DG:** *The CC, ROS, and PFSH may be listed as separate elements of history, or they may be included in the description of the history of the present illness.*

•**DG:** *A ROS and/or a PFSH obtained during an earlier encounter does not need to be rerecorded if there is evidence that the physician reviewed and updated the previous information. This may occur when a physician updates his or her own record or in an institutional setting or group practice where many physicians use a common record. The review and update may be documented by*
- *Describing any new ROS and/or PFSH information or noting there has been no change in the information*
- *Noting the date and location of the earlier ROS and/or PFSH*

•**DG:** *The ROS and/or PFSH may be recorded by ancillary staff or on a form completed by the patient. To document that the physician reviewed the information, there must be a notation supplementing or confirming the information recorded by others.*

•**DG:** *If the physician is unable to obtain a history from the patient or other source, the record should describe the patient's condition or other circumstance that precludes obtaining a history.*

Definitions and specific documentation guidelines for each of the elements of history are listed below.

Chief Complaint (CC)

The CC is a concise statement describing the symptom, problem, condition, diagnosis, physician-recommended return, or other factor that is the reason for the encounter.

•**DG:** *The medical record should clearly reflect the chief complaint.*

Examples: Patient is here for follow-up after completing antibiotics.
Patient presents for a refill on her asthma medication.

History of Present Illness (HPI)

The HPI is a chronological description of the development of the patient's present illness from the first sign and/or symptom or from the previous encounter to the present. It includes the following elements:
- Location (*right ear, big toe, head, right lower abdomen*)
- Duration (*2 days, since last night, 1 week*)
- Timing (*persistent, occasionally, twice a week, recurrent, daily, 15 minutes after…*)
- Quality (*dull, clear, cloudy, thick, throbbing*)
- Severity (*moderate, pain scale [1–10], low grade, progressive, improving, worsening*)
- Context (*occurred when awoke from nap, while playing soccer, fell from tree*)
- Modifying factors (*took acetaminophen without relief, improved with albuterol treatment*)
- Associated signs and symptoms (*blurred vision with headache, coughing with runny nose, nausea with vomiting*)

Brief and **extended** HPIs are distinguished by the amount of detail needed to accurately characterize the clinical problem(s).

AAP commentary is indicated by green tint and italic sans serif body type.

A **brief** HPI consists of one to three elements of the HPI.

•DG: *The medical record should describe one to three elements of the present illness (HPI).*

An **extended** HPI for **1995 DG** consists of four or more elements of the HPI.

•DG 1995: *The medical record should describe four or more elements of the present illness (HPI) or associated co-morbidities.*

An extended HPI for 1997 DG consists of at least four elements of the HPI or the status of at least three chronic or inactive conditions.

•DG 1997: *The medical record should describe at least four elements of the present illness (HPI), or the status of at least three chronic or inactive conditions.*

* *The HPI must be obtained and documented by the physician. Documentation guidelines do not state this; however, it is inferred. If the HPI is documented only by ancillary staff, it is not used in determining the level of history for code selection.*

* *If the HPI summarizes the status of chronic conditions, include information such as current medications and their effects, a description of the patient's present condition, and patient compliance with treatment plans.*

Review of Systems (ROS)

A ROS is an inventory of body systems obtained through a series of questions seeking to identify signs and/or symptoms that the patient may be experiencing or has experienced.

For purposes of ROS, the following systems are recognized:

* Constitutional symptoms (eg, fever, weight loss)
* Eyes
* Ears, nose, mouth, throat
* Cardiovascular
* Respiratory
* Gastrointestinal
* Genitourinary
* Musculoskeletal
* Integumentary (skin and/or breast)
* Neurological
* Psychiatric
* Endocrine
* Hematologic/lymphatic
* Allergic/immunologic

A **problem-pertinent** ROS inquires about the system directly related to the problem(s) identified in the HPI.

•DG: *The patient's positive responses and pertinent negatives for the system related to the problem should be documented.*

An **extended** ROS inquires about the system directly related to the problem(s) identified in the HPI and a limited number of additional systems.

•DG: *The patient's positive responses and pertinent negatives for two to nine systems should be documented.*

A **complete** ROS inquires about the system(s) directly related to the problem(s) identified in the HPI plus all additional body systems.

•DG: *At least 10 organ systems must be reviewed. Those systems with positive or pertinent negative responses must be individually documented. For the remaining systems, a notation indicating all other systems are negative is permissible. In the absence of such a notation, at least 10 systems must be individually documented.*

* *Documentation should clarify any conflicting information between the ROS completed by patient, family, or ancillary staff and the physician's documentation of the patient presentation (eg, ROS is negative for musculoskeletal complaints, but HPI says patient has pain in right knee).*

AAP commentary is indicated by green tint and italic sans serif body type.

Chapter 6: Evaluation and Management Documentation Guidelines

- *Appropriate documentation for a complete ROS (at least 10 of 14 systems) might include a checklist with documentation of "negative" or the pertinent response for each system. If a checklist is not used, documentation might indicate pertinent responses and "otherwise negative or unremarkable for all systems," pertinent responses and "all other systems reviewed and negative," or "complete ROS unchanged from previous review dated _____." Documentation of "ROS negative" is not sufficient.*

- *An ROS does not have to be recorded again on a subsequent encounter if there is documentation that the physician reviewed or updated a previous version. Documentation to reflect the subsequent review might be "ROS unchanged from most recent visit dated _____." (Tip: When history is pulled forward in the electronic health record [EHR] from a previous encounter, physicians must attest that the information has been reviewed and updated. Inconsistencies between the history pulled forward and the remainder of the encounter note may fail to represent the patient presentation and level of E/M service provided.)*

- *If a separate patient history form is used (eg, new patient history), the physician must sign and date the form to reflect his or her review. Pertinent responses to the ROS or PFSH may be documented on a separate history form, a progress note, or the signed history form.*

- *If the physician is unable to obtain a history, the record must describe the circumstance that precludes obtaining the history. In that circumstance, the history may be considered as comprehensive. For example, a child is transferred to the emergency department of a children's hospital and her parents are transferred to another facility following an accident. In this circumstance, if the accepting physician documents this limitation and any history obtained from available past medical records or the medical transport team, the history is considered comprehensive.*

- *The distinction between an HPI and ROS is often confusing. The HPI and ROS are obtained for different reasons and both contribute to the level of history performed in the selection of an E/M service code.*

- *Documentation guidelines do not directly state that a comment made under the HPI cannot be counted again in the ROS when it is repeated. However, most coders and payers will refer to this as "double-dipping."*

    Example: HPI: "abdominal pain for 3 days"; ROS: "abdominal pain." Think about the context in which the information was obtained. If the information was gathered as a description of the development of the problem, consider it as HPI. If the information was obtained to help further define the scope of the problem, consider the information as part of the ROS. Example: HPI: "lower abdominal pain for 3 days without nausea, vomiting, constipation"; ROS: "not associated with eating or exercise; intermittent dysuria; denies fever."

Past, Family, and/or Social History (PFSH)

The PFSH consists of a review of three areas

- Past history (the patient's past experiences with illnesses, operations, injuries, and treatments)
- Family history (a review of medical events in the patient's family, including diseases that may be hereditary or place the patient at risk)
- Social history (an age-appropriate review of past and current activities)
- *Like the ROS, the PFSH may be recorded by the patient or caregiver, clinical staff, or physician. When recorded by someone other than the physician, the physician should review and correct, clarify, or supplement, as needed, the documented information.*
- *The PFSH is considered a single element of the overall history.*
- *Notation of allergies without current complaint and current medications are counted as past history.*

For the categories of subsequent hospital care, follow-up inpatient consultations and subsequent nursing facility care, *CPT* requires only an "interval" history. It is not necessary to record information about the PFSH.

AAP commentary is indicated by green tint and italic sans serif body type.

Table 6-3. The Elements of History

History Components	Description	Elements
Chief complaint (CC)	The stated purpose or reason for the encounter (usually a quote of the patient's or parent's words)	Although not a defined element, a CC is required as part of the history documentation for all levels.
History of present illness (HPI)	Description of the development of the present illness from the onset of the problem or symptom or from the previous encounter to the present; described with 8 specified elements or a summary of the status of 3 or more chronic or inactive conditions	◉ Location (specific anatomic site) ◉ Duration (period from onset of sign/symptom to present) ◉ Timing (number or frequency of occurrences of sign/symptom within the time that patient has experienced the sign/symptom) ◉ Quality (characterizations of sign/symptom) ◉ Severity (acuteness or intensity of sign/symptom) ◉ Context (circumstances or situation in which sign/symptom occurred) ◉ Modifying factors (effort taken to change the sign/symptom and its effect) ◉ Associated signs and symptoms (other related or additional signs/symptoms) *Alternatively,* Status of each of 3 or more chronic or inactive conditions (stated in 1997 guidelines, allowed under either guideline)
Review of systems (ROS)	A series of questions asked to identify signs or symptoms experienced by the patient and to more clearly define the problem to help in establishing a diagnosis(es) and management options	◉ Constitutional (eg, fever, weight loss) ◉ Eyes ◉ Ears, nose, mouth, and throat ◉ Cardiovascular ◉ Respiratory ◉ Gastrointestinal ◉ Genitourinary ◉ Musculoskeletal ◉ Integumentary (skin or breast) ◉ Neurologic ◉ Psychiatric ◉ Endocrine ◉ Hematologic/lymphatic ◉ Allergic/immunologic
Past, family, and social history (PFSH)	Review of medical/surgical history Review of medical events in the patient's family that may place a patient at risk Age-appropriate review of activities	Illnesses, injuries, treatments, surgeries, hospitalizations, current medications, allergies, age-appropriate immunization status, age-appropriate feeding or dietary status, pregnancy and birth history (weight, Apgar score), developmental history Health status or cause of death of family members, specific diseases of family members, hereditary disorders in the family Living arrangements; use of drugs, alcohol, and tobacco by patient or caregiver; education level; sexual history; domestic violence; other relevant social factors

AAP commentary is indicated by green tint and italic sans serif body type.

Chapter 6: Evaluation and Management Documentation Guidelines

A **pertinent** PFSH is a review of the history area(s) directly related to the problem(s) identified in the HPI.

•*DG:*   *At least one specific item from **any** of the three history areas must be documented for a pertinent PFSH.*

A *complete* PFSH is a review of two or all three of the PFSH history areas, depending on the category of the E/M service. A review of all three history areas is required for services that by their nature include a comprehensive assessment or reassessment of the patient. A review of two of the three history areas is sufficient for other services.

•*DG:*   *At least one specific item from **two** of the three history areas must be documented for a complete PFSH for the following categories of E/M services: office or other outpatient services, established patient; emergency department; subsequent nursing facility care; domiciliary care, established patient; and home care, established patient.*

•*DG:*   *At least one specific item from **each** of the three history areas must be documented for a complete PFSH for the following categories of E/M services: office or other outpatient services, new patient; hospital observation services; hospital inpatient services, initial care; consultations; comprehensive nursing facility assessments; domiciliary care, new patient; and home care, new patient.*

Establishing the Level of History Performed

The patient history may be problem focused, expanded problem focused, detailed, or comprehensive. Table 6-3 lists required documentation elements for each level of history. To select a particular level of history, all elements of CC, HPI, ROS, and PFSH required for that level must be met.

For example, consider a 13-year-old established patient.

◉ **Problem focused:** *"Here for stomachache. Stomach has hurt for 2 days."*
  ❖ **CC:** *stomachache*
  ❖ **HPI:** *location—stomach, duration—2 days*

◉ **Expanded problem focused:** *"Here for stomachache. Stomach has hurt for 2 days. No diarrhea or constipation."*
  ❖ **CC:** *stomachache*
  ❖ **HPI:** *location—stomach, duration—2 days*
  ❖ **ROS:** *gastrointestinal (GI)*

◉ **Detailed:** *"Here for stomachache. Stomach has hurt on and off for a few months. Pain occurs primarily after eating, worsening over the last few days. No fever, diarrhea, or vomiting; last menstrual period 2 weeks ago and normal. Takes no medication; no known allergies."*
  ❖ **CC:** *stomachache*
  ❖ **HPI:** *location—stomach, timing—on and off, duration—few months, context—after eating, severity—worsening*
  ❖ **ROS:** *constitutional, GI, genitourinary (GU)*
  ❖ **PFSH:** *past medical—no medications, no allergies*

◉ **Comprehensive:** *"Here for stomachache. Stomach has hurt on and off for a few months. Pain occurs primarily after eating, worsening over the last few days. No fever, diarrhea, or vomiting; last menstrual period 2 weeks ago and normal; no rashes; no injuries; all other systems reviewed and negative. Takes no medication, no known allergies, no exposure to illness, has excellent grades and enjoys school. Family history negative for abdominal problems or headaches."*
  ❖ **CC:** *stomachache*
  ❖ **HPI:** *location—stomach, timing—on and off, duration—few months, context—after eating, severity—worsening*
  ❖ **ROS:** *constitutional, GI, GU, skin, all others negative*
  ❖ **PFSH:** *medical—no medications, no allergies, no exposure to illness; family—negative for abdominal or headache; social—excellent grades, enjoys school*

AAP commentary is indicated by green tint and italic sans serif body type.

Table 6-4. Levels of Physical Examination		
Level of Examination	**1995 Guidelines**	**1997 Guidelines**
Problem focused	Limited examination of the affected area or system	Performance and documentation of 1–5 elements identified by a bullet (●) in 1 or more areas or systems
Expanded problem focused	Limited examination of the affected body area or organ system and other symptomatic or related organ system(s)	Performance and documentation of at least 6 elements identified by a bullet (●) in 1 or more areas or systems
Detailed	Extended examination of the affected body area(s) and other symptomatic or related organ system(s)	Multisystem examination—Performance and documentation of at least 2 elements identified by a bullet (●) in at least 6 areas or systems or at least 12 elements identified by a bullet (●) in at least 2 areas or systems Single organ system examination—at least 12 elements identified by a bullet (●) (Eye and psychiatric examinations require only 9.)
Comprehensive	General multisystem examination (requires 8 or more organ systems) or a complete examination of a single organ system	Multisystem examination—Examination of at least 9 organ systems or body areas with performance of all elements identified by a bullet (●) in each area/system examined Documentation is expected for at least 2 elements identified by a bullet (●) of each area(s) or system(s). Single organ system examination—Performance of all elements identified by a bullet (●) and documentation of every element in each box with a shaded border and at least one element in a box with an unshaded border

B. Examination

1995 Guidelines for Documentation of Examination
The main distinction between the 1995 and 1997 documentation guidelines lie in the documentation of examination. Table 6-4 outlines the differences. (See next page for details on the 1997 examination guidelines.)

The levels of E/M services are based on four types of examination that are defined as follows:

- **Problem Focused**—a limited examination of the affected body area or organ system.
- **Expanded Problem Focused**—a limited examination of the affected body area or organ system and other symptomatic or related organ system(s).
- **Detailed**—an extended examination of the affected body area(s) and other symptomatic or related organ system(s).
- **Comprehensive**—a general multisystem examination or complete examination of a single organ system.

For purposes of examination, the following **body areas** are recognized:

- Head, including face
- Neck
- Chest, including breasts and axillae
- Abdomen
- Genitalia, groin, buttocks

AAP commentary is indicated by green tint and italic sans serif body type.

Chapter 6: Evaluation and Management Documentation Guidelines

☉ Back, including spine

☉ Each extremity

For purposes of examination, the following **organ systems** are recognized:

☉ Constitutional (eg, vital signs, general appearance)

☉ Eyes

☉ Ears, nose, mouth, throat

☉ Cardiovascular

☉ Respiratory

☉ Gastrointestinal

☉ Genitourinary

☉ Musculoskeletal

☉ Skin

☉ Neurological

☉ Psychiatric

☉ Hematologic/lymphatic/immunologic

The extent of examinations performed and documented is dependent upon clinical judgment and the nature of the presenting problem(s). They range from limited examinations of single body areas to general multisystem or complete single organ system examinations.

•DG: *Specific abnormal and relevant negative findings of the examination of the affected or symptomatic body area(s) or organ system(s) should be documented. A notation of "abnormal" without elaboration is insufficient.*

•DG: *Abnormal or unexpected findings of the examination of the unaffected or asymptomatic body area(s) or organ system(s) should be described.*

•DG: *A brief statement or notation indicating "negative" or "normal" is sufficient to document normal findings related to unaffected area(s) or asymptomatic organ system(s).*

•DG: *The medical record for a general multisystem examination should include findings about eight or more of the 12 organ systems.*

There is no clear guidance on the distinction between a limited examination versus an extended examination. Unfortunately, this leaves room for subjectivity. The CMS remains silent on this issue; however, some audit programs have attempted to quantify this.

1997 Guidelines for Documentation of Examination

The levels of E/M services are based on four types of examination

☉ **Problem Focused**—a limited examination of the affected body area or organ system.

☉ **Expanded Problem Focused**—a limited examination of the affected body area or organ system and any other symptomatic or related body area(s) or organ system(s).

☉ **Detailed**—an extended examination of the affected body area(s) or organ system(s) and any other symptomatic or related body area(s) or organ system(s).

☉ **Comprehensive**—a general multisystem examination or complete examination of a single organ system and other symptomatic or related body area(s) or organ system(s).

These types of examinations have been defined for general multisystem and the following single organ systems:

☉ Cardiovascular

☉ Ears, nose, mouth, throat

☉ Eyes

☉ Genitourinary (female)

☉ Genitourinary (male)

☉ Hematologic/lymphatic/immunologic

☉ Musculoskeletal

☉ Neurological

- Psychiatric
- Respiratory
- Skin

A general multisystem examination or a single organ system examination may be performed by any physician regardless of specialty. The type (general multisystem or single organ system) and content of examination are selected by the examining physician and are based upon clinical judgment, the patient's history, and the nature of the presenting problem(s).

The content and documentation requirements for each type and level of the 1997 examination are summarized below and described in detail in tables beginning on page 132. In the tables, organ systems and body areas recognized by *CPT* for purposes of describing examinations are shown in the left column. The content, or individual elements, of the examination pertaining to that body area or organ system are identified by bullets (•) in the right column.

Parenthetical examples, "(eg, ...)", have been used for clarification and to provide guidance regarding documentation. Documentation for each element must satisfy any numeric requirements (such as "Measurement of *any three of the following seven...*") included in the description of the element. Elements with multiple components but with no specific numeric requirement (such as "Examination of *liver* and *spleen*") require documentation of at least one component. It is possible for a given examination to be expanded beyond what is defined here. When that occurs, findings related to the additional systems and/or areas should be documented.

- **•DG:** *Specific abnormal and relevant negative findings of the examination of the affected or symptomatic body area(s) or organ system(s) should be documented. A notation of "abnormal" without elaboration is insufficient.*

- **•DG:** *Abnormal or unexpected findings of the examination of any asymptomatic body area(s) or organ system(s) should be described.*

- **•DG:** *A brief statement or notation indicating "negative" or "normal" is sufficient to document normal findings related to unaffected area(s) or asymptomatic organ system(s).*

General Multisystem Examinations

General multisystem examinations are described in detail in **Table 6-5**. To qualify for a given level of multisystem examination, the following content and documentation requirements should be met:

- **Problem-Focused Examination**—should include performance and documentation of one to five elements identified by a bullet (•) in one or more organ system(s) or body area(s).
- **Expanded Problem-Focused Examination**—should include performance and documentation of at least six elements identified by a bullet in one or more organ system(s) or body area(s).
- **Detailed Examination**—should include at least six organ systems or body areas. For each system/area selected, performance and documentation of at least two elements identified by a bullet is expected. Alternatively, a detailed examination may include performance and documentation of at least 12 elements identified by a bullet in two or more organ systems or body areas.
- **Comprehensive Examination**—should include at least nine organ systems or body areas. For each system/area selected, all elements of the examination identified by a bullet should be performed, unless specific directions limit the content of the examination. For each area/system, documentation of at least two elements identified by a bullet is expected.

AAP commentary is indicated by green tint and italic sans serif body type.

Table 6-5. General Multisystem Examination

System/Body Area	Elements of Examination
Constitutional	• Measurement of **any three of the following seven** vital signs: 1) sitting or standing blood pressure, 2) supine blood pressure, 3) pulse rate and regularity, 4) respiration, 5) temperature, 6) height, 7) weight (may be measured and recorded by ancillary staff) • General appearance of patient (eg, development, nutrition, body habitus, deformities, attention to grooming)
Eyes	• Inspection of conjunctivae and lids • Examination of pupils and irises (eg, reaction to light and accommodation, size and symmetry) • Ophthalmoscopic examination of optic discs (eg, size, C/D ratio, appearance) and posterior segments (eg, vessel changes, exudates, hemorrhages)
Ears, Nose, Mouth, and Throat	• External inspection of ears and nose (eg, overall appearance, scars, lesions, masses) • Otoscopic examination of external auditory canals and tympanic membranes • Assessment of hearing (eg, whispered voice, finger rub, tuning fork) • Inspection of nasal mucosa, septum, and turbinates • Inspection of lips, teeth, and gums • Examination of oropharynx: oral mucosa, salivary glands, hard and soft palates, tongue, tonsils, and posterior pharynx
Neck	• Examination of neck (eg, masses, overall appearance, symmetry, tracheal position, crepitus) • Examination of thyroid (eg, enlargement, tenderness, mass)
Respiratory	• Assessment of respiratory effort (eg, intercostal retractions, use of accessory muscles, diaphragmatic movement) • Percussion of chest (eg, dullness, flatness, hyperresonance) • Palpation of chest (eg, tactile fremitus) • Auscultation of lungs (eg, breath sounds, adventitious sounds, rubs)

Cardiovascular	• Palpation of heart (eg, location, size, thrills)
	• Auscultation of heart with notation of abnormal sounds and murmurs
	Examination of:
	  • Carotid arteries (eg, pulse amplitude, bruits)
	  • Abdominal aorta (eg, size, bruits)
	  • Femoral arteries (eg, pulse amplitude, bruits)
	  • Pedal pulses (eg, pulse amplitude)
	  • Extremities for edema and/or varicosities

Chest (Breasts)	• Inspection of breasts (eg, symmetry, nipple discharge) • Palpation of breasts and axillae (eg, masses or lumps, tenderness)
Gastrointestinal (Abdomen)	• Examination of abdomen with notation of presence of masses or tenderness • Examination of liver and spleen • Examination for presence or absence of hernia • Examination (when indicated) of anus, perineum, and rectum, including sphincter tone, presence of hemorrhoids, rectal masses • Obtain stool sample for occult blood test when indicated
Genitourinary	*Male* • Examination of the scrotal contents (eg, hydrocele, spermatocele, tenderness of cord, testicular mass) • Examination of the penis • Digital rectal examination of prostate gland (eg, size, symmetry, nodularity, tenderness)

AAP commentary is indicated by green tint and italic sans serif body type.

System/Body Area	Elements of Examination

Table 6-5. General Multisystem Examination (*continued*)

System/Body Area	Elements of Examination

Genitourinary (*continued*)	*Female*
	• Pelvic examination (with or without specimen collection for smears and cultures) including
	  • Examination of external genitalia (eg, general appearance, hair distribution, lesions) and vagina (eg, general appearance, estrogen effect, discharge, lesions, pelvic support, cystocele, rectocele)
	  • Examination of urethra (eg, masses, tenderness, scarring)
	  • Examination of bladder (eg, fullness, masses, tenderness)
	  • Cervix (eg, general appearance, lesions, discharge)
	  • Uterus (eg, size, contour, position, mobility, tenderness, consistency, descent, or support)
	  • Adnexa/parametria (eg, masses, tenderness, organomegaly, nodularity)

Lymphatic	Palpation of lymph nodes in **two or more** areas: • Neck • Axillae • Groin • Other
Musculoskeletal	• Examination of gait and station • Inspection and/or palpation of digits and nails (eg, clubbing, cyanosis, inflammatory conditions, petechiae, ischemia, infections, nodes) Examination of joints, bones, and muscles of **one or more of the following six areas:** 1) head and neck; 2) spine, ribs, and pelvis; 3) right upper extremity; 4) left upper extremity; 5) right lower extremity; and 6) left lower extremity. The examination of a given area includes: • Inspection and/or palpation with notation of presence of any misalignment, asymmetry, crepitation, defects, tenderness, masses, effusions • Assessment of range of motion with notation of any pain, crepitation, or contracture • Assessment of stability with notation of any dislocation (luxation), subluxation, or laxity • Assessment of muscle strength and tone (eg, flaccid, cog wheel, spastic) with notation of any atrophy or abnormal movements
Skin	• Inspection of skin and subcutaneous tissue (eg, rashes, lesions, ulcers) • Palpation of skin and subcutaneous tissue (eg, induration, subcutaneous nodules, tightening)
Neurological	• Test cranial nerves with notation of any deficits • Examination of deep tendon reflexes with notation of pathological reflexes (eg, Babinski) • Examination of sensation (eg, by touch, pin, vibration, proprioception)
Psychiatric	• Description of patient's judgment and insight Brief assessment of mental status including: • Orientation to time, place, and person • Recent and remote memory • Mood and affect (eg, depression, anxiety, agitation)

AAP commentary is indicated by green tint and italic sans serif body type.

Single Organ System Examinations

The single organ system examinations recognized by *CPT* are described in detail in the tables starting on the next page. Variations among these examinations in the organ systems and body areas identified in the left columns and in the elements of the examinations described in the right columns reflect differing emphases among specialties. To qualify for a given level of single organ system examination, the following content and documentation requirements should be met:

- **Problem-Focused Examination**—should include performance and documentation of one to five elements identified by a bullet, whether in a shaded or unshaded area.
- **Expanded Problem-Focused Examination**—should include performance and documentation of at least six elements identified by a bullet, whether in a shaded or unshaded area.
- **Detailed Examination**—examinations other than the eye and psychiatric examinations should include performance and documentation of at least 12 elements identified by a bullet, whether in a shaded or unshaded area.
    - ❖ Eye and psychiatric examinations should include the performance and documentation of at least nine elements identified by a bullet, whether in a shaded or unshaded area.
- **Comprehensive Examination**—should include performance of all elements identified by a bullet, whether in a shaded or unshaded area. Documentation of every element in a shaded area and at least one element in each category in each unshaded area is expected.

1997 Content and Documentation Requirements for All Single Organ System Exams	
Level of Exam	**Perform and Document**
Problem Focused	**One to five** elements identified by a bullet - whether in a box with a shaded or unshaded border.
Expanded Problem Focused	**At least six** elements identified by a bullet - whether in a box with a shaded or unshaded border.
Detailed	**At least 12** elements identified by a bullet – whether in a box with a shaded or unshaded border.
Comprehensive	Perform **all** elements identified by a bullet; document every element in each shaded area and at least one element in each category in each unshaded area.

AAP commentary is indicated by green tint and italic sans serif body type.

Cardiovascular Examination	
System/Body Area	**Elements of Examination**
Constitutional	• Measurement of **any three of the following seven** vital signs: 1) sitting or standing blood pressure, 2) supine blood pressure, 3) pulse rate and regularity, 4) respiration, 5) temperature, 6) height, 7) weight (may be measured and recorded by ancillary staff) • General appearance of patient (eg, development, nutrition, body habitus, deformities, attention to grooming)
Eyes	• Inspection of conjunctivae and lids (eg, xanthelasma)
Ears, Nose, Mouth, and Throat	• Inspection of teeth, gums, and palate • Inspection of oral mucosa with notation of presence of pallor or cyanosis
Neck	• Examination of jugular veins (eg, distension; a, v, or cannon a waves) • Examination of thyroid (eg, enlargement, tenderness, mass)
Respiratory	• Assessment of respiratory effort (eg, intercostal retractions, use of accessory muscles, diaphragmatic movement) • Auscultation of lungs (eg, breath sounds, adventitious sounds, rubs)
Cardiovascular	• Palpation of heart (eg, location, size, and forcefulness of the point of maximal impact; thrills; lifts; palpable S3 or S4) • Auscultation of heart including sounds, abnormal sounds, and murmurs • Measurement of blood pressure in two or more extremities when indicated (eg, aortic dissection, coarctation) Examination of • Carotid arteries (eg, waveform, pulse amplitude, bruits, apical-carotid delay) • Abdominal aorta (eg, size, bruits) • Femoral arteries (eg, pulse amplitude, bruits) • Pedal pulses (eg, pulse amplitude) • Extremities for peripheral edema and/or varicosities
Gastrointestinal (Abdomen)	• Examination of abdomen with notation of presence of masses or tenderness • Examination of liver and spleen • Obtain stool sample for occult blood from patients who are being considered for thrombolytic or anti-coagulant therapy
Musculoskeletal	• Examination of the back with notation of kyphosis or scoliosis • Examination of gait with notation of ability to undergo exercise testing and/or participation in exercise programs • Assessment of muscle strength and tone (eg, flaccid, cog wheel, spastic) with notation of any atrophy and abnormal movements
Extremities	• Inspection and palpation of digits and nails (eg, clubbing, cyanosis, inflammation, petechiae, ischemia, infections, Osler's nodes)
Skin	• Inspection and/or palpation of skin and subcutaneous tissue (eg, stasis dermatitis, ulcers, scars, xanthomas)
Neurological/ Psychiatric	Brief assessment of mental status including: • Orientation to time, place, and person • Mood and affect (eg, depression, anxiety, agitation)
System/Body Areas Not Required: Head and Face, Chest (Breasts), Genitourinary (Abdomen), and Lymphatic	

Chapter 6: Evaluation and Management Documentation Guidelines

AAP commentary is indicated by green tint and italic sans serif body type.

Chapter 6: Evaluation and Management Documentation Guidelines

Ear, Nose, and Throat Examination	
System/Body Area	**Elements of Examination**
Constitutional	• Measurement of **any three of the following seven** vital signs: 1) sitting or standing blood pressure, 2) supine blood pressure, 3) pulse rate and regularity, 4) respiration, 5) temperature, 6) height, 7) weight (may be measured and recorded by ancillary staff) • General appearance of patient (eg, development, nutrition, body habitus, deformities, attention to grooming) • Assessment of ability to communicate (eg, use of sign language or other communication aids) and quality of voice
Head and Face	• Inspection of head and face (eg, overall appearance, scars, lesions, and masses) • Palpation and/or percussion of face with notation of presence or absence of sinus tenderness • Examination of salivary glands • Assessment of facial strength
Eyes	• Test ocular motility including primary gaze alignment
Ears, Nose, Mouth, and Throat	• Otoscopic examination of external auditory canals and tympanic membranes including pneumo-otoscopy with notation of mobility of membranes • Assessment of hearing with tuning forks and clinical speech reception thresholds (eg, whispered voice, finger rub) • External inspection of ears and nose (eg, overall appearance, scars, lesions, and masses) • Inspection of nasal mucosa, septum, and turbinates • Inspection of lips, teeth, and gums • Examination of oropharynx: oral mucosa, hard and soft palates, tongue, tonsils, and posterior pharynx (eg, asymmetry, lesions, hydration of mucosal surfaces) • Inspection of pharyngeal walls and pyriform sinuses (eg, pooling of saliva, asymmetry, lesions) • Examination by mirror of larynx including the condition of the epiglottis, false vocal cords, true vocal cords, and mobility of larynx (use of mirror not required in children) • Examination by mirror of nasopharynx including appearance of the mucosa, adenoids, posterior choanae, and eustachian tubes (use of mirror not required in children)
Neck	• Examination of neck (eg, masses, overall appearance, symmetry, tracheal position, crepitus) • Examination of thyroid (eg, enlargement, tenderness, mass)
Respiratory	• Inspection of chest including symmetry, expansion, and/or assessment of respiratory effort (eg, intercostal retractions, use of accessory muscles, diaphragmatic movement) • Auscultation of lungs (eg, breath sounds, adventitious sounds, rubs)
Cardiovascular	• Auscultation of heart with notation of abnormal sounds and murmurs • Examination of peripheral vascular system by observation (eg, swelling, varicosities) and palpation (eg, pulses, temperature, edema, tenderness)
Lymphatic	• Palpation of lymph nodes in neck, axillae, groin, and/or other location

Neurological/ Psychiatric	• Test cranial nerves with notation of any deficits
	Brief assessment of mental status including:
	   • Orientation to time, place, and person
	   • Mood and affect (eg, depression, anxiety, agitation)

System/Body Areas Not Required: Chest (Breasts), Gastrointestinal (Abdomen), Genitourinary, Musculoskeletal, Extremities, and Skin	

AAP commentary is indicated by green tint and italic sans serif body type.

Eye Examination

System/Body Area	Elements of Examination
Eyes	• Test visual acuity (does not include determination of refractive error) • Gross visual field testing by confrontation • Test ocular motility including primary gaze alignment • Inspection of bulbar and palpebral conjunctivae • Examination of ocular adnexae including lids (eg, ptosis or lagophthalmos), lacrimal glands, lacrimal drainage, orbits, and preauricular lymph nodes • Examination of pupils and irises including shape, direct and consensual reaction (afferent pupil), size (eg, anisocoria), and morphology • Slit lamp examination of the corneas including epithelium, stroma, endothelium, and tear film • Slit lamp examination of the anterior chambers including depth, cells, and flare • Slit lamp examination of the lenses including clarity, anterior and posterior capsule, cortex, and nucleus • Measurement of intraocular pressures (except in children and patients with trauma or infectious disease) Ophthalmoscopic examination through dilated pupils (unless contraindicated) of: • Optic discs including size, C/D ratio, appearance (eg, atrophy, cupping, tumor elevation), and nerve fiber layer • Posterior segments including retina and vessels (eg, exudates and hemorrhages)
Respiratory	• Inspection of chest including symmetry, expansion, and/or assessment of respiratory effort (eg, intercostal retractions, use of accessory muscles, diaphragmatic movement) • Auscultation of lungs (eg, breath sounds, adventitious sounds, rubs)
Neurological/ Psychiatric	Brief assessment of mental status including: • Orientation to time, place, and person • Mood and affect (eg, depression, anxiety, agitation)

System/Body Areas Not Required: Constitutional; Head and Face; Ears, Nose, Mouth, and Throat; Neck; Cardiovascular; Chest (Breasts); Genitourinary; Lymphatic; Musculoskeletal; Extremities; and Skin Extremities and Skin

Genitourinary Examination

System/Body Area	Elements of Examination
Constitutional	• Measurement of **any three of the following seven** vital signs: 1) sitting or standing blood pressure, 2) supine blood pressure, 3) pulse rate and regularity, 4) respiration, 5) temperature, 6) height, 7) weight (may be measured and recorded by ancillary staff) • General appearance of patient (eg, development, nutrition, body habitus, deformities, attention to grooming)
Neck	• Examination of neck (eg, masses, overall appearance, symmetry, tracheal position, crepitus) • Examination of thyroid (eg, enlargement, tenderness, mass)
Respiratory	• Assessment of respiratory effort (eg, intercostal retractions, use of accessory muscles, diaphragmatic movement) • Auscultation of lungs (eg, breath sounds, adventitious sounds, rubs)
Cardiovascular	• Auscultation of heart with notation of abnormal sounds and murmurs • Examination of peripheral vascular system by observation (eg, swelling, varicosities) and palpation (eg, pulses, temperature, edema, tenderness)
Chest (Breasts)	[See Genitourinary (female)]

AAP commentary is indicated by green tint and italic sans serif body type.

Chapter 6: Evaluation and Management Documentation Guidelines

Genitourinary Examination (*continued*)	
System/Body Area	**Elements of Examination**
Gastrointestinal (Abdomen)	• Examination of abdomen with notation of presence of masses or tenderness • Examination for presence or absence of hernia • Examination of liver and spleen • Obtain stool sample for occult blood test when indicated
Genitourinary	*Male* • Inspection of anus and perineum Examination (with or without specimen collection for smears and cultures) of genitalia including: • Scrotum (eg, lesions, cysts, rashes) • Epididymides (eg, size, symmetry, masses) • Testes (eg, size, symmetry, masses) • Urethral meatus (eg, size, location, lesions, discharge) • Penis (eg, lesions, presence or absence of foreskin, fore-skin retractability, plaque, masses, scarring, deformities) Digital rectal examination including: • Prostate gland (eg, size, symmetry, nodularity, tenderness) • Seminal vesicles (eg, symmetry, tenderness, masses, enlargement) • Sphincter tone, presence of hemorrhoids, rectal masses *Female* Includes **at least seven of the following 11** elements identified by bullets: • Inspection and palpation of breasts (eg, masses or lumps, tenderness, symmetry, nipple discharge) • Digital rectal examination including sphincter tone, presence of hemorrhoids, rectal masses Pelvic examination (with or without specimen collection for smears and cultures) including: • External genitalia (eg, general appearance, hair distribution, lesions) • Urethral meatus (eg, size, location, lesions, prolapse) • Urethra (eg, masses, tenderness, scarring) • Bladder (eg, fullness, masses, tenderness) • Vagina (eg, general appearance, estrogen effect, discharge, lesions, pelvic support, cystocele, rectocele) • Cervix (eg, general appearance, lesions, discharge) • Uterus (eg, size, contour, position, mobility, tenderness, consistency, descent, or support) • Adnexa/parametria (eg, masses, tenderness, organomegaly, nodularity) • Anus and perineum
Lymphatic	• Palpation of lymph nodes in neck, axillae, groin, and/or other location
Skin	• Inspection and/or palpation of skin and subcutaneous tissue (eg, rashes, lesions, ulcers)
Neurological/ Psychiatric	Brief assessment of mental status including: • Orientation (eg, time, place, and person) • Mood and affect (eg, depression, anxiety, agitation)
System/Body Areas Not Required: Head and Face; Eyes; Ears, Nose, Mouth, and Throat; Musculoskeletal; and Extremities	

AAP commentary is indicated by green tint and italic sans serif body type.

Hematologic/Lymphatic/Immunologic Examination

System/Body Area	Elements of Examination
Constitutional	• Measurement of **any three of the following seven** vital signs: 1) sitting or standing blood pressure, 2) supine blood pressure, 3) pulse rate and regularity, 4) respiration, 5) temperature, 6) height, 7) weight (may be measured and recorded by ancillary staff) • General appearance of patient (eg, development, nutrition, body habitus, deformities, attention to grooming)
Head and Face	• Palpation and/or percussion of face with notation of presence or absence of sinus tenderness
Eyes	• Inspection of conjunctivae and lids
Ears, Nose, Mouth, and Throat	• Otoscopic examination of external auditory canals and tympanic membranes • Inspection of nasal mucosa, septum, and turbinates • Inspection of teeth and gums • Examination of oropharynx (eg, oral mucosa, hard and soft palates, tongue, tonsils, posterior pharynx)
Neck	• Examination of neck (eg, masses, overall appearance, symmetry, tracheal position, crepitus) • Examination of thyroid (eg, enlargement, tenderness, mass)
Respiratory	• Assessment of respiratory effort (eg, intercostal retractions, use of accessory muscles, diaphragmatic movement) • Auscultation of lungs (eg, breath sounds, adventitious sounds, rubs)
Cardiovascular	• Auscultation of heart with notation of abnormal sounds and murmurs • Examination of peripheral vascular system by observation (eg, swelling, varicosities) and palpation (eg, pulses, temperature, edema, tenderness)
Gastrointestinal (Abdomen)	• Examination of abdomen with notation of presence of masses or tenderness • Examination of liver and spleen
Lymphatic	• Palpation of lymph nodes in neck, axillae, groin, and/or other location
Extremities	• Inspection and palpation of digits and nails (eg, clubbing, cyanosis, inflammation, petechiae, ischemia, infections, nodes)
Skin	• Inspection and/or palpation of skin and subcutaneous tissue (eg, rashes, lesions, ulcers, ecchymoses, bruises)
Neurological/ Psychiatric	Brief assessment of mental status including: • Orientation to time, place, and person • Mood and affect (eg, depression, anxiety, agitation)
System/Body Areas Not Required: Chest (Breasts), Genitourinary, and Musculoskeletal	

AAP commentary is indicated by green tint and italic sans serif body type.

Chapter 6: Evaluation and Management Documentation Guidelines

Musculoskeletal Examination	
System/Body Area	**Elements of Examination**
Constitutional	• Measurement of **any three of the following seven** vital signs: 1) sitting or standing blood pressure, 2) supine blood pressure, 3) pulse rate and regularity, 4) respiration, 5) temperature, 6) height, 7) weight (may be measured and recorded by ancillary staff) • General appearance of patient (eg, development, nutrition, body habitus, deformities, attention to grooming)
Cardiovascular	• Examination of peripheral vascular system by observation (eg, swelling, varicosities) and palpation (eg, pulses, temperature, edema, tenderness)
Lymphatic	• Palpation of lymph nodes in neck, axillae, groin, and/or other location
Musculoskeletal	• Examination of gait and station Examination of joint(s), bone(s), and muscle(s)/tendon(s) of **four of the following six** areas: 1) head and neck; 2) spine, ribs, and pelvis; 3) right upper extremity; 4) left upper extremity; 5) right lower extremity; and 6) left lower extremity. The examination of a given area includes: • Inspection, percussion, and/or palpation with notation of any misalignment, asymmetry, crepitation, defects, tenderness, masses, or effusions • Assessment of range of motion with notation of any pain (eg, straight leg raising), crepitation, or contracture • Assessment of stability with notation of any dislocation (luxation), subluxation, or laxity • Assessment of muscle strength and tone (eg, flaccid, cog wheel, spastic) with notation of any atrophy or abnormal movements *Note:* For the comprehensive level of examination, all four of the elements identified by a bullet must be performed and documented for each of four anatomic areas. For the three lower levels of examination, each element is counted separately for each body area. For example, assessing range of motion in two extremities constitutes two elements.
Extremities	[See Musculoskeletal and Skin]
Skin	• Inspection and/or palpation of skin and subcutaneous tissue (eg, scars, rashes, lesions, cafe-au-lait spots, ulcers) in **four of the following six** areas: 1) head and neck, 2) trunk, 3) right upper extremity, 4) left upper extremity, 5) right lower extremity, and 6) left lower extremity. *Note:* For the comprehensive level, the examination of all four anatomic areas must be performed and documented. For the three lower levels of examination, each body area is counted separately. For example, inspection and/or palpation of the skin and subcutaneous tissue of two extremities constitutes two elements.
Neurological/ Psychiatric	• Test coordination (eg, finger/nose, heel/knee/shin, rapid alternating movements in the upper and lower extremities, evaluation of fine motor coordination in young children) • Examination of deep tendon reflexes and/or nerve stretch test with notation of pathological reflexes (eg, Babinski) • Examination of sensation (eg, by touch, pin, vibration, proprioception) Brief assessment of mental status including: • Orientation to time, place, and person • Mood and affect (eg, depression, anxiety, agitation)
System/Body Areas Not Required: Head and Face; Eyes; Ears, Nose, Mouth, and Throat; Neck; Respiratory; Chest (Breasts); Gastrointestinal (Abdomen); and Genitourinary	

AAP commentary is indicated by green tint and italic sans serif body type.

Neurological Examination	
System/Body Area	**Elements of Examination**
Constitutional	• Measurement of **any three of the following seven** vital signs: 1) sitting or standing blood pressure, 2) supine blood pressure, 3) pulse rate and regularity, 4) respiration, 5) temperature, 6) height, 7) weight (may be measured and recorded by ancillary staff) • General appearance of patient (eg, development, nutrition, body habitus, deformities, attention to grooming)
Eyes	• Ophthalmoscopic examination of optic discs (eg, size, C/D ratio, appearance) and posterior segments (eg, vessel changes, exudates, hemorrhages)
Cardiovascular	• Examination of carotid arteries (eg, pulse amplitude, bruits) • Auscultation of heart with notation of abnormal sounds and murmurs • Examination of peripheral vascular system by observation (eg, swelling, varicosities) and palpation (eg, pulses, temperature, edema, tenderness)

Musculoskeletal	• Examination of gait and station
	Assessment of motor function including:
	  • Muscle strength in upper and lower extremities
	  • Muscle tone in upper and lower extremities (eg, flaccid, cog wheel, spastic) with notation of any atrophy or abnormal movements (eg, fasciculation, tardive dyskinesia)

Extremities	[See Musculoskeletal]

Neurological	Evaluation of higher integrative functions including:
	  • Orientation to time, place, and person
	  • Recent and remote memory
	  • Attention span and concentration
	  • Language (eg, naming objects, repeating phrases, spontaneous speech)
	  • Fund of knowledge (eg, awareness of current events, past history, vocabulary)
	Test the following cranial nerves:
	  • 2nd cranial nerve (eg, visual acuity, visual fields, fundi)
	  • 3rd, 4th, and 6th cranial nerves (eg, pupils, eye movements)
	  • 5th cranial nerve (eg, facial sensation, corneal reflexes)
	  • 7th cranial nerve (eg, facial symmetry, strength)
	  • 8th cranial nerve (eg, hearing with tuning fork, whispered voice, and/or finger rub)
	  • 9th cranial nerve (eg, spontaneous or reflex palate movement)
	  • 11th cranial nerve (eg, shoulder shrug strength)
	  • 12th cranial nerve (eg, tongue protrusion)
	• Examination of sensation (eg, by touch, pin, vibration, proprioception)
	• Examination of deep tendon reflexes in upper and lower extremities with notation of pathological reflexes (eg, Babinski)
	• Test coordination (eg, finger/nose, heel/knee/shin, rapid alternating movements in the upper and lower extremities, evaluation of fine motor coordination in young children)

System/Body Areas Not Required: Head and Face; Ears, Nose, Mouth, and Throat; Neck; Respiratory; Chest (Breasts); Gastrointestinal (Abdomen); Genitourinary; Lymphatic; Skin; and Psychiatric

AAP commentary is indicated by green tint and italic sans serif body type.

Psychiatric Examination	
System/Body Area	**Elements of Examination**
Constitutional	• Measurement of **any three of the following seven** vital signs: 1) sitting or standing blood pressure, 2) supine blood pressure, 3) pulse rate and regularity, 4) respiration, 5) temperature, 6) height, 7) weight (may be measured and recorded by ancillary staff) • General appearance of patient (eg, development, nutrition, body habitus, deformities, attention to grooming)
Musculoskeletal	• Assessment of muscle strength and tone (eg, flaccid, cog wheel, spastic) with notation of any atrophy and abnormal movements • Examination of gait and station
Psychiatric	• Description of speech including: rate, volume, articulation, coherence, and spontaneity with notation of abnormalities (eg, perseveration, paucity of language) • Description of thought processes including: rate of thoughts (eg, logical vs. illogical, tangential), abstract reasoning, and computation • Description of associations (eg, loose, tangential, circumstantial, intact) • Description of abnormal or psychotic thoughts including hallucinations, delusions, pre-occupation with violence, homicidal or suicidal ideation, and obsessions • Description of the patient's judgment (eg, concerning everyday activities and social situations) and insight (eg, concerning psychiatric condition) Complete mental status examination including: • Orientation to time, place, and person • Recent and remote memory • Attention span and concentration • Language (eg, naming objects, repeating phrases) • Fund of knowledge (eg, awareness of current events, past history, vocabulary) • Mood and affect (eg, depression, anxiety, agitation, hypomania, lability)
System/Body Areas Not Required: Head and Face; Eyes; Ears, Nose, Mouth, and Throat; Neck; Respiratory; Cardiovascular; Chest (Breasts); Gastrointestinal (Abdomen); Genitourinary; Lymphatic; Extremities; Skin; and Neurological	

AAP commentary is indicated by green tint and italic sans serif body type.

Respiratory Examination

System/Body Area	Elements of Examination
Constitutional	• Measurement of **any three of the following seven** vital signs: 1) sitting or standing blood pressure, 2) supine blood pressure, 3) pulse rate and regularity, 4) respiration, 5) temperature, 6) height, 7) weight (may be measured and recorded by ancillary staff) • General appearance of patient (eg, development, nutrition, body habitus, deformities, attention to grooming)
Ears, Nose, Mouth, and Throat	• Inspection of nasal mucosa, septum, and turbinates • Inspection of teeth and gums • Examination of oropharynx (eg, oral mucosa, hard and soft palates, tongue, tonsils, and posterior pharynx)
Neck	• Examination of neck (eg, masses, overall appearance, symmetry, tracheal position, crepitus) • Examination of thyroid (eg, enlargement, tenderness, mass) • Examination of jugular veins (eg, distension; a, v, or cannon a waves)
Respiratory	• Inspection of chest with notation of symmetry and expansion • Assessment of respiratory effort (eg, intercostal retractions, use of accessory muscles, diaphragmatic movement) • Percussion of chest (eg, dullness, flatness, hyper-resonance) • Palpation of chest (eg, tactile fremitus) • Auscultation of lungs (eg, breath sounds, adventitious sounds, rubs)
Cardiovascular	• Auscultation of heart including sounds, abnormal sounds, and murmurs • Examination of peripheral vascular system by observation (eg, swelling, varicosities) and palpation (eg, pulses, temperature, edema, tenderness)
Gastrointestinal (Abdomen)	• Examination of abdomen with notation of presence of masses or tenderness • Examination of liver and spleen
Lymphatic	• Palpation of lymph nodes in neck, axillae, groin, and/or other location
Musculoskeletal	• Assessment of muscle strength and tone (eg, flaccid, cog wheel, spastic) with notation of any atrophy and abnormal movements • Examination of gait and station
Extremities	• Inspection and palpation of digits and nails (eg, clubbing, cyanosis, inflammation, petechiae, ischemia, infections, nodes)
Skin	• Inspection and/or palpation of skin and subcutaneous tissue (eg, rashes, lesions, ulcers)
Neurological/ Psychiatric	Brief assessment of mental status including: • Orientation to time, place, and person • Mood and affect (eg, depression, anxiety, agitation)

System/Body Areas Not Required: Head and Face, Eyes, Chest (Breasts), and Genitourinary

Chapter 6: Evaluation and Management Documentation Guidelines

AAP commentary is indicated by green tint and italic sans serif body type.

Chapter 6: Evaluation and Management Documentation Guidelines

System/Body Area	Elements of Examination
Skin Examination	
Constitutional	• Measurement of **any three of the following seven** vital signs: 1) sitting or standing blood pressure, 2) supine blood pressure, 3) pulse rate and regularity, 4) respiration, 5) temperature, 6) height, 7) weight (may be measured and recorded by ancillary staff) • General appearance of patient (eg, development, nutrition, body habitus, deformities, attention to grooming)
Eyes	• Inspection of conjunctivae and lids
Ears, Nose, Mouth, and Throat	• Inspection of lips, teeth, and gums • Examination of oropharynx (eg, oral mucosa, hard and soft palates, tongue, tonsils, posterior pharynx)
Neck	• Examination of thyroid (eg, enlargement, tenderness, mass)
Cardiovascular	• Examination of peripheral vascular system by observation (eg, swelling, varicosities) and palpation (eg, pulses, temperature, edema, tenderness)
Gastrointestinal (Abdomen)	• Examination of liver and spleen • Examination of anus for condyloma and other lesions
Lymphatic	• Palpation of lymph nodes in neck, axillae, groin, and/or other location
Extremities	• Inspection and palpation of digits and nails (eg, clubbing, cyanosis, inflammation, petechiae, ischemia, infections, nodes)
Skin	• Palpation of scalp and inspection of hair of scalp, eyebrows, face, chest, pubic area (when indicated), and extremities Inspection and/or palpation of skin and subcutaneous tissue (eg, rashes, lesions, ulcers, susceptibility to and presence of photo damage) in **eight of the following 10** areas: • Head, including face • Neck • Chest, including breasts and axillae • Abdomen • Genitalia, groin, buttocks • Back • Right upper extremity • Left upper extremity • Right lower extremity • Left lower extremity Note: For the comprehensive level, the examination of at least eight anatomic areas must be performed and documented. For the three lower levels of examination, each body area is counted separately. For example, inspection and/or palpation of the skin and subcutaneous tissue of the right upper extremity and the left upper extremity constitutes two elements. • Inspection of eccrine and apocrine glands of skin and subcutaneous tissue with identification and location of any hyperhidrosis, chromhidroses, or bromhidrosis
Neurological/ Psychiatric	Brief assessment of mental status including: • Orientation to time, place, and person • Mood and affect (eg, depression, anxiety, agitation)
System/Body Areas Not Required: Head and Face, Respiratory, Chest (Breasts), Genitourinary, and Musculoskeletal	

AAP commentary is indicated by green tint and italic sans serif body type.

C. Documentation of the Complexity of Medical Decision-making

The levels of E/M services recognize four types of medical decision-making (straightforward, low complexity, moderate complexity, and high complexity). Medical decision-making refers to the complexity of establishing a diagnosis and/or selecting a management option as measured by

1. The number of possible diagnoses and/or the number of management options that must be considered

2. The amount and/or complexity of medical records, diagnostic tests, and/or other information that must be obtained, reviewed, and analyzed

3. The risk of significant complications, morbidity, and/or mortality, as well as co-morbidities, associated with the patient's presenting problem(s), the diagnostic procedure(s), and/or the possible management options.

Table 6-6 shows the progression of the elements required for each level of medical decision-making. To qualify for a given type of decision-making, **two of the three elements in the table must be either met or exceeded.**

Each of the elements of medical decision-making is described below.

Number of Diagnoses or Management Options

The number of possible diagnoses and/or the number of management options that must be considered is based on the number and types of problems addressed during the encounter, the complexity of establishing a diagnosis, and the management decisions that are made by the physician.

Generally, decision-making with respect to a diagnosed problem is easier than that for an identified but undiagnosed problem. The number and type of diagnostic tests employed may be an indicator of the number of possible diagnoses. Problems that are improving or resolving are less complex than those that are worsening or failing to change as expected. The need to seek advice from others is another indicator of complexity of diagnostic or management problems.

•*DG: For each encounter, an assessment, clinical impression, or diagnosis should be documented. It may be explicitly stated or implied in documented decisions regarding management plans and/or further evaluation.*

☀ *For a presenting problem with an established diagnosis the record should reflect whether the problem is: (a) improved, well controlled, resolving, or resolved; or (b) inadequately controlled, worsening, or failing to change as expected.*

☀ *For a presenting problem without an established diagnosis, the assessment or clinical impression may be stated in the form of a differential diagnoses or as "possible," "probable," or "rule out" (R/O) diagnoses.*

•*DG: The initiation of, or changes in, treatment should be documented. Treatment includes a wide range of management options including patient instructions, nursing instructions, therapies, and medications.*

•*DG: If referrals are made, consultations requested, or advice sought, the record should indicate to whom or where the referral or consultation is made or from whom the advice is requested.*

Amount and/or Complexity of Data to Be Reviewed

The amount and/or complexity of data to be reviewed is based on the types of diagnostic testing ordered or reviewed. A decision to obtain and review old medical records and/or obtain history from sources other than the patient increases the amount and complexity of data to be reviewed.

Discussion of contradictory or unexpected test results with the physician who performed or interpreted the test is an indication of the complexity of data being reviewed. On occasion the physician who ordered a test may personally review the image, tracing, or specimen to supplement information from the physician who prepared the test report or interpretation; this is another indication of the complexity of data being reviewed.

•*DG: If a diagnostic service (test or procedure) is ordered, planned, scheduled, or performed at the time of the E/M encounter, the type of service (eg, lab or x-ray) should be documented.*

•*DG: The review of lab, radiology, and/or other diagnostic tests should be documented. An entry in a progress note such as "WBC elevated" or "chest x-ray unremarkable" is acceptable. Alternatively, the review may be documented by initialing and dating the report containing the test results.*

•*DG:*   *A decision to obtain old records or to obtain additional history from the family, caretaker, or other source to supplement that obtained from the patient should be documented.*

•*DG:*   *Relevant findings from the review of old records and/or the receipt of additional history from the family, caretaker, or other source should be documented. If there is no relevant information beyond that already obtained, that fact should be documented. A notation of "old records reviewed" or "-additional history obtained from family" without elaboration is insufficient.*

•*DG:*   *The results of discussion of laboratory, radiology, or other diagnostic tests with the physician who performed or interpreted the study should be documented.*

•*DG:*   *The direct visualization and independent interpretation of an image, tracing, or specimen previously or subsequently interpreted by another physician should be documented.*

Risk of Significant Complications, Morbidity, and/or Mortality

The risk of significant complications, morbidity, and/or mortality is based on the risks associated with the presenting problem(s), the diagnostic procedure(s), and the possible management options.

•*DG:*   *Co-morbidities/underlying diseases or other factors that increase the complexity of medical decision making by increasing the risk of complications, morbidity, and/or mortality should be documented.*

•*DG:*   *If a surgical or invasive diagnostic procedure is ordered, planned, or scheduled at the time of the E/M encounter, the type of procedure (eg, laparoscopy) should be documented.*

•*DG:*   *If a surgical or invasive diagnostic procedure is performed at the time of the E/M encounter, the specific procedure should be documented.*

•*DG:*   *The referral for or decision to perform a surgical or invasive diagnostic procedure on an urgent basis should be documented or implied.*

The following table may be used to help determine whether the risk of significant complications, morbidity, and/or mortality is **minimal**, **low**, **moderate**, or **high**. Because the determination of risk is complex and not readily quantifiable, the table includes common clinical examples rather than absolute measures of risk. The assessment of risk of the presenting problem(s) is based on the risk related to the disease process anticipated between the present encounter and the next one. The assessment of risk of selecting diagnostic procedures and management options is based on the risk during and immediately following any procedures or treatment. *The highest level of risk in any one category (presenting problem(s), diagnostic procedure(s), or management options) determines the overall risk.*

CMS Table of Risk			
Level of Risk	**Presenting Problem(s)**	**Diagnostic Procedure(s) Ordered**	**Management Options Selected**
Minimal	⚙ One self-limited or minor problem (eg, cold, insect bite, tinea corporis)	⚙ Laboratory tests requiring venipuncture ⚙ Chest x-rays ⚙ EKG/EEG ⚙ Urinalysis ⚙ Ultrasound, eg, echocardiography ⚙ KOH prep	⚙ Rest ⚙ Gargles ⚙ Elastic bandages ⚙ Superficial dressings
Low	⚙ Two or more self-limited or minor problems ⚙ One stable chronic illness (eg, well-controlled hypertension, non–insulin-dependent diabetes, cataract, benign prostatic hyperplasia) ⚙ Acute uncomplicated illness or injury (eg, cystitis, allergic rhinitis, simple sprain)	⚙ Physiologic tests not under stress (eg, pulmonary function tests) ⚙ Non-cardiovascular imaging studies with contrast (eg, barium enema) ⚙ Superficial needle biopsies ⚙ Clinical laboratory tests requiring arterial puncture ⚙ Skin biopsies	⚙ Over-the-counter drugs ⚙ Minor surgery with no identified risk factors ⚙ Physical therapy ⚙ Occupational therapy ⚙ Intravenous fluids without additives

AAP commentary is indicated by green tint and italic sans serif body type.

CMS Table of Risk (*continued*)

Level of Risk	Presenting Problem(s)	Diagnostic Procedure(s) Ordered	Management Options Selected
Moderate	◉ One or more chronic illnesses with mild exacerbation, progression, or side effects of treatment ◉ Two or more stable chronic illnesses ◉ Undiagnosed new problem with uncertain prognosis (eg, lump in breast) ◉ Acute illness with systemic symptoms (eg, pyelonephritis, pneumonitis, colitis) ◉ Acute complicated injury (eg, head injury with brief loss of consciousness)	◉ Physiologic tests under stress (eg, cardiac stress test, fetal contraction stress test) ◉ Diagnostic endoscopies with no identified risk factors ◉ Deep needle or incisional biopsy ◉ Cardiovascular imaging studies with contrast and no identified risk factors (eg, arteriogram, cardiac catheterization) ◉ Obtain fluid from body cavity (eg, lumbar puncture, thoracentesis, culdocentesis)	◉ Minor surgery with identified risk factors ◉ Elective major surgery (open, percutaneous, or endoscopic) with no identified risk factors ◉ Prescription drug management ◉ Therapeutic nuclear medicine ◉ Intravenous fluids with additives ◉ Closed treatment of fracture or dislocation without manipulation
High	◉ One or more chronic illnesses with severe exacerbation, progression, or side effects of treatment ◉ Acute or chronic illnesses or injuries that pose a threat to life or body function (eg, multiple trauma, acute myocardial infarction, pulmonary embolus, severe respiratory distress, progressive severe rheumatoid arthritis, psychiatric illness with potential threat to self or others, peritonitis, acute renal failure) ◉ An abrupt change in neurologic status (eg, seizure, transient ischemic attack, weakness, sensory loss)	◉ Cardiovascular imaging studies with contrast with identified risk factors ◉ Cardiac electrophysiologic tests ◉ Diagnostic endoscopies with identified risk factors ◉ Discography	◉ Elective major surgery (open, percutaneous, or endoscopic) with identified risk factors ◉ Emergency major surgery (open, percutaneous, or endoscopic) ◉ Parenteral controlled substances ◉ Drug therapy requiring intensive monitoring for toxicity ◉ Decision not to resuscitate or to deescalate because of poor prognosis

*Therefore, in the event of an encounter resulting in **multiple** diagnoses/management options,* **limited** *data and* **moderate risk** *lead to* **overall** **moderate complexity** *for MDM (Table 6-6).*

Table 6-6. Determining Medical Decision-making

Number of Diagnoses or Management Options	Amount and/or Complexity of Data to Be Reviewed	Risk of Significant Complications, Morbidity, and/or Mortality	Type of Decision-Making
Minimal	*Minimal or none*	*Minimal*	*Straightforward*
Limited	*Limited*	*Low*	*Low complexity*
Multiple	*Moderate*	*Moderate*	*Moderate complexity*
Extensive	*Extensive*	*High*	*High complexity*

AAP commentary is indicated by green tint and italic sans serif body type.

D. Documentation of an Encounter Dominated by Counseling or Coordination of Care

In the case where counseling and/or coordination of care dominates (more than 50%) the physician/patient and/or family encounter (face-to-face time in the office or other outpatient setting or floor/unit time in the hospital or nursing facility), time is considered the key or controlling factor to qualify for a particular level of E/M services.

•**DG:**   *If the physician elects to report the level of service based on counseling and/or coordination of care, the total length of time of the encounter (face-to-face or floor time, as appropriate) should be documented and the record should describe the counseling and/or activities to coordinate care.*

Split/Shared E/M Services

A split/shared E/M service is one in which a physician and a QHP from the same group practice each personally perform a medically necessary and substantive portion of one or more face-to-face E/M encounters on the same date. A portion of the key components of the service must be provided face-to-face by the physician to report under the physician's National Provider Identifier (NPI). Split/shared services were defined and implemented for services to Medicare beneficiaries. Private payers may adopt the same or a similar policy. The split/shared concept is applied differently for inpatient services than for services in the office or clinic setting.

❁   In the office or clinic setting, split/shared E/M services must meet incident-to requirements for the service to be reported under the physician's NPI. Incident-to services require the physician's presence in the office suite at the time of the QHP service and that the QHP provides care only in accordance with a physician's established care plan for the patient. See Chapter 13, Allied Health and Clinical Staff Services, for more information on incident-to services.

Example

The patient history and a portion of the examination are provided in the office by a nurse practitioner for an established patient in continuation of a physician's previously documented plan of care for irritable bowel syndrome. The physician is consulted about concerns regarding increased GI symptoms, sees the patient face-to-face, performs a more detailed examination, and documents the assessment and plan of care. The total service may be reported under the physician's NPI because incident-to provisions have been met and both professionals provided face-to-face services.

❁   When a hospital inpatient/hospital outpatient (on campus outpatient hospital or off campus outpatient hospital) or emergency department E/M is shared between a physician and an NPP from the same group practice and the physician provides any face-to-face portion of the E/M encounter with the patient, the service may be billed under either the physician or the NPP. However, if there was no face-to-face encounter between the patient and the physician (eg, even if the physician participated in the service by only reviewing the patient's medical record), then the service may only be billed under the NPP. Payment will be made at the appropriate physician fee schedule rate based on the reporting provider entered on the claim.

The following conditions apply to all split/shared services:

❁   *The physician and QHP must document and sign their portion of the service. A physician cannot merely sign off on the documentation of the QHP's work.*

❁   *If the E/M service is reported based on counseling and/or coordination of care, only the physician's time is used to select the level of service. The physician must document his or her total time spent in counseling and/or coordination of care and a summary of the issues discussed or coordination of care provided.*

❁   *Critical care is never a split/shared service because critical care services reflect the work of only one individual.*

❁   *Split/shared billing does not apply in the nursing or skilled nursing facility settings.*

AAP commentary is indicated by green tint and italic sans serif body type.

More E/M Documentation and Coding Tips

- When using an EHR system, it is important that the documentation for each encounter is unique and reflects the purpose and activity of that encounter. Use of documentation features, such as carryforward of prior history, copy and paste, and auto-completion, may lead to inaccurate documentation and wrong code assignment. (See Coding Conundrum: Pitfalls of Electronic Health Record Coding in Chapter 5, Preventing Fraud and Abuse: Compliance, Audits, and Paybacks, for more on this topic.)

- Ideally, physicians in a group practice should be consistent in their documentation policies. However, if documentation practices differ between physicians, have those differences documented in the practice's written policies.

- The code selected for a new patient will often be one level lower than for an established patient for the same amount of work. However, the Medicare relative value units are higher for new patient visits, compensating the physician for the extra work required.

- The American Academy of Pediatrics (AAP) has developed forms that promote good documentation of office or outpatient visits. Examples can be ordered from the AAP by calling 888/227-1770 or visiting http://shop.aap.org.

Guidelines for Reporting E/M Services Under Teaching Physician Guidelines

- A teaching physician may bill for resident or fellow services if the teaching physician personally performs the key components (history, physical examination, and MDM) of the service, performs the key components jointly with a resident, or personally observes the resident performing the key or critical components.

- The level of service billed will be dependent on the level of work performed and documented by the resident and the teaching physician in combination or by the teaching physician if seen independent of the resident.

- Any contribution and participation of a student to the performance of a billable service (other than the ROS and/or PFSH, which are not separately billable but are taken as part of an E/M service) must be performed in the physical presence of a teaching physician or a resident in a service meeting the requirements set forth in this section for teaching physician billing.

- Students may document services in the medical record. However, the teaching physician must verify in the medical record all student documentation or findings, including history, physical examination, and/or MDM. The teaching physician must personally perform (or re-perform) the physical examination and MDM activities of the E/M service being billed but may verify any student documentation in the medical record, rather than re-documenting this work (new guidance in 2018).

- The teaching physician must document that he or she personally performed the service or was physically present (in the same room as the patient) during the key or critical portions of the service performed by the resident and participated in the management of the patient. The selected key or critical portion of the visit is at the discretion of the physician.

- Time-based services (eg, face-to-face prolonged services, critical care, hospital discharge management) can only be billed when the teaching physician is present for the time required by the description of service. This also applies to E/M visits when time is considered the key component in the selection of the E/M code (>50% of the total face-to-face visit was spent counseling and/or coordinating care). The total time spent by the teaching physician must be documented.

- The teaching physician must document the key or critical part of the service personally performed, link his or her documentation back to the resident's note, and document that the care plan was reviewed and approved. It is not necessary to repeat the resident's documentation. However, the teaching physician documentation must be linked to the resident's note and all exceptions to the resident's findings must be documented. A signature alone is not acceptable documentation.

AAP commentary is indicated by green tint and italic sans serif body type.

- Medicare guidelines stipulate that when documenting in an EHR, the teaching physician may use a macro (eg, predetermined text) as the required personal documentation if it is personally entered by the teaching physician. The resident or teaching physician must enter customized information to support medical necessity. If the resident and teaching physician use macros, the documentation is not sufficient.

Examples

- The resident admits a 2-month-old at 10:30 pm. The teaching physician's initial visit is performed the following morning at 8:00 am. The teaching physician reports an initial hospital care service based on the work personally performed that morning.
- The teaching physician sees the same patient for follow-up inpatient care subsequent to the resident's visit.
- The teaching physician and resident jointly admit or perform a subsequent visit on the same patient.
- The teaching physician performs the subsequent inpatient visit jointly with the resident.

Unacceptable	Minimal Documentation Required
Countersignature	"I performed a history and physical exam of the patient. Findings are consistent with Resident's note. Discussed patient's management with Resident and agree with his documented findings and plan of care." Signature
"Agree with above." Signature "Rounded, reviewed, agree." Signature	"I saw and evaluated the patient. I agree with the findings and the plan of care as documented in Resident's note." Signature
"Patient seen with resident and evaluated." Signature "Seen and agree." Signature	"I saw the patient with Resident and agree with Resident's findings and plans as written." Signature
"Discussed with resident." Signature	"I was present with Resident during the history and exam. I discussed the case with Resident and agree with the findings and plan as documented in Resident's note." Signature

Primary Care Exception Rule

The primary care exception rule (PCER) in the teaching physician guidelines allows teaching physicians to bill for services provided by residents under their supervision who have completed at least 6 months of approved graduate medical education (GME).

- To qualify for this exception, services must be provided in a teaching hospital ambulatory care center or clinic. If the services are provided outside a hospital, there must be a written agreement with the teaching hospital that includes a contract outlining the payment for the teaching services or written documentation that the services will be "donated." In general, this exception cannot be applied in a private physician's office.
- Preventive medicine visit codes are not included in the Medicare exception at this time. Some state Medicaid programs have granted the exemption for preventive medicine services to established patients.
- No more than 4 residents can be supervised at a time by a teaching physician. This may include residents with fewer than 6 months in a GME-approved residency program in the mix of 4 residents under the teaching physician's supervision. However, the teaching physician must be physically present for the critical or key portions of services furnished by the resident with fewer than 6 months in a GME-approved residency program. That is, the primary care exception does not apply in the case of the resident with fewer than 6 months in a GME-approved residency program.
- Patients seen should consider this practice as their primary location for health care.
- The teaching physician
  - ❖ Must be physically present in the clinic or office and immediately available to the residents and may not have other responsibilities (including supervising other personnel or seeing patients).
  - ❖ Must review the care provided (history, findings on physical examination, assessment, and treatment plan) during or immediately after each visit. The documentation must reflect the teaching physician's participation in the review and direction of the services performed.

AAP commentary is indicated by green tint and italic sans serif body type.

❖ May only report codes **99201–99203** for new patient visits or **99211–99213** for established patient visits. If a higher-level E/M service is necessary and performed, the teaching physician must personally participate in the care of the patient as outlined in the guidelines. As always, code selection is based on the E/M code descriptions and documentation guidelines.

The AAP continues to advocate for the preventive medicine service codes (99381–99385 and 99391–99395) to be included under the PCER. In some instances, state Medicaid plans already consider preventive medicine service codes as part of their primary care exception, so be sure to check with your payers. Look for updates in AAP Pediatric Coding Newsletter™.

You can access the updated guidelines addressing the PCER at www.aap.org/cfp (access code AAPCFP24) or https://www.cms.gov/Regulations-and-Guidance/Guidance/Transmittals/downloads/R2247CP.pdf.

> |||||||| **Coding Pearl** ||||||||
>
> Preventive medicine visit codes are not included in the Medicare primary care exception rule at this time despite continued advocacy from the American Academy of Pediatrics.

Example

➤ The teaching physician is supervising the resident in the clinic under the primary care exception. A child is diagnosed with acute otitis media. An expanded-level history and physical examination are performed with MDM of low complexity.

Unacceptable	Acceptable
Countersignature	"I reviewed Resident's note and agree with Resident's findings and plans as written." Signature "I reviewed Resident's note and agree but will refer to ENT for consultation." Signature

Reporting Procedures Under Teaching Physician Guidelines

Refer to Chapter 19, Common Surgical Procedures and Sedation in Facility Settings, for the teaching physician guidelines for billing surgical, high-risk, or other complex procedures.

AAP commentary is indicated by green tint and italic sans serif body type.

Part 2:
Primarily for the Office and Other Outpatient Settings

Part 2: Primarily for the Office and Other Outpatient Settings

Evaluation and Management Services in the Office and Outpatient Clinics

Contents

Chapter 7: Evaluation and Management Services in the Office and Outpatient Clinics

Codes discussed in this chapter are used chiefly in the office and outpatient clinic settings. Other sites of service for which office and other outpatient evaluation and management (E/M) and consultation codes are reported include an urgent care facility, hospital observation by other than the attending physician, and care in the emergency department (ED) in conjunction with care by an ED physician. See the E/M Services in Urgent Care Facilities section later in this chapter for more information on reporting E/M services in urgent care settings.

Selecting the Appropriate Evaluation and Management (E/M) Codes

This chapter includes tables with descriptions of the required key components (ie, history, physical examination, medical decision-making [MDM], and, if appropriate, time) for all the E/M services that are reported in the office and outpatient clinic settings. **Table 7-1** provides the key components and specific details on required elements within each level of history and physical examination (eg, problem focused, expanded) and MDM (eg, straightforward, moderate) of an E/M code. Refer to this table when using some of the other tables in this chapter. These tables can be downloaded at www.aap.org/cfp (access code AAPCFP24).

Note: All E/M code descriptors and their specific instructions exclude references to provider/professional type, whenever not essential. When the word "physician" is included in the code descriptor, it includes qualified health care professionals (QHPs).

See Chapter 6, Evaluation and Management Documentation Guidelines, for a detailed description of the guidelines and components of E/M services with documentation requirements and tips.

> |||||||| **Coding Pearl** ||||||||
>
> Although much of the focus of this chapter is on selecting a level of service based on key components documented, medical necessity is the overarching criteria for determining which level of service is reported. Physicians should not select a code based on performance and documentation of history or examination components that were not clinically indicated by the nature of the patient presentation.

Office and Other Outpatient Visits (99201–99205, 99211–99215)

Codes **99201–99205** and **99212–99215** are reported when services are provided in an outpatient setting (eg, physician office, outpatient hospital clinic, walk-in urgent care clinic, health department clinic).

* The place of service code (eg, **11**, office; **22**, on campus—outpatient hospital) is used to indicate whether office or other outpatient services are provided in a facility or non-facility setting. (See Chapter 4, The Business of Medicine: Working With Current and Emerging Payment Systems, for more information on place of service codes.)

> |||||||| **Coding Pearl** ||||||||
>
> When reporting office or other outpatient services, place of service codes may affect payment. Never report place of service code **11** (office) for care in a hospital clinic or other facility.

* Codes are subcategorized into *new patient* and *established patient* visits.
* New patient E/M visits (**99201–99205**) require performance and documentation of all 3 key components unless billing based on time. The patient must also meet the *Current Procedural Terminology (CPT®)* criteria for a new patient. See Chapter 6, Evaluation and Management Documentation Guidelines, for information on new versus established patient.
* Established patient visits (**99212–99215**) are reported based on the performance and documentation of 2 of the 3 key components unless billing based on time. Some payers require selection of the level of service based on the performed and documented MDM and either history or examination.
* Code **99211** is used to report E/M services that do not require a physician's presence but are usually performed incident to the physician. (See Chapter 13, Allied Health and Clinical Staff Services, for more information on incident-to services.) There are no required key components. Physicians and other QHPs should not report **99211** for face-to-face encounters with patients.

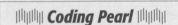

Chapter 7: Evaluation and Management Services in the Office and Outpatient Clinics

Chapter 7: Evaluation and Management Services in the Office and Outpatient Clinics

Table 7-1. Evaluation and Management Key Components				
History (must meet or exceed HPI, ROS, and PFSH)	**Problem Focused** HPI: 1–3 elements ROS: 0 PFSH: 0	**Expanded Problem Focused** HPI: 1–3 elements ROS: 1 PFSH: 0	**Detailed** HPI: 4+ elements or status of 3 chronic or inactive conditions ROS: 2–9 PFSH: 1	**Comprehensive** HPI: 4+ elements or status of 3 chronic or inactive conditions ROS: 10+ PFSH: 2 (established patient) or 3 (new patient)
Physical Examination	**Problem Focused** 1995: 1 body area/organ system 1997: Performance and documentation of 1–5 elements identified by a bullet (●) in ≥1 areas or systems	**Expanded Problem Focused** 1995: Limited examination—affected body area/organ system and other related areas/systems 1997: Performance and documentation of at least 6 elements identified by a bullet (●) in ≥1 areas or systems	**Detailed** 1995: Extended examination—affected body area(s) and other symptomatic or related organ system(s) 1997: Performance and documentation of at least 2 elements identified by a bullet (●) in at least 6 areas or systems or at least 12 elements identified by a bullet (●) in at least 2 areas or systems	**Comprehensive** 1995: 8+ organ systems or complete examination of a single organ system 1997: <u>Multisystem examination</u>—9 systems or areas with performance of all elements identified by a bullet (●) in each area/system examined Documentation of at least 2 elements identified by a bullet (●) of each area(s) or system(s) <u>Single organ system examination</u>—Performance of all elements identified by a bullet (●) and documentation of every element in box with shaded border and at least 1 element in box with unshaded border
Medical Decision-making (must meet 2 of diagnoses/ options, data, and risk)	**Straightforward** Presenting problem: Usually self-limited or minor severity # diagnoses/ options: Minimal Data: Minimal Risk: Minimal	**Low Complexity** Presenting problem: Usually moderate severity # diagnoses/options: Limited Data: Limited Risk: Low	**Moderate Complexity** Presenting problem: Usually moderate to high severity # diagnoses/ options: Multiple Data: Moderate Risk: Moderate	**High Complexity** Presenting problem: Usually moderate to high severity # diagnoses/options: Extensive Data: Extensive Risk: High

Abbreviations: HPI, history of present illness; PFSH, past, family, and social history; ROS, review of systems.

- Any service with its own code (eg, immunizations, laboratory procedures) should be reported in addition to E/M visit codes when performed as a separate service and documented. (Modifiers may be necessary; see Chapter 2, Modifiers and Coding Edits, for more information.) See also discussion of E/M services on the same date as a procedure in Chapter 10, Surgery, Infusion, and Sedation in the Outpatient Setting.
- Time may be used as the key controlling factor in the selection of the code, when appropriate, in lieu of key components. To report based on time, counseling and/or coordination of care must account for more than 50% of the face-to-face time with the patient.
  - ❖ Billing based on time requires documentation of the total face-to-face time (may be approximate) and the percentage or number of minutes spent in counseling and/or coordination of care. For example, "I spent 40 minutes with the patient; 25 minutes was spent in discussion of the diagnosis of asthma and management options, as documented above."
  - ❖ CPT® instructs that time is met when the midpoint is passed. In other words, select the code where the typical time is closest to the total face-to-face time of service. Other payers may require that the typical time specified for a service be met or exceeded.

Example

> **An established patient office visit includes 20 minutes of physician face-to-face time with more than 50% spent in counseling.** The actual time of 20 minutes falls exactly at the midpoint between code 99213 (typical time 15 minutes) and code 99214 (typical time 25 minutes), so the midpoint was not passed. The appropriate code for this encounter would be 99213. If the office visit was 21 minutes of physician face-to-face time, code 99214 would be the appropriate code.
>
> See Chapter 1, The Basics of Coding, for specific guidelines to follow when reporting an E/M service based on time.

Use **Table 7-2** to guide you in the selection of the appropriate codes in the following clinical examples. Clinical vignettes are provided to illustrate correct coding applications and are not intended to offer advice on the practice of medicine.

The examples included here and throughout the chapter are based on the 1995 E/M documentation guidelines. Medical decision-making is listed before history and physical examination because some payers require that the level of MDM be 1 of the 2 key components met to support the level of service for an established patient encounter. See the Examination in the Evaluation and Management Guidelines: 1995 or 1997 box later in this chapter for an example based on the 1997 guidelines.

> ### ~ More From the AAP ~
>
> Read more about reporting evaluation and management services based on time in the March 2016 *AAP Pediatric Coding Newsletter*™ at http://coding.aap.org (subscription required).

Examples

> **A 2-year-old patient is seen with chief complaint of vomiting and diarrhea.**
>
> *History:* Vomited twice and watery diarrhea 3 times since last evening; a little fussy. No fever. Drank some juice this morning but ate only a few bites of oatmeal. Voided at least twice this morning, but less than usual output.
>
> History of present illness (HPI), including
> - Duration: Since last evening
> - Quality: Watery diarrhea
> - Associated signs/symptoms: A little fussy; vomiting with diarrhea
>
> Review of 3 systems
> - Constitutional: No fever
> - Gastrointestinal: Drank some juice but ate only a few bites of oatmeal
> - Urinary: Voided at least twice this morning, but less than usual output

Table 7-2. Office Visit Codes

New Patient Key Components (For a description of key components, see Table 7-1.)
3 of 3 key components must be performed to at least the degree specified for the code.

CPT® Code/Time[a]	Medical Decision-making	History (chief complaint required for each level)	1995 Examination[b]
99201 10 min	Straightforward PP: Usually self-limited or minor severity	HPI: 1–3; ROS: 0; PFSH: 0	1 body area/ system
99202 20 min	Straightforward PP: Usually low to moderate severity	HPI: 1–3; ROS: 1; PFSH: 0	2–7 limited
99203 30 min	Low complexity PP: Usually moderate severity	HPI: ≥4 or 3 chronic conditions; ROS: 2–9; PFSH: 1/3	2–7 detailed
99204 45 min	Moderate complexity PP: Usually moderate to high severity	HPI: ≥4 or 3 chronic conditions; ROS: ≥10; PFSH: 3/3	≥8 body areas/ systems
99205 60 min	High complexity PP: Usually moderate to high severity	HPI: ≥4 or 3 chronic conditions; ROS: ≥10; PFSH: 3/3	≥8 body areas/ systems

Established Patient Key Components (For a description of key components, see Table 7-1.)
2 of 3 key components must be performed to at least the degree specified for the code. Some payers may require medical decision-making as 1 of the 2 components performed and documented.

CPT® Code/Time[a]	Medical Decision-making	History (chief complaint required for each level)	1995 Examination[b]
99211 5 min	Not required; may not require the presence of a physician PP: Usually minimal severity	Not required	Not required
99212 10 min	Straightforward PP: Usually self-limited or minor severity	HPI: 1–3; ROS: 0; PFSH: 0	1 body area/ system
99213 15 min	Low complexity PP: Usually moderate severity	HPI: 1–3; ROS: 1; PFSH: 0	2–7 limited
99214 25 min	Moderate complexity PP: Usually moderate to high severity	HPI: ≥4 or 3 chronic conditions; ROS: 2–9; PFSH: 1/3	2–7 detailed
99215 40 min	High complexity PP: Usually moderate to high severity	HPI: ≥4 or 3 chronic conditions; ROS: ≥10; PFSH: 2/3	≥8 body areas/ symptoms

Abbreviations: CPT, Current Procedural Terminology; *HPI, history of present illness; PFSH, past, family, and social history; PP, presenting problem; ROS; review of systems.*

[a] *Typical time is an average and represents a range of times that may be higher or lower depending on clinical circumstances. The presenting problem is considered to be a contributory factor and does not need to be present to the degree specified.*

[b] *Number of body areas or organ systems examined; see **Table 7-1** for details and examination requirements based on 1997 documentation guidelines.*

Physical examination: 4 organ systems documented (a limited examination of the affected body area or organ system and other symptomatic or related organ system[s])

- Constitutional
- Cardiovascular
- Respiratory
- Gastrointestinal

Assessment/plan: Acute noninfectious gastroenteritis. Mother is told to give fluids to patient, watch for dehydration, and call if no improvement or condition worsens.

MDM: Low complexity (acute uncomplicated illness and low risk) *History:* Expanded problem focused (brief HPI and review of 3 systems) *Physical examination:* Expanded problem focused (a limited examination of the affected body area or organ system and other symptomatic or related organ system[s])	***International Classification of Diseases, 10th Revision, Clinical Modification (ICD-10-CM)*** **K52.9** (noninfectious gastroenteritis and colitis, unspecified)
	CPT® **New Patient** **Established Patient** **99202** **99213**

Teaching Point: The level of service for new patient visits must be supported by all 3 key components, while the level of service for the established patient encounter requires meeting 2 of 3 key components. Although low-complexity MDM would support code **99203**, detailed history and examination are required to support this level of service. Although only 2 of 3 key components are required to support **99213**, all 3 were met.

Physicians participating in quality initiatives may elect to additionally report *CPT* Category II performance measure codes to indicate specific elements of care were provided (eg, **2030F**, hydration status documented, normally hydrated, and **4058F**, pediatric gastroenteritis education provided to caregiver). Category II codes are not used for direct fee-for-service payment. For more on Category II codes, see Chapter 3, Coding to Demonstrate Quality and Value.

➤ **The 2-year-old patient from the previous example is seen later the same day by another pediatrician in the same group practice due to continued vomiting and diarrhea and concerns of dehydration.** The physician reviews the documentation from the visit earlier that day and obtains an interval history, including documentation of multiple episodes of vomiting within minutes of fluid intake, lack of appetite, and continued loose, watery stools. Review of systems (ROS) is updated to include 4 additional systems. Past medical history is reviewed, including previous urinary tract infections and up-to-date immunization status. Social and family history is negative for recent illness in family or known infectious contacts at child care. Examination includes constitutional; eyes, ears, nose, and throat; cardiovascular; respiratory; abdomen; and extremities. Urinalysis is performed, and the result is negative. The physician directs a nurse to provide oral rehydration per a time-based rehydration plan and reassess the patient periodically until completed. On completion of the rehydration plan, the physician reevaluates the patient, who is now tolerating fluids and showing overall improvement. The patient is discharged to home from the office. Diagnoses are lethargy and dehydration due to noninfectious gastroenteritis.

Combined key components of the 2 encounters *MDM:* Moderate complexity (established problem worsening with manifestations and moderate risk) *History:* Detailed (≥4 HPI and review of 7 systems; past, family, and social history [PFSH]) *Physical examination:* Detailed (expanded examination of the affected and related organ systems or body areas)	***ICD-10-CM*** **K52.9** (noninfectious gastroenteritis and colitis, unspecified) **E86.0** (dehydration) **R53.83** (other fatigue, lethargy)
	CPT **New Patient** **Established Patient** **99203** **99214**

Teaching Point: The combined work of the 2 encounters is reported as a single E/M service (typically by the physician who provided the greater portion of the service). The level of service is based on the combined history, examination, and MDM of the physicians. If more than 50% of the combined face-to-face time of the 2 encounters was spent in counseling and/or coordination of care, the level of service could be selected based on time (eg, typical time for **99215** is 40 minutes).

Time spent by clinical staff providing oral rehydration services may be separately reportable if the total accumulated clinical staff time for this service is greater than 45 minutes beyond the typical time of the related physician E/M service. See discussion of prolonged clinical staff service codes **99415** and **99416** later in this chapter.

➤ **A 12-year-old boy presents for management of medications prescribed for predominantly hyperactive attention-deficit/hyperactivity disorder (ADHD).** Medication was prescribed 3 weeks earlier.

History: No improvement was seen after starting medication; continues to disrupt class, fidgeting more, and unable to focus on work; occasional trouble sleeping, loss of appetite, and no diarrhea. No changes in his school or home environment.

Behavioral rating scales: Parent National Institute for Children's Health Quality (NICHQ) Vanderbilt ADHD scale is strongly positive for inattention and hyperactivity; teacher NICHQ Vanderbilt scale is also strongly positive for inattention and hyperactivity. Neither rating scale by either observer showed changes from pre-treatment behaviors.

Physical examination: 3 organ systems documented (constitutional [weight, height, and blood pressure documented], cardiovascular, psychiatric [mental status]).

Assessment/plan: New medication is prescribed, old discontinued; follow up in 2 weeks. Twenty-five minutes is spent discussing side effects of the medication, behavior modifications, changes at school, and when psychiatric referral may be needed. Total visit time is 35 minutes.

The physician documents that 35 minutes was spent face-to-face with the child and guardian and 25 minutes of that was spent on counseling. A summary of the issues discussed is documented. Time (35 minutes face-to-face) is the key controlling factor.	**ICD-10-CM** **F90.1** (ADHD, predominantly hyperactive) **CPT®** **New Patient** **Established Patient** **99203 25** (30 minutes) **99215 25** (40 minutes) **96127** × 2 (brief behavioral and emotional assessment, with scoring and documentation, per instrument [2 scales reviewed])

Teaching Point: Because more than 50% of the physician's 35-minute face-to-face time was spent in counseling and/or coordinating care, code selection may be based on time rather than key components. Per *CPT* instruction, when the physician's total face-to-face time falls between the typical times of 2 codes, report the code with the closest typical time. (Some state Medicaid programs may require that the typical time assigned to a code be met or exceeded.)

Health plans may include follow-up care for children aged 6 to 12 years with ADHD in the collection of Healthcare Effectiveness Data and Information Set (HEDIS) measurement. Office visits linked to an *ICD-10-CM* code for ADHD would prompt payer identification of the visit provided within 30 days of when the first ADHD medication was dispensed (performance measure for ADHD). This measure also calls for 2 additional follow-up visits within the 31 to 300 days after start of medication for patients who remain on the medication for at least 210 days. When *ICD-10-CM* and *CPT* codes provide information necessary for measurement, time-consuming manual chart review might be avoided. For more on HEDIS, see Chapter 3, Coding to Demonstrate Quality and Value.

> |||||||| **Coding Pearl** ||||||||
>
> When reporting code **96127**, National Correct Coding Initiative edits may require reporting of 2 units of service per claim line. Modifier **59** is appended to the second claim line to indicate the additional units of service are for separately completed screening instruments.

➤ **A 5-year-old is seen by an office nurse in follow-up to a physician office visit 3 days earlier at which nonbullous impetigo was diagnosed and a topical antibiotic was prescribed.** The area of infection shows improvement, and the child's temperature is normal. Based on the physician's orders, the nurse advises the parents to continue the antibiotic until the skin is clear and completes a form provided by the child's school indicating the child has improved sufficiently to return to class.

History: Here for follow-up of nonbullous impetigo per Dr Good's order. Started antibiotic ointment on Monday evening. Mother reports no fever and feels the sores are healing quickly. Needs form completed for return to school.

Physical assessment: Small area of sores remains. Temperature is 36.8°C (98.2°F).

Plan: Discussed with Dr Good. Mother is told to continue antibiotic ointment until all sores are gone. Form completed. Call if no improvement or condition worsens.

Office or other outpatient visit for the E/M of an established patient that may not require the presence of a physician or other QHP. Usually, the presenting problem(s) is minimal. Typically, 5 minutes are spent performing or supervising these services.	***ICD-10-CM*** **L01.01** (non-bullous impetigo)
	CPT® **99211**

➤ **A 5-year-old is seen by an office nurse in follow-up to a physician office visit 3 days earlier at which nonbullous impetigo was diagnosed and a topical antibiotic was prescribed.** The area of infection shows improvement and the child's temperature is normal, but the nurse is not sure if improvement is sufficient for return to class. The physician provides a face-to-face E/M service and advises the parents to continue the antibiotic until the skin is clear and completes a form provided by the child's school indicating the child has improved sufficiently to return to class.

History: No complaints. No fever. Has followed instructions in using antibiotic ointment.

Physical examination: Small area of sores remains but otherwise healing well with no indication of complications.

Assessment/plan: Resolving impetigo. Instructed patient's mother to continue antibiotic ointment until all sores are gone. Return to school form completed. Call if no improvement or condition worsens.

> **⠀⠀ Coding Pearl ⠀⠀**
>
> Do not code diagnoses documented as "possible" or other similar terms indicating uncertainty. Rather, code the condition(s) to the highest degree of clinical certainty for that encounter/visit, such as symptoms, signs, abnormal test results, or other reason for the visit. In addition, you do not need to have a positive test result to diagnose a condition.

MDM: Straightforward *History:* Problem focused *Physical examination:* Problem focused	***ICD-10-CM*** **L01.01** (non-bullous impetigo)
	CPT **99212**

➤ **A 13-year-old girl is seen with complaints of severe headaches.**

History: Throbbing headaches on left side of face and head a few times over the last few months, each lasting about 24 hours. Has nausea but no vomiting. No family history of migraines; doing well in school; no known allergies. No specific triggers noted. Headaches do not awaken from sleep and intensity does not seem to be increasing. Naproxen and acetaminophen have not been effective.

Review of systems: Last menstrual period 2 weeks ago; no gastrointestinal complaints other than nausea with headaches; appetite normal; no complaints of visual disturbance or eye problems; neurologic normal other than headaches; denies stress, worry, or fatigue and is negative for all other systems.

(History level is comprehensive with chief complaint of severe headaches; extended HPI—location [left side of face and head], duration [about 24 hours], quality [throbbing], duration [over last few months], associated signs and symptoms [nausea, no vomiting], and modifying factors [unrelieved by over-the-counter medication]; complete ROS—systems directly related to problems identified in HPI and all other body systems; and PFSH with one element each of past [no allergies], family [no history of migraines], and social history [doing well in school].)

Physical examination: Detailed examination of the neurologic system with additional 4 organ systems documented.

(The level of physical examination is detailed based on 1995 guidelines requiring an extended examination of the affected body area or organ system [neurologic] and other symptomatic or related organ system[s]. See the Examination in the Evaluation and Management Guidelines: 1995 or 1997 box later in this chapter for examination requirements when using 1997 E/M guidelines.)

Assessment/plan: Headaches, possible migraine. Given headache diary to complete and counseled on triggers and treatment of migraines. Follow-up visit is scheduled.

(The level of MDM is moderate, as the problem is an undiagnosed new problem and the risk is moderate [undiagnosed new problem].)

MDM: Moderate complexity *History:* Comprehensive *Physical examination:* Detailed	**ICD-10-CM** **R51** (headache) **R11.0** (nausea without vomiting)
	CPT® **New Patient** **Established Patient** 99203 99214

Teaching Point: If the physician spent more than 50% of the face-to-face time of this visit counseling the patient and caregiver on questions and concerns (eg, possibility of tumor, indications for imaging studies), the service may be reported based on time spent counseling and/or coordinating care. Documentation should include sufficient detail about the nature of the counseling and/or coordination of care (eg, discussed mother's concerns about possible tumor and lack of indications for imaging or other diagnostic testing) and both the total face-to-face time of the visit and the portion spent in counseling and/or coordination of care (percentage or amount of time).

Telephone Services (99441–99443, 98966–98968)

99441   Telephone E/M service by a physician or other qualified health care professional who may report E/M services provided to an established patient, parent, or guardian not originating from a related E/M service provided within the previous 7 days nor leading to an E/M service or procedure within the next 24 hours or soonest available appointment; 5–10 minutes of medical discussion

99442   11–20 minutes of medical discussion

99443   21–30 minutes of medical discussion

98966   Telephone assessment and management services provided by a qualified nonphysician health care professional to an established patient, parent, or guardian not originating from related assessment and management service provided within the previous 7 days nor leading to an assessment and management service or procedure within the next 24 hours or soonest available appointment; 5–10 minutes of medical discussion

98967   11–20 minutes of medical discussion

98968   21–30 minutes of medical discussion

Telephone services (99441–99443) are non–face-to-face E/M services provided to a patient using the telephone by a physician or other QHP who may report E/M services. Codes 98966–98968 are used to report telephone assessment and management services by qualified nonphysician health care professionals who may not report E/M services.

Guidelines for reporting of telephone assessment and management services (98966–98968) are the same as those for physician and QHP telephone E/M service (99441–99443).

Most payers consider telephone services bundled to other E/M services and will pay for these services. Verify payer guidelines before reporting. Contracts with payers may prohibit billing the patient for services that are denied as bundled.

Examination in the Evaluation and Management Guidelines: 1995 or 1997

The examination of a 13-year-old girl with complaints of severe headache in the example on page 163 indicated that a detailed examination was reported based on the 1995 examination guidelines (an extended examination of the affected body area or organ system [neurologic] and other symptomatic or related organ system[s]). The following examples[a] demonstrate elements of a detailed examination based on the 1997 documentation guidelines using the multisystem or single-organ (neurologic) examination. See Chapter 6, Evaluation and Management Documentation Guidelines, for more on the 1997 examination guidelines.

1997 Multisystem examination: Performance and documentation of at least 2 elements identified by a bullet (●) in at least 6 organ systems or body areas *or* performance and documentation of at least 12 elements identified by a bullet (●) in ≥2 organ systems or body areas

Constitutional
- Temperature, pulse rate and regularity, blood pressure
- General appearance

Eyes
- Examination of pupils and irises (eg, reaction to light and accommodation, size and symmetry)
- Ophthalmoscopic examination of optic discs (eg, size, cup to disc ratio, appearance) and posterior segments (eg, vessel changes, exudates, hemorrhages)

Ears, Nose, Mouth, Throat
- Otoscopic examination of auditory canals and tympanic membranes
- Inspection of nasal mucosa, septum, and turbinates

Neck
- Examination of neck (eg, masses, overall appearance, symmetry, tracheal position, crepitus)

Cardiovascular
- Auscultation of heart with notation of abnormal sounds and murmurs

Gastrointestinal
- Examination of liver and spleen

Musculoskeletal
- Assessment of muscle strength and tone (eg, flaccid, cog wheel, spastic) with notation of any atrophy or abnormal movements

Skin
- Inspection of skin and subcutaneous tissue (eg, rashes, lesions, ulcers)

Neurologic
- Test cranial nerves with notation of any deficits

Psychiatric
- Brief assessment of mental status, including orientation to time, place, and person; recent and remote memory; mood and affect (eg, depression, anxiety, agitation)

1997 Single organ system examination: Performance and documentation of at least 12 elements identified by a bullet (●), whether in a box with a shaded or unshaded border (See guidelines for exceptions for eye and psychiatric examinations.)

Constitutional
- Temperature, pulse rate and regularity, blood pressure
- General appearance

Eyes
- Ophthalmic examination of optic discs and posterior segments

Cardiovascular
- Auscultation of heart with notation of abnormal sounds and murmurs

Musculoskeletal
- Muscle strength in upper and lower extremities
- Muscle tone in upper and lower extremities (eg, flaccid, cog wheel, spastic) with notation of any atrophy or abnormal movements (eg, fasciculation, tardive dyskinesia)

Neurologic
- Orientation
- Attention span
- Concentration
- Language
- Third, fourth, and sixth cranial nerves (eg, pupils, eye movements)
- Test coordination (eg, finger/nose, heel/knee/shin, rapid alternating movements in the upper and lower extremities, evaluation of fine motor coordination in young children)

[a] *Example only; documentation elements may vary. The guidelines were developed for the adult population. Physicians and coders should recognize that different or additional information may be included in the pediatric population (eg, examination of head circumference in children).*

See Chapter 20, Digital Medicine Services: Technology-Enhanced Care Delivery, for information on coding for services provided via digital technology (eg, e-mail, real-time synchronous audio-visual technology).

Examples

➤ **A 6-month-old was seen in the office 3 days ago for treatment of otitis media.** Mother calls to discuss problems with diarrhea. The discussion of antibiotic-associated diarrhea, probiotics, and symptoms that may require change in treatment lasts for 10 minutes.

Code **99441** cannot be reported because it is related to the E/M visit performed within the previous 7 days.

➤ **Mother calls because her 12-year-old has poison ivy after being in the woods 2 days ago.** Physician spends 10 minutes confirming poison ivy and prescribing a treatment plan.

ICD-10-CM	CPT®
L23.7 (allergic contact dermatitis due to plants, except food)	**99441** (physician telephone E/M, 5–10 minutes)

➤ **Father calls to discuss son's anxiety since his mother left for a tour of duty.** Physician spends 20 minutes discussing how the father can help with the child's anxiety.

ICD-10-CM	CPT
F43.22 (adjustment disorder with anxiety) **Z63.31** (absence of family member due to military deployment)	**99442** (physician telephone E/M, 11–20 minutes)

See Chapter 12, Managing Chronic and Complex Conditions, for more information on when telephone services may be separately reported.

Office or Other Outpatient Consultations (99241–99245)

Codes **99241–99245** are used to report consultations provided in the physician's office or in an outpatient or other ambulatory facility, including hospital observation services, home services, domiciliary, rest home, custodial care, or ED. (See Chapter 16, Noncritical Hospital Evaluation and Management Services, to learn the reporting guidelines for inpatient consultations.)

The Medicare program no longer covers consultation codes **99241–99245** but has guidelines for reporting the services with office or outpatient E/M codes **99201–99215**. Check with your state Medicaid program and commercial payers to learn their coding policies regarding consultation codes.

Consultations are defined by *CPT®* as services provided by a physician at the request of another physician or "other appropriate source" to provide advice or opinion about the management or evaluation of a specific problem or to determine whether to accept responsibility for ongoing management of the patient's entire care or for the care of a specific condition/problem. The "other appropriate source" is not explicitly defined in *CPT*. It may mean any interested source (eg, schools, juvenile court, attorney, psychologist, dentist, physician extender, occupational therapist).

Guidelines for reporting consultations include

⚬ A physician or other appropriate source must request the consultation for opinion and/or advice.
Consultations may be requested of a child's primary care physician by other physicians or sources, such as a school counselor or coach.

- Documentation must include
  - The request (written or verbal from the consultant; if verbal, still must be documented).
  - Name of the requesting physician or other appropriate source who requested the consultation.
  - Reason or need for the consultation (advice or opinion requested).
  - Opinion, recommendations, and services performed or ordered.
  - Written report back to the requesting physician or other appropriate source. A copy of the report must be maintained in the medical record. The report may be in letter form, a copy of the progress note, or a completed form (eg, preoperative form, consultation report). In a large group practice with shared medical records, it is acceptable to include the consultant's report as part of the documentation, and a separate letter or report is not required.
  - The requesting physician or other appropriate source must also document the request (even if it is a verbal request) for consultation in his or her patient medical record. This is not required by *CPT*, but some payers have adopted this policy to assist in review of records where it is unclear that consultation (ie, advice or opinion) was requested in lieu of a transfer of care for a particular problem.
- The consultant may initiate diagnostic or therapeutic services at the same or subsequent visit. Any identifiable procedures performed on or after the date of initial consultation (eg, endoscopy, cardiac catheterization, biopsy) should be reported separately.
- The management of the patient remains with the requesting or attending physician and is released in whole or in part only by the written notation of the requesting or attending physician in the medical record.
- Physicians in a group practice can provide consultations at the request of another member of the same practice if they are a different specialty or have an expertise in a specific medical area. For example, you may refer a patient to your partner, who has expertise in the treatment of asthma and is an allergist.
- Consultations for preoperative clearance may be reported when the surgeon requests an opinion and/or advice and a written report is sent to the requesting physician. Be aware of Medicaid program and commercial payer guidelines—some do not allow preoperative clearance consultations.
- Follow-up visits that are initiated by the physician consultant are reported using codes for established patients appropriate to the place of service (office, home, domiciliary, rest home, custodial care).
- If an additional request for an opinion or advice on the same or a new problem is received from the attending physician and documented, the office consultation codes may be used again.
- Consultations mandated by a third party (eg, payer, regulatory authority) are reported with modifier 32.

> **Coding Pearl**
>
> Do not report a consultation code for an encounter requested by a patient or parent/guardian.

Examples

Use **Table 7-3** to determine the appropriate consultation codes in the following examples:

> **A 3-month-old with a right indirect inguinal hernia is seen by the pediatric general surgeon for evaluation of the need for repair at the request of the primary care physician.** A comprehensive history and detailed physical examination are performed.
>
>   *Assessment/plan:* Surgery is scheduled. Patient will have preoperative laboratory testing performed at the primary care physician's office. A letter with these recommendations is sent to the primary care physician.

MDM: Moderate complexity (new problem, laboratory tests ordered, high risk for surgery due to age) *History:* Comprehensive *Physical examination:* Detailed	**ICD-10-CM** **K40.90** (inguinal hernia, without mention of obstruction or gangrene, unilateral or unspecified)
	CPT® **99243** or, if payer does not recognize consultations, **New Patient** **Established Patient** **99203** **99214**

Teaching Point: When a decision for surgery is made during an E/M service on the day before or day of a procedure, it may be necessary to append modifier **57**, decision for surgery, to indicate the service should not be included in the global period for the procedure. (See Chapter 2, Modifiers and Coding Edits, for more information on modifier **57** and the global period for procedures.)

Table 7-3. New or Established Office/Outpatient Consultation Codes (99241–99245)

Key Components (For a description of key components, see Table 7-1.)
3 of 3 key components must be performed to at least the degree specified under the code.

CPT® Code/Timeª	Medical Decision-making	History (chief complaint required for each level)	1995 Examinationᵇ
99241 15 min	Straightforward PP: Usually self-limited or minor	HPI: 1–3; ROS: 0; PFSH: 0	1 body area/ system
99242 30 min	Straightforward PP: Usually low to moderate severity	HPI: 1–3; ROS: 1; PFSH: 0	2–7 limited
99243 40 min	Low complexity PP: Usually moderate severity	HPI: ≥4 or 3 chronic conditions; ROS: 2–9; PFSH: 1/3	2–7 detailed
99244 60 min	Moderate complexity PP: Usually moderate to high severity	HPI: ≥4 or 3 chronic conditions; ROS: ≥10; PFSH: 3/3	≥8 body areas/ systems
99245 80 min	High complexity PP: Usually moderate to high severity	HPI: ≥4 or 3 chronic conditions; ROS: ≥10; PFSH: 3/3	≥8 body areas/ systems

Abbreviations: CPT, Current Procedural Terminology; *HPI, history of present illness; PFSH, past, family, or social history; PP, presenting problem; ROS; review of systems.*

ª *Typical time is an average and represents a range of times that may be higher or lower depending on clinical circumstances. The presenting problem is considered to be a contributory factor and does not need to be present to the degree specified.*

ᵇ *Number of body areas or organ systems examined; see **Table 7-1** for details.*

➤ **A 5-year-old boy is referred from his family physician for opinion and recommendations for the treatment of sickle cell anemia.** A comprehensive history and physical examination are performed. Recent laboratory test results are reviewed, and a recent chest radiograph is independently visualized. The child reports minimal pain and no ED visits in the last year. A written report is sent back to the referring family physician with recommendations of dosage and monitoring of hydroxyurea therapy.

MDM: Moderate complexity (new problem with no additional workup, review of laboratory results and independent visualization of chest radiograph, high risk of prescription drug therapy requiring intensive monitoring for toxicity) *History:* Comprehensive *Physical examination:* Comprehensive	***ICD-10-CM*** D57.1 (sickle cell disease without crisis)
	CPT 99244 or, if payer does not recognize consultations, **New Patient** 99204 **Established Patient** 99215

Teaching Point: If a payer requires MDM as 1 of the 2 key components to support the level of service for an established patient office or other outpatient E/M encounter, moderate-complexity MDM would support code **99214** rather than **99215**. High-complexity MDM would require 2 of the following 3 conditions: new problem with additional workup planned; extended amount and/or complexity of medical records, diagnostic tests, and/or other information that must be obtained, reviewed, and analyzed; or high risk (eg, acute or chronic illness or injuries that may pose a threat to life or bodily function [eg, myocardial infarction, embolus]). Although high risk is supported by monitoring for drug toxicity (blood cell counts related to hydroxyurea therapy), the other 2 elements of MDM are not supportive of high-complexity MDM.

➤ **A 6-year-old is seen at the request of his surgeon for preoperative clearance prior to an adenoidectomy and tonsillectomy.** The child has had 6 episodes of streptococcal tonsillitis in the past 15 months, with one episode that resulted in a peritonsillar abscess that required surgical drainage. He has seasonal allergies and persistent asthma, takes montelukast and inhaled corticosteroids daily, and is allergic to penicillin. A comprehensive history and physical examination are performed and the results of the complete blood cell count and coagulation profile that was ordered by the surgeon are reviewed. The child is determined to be at standard anesthetic risk for the surgery. Medical record documentation includes the request for the consultation, findings, and a copy of the written report that is sent to the requesting physician. Diagnoses are preoperative examination, chronic tonsillitis with history of peritonsillar abscess, and mild persistent asthma.

MDM: Low complexity *History:* Comprehensive *Physical examination:* Comprehensive	**ICD-10-CM** **Z01.818** (preoperative examination, unspecified) **J35.01** (chronic tonsillitis) **Z87.09** (personal history of diseases of respiratory system) **J45.30** (mild persistent asthma, uncomplicated)
	CPT® **99243** or, if payer does not recognize consultations, **New Patient** **Established Patient** **99203** **99214**

Teaching Point: In this scenario, if the patient did not have a chronic (respiratory) problem or other preexisting risk factors, some payers may not allow the consultation. A straightforward preoperative physical examination may not qualify as a consultation. The comprehensive history and physical examination described in this example could be used to support reporting of code **99215** for an established patient based on the *CPT* requirement of 2 of 3 key components. However, physicians should always consider medical necessity (eg, was the level of examination performed reasonable in relation to reason for encounter) and overall complexity of the service when selecting a level of service. Medical decision-making was low for the patient with 3 or more stable conditions, laboratory results reviewed, and elective major surgery planned. Some payers require MDM as 1 of the 2 required components for established patient visits.

> ||||||| *Coding Pearl* |||||||
>
> For patients receiving preoperative evaluations only, sequence first a code from subcategory **Z01.81**, encounter for preprocedural examinations. Assign additional codes for the condition to describe the reason for the surgery and any findings related to the preoperative evaluation.

Reporting to Payers That Follow Medicare Consultation Guidelines

It is important to check with your major payers to determine if they have adopted the Medicare policy or if they have established their own policy and guidelines for reporting consultations. You can access the American Academy of Pediatrics (AAP) position on Medicare consultation policy at www.aap.org/cfp (access code AAPCFP24).

* See Chapter 16, Noncritical Hospital Evaluation and Management Services, for Medicare requirements for reporting consultations performed in the hospital setting.
* Consultations performed on patients in the office or outpatient setting are reported with the office or outpatient E/M codes **99201–99215** to payers that do not accept the consultation codes.
  * If the patient is new to the consulting physician (ie, has not received any face-to-face professional services from the physician or another physician of the same specialty who belongs to the same group practice within the past 3 years), code **99201–99205** is reported based on the performance and documentation of the required key components or time, if appropriate.
  * If the patient does not meet the requirements of a new patient, an established patient office or outpatient E/M code (**99211–99215**) is reported.

☀ If the service is provided in the ED, ED codes **99281–99285** are reported.

☀ The referring physician must document the request for consultation in his or her medical record, and the consulting physician must document the request and communicate the results back to the referring physician.

Coding Conundrum: Consultation or Transfer of Care?

Consultation codes (**99241–99245, 99251–99255**) should not be reported by the physician who has agreed to accept transfer of care (ie, takes over the responsibility of management of the patient's entire care, or the care of a specific condition or problem, at the request of another physician) before an initial evaluation. Consultation codes are appropriate to report if the decision to accept transfer of care cannot be made until after the initial consultation evaluation, regardless of site of service. Any services that constitute transfer of care are reported with the appropriate new or established patient codes for office or other outpatient visits, domiciliary services, rest home services, or home services. The medical record should reflect the transfer of care to the service of the receiving physician.

Examples

Consultation	Transfer of Care
Primary Care Pediatrician to Specialist	**Pediatrician to Endocrinologist**
"Consultation <u>requested for opinion</u> regarding treatment of 8-year-old with multiple joint pain, + rheumatoid factor, limited range of motion, malaise, and fatigue."	*"Please <u>accept ongoing care</u> of type 1 diabetes."* Subsequent to a consultation, the physician accepts the responsibility of ongoing management of the patient or care for the specific condition or problem.
Specialist to Pediatrician	
Written summary of findings and recommended treatment plan for treatment of juvenile idiopathic arthritis sent. Consulting physician is unable to accept the responsibility of ongoing management for the specific condition or problem until he or she has performed an E/M service.	**Endocrinologist to Pediatrician** *"Thank you for referring this patient to us for the management of her type 1 diabetes. Attached for your records is a copy of initial encounter note."* Transferring physician no longer provides care for the management of a patient or for those problems for which another physician has agreed to accept.
Pediatrician to Specialist	
"Consultation requested for consideration of assuming management of juvenile idiopathic arthritis on this 8-year-old patient."	
Specialist to Pediatrician	
Written summary of findings and agreement to assume ongoing care of the problem.	

Critical Care (99291, 99292)

Critical care services provided in the office or outpatient setting are reported with hourly critical care codes (**99291** and **99292**) regardless of the patient's age. If the same patient requires outpatient and inpatient critical care services on the same day, the physician or a physician of the same group and specialty would report his or her services based on where the services were provided as well as the patient's age. See Chapter 18, Critical and Intensive Care, for reporting guidelines.

Example

➤ A 3-year-old girl is seen with complaints of shortness of breath and wheezing at the pediatrician's office. She has moderate persistent childhood asthma. The patient goes into respiratory failure with hypoxia, and vital signs are deteriorating. The physician initiates critical care. An ambulance is called, and the physician continues critical care services until the transport team accepts care of the patient. The total time for critical care services provided in the office was 35 minutes. The patient is admitted to the pediatric intensive care unit at the local university hospital under a pediatric intensivist. The pediatrician provides no more hands-on care for the patient that day and reports outpatient critical care services with a diagnosis of respiratory failure due to status asthmaticus. Documentation includes the critical nature of the patient's condition, the care provided, and the total time spent in critical care dedicated to this patient.

ICD-10-CM	CPT®
J96.01 (acute respiratory failure with hypoxia) J45.42 (moderate persistent asthma with status asthmaticus)	99291 (critical care, first 30–74 minutes)

Teaching Point: If the same physician or physician of the same specialty and group practice provided outpatient and inpatient critical care services on the same calendar date, due to the patient's age, only the per-day critical care code (**99475**, initial inpatient pediatric critical care, per day, for the E/M of a critically ill infant or young child, 2–5 years of age) would be reported. Had the patient been 6 years or older, the time spent in outpatient critical care would be combined with time spent in the inpatient setting.

E/M Services in Urgent Care Facilities

The Centers for Medicare & Medicaid Services describes an *urgent care facility* as a location, distinct from a hospital ED, an office, or a clinic, whose purpose is to diagnose and treat illness or injury for unscheduled, ambulatory patients seeking immediate medical attention. However, *CPT®* does not include codes specific to E/M services provided at an urgent care facility. Office and other outpatient E/M codes (**99201–99215**) are typically reported. The site of service is differentiated from a physician office by the place of service code (eg, **20** for urgent care facility; **11** for office). Some physician practices operate a primary care pediatric practice and an urgent care center in the same location but with different tax identification numbers and insurance contracts for each. Physicians should consult a health care attorney for assistant in establishing an urgent care practice and contracting with payers to cover the additional overhead costs often applicable to urgent care (eg, extended staffing, radiology, procedural services).

Additional codes that may be applicable to E/M services in an urgent care facility include the after-hours service codes discussed later in this chapter and Healthcare Common Procedure Coding System (HCPCS) code **S9088** (services provided in an urgent care center). Code **S9088** is listed in addition to the codes for other services provided. Some urgent care clinics also contract to bill all services under code **S9083** (global fee urgent care centers).

> ||||||||| *Coding Pearl* |||||||||
>
> Urgent care facilities are not emergency departments as defined in *Current Procedural Terminology®* (an organized hospital-based facility for the provision of unscheduled episodic services to patients who present for immediate medical attention and available 24 hours a day.). Codes **99281–99285** are not reported for urgent care evaluation and management services.

It is imperative to know your contractual agreements for coding and billing as an urgent care facility or clinic versus a primary care practice, as rates of payment are typically higher for urgent care facilities and so, too, are patient co-pays. Billing and payment also vary for those urgent care facilities owned by hospitals, and guidance on billing and coding for these locations should be obtained from the hospital's compliance officer or other administrative personnel.

After-hours Services (99050–99060)

Codes **99050–99060** are used to report services that are provided after hours or on an emergency basis and are an adjunct to the basic E/M service provided.

Third-party payers will have specific policies for coverage and payment. Some carriers pay practices for extended hours because they recognize the cost benefit they realize from decreased urgent care and ED visits. Communicate with individual payers to understand their definition or interpretation of the service and their coverage and payment policies. As part of this negotiation and education process, it is important to demonstrate the cost savings recognized by the payer for these adjunct services. If appropriate, more than one adjunct code may be reported on the same day of service (eg, **99058** and **99051**). However, most payers will pay only for the use of a single special services code per encounter and may manually review, question, or deny payment for a claim with multiple after-hours codes.

After-hours service codes are used by physicians or other QHPs (under their state scope of practice and when billing with their own National Provider Identifier) to identify the services that are adjunct to the basic services rendered. These codes

<table>
<tr><td>

* Describe the special circumstances under which a basic procedure is performed.
* Are only reported in addition to an associated basic service (eg, E/M, fracture care).
* Are reported without a modifier appended to the basic service because they only further describe the services provided.

</td><td>

~ More From the AAP ~

For more information on reporting care during atypical office hours, see "Coding for Special Services In and Out of the Office" in the May 2018 *AAP Pediatric Coding Newsletter*™ at https://coding.aap.org (subscription required).

</td></tr>
</table>

99050   Service(s) provided in office at times other than regularly scheduled office hours, or days when the office is normally closed (eg, holidays, Saturday, Sunday), in addition to basic service

* Office hours must be posted. *CPT*® does not define a holiday or posted office hours. While most commonly applied to evening, weekend, or holiday hours, code **99050** could be applied to services provided at the patient request on a weekday provided the office is typically closed on that day.
* Code **99050** is *not* reported when a physician or other QHP is behind schedule and sees patients after posted office hours.
* The service must be requested by the patient, and the physician or other QHP must agree to see the patient.
* Documentation must indicate the time and date of the encounter and the request to be seen outside of normal posted hours.

99051   Service(s) provided in the office during regularly scheduled evening, weekend, or holiday office hours, in addition to basic service

* Regularly scheduled office hours must be posted.
* Documentation must include the time and date of the encounter.
* Evenings and holidays are not defined by *CPT*, but holidays can generally refer to national and/or state holidays, and evenings are generally 6:00 pm and later. Check with payers for coverage and/or ability to bill patients these charges under the health plan contract.

99053   Services(s) provided between 10:00 pm and 8:00 am at 24-hour facility, in addition to basic service
* Documentation must include the time and date of the encounter.
* Use the appropriate place of service code.

99056   Service(s) typically provided in the office, provided out of the office at request of patient, in addition to basic service
* It is not appropriate for an ED physician to report code **99056**.
* Documentation should include the patient's request to be seen outside of the office.

99058   Service(s) provided on an emergency basis in the office, which disrupts other scheduled office services, in addition to basic service
* Report when an office patient's condition, in the clinical judgment of the physician, warrants the physician interrupting care of another patient to deal with the emergency.
* Code **99058** may not be reported when patients are simply fit into the schedule or for walk-ins.
* Document that the patient was seen immediately and the reason for the emergent care.

99060   Service(s) provided on an emergency basis, out of the office, which disrupts other scheduled office services, in addition to basic service
* Documentation should indicate that the physician was called away during scheduled office hours to attend to a patient in another location (eg, ED).

Examples

➤ **A child is seen for severe exacerbation of moderate persistent asthma on a Saturday at 9:00 am.** The child arrives 30 minutes prior to their scheduled time and is immediately taken to an examination room by the triage nurse, and the physician disrupts his schedule to see the child urgently. The office is open on Saturday mornings from 8:00 am to 12:00 noon.

ICD-10-CM	CPT®
J45.41 (moderate persistent asthma with acute exacerbation)	99201–99215 (new or established office E/M) 99058 (service provided on an emergency basis in office, disrupting other scheduled services) 99051 (service provided in office during regularly scheduled weekend hours)

Teaching Point: If the Saturday hours were for walk-in visits only (ie, no scheduled appointments), code **99058** would not be reported. Note that if the patient is admitted to observation or inpatient hospital care on the same date by the same physician or a physician or other QHP of the same specialty and same group practice, all services on the same date are included in the code selection for initial observation or initial hospital care.

➤ **A pediatric clinic offers urgent care appointments 3 evenings a week with staffing by nonphysician qualified health care professionals (ie, nurse practitioners, physician assistants) working under general supervision.** A patient who has been seen at the clinic by Dr A within the last year is seen in the evening clinic by a nurse practitioner who documents an expanded problem-focused history and examination with low-complexity MDM with diagnosis of upper respiratory infection.

ICD-10-CM	CPT
J06.9 (acute upper respiratory infection, unspecified)	99213 (established office E/M) 99051 (service provided in office during regularly scheduled weekend hours)

Teaching Point: Because the office offers regularly scheduled evening hours, code **99051** is reported. The patient is established because *CPT* instructs that QHPs are considered to be of the same specialty as the physicians with whom they work in a group practice.

Prolonged Services

Prolonged Service With Direct Patient Contact (99354, 99355)

+99354   Prolonged evaluation and management or psychotherapy service(s) (the service beyond the typical service time) in the office or other outpatient setting requiring direct patient contact; first hour

+99355   each additional 30 minutes

Prolonged service codes **99354** and **99355** are used to report 30 minutes or more of a physician's or QHP's prolonged face-to-face E/M service provided on the same date as designated office or other E/M services that have a typical or designated time published in *CPT,* in conjunction with psychotherapy of 60 minutes or more (**90837**), or in conjunction with family psychotherapy (conjoint psychotherapy) (with patient), 50 minutes (**90847**).

Code **99354** and **99355** may *not* be reported with initial- or subsequent-day observation care services (**99218–99220** and **99224–99226**). The American Medical Association has clarified that although observation care services are performed in an "outpatient" setting, intraservice times for the observation care codes are defined as unit or floor time rather than face-to-face time as required in the office or outpatient setting. Chapter

16, Noncritical Hospital Evaluation and Management Services, addresses reporting prolonged services performed in the observation and inpatient hospital setting (**99356**, **99357**).

Here are guidelines for reporting direct (face-to-face) physician or other QHP prolonged services when performed in the office or outpatient setting.

- Use codes **99354** and **99355** in conjunction with E/M codes **99201–99215**, **99241–99245**, **99324–99337**, and **99341–99350** or psychotherapy codes **90837** (psychotherapy, 60 minutes with patient and/or family member) and **90847** (family psychotherapy [conjoint psychotherapy] [with patient present], 50 minutes).
- Only the time spent face-to-face between the physician or other QHP and the patient/family may be reported.
- Time does not have to be continuous but is reported for services provided in a calendar day.
- Reported with any level E/M service that is assigned a typical time.
- When an E/M service is reported using time as the key or controlling factor (>50% of the total face-to-face time was spent in counseling and/or coordination of care), prolonged service can be reported only when the prolonged service exceeds 30 minutes beyond the highest level of E/M service (eg, **99205**, **99245**).
- The start and stop times of and medical necessity for the service must be documented.
- The first-hour prolonged service code (**99354**) is reported for the total duration of prolonged service of 30 (minimum) to 74 minutes' duration on a given day of service. Prolonged service of less than 30 minutes is included in the E/M service performed (eg, **99203**) and may not be reported separately (**Table 7-4**).
- Each additional 30 minutes beyond the first hour (**99355**) is reported. Code **99355** may be used to report the final 15 to 30 minutes of prolonged service on a given date.
- Less than 15 minutes beyond the first hour or less than 15 minutes beyond the final 30 minutes is not reported separately.
- Time spent providing separately reported services/procedures (eg, inhalation therapy) is not counted toward the prolonged service time.
- Codes for prolonged service by a physician or QHP are never reported in conjunction with prolonged service provided by clinical staff (**99415**, **99416**).

> ||||||||||| **Coding Pearl** |||||||||||
>
> Codes **99354** and **99355** may not be reported with initial- or subsequent-day observation care services (**99218–99220** and **99224–99226**). Refer to the inpatient/observation setting prolonged services codes (**99356**, **99357**) in Chapter 16.

Table 7-4 illustrates time requirements for reporting **99354** and **99355** and prolonged service before and/or after direct patient contact (**99358**, **99359**).

Table 7-4. How to Code Prolonged Services (Office or Outpatient)

Total Duration of Prolonged Services, min (Time begins after typical time of related E/M service.)	Code(s)
<30	Not reported separately
30–74	**99354** or **99358** × 1 (First hour includes 30–74 min beyond the typical time of the related E/M service.)
75–104	**99354** or **99358** × 1 (first 74 min) AND **99355** or **99359** × 1 (75–104 min)
≥105 (≥1 h 45 min)	**99354** or **99358** × 1 (first 74 min) AND **99355** or **99359** × 2 (1 unit for 75–104 min and 1 for 105–134 min) or more for each additional 30 or final 15–30 min

Abbreviation: E/M, evaluation and management.

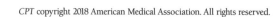

Examples

➤ **A 9-month-old previously healthy infant is seen in follow-up for failure to gain weight and increasing irritability with recurrent bouts of constipation.** A comprehensive history and detailed physical examination are performed. Medical decision-making is moderate. Because of a family history of gluten intolerance, the physician wants to refer the child to a pediatric gastroenterologist. The parents are resistant to the referral. A total of 35 minutes was spent providing the key components of the face-to-face E/M service and another 30 minutes was spent counseling the parents.

Office/outpatient visit Prolonged service of 30–74 minutes	*ICD-10-CM* **R62.51** (failure to thrive, child) **K59.00** (constipation, unspecified) **R45.4** (irritability and anger)
	CPT® **99214** (25 minutes typical time) **99354** (additional 40 minutes)

Teaching Point: The total face-to-face time of this visit was 65 minutes, with 30 minutes spent counseling. Because the time spent counseling does not exceed 50% of the total face-to-face time, the E/M is not reported based on time. Code **99214** is supported by the comprehensive history, detailed physical examination, and moderate MDM. Code **99354** is supported by the prolonged 40 minutes of face-to-face service that extended beyond the typical time of 25 minutes assigned to code **99214**.

➤ **A 9-month-old previously healthy infant is seen in follow-up for failure to gain weight and increasing irritability with recurrent bouts of constipation.** A comprehensive history and detailed physical examination are performed. Medical decision-making is moderate. Because of a family history of gluten intolerance, the physician wants to refer the infant to a pediatric gastroenterologist. The parents are resistant to the referral. A total of 35 minutes was spent providing the face-to-face E/M service and another 40 minutes was spent counseling the parents.

Office/outpatient visit Prolonged service of 30–74 minutes	*ICD-10-CM* **R62.51** (failure to thrive, child) **K59.00** (constipation, unspecified) **R45.4** (irritability and anger)
	CPT® **99215** (40 minutes typical time) **99354** (additional 35 minutes)

Teaching Point: The total face-to-face time spent by the physician was 75 minutes, with more than half spent in counseling and/or coordination of care. Code **99215** with a typical time of 40 minutes may be reported using time spent counseling as the key or controlling factor. The face-to-face time exceeds the typical time of 40 minutes and supports 1 unit of prolonged service with direct patient contact. When an E/M service is reported using time as the key or controlling factor (>50% of the total face-to-face time was spent in counseling and/or coordination of care), prolonged service can be reported only when the prolonged service exceeds 30 minutes beyond the highest level of E/M service (eg, **99205**, **99245**).

➤ **A 6-year-old established patient is seen for acute exacerbation of mild persistent asthma.** An expanded problem-focused history and physical examination are performed, and MDM is moderately complex. Pulse oximetry is performed and indicative of moderate asthma exacerbation. The patient receives 2 nebulizer treatments and is reexamined by the physician after each treatment. The physician spends a total of 20 minutes providing face-to-face care. The child returns later that afternoon and is examined. Two additional

Chapter 7: Evaluation and Management Services in the Office and Outpatient Clinics

nebulizer treatments are administered. The physician documents the initial care, each subsequent reevaluation following treatments, the subsequent care, the assessment, and the plan. A total of 80 minutes is spent in face-to-face E/M services (not including the time spent providing nebulizer treatments).

Office/outpatient visit Prolonged service of 30 minutes	**ICD-10-CM** **J45.31** (acute exacerbation of mild persistent asthma)
	CPT **99214** (25 minutes average time) **99354** (additional 55 minutes) **94640 76** × 4 (nebulizer treatments) **94760** (noninvasive ear or pulse oximetry for oxygen saturation; single determination)

Teaching Point: Time spent performing separately reported services, such as nebulizer treatments, is not counted toward the time of prolonged E/M service. The initial 25 minutes of service is included in code **99214**; prolonged service time is counted from that point forward (ie, it takes a total time of at least 55 minutes to report prolonged service in conjunction with code **99214**). Code **99355** would be additionally reported when time reaches 75 minutes or more beyond the 25 minutes assigned to **99214**.

CPT stipulates that modifier **76** (repeat procedure) be used to report multiple nebulizer treatments. At time of publication, Medicaid National Correct Coding Initiative policy does not allow for the reporting of multiple **94640** codes for the same encounter.

Prolonged Service Without Direct Patient Contact (99358, 99359)

99358   Prolonged evaluation and management service before and/or after direct patient care; first hour

+99359   each additional 30 minutes (Use in conjunction with code **99358**.)

Prolonged service without direct patient contact (ie, non–face-to-face) is reported when a physician provides prolonged service that does not involve face-to-face care. The prolonged service must relate to a service and patient where direct (face-to-face) patient care has occurred or will occur and to ongoing patient management. Only time spent by a physician or other QHP may be counted toward the time of prolonged service. Prolonged service of less than 30 minutes on a given date is not separately reported. Report code **99359** for 15 or more minutes beyond the first hour or the last full 30-minute period of prolonged service. See Chapter 12, Managing Chronic and Complex Conditions, for more information and another coding example.

Examples

➤ **A child is seen in the physician's office with several months of recurring ill-defined symptoms.** Tests are ordered. On a later date, when the physician receives the test results, she spends 30 minutes reviewing the results in light of the patient's signs and symptoms and researching options for further investigating the cause of the patient's symptoms. Code **99358** may be reported based on *CPT®* instruction. The date of service is the date that the physician reviews the results and researches further potential causes for the patient's symptoms. Unless directed by a payer, it is not necessary to submit charges for prolonged service without direct patient contact on the same claim as a face-to-face service.

➤ **A child is seen in the pediatrician's office following hospital discharge.** The child has Down syndrome with recurrent pneumonia, asthma, and gastroesophageal reflux. The face-to-face time of the visit (30 minutes) is predominantly spent in counseling the mother on the need for follow-up with a pulmonologist, a gastroenterologist, and an immunologist. The next day, the pediatrician spends 35 minutes calling each of the subspecialty physicians to provide history and arrange referrals. An additional 5 minutes is spent on the phone with the child's mother advising of the referrals made and answering questions about ongoing care.

Mother will follow up with the pediatrician in 1 week. Code **99214** is reported for the face-to-face visit, and code **99358** is reported for the pediatrician's time spent in non–face-to-face prolonged service on the next day.

Prolonged Clinical Staff Service (99415, 99416)

+99415   Prolonged clinical staff service (the service beyond the typical service time) during an evaluation and management service in the office or outpatient setting, direct patient contact with physician supervision; first hour

+99416   each additional 30 minutes

Codes **99415** and **99416** are used to report 45 minutes or more of clinical staff time spent face-to-face providing care to a patient under the supervision of a physician or other QHP who has provided an office or other outpatient E/M service at the same session. *Never report both* prolonged service by a physician or other QHP (**99354, 99355**) and prolonged clinical staff services together. Codes **99415** and **99416** were assigned relative value units (RVUs) based only on clinical staff's intraservice time, as the preservice and post-service times were considered to be included in the value of the related E/M service. Relative value units (non-facility practice expense only) assigned are 0.27 for **99415** and 0.13 for **99416**.

The following guidelines apply to reporting of prolonged clinical staff services:

* Prolonged clinical staff services are reported only in conjunction with E/M services in the office or other outpatient setting. Report **99415** and **99416** in addition to office or other outpatient E/M codes **99201–99215**.
* Supervision must be provided by a physician or other QHP during the provision of prolonged clinical staff services.
* Prolonged clinical staff services are reported only when the face-to-face time spent by clinical staff is 45 minutes or more beyond the typical time of the related E/M service on the same date. (See **Table 7-2** for typical times assigned to office and other outpatient services.)
* Do not report prolonged service of less than 45 minutes beyond the typical time of the related E/M service.
* The total time of and medical necessity for the service must be documented.
* Time spent providing separately reported services, such as intravenous medication administration or inhalation treatment, is not counted toward the time of prolonged service.
* It is not required that the clinical staff time be continuous, but each episode of face-to-face time should be documented.
* Report code **99416** for each additional 30 minutes of clinical staff time beyond the first hour and for the last 15 to 30 minutes of prolonged clinical staff service. Do not report **99416** for less than 15 minutes beyond the first hour or last 30-minute period.

Table 7-5 shows the time requirements for reporting codes **99415** and **99416**.

Table 7-5. How to Code Prolonged Clinical Staff Services

Total Duration of Prolonged Services, min	Code(s)
<45	Not reported separately
45–74	**99415** × 1 (First hour includes 45–74 min beyond the typical time of the related E/M service.)
75–104	**99415** × 1 (first 45–74 min) AND **99416** × 1 (from 75–104 min beyond typical time of related E/M service)
≥105 (≥1 h 45 min)	**99415** × 1 (first 45–74 min) AND **99416** × 2 (1 unit for 75–104 min and 1 unit for 105–134 min) or more for each additional 30 min or last period of 15–30 min

Abbreviation: E/M, evaluation and management.

Examples

➤ **A child is seen for diarrhea and concerns of dehydration.** The physician diagnoses moderate dehydration due to viral gastroenteritis. Oral rehydration is ordered. The physician completes her documentation and selects code **99214** for service to this established patient. The physician remains in the office suite while a nurse delivers and monitors a time-based oral rehydration plan using an electrolyte solution. The nurse's total direct care time is 2 hours. The first 25 minutes are included in the practice expense of the physician service (**99214**). The additional 95 minutes following the physician's service are reported as prolonged clinical staff service.

E/M service by physician Prolonged clinical staff time	**ICD-10-CM** **A08.4** (viral intestinal infection, unspecified) **E86.0** (dehydration)
	CPT® **99214** (typical time of 25 minutes) **99415** × 1 (first hour) and **99416** × 1 (final 30-minute period)

Teaching Point: *CPT* instructs that prolonged clinical staff time begins 45 minutes after the typical time of the E/M service provided by the physician. In this scenario, the typical time of the physician service is 25 minutes, so prolonged clinical staff time is not reported until clinical staff have spent at least 70 minutes in face-to-face patient care. The final 5 minutes beyond the last 30-minute period reported with code **99416** is not separately reported, as only time of 15 to 30 minutes beyond the previous period is reported.

➤ **A new patient who has been vomiting for 2 days is seen in the physician's office.** After evaluation by a physician, she is given antipyretics and fluids and then monitored and reexamined by clinical staff for a total face-to-face clinical staff time of 90 minutes. At the end of 90 minutes, the physician returns to the examination room and provides final instruction to the mother before releasing the child. The physician service includes a comprehensive history and examination with moderate-complexity MDM (**99204** based on key components). Physician face-to-face time was 35 minutes, with 10 minutes spent in counseling and coordination of care.

E/M service by physician Prolonged clinical staff time	**ICD-10-CM** **K52.9** (gastroenteritis, unspecified)
	CPT® **99204** (typical time of 45 minutes) **99415** × 1 (first hour)

Teaching Point: Prolonged service by clinical staff under physician supervision is reported rather than the physician's prolonged service, as the physician's face-to-face time did not exceed the typical time of code **99204** (established based on key components).

➤ **A physician provides treatment to an established patient with acute exacerbation of moderate persistent asthma.** Over the course of 2 hours, the patient is given fluids (oral) for mild dehydration and oxygen as needed, oral steroids, and 3 inhaled bronchodilators. Documentation supports a detailed history, detailed examination, and moderate-complexity MDM and total face-to-face time by the physician of 65 minutes. Clinical staff also document 60 minutes of direct patient care (eg, providing nebulizer treatments) following the physician's E/M service.

E/M service by physician Prolonged physician service	*ICD-10-CM* **J45.41** (acute exacerbation of moderate persistent asthma) **E86.0** (dehydration)
	CPT® **99214** (typical time of 25 minutes) **99354** (additional 40 minutes) **94640 76** × 3 (nebulizer treatments)

Teaching Point: The physician's service described includes code **99214**, office or other outpatient encounter, and 1 unit of prolonged service with direct patient contact (**99354**). Prolonged clinical staff service is not reported on the same date as prolonged service by a physician or QHP, and time spent providing separately reported services (eg, nebulizer treatment) is not included in prolonged service time.

Supplies related to services such as nebulizer treatment are included in the practice expense RVUs assigned to each code. If a payer does not base payment on RVUs, supplies may be separately reported with code **99070** (supplies and materials [except spectacles], provided by the physician or other QHP over and above those usually included with the office visit or other services rendered [list drugs, trays, supplies, or materials provided]) or specific HCPCS codes (eg, **A7003**, administration set, with small volume nonfiltered pneumatic nebulizer, disposable).

E/M Services and Care of Children With Chronic Medical Conditions

As electronic communications and adoption of the principles of the medical home have increased, so has the need for codes that capture services beyond the traditional face-to-face visit. See Chapter 12, Managing Chronic and Complex Conditions, for information on reporting E/M services provided to patients with chronic and/or complex health conditions. Chapter 12 includes information on services such as

- Chronic care management (**99487, 99489, 99490**)
- Transitional care management services (**99495** and **99496**)
- Medical team conferences (**99366–99368**)
- Care plan oversight (**99339, 99340**; **99374–99380**)

See also Chapter 20, Digital Medicine Services: Technology-Enhanced Care Delivery, for information on telemedicine services and Chapter 13, Allied Health and Clinical Staff Services, for information on services provided by nonphysician health care providers (eg, psychologist, nutritionist).

Continuum Models for Otitis Media, Attention-Deficit/Hyperactivity Disorder, and Asthma

Continuum Model for Otitis Media			
Code selection at any level above 99211 may be based on time when documentation states that more than 50% of the total face-to-face time of the encounter is spent in counseling and/or coordination of care. Select the code with the typical time closest to the total face-to-face time.			
CPT® Code Vignette	**History**	**Physical Examination (systems)**	**Medical Decision-making (diagnoses, data, risk)**
99211 Clinical staff evaluations Follow-up on serous fluid or hearing loss with tympanogram (Be sure to code tympanogram [92567] and/or audiogram [92551 series] in addition to 99211.)	No specific key components required. Must indicate continuation of physician's plan of care, medical necessity, assessment, and/or education provided. CC: Follow-up on serous fluid OR on hearing loss. HPI: Mom reports medication completed and previous symptoms resolved. Assessment: Problem resolved. Follow-up with physician for recommended preventive service.		
99212 Follow-up otitis media, uncomplicated	**Problem focused** CC: Follow-up otitis media HPI: History of treatment, difficulties with medication, hearing status	**Problem focused** 1. ENMT	**Straightforward** 1. One established problem, improved 2. No tests ordered/data reviewed 3. Risk: No need for further follow-up
99213 2-year-old presents with tugging at her right ear. Afebrile. Mild otitis media.	**Problem focused** CC: Tugging at right ear HPI: Duration, associated signs/symptoms, and home management, including over-the-counter medications, and response ROS: Constitutional, eyes, ENMT, gastrointestinal, genitourinary	**Expanded problem focused** 1. ENMT 2. Conjunctiva 3. Overall appearance	**Low complexity** 1. Minor problem 2. No tests ordered/data reviewed 3. Risk: Observation and nonprescription analgesics
99214 Infant presents for suspected third episode of otitis media within 3 months. Infant presents with fever and cough.	**Detailed** CC: Fever and cough, suspected otitis media HPI: Duration, severity of fever, other symptoms, modifying factor (medication) ROS: Constitutional, eyes, ENMT, respiratory, gastrointestinal, urinary PSFH: Allergies, frequency of similar infection in past and response to treatment, environmental factors (eg, tobacco exposure, child care), immunization status	**Detailed** 1. Constitutional 2. Eyes 3. ENMT 4. Lungs 5. Skin	**Moderate complexity** 1. Established problem, not responding to management 2. Hearing evaluation planned 3. Risk: Prescription drug management

Continuum Model for Otitis Media (*continued*)

Code selection at any level above 99211 may be based on time when documentation states that more than 50% of the total face-to-face time of the encounter is spent in counseling and/or coordination of care. Select the code with the typical time closest to the total face-to-face time.

CPT® Code Vignette	History	Physical Examination (systems)	Medical Decision-making (diagnoses, data, risk)
99215 3-month-old presents with high fever, vomiting, irritability.	Detailed CC: Fever, vomiting, irritability HPI: Severity of fever, quality of irritability, duration of symptoms, and modifying factors ROS: Constitutional, eyes, ENMT, respiratory, gastrointestinal, genitourinary PFSH: Medications, allergies, frequency of similar infection in past and response to treatment, environmental factors (eg, tobacco exposure, child care)	Comprehensive 1. Overall appearance, hydration status 2. Head 3. Eyes 4. ENMT 5. Neck 6. Cardiovascular 7. Respiratory 8. Skin	High complexity 1. New problem with additional work-up planned. 2. Tests ordered: Complete blood cell count with differential, blood culture, blood urea nitrogen, creatinine, electrolytes, urinalysis with culture, chest radiograph, and possible lumbar puncture. 3. Risk: Consider admission to NICU.
99214 or 99215 NOTE: Depending on the variables (ie, time), this example could be reported as 99214 or 99215. Extended evaluation of child with chronic or recurrent otitis media	Documentation of total face-to-face time and >50% of time spent in extensive discussion of treatment options, including, but not limited to 1. Continued episodic treatment with antibiotics 2. Myringotomy and tube placement 3. Adenoidectomy 4. Allergy evaluation 5. Steroid therapy with weighing of risk to benefit ratio of various therapies NOTE: Time is the key factor when counseling and/or coordination of care are more than 50% of the face-to-face time with the patient. For 99214, the total visit time would be 25 minutes; for 99215, the total time is 40 minutes. You must document time spent on counseling and/or coordination of care and include the areas discussed.		

Abbreviations: CC, chief complaint; CPT, Current Procedural Terminology; ENMT, ears, nose, throat, mouth; HPI, history of present illness; PFSH, past, family, and social history; ROS, review of systems.

Continuum Model for Attention-Deficit/Hyperactivity Disorder

Code selection at any level above 99211 may be based on time when documentation states that more than 50% of the total face-to-face time of the encounter is spent in counseling and/or coordination of care. Select the code with the typical time closest to the total face-to-face time.

CPT® Code Vignette	History	Physical Examination (systems)	Medical Decision-making (2 of 3 diagnoses, data, risk)
99211 Nurse visit to check growth or blood pressure prior to renewing prescription for psychoactive drugs	No specific key components required. Must indicate continuation of physician's plan of care, medical necessity, assessment, and/or education provided. CC: Check growth or blood pressure. HPI: Existing medications and desired/undesired effects. Documentation of height, weight, and blood pressure. Assessment: Doing well. Obtained physician approval for prescription refill. Keep appointment with physician in 1 month.		

Continuum Model for Attention-Deficit/Hyperactivity Disorder (*continued*)

Code selection at any level above 99211 may be based on time when documentation states that more than 50% of the total face-to-face time of the encounter is spent in counseling and/or coordination of care. Select the code with the typical time closest to the total face-to-face time.

CPT® Code Vignette	History	Physical Examination (systems)	Medical Decision-making (2 of 3 diagnoses, data, risk)
99212 (Typical time: 10 min) Visit to recheck recent weight loss in patient with established ADHD otherwise stable on stimulant medication	**Problem focused** CC: Weight loss, ADHD HPI: Appetite, signs and symptoms, duration since last weight check	**Problem focused** 1. Constitutional (weight, blood pressure, overall appearance)	**Straightforward** 1. Stable established problem 2. No tests ordered/data reviewed 3. Risk: 1 chronic illness with side effects of treatment and prescription drug management
99213 (Typical time: 15 min) 3- to 6-month visit for child with ADHD who is presently doing well using medication and without other problems	**Expanded problem focused** CC: ADHD HPI: Effect of medication on appetite, mood, sleep, quality of schoolwork (eg, review report cards) ROS: Neurologic (no tics) PFSH: Review of medications	**Expanded problem focused** 1. Constitutional (temperature, weight, blood pressure) 2. Neurologic 3. Psychiatric (alert and oriented, mood and affect)	**Low complexity** 1. Stable established problem 2. Data reviewed: Rating scale results and feedback materials from teacher 3. Risk: Prescription drug management *or* Time: Documented faced-to-face time and >50% spent in counseling and/or coordination and context of discussion of 6-month treatment plan with adjustment of medication
99214 (Typical time: 25 min) Follow-up evaluation of an established patient with ADHD with failure to improve on medication and/or weight loss and new symptoms of depression	**Detailed** CC: ADHD with failure to improve HPI: Signs and symptoms since start of medication; modifying factors; quality of schoolwork (eg, review report cards) ROS: Gastrointestinal and psychiatric PFSH: Current medications; allergies; school attendance; substance use	**Detailed** 1. General multisystem examination with details of affected systems (2–7 systems in all) or detailed single organ system examination of neurologic system	**Moderate complexity** 1. Established problem, not improving with current therapy, and new problem without additional workup planned 2. Data reviewed: Rating scale results and feedback materials from teacher; depression screening score 3. Risk: Prescription drug management *or* Time: Documented face-to-face time with >50% spent in discussion of possible interventions, including, but not limited to a. Educational intervention b. Alteration in medications c. Obtaining drug levels d. Psychiatric intervention e. Behavioral modification program

Continuum Model for Attention-Deficit/Hyperactivity Disorder (*continued*)

Code selection at any level above 99211 may be based on time when documentation states that more than 50% of the total face-to-face time of the encounter is spent in counseling and/or coordination of care. Select the code with the typical time closest to the total face-to-face time.

CPT® Code Vignette	History	Physical Examination (systems)	Medical Decision-making (2 of 3 diagnoses, data, risk)
99215 (Typical time: 40 min) Initial evaluation of an established patient experiencing difficulty in classroom, home, or social situation and suspected of having ADHD	**Comprehensive** CC: Difficulty in school, home, and social situations HPI: Signs and symptoms, duration, modifying factors, severity ROS: Constitutional, eyes, ENMT, cardiovascular, respiratory, musculoskeletal, integumentary, neurological, psychiatric, endocrine	Comprehensive examination of ≥8 systems or comprehensive neurologic/psychiatric examination (1997 guidelines	**High complexity** 1. New problem with additional workup 2. Tests ordered and data reviewed: ADHD assessment instruments; history obtained from parents; and case discussion with another provider (eg, school counselor) 3. Risk: Undiagnosed new problem

Abbreviations: ADHD, attention-deficit/hyperactivity disorder; CC, chief complaint; CPT, Current Procedural Terminology; ENMT, ears, nose, mouth, throat; HPI, history of present illness; PFSH, past, family, and social history; ROS, review of systems.

Continuum Model for Asthma

Code selection at any level above 99211 may be based on time when documentation states that more than 50% of the total face-to-face time of the encounter is spent in counseling and/or coordination of care. Select the code with the typical time closest to the total face-to-face time.

CPT® Code Vignette	History	Physical Examination	Medical Decision-making
99211 Nurse reviews medication list and use and obtains a peak expiratory flow rate for a well 10-year-old established patient. Nurse reviews disease management protocol with mother and child, including acute exacerbations.	No specific key components required. Must indicate continuation of physician's plan of care, medical necessity, assessment, and/or education provided. CC: Asthma care plan review. Documentation of medications, peak expiratory flow, education topics reviewed, and questions answered.		
99212 (Typical time: 10 min) An 8-year-old with stable asthma presents to get the influenza vaccine and parent has a question about a prior influenza vaccine reaction.	**Problem focused** CC: Needs influenza immunization HPI: Description of reaction to prior vaccine	**Problem focused** Constitutional (general appearance)	**Straightforward** 1. Minor problem 2. No tests ordered/data reviewed 3. Risk: Stable chronic condition

Continuum Model for Asthma (*continued*)

Code selection at any level above 99211 may be based on time when documentation states that more than 50% of the total face-to-face time of the encounter is spent in counseling and/or coordination of care. Select the code with the typical time closest to the total face-to-face time.

CPT® Code Vignette	History	Physical Examination	Medical Decision-making
99213 (Typical time: 15 min) A 7-year-old with stable persistent asthma who is using a metered-dose steroid inhaler with β-agonist as needed returns for follow-up with complaint of insect bite on finger.	**EPF** CC: Asthma HPI: Associated signs and symptoms, timing, severity, context ROS: ENMT, respiratory, integumentary	**EPF** Examination of constitutional, ENMT, cardiovascular, and respiratory systems	**Low complexity** 1. Stable chronic problem and minor complaint 2. Review of asthma control test; ordered/performed spirometry 3. Risk: Prescription drug management
99214 (Typical time: 25 min) An 8-year-old with unstable asthma is examined because of an acute exacerbation of the disease; already receiving inhaled albuterol and inhaled steroids by metered-dose inhaler.	**Detailed** CC: Asthma symptoms HPI: Symptoms, duration, modifying factors, severity ROS: Constitutional, eyes, ENMT, respiratory PFSH: Medications, allergies	**Detailed** Examination of constitutional, ENMT, head and neck (musculoskeletal), lymphatic, respiratory, and cardiovascular systems	**Moderate complexity** 1. Established problem, worsening 2. Tests ordered: Pulse oximetry and pre- and post-bronchodilator spirometry done 3. Risk: Chronic illness with mild exacerbation
99215 (Typical time: 40 min) A 1-year-old known to have recurrent wheezing following respiratory syncytial virus bronchiolitis has had increasingly frequent attacks during the past 2 months. New infiltrates are revealed by chest radiograph. Cystic fibrosis is suspected. A sweat test is ordered.	**Comprehensive** CC: Wheezing attacks HPI: Context, severity, timing, modifying factors ROS: Constitutional, eyes, ENMT, cardiovascular, respiratory, gastrointestinal, genitourinary, integumentary, hematologic/lymphatic, allergic/immunologic PFSH: Medications, allergies, past illness, medical history of parents specific to genetic risk	**Comprehensive** As in 99214, plus examination of eyes, integumentary, and gastrointestinal systems	**High complexity** 1. Established problem, worsening. 2. Data reviewed and tests ordered: Laboratory data and radiology results reviewed; consult with pulmonologist by telephone; sweat test ordered. 3. Risk: Undiagnosed new problem with uncertain prognosis.

Abbreviations: CC, chief complaint; CPT, Current Procedural Terminology; ENMT, ears, nose, mouth, throat; EPF, expanded problem focused; HPI, history of present illness; PFSH, past, family, and social history; ROS, review of systems.

Evaluation and Management Services in Home or Nursing Facility Settings

Contents

Chapter 8: Evaluation and Management Services in Home or Nursing Facility Settings

Selecting the Appropriate Evaluation and Management Codes

This chapter includes tables with descriptions of the required key components (ie, history, physical examination, medical decision-making [MDM], and, if appropriate, time) for all the evaluation and management (E/M) services that are reported in the home, nursing facility and domiciliary, and rest home settings. **Table 8-1** provides the key components and specific details on required elements within each level of history and physical examination (eg, problem focused, expanded) and MDM (eg, straightforward, moderate) of an E/M code. Refer to this table when using some of the other tables in this chapter. These tables can be downloaded at www.aap.org/cfp (access code AAPCFP24).

Note: All E/M code descriptors and their specific instructions reflect the exclusion of references to provider/professional type, whenever not essential, throughout the code set. When the word "physician" is included in a code descriptor, a qualified health care professional (QHP) working within his or her scope of practice may also provide the service.

See Chapter 6, Evaluation and Management Documentation Guidelines, for a detailed description of the guidelines and components of E/M services with documentation requirements and tips.

* Time may be used as the key controlling factor in the selection of the code, when appropriate, in lieu of key components. To report based on time, counseling and/or coordination of care must account for more than 50% of the face-to-face time with the patient.
  * Billing based on time requires documentation of the total face-to-face time (may be approximate) and the percentage or number of minutes spent in counseling and/or coordination of care.
  * *Current Procedural Terminology* (*CPT*®) instructs that time is met when the midpoint is passed. Other payers may require that the typical time specified for a service be met or exceeded.
  * See Chapter 1, The Basics of Coding, for specific guidelines to follow when reporting an E/M service based on time.

The examples included here and throughout the chapter are based on the 1995 E/M documentation guidelines. Medical decision-making is listed before history and physical examination because some payers require that the level of MDM be 1 of the 2 key components met to support the level of service for an established patient encounter. **Table 8-1** highlights the requirements for the history, examination (1995 or 1997), and MDM.

Medical necessity for the extent of history, examination, and MDM should be evident in the documentation for each encounter. Consider only the medically necessary services when selecting the level of E/M service.

> ## ~ More From the AAP ~
>
> Read more about reporting evaluation and management services based on time in the March 2016 *AAP Pediatric Coding Newsletter*™ at http://coding.aap.org (subscription required).

Home Care Services (99341–99350)

* Home visits are reported with place of service code 12 (home location, other than hospital or other facility, where patient receives care in a private residence). For purposes of reporting home visits, *home* may be defined as a private residence, temporary lodging, or short-term accommodation (eg, hotel, campground, hostel, cruise ship). Medicaid plans may vary in sites of service reported as home visits. For example, some states consider visits to patients in state medical facilities to be home visits.
* Do not report home visit codes for visits to patients in residential facilities or group homes. See codes for domiciliary, rest home, or custodial care services (99324–99328 and 99334–99337).
* Code selection is based on the performance and documentation of the required key components or time if more than 50% of the time is spent in counseling and/or coordination of care, as seen in **tables 8-2 and 8-3**.
* Travel time to and from a patient's home is assumed to be in the level of care, just as travel time to and from the hospital is included in hospital care codes and is not counted in the time spent. However, if escorting a patient to a medical facility becomes necessary, code 99082 (unusual travel) is available.

Table 8-1. Evaluation and Management Key Components

History (must meet or exceed HPI, ROS, and PFSH)	Problem Focused	Expanded	Detailed	Comprehensive
	HPI: 1–3 elements ROS: 0 PFSH: 0	HPI: 1–3 elements ROS: 1 PFSH: 0	HPI: 4+ elements or status of 3 chronic or inactive conditions ROS: 2–9 PFSH: 1	HPI: 4+ elements or status of 3 chronic or inactive conditions ROS: 10+ PFSH: 2 (established patient) or 3 (new patient)
Physical Examination	Problem Focused 1995: 1 body area/organ system 1997: Performance and documentation of 1–5 elements identified by a bullet (●) in ≥1 areas or systems	Expanded 1995: Limited examination—affected body area/organ system and 1–6 other related areas/systems 1997: Performance and documentation of at least 6 elements identified by a bullet (●) in ≥1 areas or systems	Detailed 1995: Extended examination—affected body area(s) and 1–6 other symptomatic or related organ system(s) 1997: Performance and documentation of at least 2 elements identified by a bullet (●) in at least 6 areas or systems or at least 12 elements identified by a bullet (●) in at least 2 areas or systems	Comprehensive 1995: 8+ organ systems or complete examination of a single organ system 1997: <u>Multisystem examination</u>—9 systems or areas with performance of all elements identified by a bullet (●) in each area/system examined Documentation of at least 2 elements identified by a bullet (●) of each area(s) or system(s) <u>Single organ system examination</u>—Performance of all elements identified by a bullet (●) and documentation of every element in box with shaded border and at least 1 element in box with unshaded border
Medical Decision-making	Straightforward	Low Complexity	Moderate Complexity	High Complexity
(must meet 2 of diagnoses/options, data, and risk)				
Presenting Problem	Usually self-limited or minor severity	Usually moderate severity	Usually moderate to high severity	Usually moderate to high severity
# D/M Options	Minimal	Limited	Multiple	Extensive
Data	Minimal	Limited	Moderate	Extensive
Risk	Minimal	Low	Moderate	High

Abbreviations: D/M, diagnosis and management; HPI, history of present illness; PFSH, past, family, and social history; ROS, review of systems.

Table 8-2. Home Visits for New Patients

Key Components (For a description of key components, see Table 8-1.)
3 of 3 key components must be performed to at least the degree specified under the code.

CPT® Code/Timeª	Medical Decision-making	Historyᵇ	1995 Examinationᶜ
99341 20 min	Straightforward PP: Usually low severity	HPI: 1–3; ROS: 0; PFSH: 0	1 body area/ system
99342 30 min	Low complexity PP: Usually moderate severity	HPI: 1–3; ROS: 1; PFSH: 0	2–7 limited
99343 45 min	Moderate complexity PP: Usually moderate to high severity	HPI: ≥4 or 3 CC; ROS: 2–9; PFSH: 1/3	2–7 detailed
99344 60 min	Moderate complexity PP: Usually moderate to high severity	HPI: ≥4 or 3 CC; ROS: ≥10; PFSH: 3/3	≥8 body areas/ systems
99345 75 min	High complexity PP: Usually patient is unstable or has developed a new problem requiring immediate physician attention.	HPI: ≥4 or 3 CC; ROS: ≥10; PFSH: 3/3	≥8 body areas/ systems

Abbreviations: CC, chronic condition; CPT, Current Procedural Terminology; HPI, history of present illness; ROS, review of systems; PFSH, past, family, and social history; PP, presenting problem.

ª Typical time is an average and represents a range of times that may be higher or lower depending on clinical circumstances. The presenting problem is considered to be a contributory factor and does not need to be present to the degree specified.
ᵇ A chief complaint is required for all levels of history.
ᶜ Number of body areas or organ systems examined; see **Table 8-1** for details.

Table 8-3. Home Visits for Established Patients

Key Components (For a description of key components, see Table 8-1.)
2 of 3 key components must be performed to at least the degree specified under the code. Some payers may require medical decision-making as 1 of the 2 components performed and documented.

CPT® Code/Timeª	Medical Decision-making	Historyᵇ	Examinationᶜ
99347 15 min	Straightforward PP: Usually self-limited or minor	HPI: 1–3; ROS: 0; PFSH: 0	1 body area/ system
99348 25 min	Low complexity PP: Usually low to moderate severity	HPI: 1–3; ROS: 1; PFSH: 0	2–7 limited
99349 40 min	Moderate complexity PP: Usually moderate to high severity	HPI: ≥4 or 3 CC; ROS: 2–9; PFSH: 1/3	2–7 detailed
99350 60 min	Moderate to high complexity PP: Usually moderate to high severity	HPI: ≥4 or 3 CC; ROS: ≥10; PFSH: 2/3	≥8 body areas/ systems

Abbreviations: CC, chronic condition; CPT, Current Procedural Terminology; HPI, history of present illness; ROS, review of systems; PFSH, past, family, and social history; PP, presenting problem.

ª Typical time is an average and represents a range of times that may be higher or lower depending on clinical circumstances. The presenting problem is considered to be a contributory factor and does not need to be present to the degree specified.
ᵇ A chief complaint is required for all levels of history.
ᶜ Number of body areas or organ systems examined; see **Table 8-1** for details.

Chapter 8: Evaluation and Management Services in Home or Nursing Facility Settings

- Services provided by a nonphysician provider who does not have his or her own National Provider Identifier may not be billed unless the physician provides direct supervision. Refer to Chapter 13, Allied Health and Clinical Staff Services.
- Any procedures performed by the physician may be separately reported.
- Payers may have varied policies on coverage and reporting requirements for home visits and may not use Medicare incident-to guidelines. Check with them prior to reporting this service.

Example

➤ A pediatrician agrees to provide a home visit to an 8-year-old patient with autism spectrum disorder (ASD) who becomes agitated and fearful in the physician office setting. The child has had a cough and nasal congestion with clear discharge for 2 days and is not eating well. Patient had fever, which was relieved with ibuprofen. Patient may have had headache but does not verbalize pain well. Parents are concerned about a possible exposure to influenza at school. The patient did not receive the influenza immunization this season. Review of systems: poor appetite but drinking fluids, no other gastrointestinal symptoms, and good urinary output. Examination: The patient is alert, although subdued from usual presentation. Eyes: pupils equal, round, react to light; conjunctiva and eyelids normal. Ears: normal. Nose: membranes are swollen and erythematous with clear discharge. Mouth and throat: clear. Neck: supple, no lymphadenopathy. Respiratory: clear to auscultation, normal rate. Cardiovascular: normal, no murmurs. Rapid influenza testing for types A and B (test yields separate results for influenza A and B) is negative, but presentation is consistent with current influenza outbreak. Assessment: influenza with respiratory symptoms—oseltamivir prescribed. Instructions to parents: Continue symptomatic treatment and maintain hydration. The patient tolerated examination well with ASD. Eye contact and behaviors are much improved from last encounter.

International Classification of Diseases, 10th Revision, Clinical Modification (ICD-10-CM)	CPT
J11.1 (influenza with upper respiratory symptoms) F84.0 (ASD)	99349 History: detailed Examination: expanded problem focused MDM: moderate complexity 87804 QW (infectious agent antigen detection by immunoassay with direct optical observation; influenza) 87804 QW 59

Teaching Point: Many payers require documentation of medical necessity for provision of services in the home rather than the office. Inclusion of codes that limit the patient's ability to be seen in the office or outpatient clinic may help demonstrate medical necessity. Code **87804** is reported twice with modifier **59** (distinct service) because the test used yields 2 results testing separately for influenza A and influenza B. Payer guidance may vary regarding reporting of influenza testing.

Domiciliary, Rest Home, or Custodial Care Services (99324–99337)

These services are provided in a facility that provides room and board and other personal assistance services (eg, assisted living facility) (**tables 8-4 and 8-5**).

- These codes are not reported for patients residing in a private residence (see codes **99341–99350**).
- Codes **99324–99328** and **99334–99337** are reported for services provided in facilities assigned the following place of service codes: **13** (assisted living) and **14** (group home), **33** (custodial care facility), and **55** (residential substance abuse facility).
- Prolonged services provided in a domiciliary, rest home, or custodial care are reported with codes **99354** and **99355**.

Table 8-4. Domiciliary, Rest Home, or Custodial Care Services: New Patient

Key Components (For a description of key components, see Table 8-1.)

3 of 3 key components must be performed to at least the degree specified under the code.

CPT® Code/Time[a]	Medical Decision-making	History[b]	Examination[c]
99324 20 min	Straightforward PP: Usually low severity	HPI: 1–3; ROS: 0; PFSH: 0	1 body area/ system
99325 30 min	Low complexity PP: Usually moderate severity	HPI: 1–3; ROS: 1; PFSH: 0	2–7 limited
99326 45 min	Moderate complexity PP: Usually moderate to high severity	HPI: ≥4 or 3 CC; ROS: 2–9; PFSH: 1/3	2–7 detailed
99327 60 min	Moderate complexity PP: Usually high severity	HPI: ≥4 or 3 CC; ROS: ≥10; PFSH: 3/3	≥8 body areas/ systems
99328 75 min	High complexity PP: Usually patient is unstable or has developed a new problem requiring immediate physician attention.	HPI: ≥4 or 3 CC; ROS: ≥10; PFSH: 3/3	≥8 body areas/ systems

Abbreviations: CC, chronic condition; CPT, Current Procedural Terminology; HPI, history of present illness; ROS, review of systems; PFSH, past, family, and social history; PP, presenting problem.

[a] Typical time is an average and represents a range of times that may be higher or lower depending on clinical circumstances. The presenting problem is considered to be a contributory factor and does not need to be present to the degree specified.

[b] A chief complaint is required for all levels of history.

[c] Number of body areas or organ systems examined; see **Table 8-1** for details.

Table 8-5. Domiciliary, Rest Home, or Custodial Care Services: Established Patient

Key Components (For a description of key components, see Table 8-1.)

3 of 3 key components must be performed to at least the degree specified under the code. Some payers may require medical decision-making as 1 of the 2 components performed and documented.

CPT® Code/Time[a]	Medical Decision-making	History[b]	Examination[c]
99334 15 min	Straightforward PP: Usually self-limited to minor	HPI: 1–3; ROS: 0; PFSH: 0	1 body area/ system
99335 25 min	Low complexity PP: Usually low to moderate severity	HPI: 1–3; ROS: 1; PFSH: 0	2–7 limited
99336 40 min	Moderate complexity PP: Usually moderate to high severity	HPI: ≥4 or 3 CC; ROS: 2–9; PFSH: 1/3	2–7 detailed
99337 60 min	Moderate to high complexity PP: Usually moderate to high severity; patient may be unstable or develop new problem requiring immediate attention.	HPI: ≥4 or 3 CC; ROS: ≥10; PFSH: 2/3	≥8 body areas/ systems

Abbreviations: CC, chronic condition; CPT, Current Procedural Terminology; HPI, history of present illness; ROS, review of systems; PFSH, past, family, and social history; PP, presenting problem.

[a] Typical time is an average and represents a range of times that may be higher or lower depending on clinical circumstances. The presenting problem is considered to be a contributory factor and does not need to be present to the degree specified.

[b] A chief complaint is required for all levels of history.

[c] Number of body areas or organ systems examined; see **Table 8-1** for details.

Example

➤ **A pediatrician agrees to provide medically necessary services to patients living at a youth ranch at the facility's infirmary.** An established patient presents with complaint of pain on the sole of the right foot. The pediatrician examines the patient's foot and finds a plantar wart on the ball of the right foot just below the fourth toe. Recommendation for over-the-counter salicylic acid treatment is relayed to the facility nursing staff. Documentation includes a problem-focused history and examination and straightforward MDM.

ICD-10-CM	CPT
B07.0 (verruca plantaris)	**99334**

Teaching Point: The place of service on this claim could be group home (**14**) or custodial care facility (**33**). It is important to verify the appropriate place of service for reporting.

Nursing Facility Care

Nursing facility care is provided to patients who require medical, nursing, or rehabilitative services above the level of custodial care but not at the level of care available in a hospital. Place of service codes for nursing facility care were created by the Medicare program to differentiate skilled nursing facility care from nursing facility care because Medicare benefits are different for patients requiring skilled nursing care. Medicaid and private payer plans may offer specific instructions on the appropriate places of service for reporting physician services provided in nursing facilities.

Place of service codes for physician services provided to patients in a nursing facility are described in **Table 8-6**.

Table 8-6. Nursing Facility Place of Service Codes	
Place of Service Code	**Description**
31	A facility which primarily provides inpatient skilled nursing care and related services to patients who require medical, nursing, or rehabilitative services but does not provide the level of care or treatment available in a hospital.
32	A facility which primarily provides to residents skilled nursing care and related services for the rehabilitation of injured, disabled, or sick persons, or, on a regular basis, health-related care services above the level of custodial care to other than individuals with intellectual disabilities.

Initial Nursing Facility Care (99304–99306)

* The level of service reported is dependent on performance and documentation of the 3 key components (history, physical examination, and MDM) or time if more than 50% of the floor or unit time is spent in counseling and/or care coordination (**Table 8-7**).
* Services are reported for a new or an established patient.
* When the patient is admitted to the nursing facility in the course of an encounter at another site of service (eg, hospital emergency department, physician's office), all E/M services provided by that physician in conjunction with that admission are considered part of the initial nursing facility care when performed on the same date as the admission or readmission.
* The nursing facility care level of service reported by the admitting physician should include services related to the admission he or she provided in the other sites of service on the same date.
* Hospital discharge or observation discharge services performed on the same date of nursing facility admission or readmission may be reported separately. When a patient is discharged from inpatient or observation status on the same date of nursing facility admission or readmission, hospital discharge services (**99238**, **99239**, or **99217**) should be reported in addition to the initial nursing facility care. (For a patient admitted and discharged from observation or inpatient status on the same date, see codes **99234–99236**)
* For nursing facility care discharge, see codes **99315** and **99316**

❖ Prolonged service provided in conjunction with a face-to-face nursing facility service is reported with codes **99356** and **99357**. For more information on these codes, see Chapter 16, Noncritical Hospital Evaluation and Management Services.

Table 8-7. Initial Nursing Facility Care: New or Established Patient

Key Components (For a description of key components, see Table 8-1.)
3 of 3 key components must be performed to at least the degree specified for each code.

CPT® Code/Timeᵃ	Medical Decision-making	Historyᵇ	Examinationᶜ
99304 25 min	Straightforward or low PP: Usually low severity	HPI: ≥4 or 3 CC; ROS: 2–9; PFSH: 1/3	2–7 detailed
99305 35 min	Moderate complexity PP: Usually moderate severity	HPI: ≥4 or 3 CC; ROS: ≥10; PFSH: 3/3	≥8 body areas/ systems
99306 45 min	High complexity PP: Usually high severity	HPI: ≥4 or 3 CC; ROS: ≥10; PFSH: 3/3	≥8 body areas/ systems

Abbreviations: *CC, chronic condition; CPT, Current Procedural Terminology; HPI, history of present illness; ROS, review of systems; PFSH, past, family, and social history; PP, presenting problem.*

ᵃ *Typical time is an average and represents a range of time that may be higher or lower depending on clinical circumstances. The presenting problem is considered to be a contributory factor and does not need to be present to the degree specified.*
ᵇ *A chief complaint is required for all levels of history.*
ᶜ *Number of body areas or organ systems examined; see **Table 8-1** for details.*

Subsequent Nursing Facility Care (99307–99310)

❖ Codes are used to report services provided to residents of nursing facilities who do not require a comprehensive assessment and/or who have not had a major, permanent change of status.

❖ Code selection is based on the performance and documentation of 2 of the 3 key components or time if more than 50% of the floor or unit time is spent in counseling and/or coordination of care (**Table 8-8**).

❖ All levels of service include reviewing the medical record and results of diagnostic studies, noting changes in the resident's status and response to management since the last visit, and reviewing and signing orders.

❖ An interval history, not requiring past, family, or social history, is used in selecting the level of history.

Table 8-8. Subsequent Nursing Facility Care

Key Components (For a description of key components, see Table 8-1.)
2 of 3 key components must be performed to at least the degree specified for each code. Some payers may require medical decision-making as 1 of the 2 components performed and documented.

CPT® Code/Timeᵃ	Medical Decision-making	Historyᵇ	Examinationᶜ
99307 10 min	Straightforward PP: Usually stable, recovering, or improving	HPI: 1–3; ROS: 0; PFSH: 0	1 body area/ system
99308 15 min	Low complexity PP: Usually responding inadequately to therapy or minor complication	HPI: 1–3; ROS: 1; PFSH: 0	2–7 limited
99309 25 min	Moderate complexity PP: Usually patient develops significant complication or new problem.	HPI: ≥4 or 3 CC; ROS: 2–9; PFSH: 0	2–7 detailed
99310 35 min	High complexity PP: Usually patient is unstable or has a new problem requiring immediate attention.	HPI: ≥4 or 3 CC; ROS: ≥10; PFSH: 0	≥8 body areas/ systems

Abbreviations: *CC, chronic condition; CPT, Current Procedural Terminology; HPI, history of present illness; ROS, review of systems; PFSH, past, family, and social history; PP, presenting problem.*

ᵃ *Typical time is an average and represents a range of times that may be higher or lower depending on clinical circumstances. The presenting problem is considered to be a contributory factor and does not need to be present to the degree specified.*
ᵇ *A chief complaint is required for all levels of history.*
ᶜ *Number of body areas or organ systems examined; see **Table 8-1** for details.*

Nursing Facility Discharge Services (99315, 99316)

* The nursing facility discharge day management codes (Table 8-9) are used to report the total time spent by a physician for the final nursing facility discharge of a patient, even if the time spent by the physician on that date is not continuous.
* The codes include, as appropriate, final patient examination and discussion of the nursing facility stay. Instructions are given to all relevant caregivers for continuing care, preparation of discharge records, prescriptions, and referral forms.
* If the work of performing the discharge management is more than 30 minutes, the total time must be documented in the medical record.

Table 8-9. Nursing Facility Discharge Services	
99315	Nursing facility discharge day management; 30 minutes or less
99316	more than 30 minutes

Annual Nursing Facility Assessment (99318)

Code 99318 is used to report a comprehensive annual assessment that includes a detailed interval history, comprehensive physical examination, and minimum data set or resident assessment instrument evaluation. The patient's and family's goals for care and preferences for medical interventions are assessed, including, if applicable, reassessment of advance directives and updates of contact information for surrogate decision-makers. Table 8-10 describes the 3 key components for code 99318.

Table 8-10. Annual Nursing Facility Assessment

Key Components (For a description of key components, see Table 8-1.)
3 of 3 key components must be performed to at least the degree specified under the code.

CPT® Code/Time[a]	Medical Decision-making	History[b]	Examination[c]
99318 30 min	Low to moderate complexity PP: Usually stable, recovering, or improving	HPI: ≥4 or 3 CC; ROS: 2–9; PFSH: 0	≥8 body areas/ systems

Abbreviations: CC, chronic condition; CPT, Current Procedural Terminology; HPI, history of present illness; ROS, review of systems; PFSH, past, family, and social history; PP, presenting problem.

[a] Typical time is an average and represents a range of times that may be higher or lower depending on clinical circumstances. The presenting problem is considered to be a contributory factor and does not need to be present to the degree specified.
[b] A chief complaint is required for all levels of history.
[c] Number of body areas or organ systems examined; see **Table 8-1** for details.

Consultations

Codes 99241–99245 are used to report consultations provided in home services, domiciliaries, rest homes, and custodial care. Please see Chapter 7, Evaluation and Management Services in the Office and Outpatient Clinics, for guidelines for reporting these codes. A summary of key components for each level is in Table 8-11.

Guidelines Used by Payers That Follow Medicare Consultation Guidelines

It is important to check with major payers to determine if they have adopted the Medicare policy or established their own policy and guidelines for reporting consultations. The American Academy of Pediatrics (AAP) position on Medicare consultation policy is available at www.aap.org/cfp (access code AAPCFP24).

- If the patient is new to the consulting physician (ie, has not received any face-to-face professional services from the physician or another physician of the same specialty who belongs to the same group practice within the past 3 years), codes for the appropriate site of service are reported based on the performance and documentation of the required key components or time, if appropriate.
  - ❖ **99341–99345** New patient home visit
  - ❖ **99324–99328** New patient domiciliary or rest home visit
  - ❖ **99304–99306** Initial nursing facility care
- If the patient does not meet the requirements of a new patient, an established patient E/M code for the site of service is reported.
  - ❖ **99347–99350** Established patient home visit
  - ❖ **99334–99336** Established patient domiciliary or rest home visit
  - ❖ **99307–99310** Subsequent nursing facility care
- The referring physician must document the request for consultation in his or her medical record, and the consulting physician must document the request and communicate the results back to the referring physician.

Table 8-11. Outpatient Consultations

Key Components (For a description of key components, see Table 8-1.)
3 of 3 key components must be performed to at least the degree specified under the code.

CPT® Code/Time[a]	Medical Decision-making	History[b]	1995 Examination[c]
99241 20 min	Straightforward PP: Usually low severity	HPI: 1–3; ROS: 0; PFSH: 0	1 body area/ system
99242 30 min	Low complexity PP: Usually moderate severity	HPI: 1–3; ROS: 1; PFSH: 0	2–7 limited
99243 45 min	Moderate complexity PP: Usually moderate to high severity	HPI: ≥4 or 3 CC; ROS: 2–9; PFSH: 1/3	2–7 detailed
99244 60 min	Moderate complexity PP: Usually moderate to high severity	HPI: ≥4 or 3 CC; ROS: ≥10; PFSH: 3/3	≥8 body areas/ systems
99245 80 min	High complexity PP: Usually patient is unstable or has developed a new problem requiring immediate physician attention.	HPI: ≥4 or 3 CC; ROS: ≥10; PFSH: 3/3	≥8 body areas/ systems

Abbreviations: CC, chronic condition; CPT, Current Procedural Terminology; HPI, history of present illness; ROS, review of systems; PFSH, past, family, and social history; PP, presenting problem.

[a] Typical time is an average and represents a range of times that may be higher or lower depending on clinical circumstances. The presenting problem is considered to be a contributory factor and does not need to be present to the degree specified.

[b] A chief complaint is required for all levels of history.

[c] Number of body areas or organ systems examined; see Table 8-1 for details.

Example

➤ **A 10-year-old boy with childhood-onset conduct disorder lives in a group home.** The boy has become more aggressive recently, and his psychologist has recommended a new medication. The child's pediatrician is consulted by the psychologist for advice on the appropriateness of the new medication in conjunction with the patient's current medications and other medical conditions. The pediatrician provides a face-to-face service at the group home and agrees with the recommended treatment. Twenty minutes is spent face-to-face with this established patient performing an expanded problem-focused history and detailed examination and discussing the risks and benefits of the new medication with the patient. The level of MDM is moderate. The medication is prescribed, and the physician spends another 10 minutes discussing the change in management with staff in the office at the group home. The total time for the pediatrician's visit is approximately 30 minutes.

ICD-10-CM	CPT®
F91.1 (conduct disorder, childhood-onset type)	The consultant reports **99242** (based on expanded problem-focused history, detailed examination, and moderate MDM) or, if the payer does not recognize consultation codes, **99336** (based on detailed examination and moderate MDM)

Teaching Point: Three of 3 key components are required for office consultations, so the expanded problem-focused history limits code selection to **99242** Time is not used for code selection because the physician documented 20 minutes with the patient but did not document that more than 50% of that time was spent in counseling and/or coordination of care. Time in the office of the group home discussing care with the staff would not be attributed to the face-to-face time of the visit.

Out-of-Office Service Add-on Codes (99050–99060)

Codes **99056–99060** are used to report services that are provided after hours or on an emergency basis and are an adjunct to the basic E/M service provided.

Third-party payers will have specific policies for coverage and payment. Communicate with individual payers to understand their definition or interpretation of the service and their coverage and payment policies. As part of this negotiation and education process, it is important to demonstrate the cost savings recognized by the payer for these adjunct services. After-hours service codes are used by physicians or other QHPs (under their state scope of practice and when billing with their own National Provider Identifier) to identify the services that are adjunct to the basic services rendered. These codes

- Describe the special circumstances under which a basic procedure is performed.
- Are only reported in addition to an associated basic service (eg, E/M, fracture care).
- Are reported without a modifier appended to the basic service because they only further describe the services provided.

99056   Service(s) typically provided in the office, provided out of the office at request of patient, in addition to basic service

- It is not appropriate for an ED physician to report code **99056.**
- Documentation should include the patient's request to be seen outside of the office.

99060   Service(s) provided on an emergency basis, out of the office, which disrupts other scheduled office services, in addition to basic service

- Documentation should indicate that the physician was called away during scheduled office hours to attend to a patient in another location (eg, emergency department).

Example

➤ **A 10-year-old is seen in her home for exacerbation of moderate persistent asthma at the request of the parents.** The pediatrician evaluates the patient, who is improved after a self-administered inhalation treatment. The child has had 2 urgent visits for exacerbation of asthma in the past 4 months. The parents and child are counseled about medication compliance and control of allergens in the home and given an action plan for home and school. The total time of the visit is 25 minutes, including 15 minutes spent in counseling. The diagnosis is exacerbation of moderate persistent asthma.

ICD-10-CM	CPT
J45.41 (moderate persistent asthma with acute exacerbation)	**99348** (established home E/M with typical time of 25 minutes) **99056** (service[s] typically provided in the office, provided out of the office at request of patient, in addition to basic service)

Teaching Point: Payers may or may not allow payment for code 99056 when services are rendered in the patient's home. The level of home visit was determined by time because more than 50% of the visit was spent in counseling and/or coordination of care.

Prolonged Services

Prolonged Service With Direct Patient Contact (99354, 99355)

+99354　　Prolonged evaluation and management or psychotherapy service(s) (the service beyond the typical service time) in the office or other outpatient setting requiring direct patient contact; first hour

+99355　　　each additional 30 minutes

Prolonged service codes 99354 and 99355 are used to report 30 minutes or more of a physician's or QHP's prolonged face-to-face E/M service provided on the same date as designated office or other E/M services that have a typical or designated time published in *CPT* or for prolonged service in conjunction with psychotherapy of 60 minutes or more (90837).

See Chapter 7, Evaluation and Management Services in the Office and Outpatient Clinics, for more information on reporting prolonged service.

Prolonged Service Without Direct Patient Contact (99358, 99359)

99358　　　Prolonged evaluation and management service before and/or after direct patient care; first hour

+99359　　　each additional 30 minutes (Use in conjunction with code 99358.)

Prolonged service without direct patient contact (ie, non–face-to-face) is reported when a physician provides prolonged service that does not involve face-to-face care. The prolonged service must relate to a service and patient where direct (face-to-face) patient care has occurred or will occur and to ongoing patient management. Only time spent by a physician or other QHP may be counted toward the time of prolonged service. Prolonged service of less than 30 minutes on a given date is not separately reported. Report code 99359 for 15 or more minutes beyond the first hour or the last full 30-minute period of prolonged service. See Chapter 12, Managing Chronic and Complex Conditions, for more information and a coding example.

CHAPTER 9

Preventive Services

Contents

Preventive Care

Preventive care is the hallmark of pediatrics. The Patient Protection and Affordable Care Act (PPACA) recognized the importance of preventive care for children, a critical provision of which ensures that most health care plans cover, *without cost sharing*, the gold standard of pediatric preventive care—the American Academy of Pediatrics (AAP) *Bright Futures: Guidelines for Health Supervision of Infants, Children, and Adolescents*, 4th Edition.

Coverage of and appropriate payment for these pediatric preventive services should, at a minimum, reflect the total relative value units (RVUs) outlined for the current year under the Medicare Resource-Based Relative Value Scale Physician Fee Schedule, inclusive of all separately reported codes for these services. Section 2713 of the PPACA includes the following 2 sets of services that must be provided to children without cost sharing:

1. The standard set of immunizations recommended by the Advisory Committee on Immunization Practices (ACIP) of the Centers for Disease Control and Prevention (CDC) with respect to the individual involved
2. Evidence-informed preventive care and screenings provided for in the comprehensive guidelines supported by the Health Resources and Services Administration (HRSA), which include
   - Bright Futures recommendations for preventive pediatric health care
   - Recommendations of the Secretary's Advisory Committee on Heritable Disorders in Newborns and Children

The Bright Futures periodicity schedule, "Recommendations for Preventive Pediatric Health Care," is a great tool to identify recommended age-appropriate services; in addition, it can be used to identify those services that can and should be reported with their own *Current Procedural Terminology* (*CPT*®) or Healthcare Common Procedure Coding System code, and it identifies appropriate diagnosis coding. This tool can be found at the end of this book as an insert or accessed online at www.aap.org/periodicityschedule.

Although all recommended preventive services are covered, physicians and practice managers should be aware of health plan policies that may affect payment.

- Specific diagnosis codes may be required to support claims adjudication under preventive medicine benefits. Be sure to link the appropriate diagnosis to each service provided (eg, code **Z71.3**, dietary counseling, may be linked to code **99401** for a risk-factor reduction counseling visit).
- Some payers bundle certain services when the services are provided on the same date. For instance, some plans will not allow separate payment for obesity counseling on the same date as a well-child examination but will cover obesity counseling when no other evaluation and management (E/M) service is provided on the same date. It is beneficial to monitor and maintain awareness of the payment policies of those plans most commonly billed by your practice. Most policies are available on payers' Web sites with notification of changes provided in payer communications, such as electronic newsletters.

Quality Initiatives and Preventive Care

Quality initiatives and measurement are becoming standard practice in health care. Many physicians have participated in quality measurement through programs such as the Centers for Medicare & Medicaid Services (CMS) Promoting Interoperability Programs and medical home recognition programs. In pediatrics, many quality measures are associated with preventive care (eg, provision of one meningococcal vaccine on or between the patient's 11th and 13th birthdays).

Quality measurement is also required of health plans funded by government programs or offered through health exchanges created to support health insurance adoption under the PPACA. These health plans must collect and submit Quality Rating System measure data to the CMS. This entails collecting clinical quality measures, including a subset of the National Committee for Quality Assurance Healthcare Effectiveness Data and Information Set (HEDIS) measures and a Pharmacy Quality Alliance measure. (See Chapter 3, Coding to Demonstrate Quality and Value, for more information on HEDIS and quality reporting.) Physicians contracting with these plans may be asked to provide evidence that quality measures

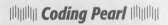

|||||||| **Coding Pearl** ||||||||

It is important to note that a request for medical records is less likely when you submit claims with procedure and diagnosis codes associated with pediatric quality measures.

Chapter 9: Preventive Services

were met through claims data or medical records. It is important to note that a request for medical records is less likely when you submit claims with procedure and diagnosis codes associated with pediatric quality measures. Examples of HEDIS measures related to preventive care include

- Percentage of members 12 to 21 years of age who had at least one comprehensive well-care visit with a primary care provider or obstetrician-gynecologist during the measurement year
- Percentage of members who were 3, 4, 5, or 6 years of age who received one or more well-child visits with a primary care provider during the measurement year
- Percentage of members who turned 15 months old during the measurement year and who had 6 or more well-child visits with a primary care provider during the first 15 months after birth
- Members 3 to 17 years of age who had an outpatient visit with a primary care provider and who had the following services in the current year:
  - Body mass index (BMI) percentile documentation
  - Counseling for nutrition
  - Counseling for physical activity

Certain preventive services, such as anticipatory guidance on healthy diet and exercise, are components of the preventive medicine service and require no additional procedure coding for payment purposes. However, associated diagnosis and procedure codes may be reported to support quality reporting initiatives. For instance, a group practice may decide to participate in a quality improvement program that requires documentation of counseling for nutrition and for physical activity at all well-child visits for children aged 3 to 17 years. *International Classification of Diseases, 10th Revision, Clinical Modification* (ICD-10-CM) codes **Z71.3** (dietary counseling) and **Z71.82** (exercise counseling) may be used in support of this effort. *ICD-10-CM* codes for BMI percentiles are reported only in conjunction with diagnosis of a related condition (eg, underweight, overweight, obesity), which is official guidance from *Coding Clinic*. *CPT* category II code **3008F** (body mass index, documented) is reported when BMI is documented without a related diagnosis.

Certain procedure codes also support quality measurement. For example, submission of claims containing codes for meningococcal (**90734**); tetanus, diphtheria, and acellular pertussis (**90715**); and 2 or 3 doses of human papillomavirus (HPV) vaccine (**90649–90651**) provided to an adolescent before the patient's 13th birthday is indicative of meeting the measure for the immunization of adolescents.

Preventive Medicine Evaluation and Management Services

Well-child or preventive medicine services are a type of E/M service and are reported with codes **99381–99395**. Most health plans provide a 100% benefit (no patient out-of-pocket cost) for the 31 recommended preventive medicine service encounters when provided by in-network providers. The selection of the pediatric-specific codes **99381–99395** is based simply on the age of the patient and whether the patient is new or established (**Table 9-1**) to the practice. In brief, an established patient has been seen (face-to-face, including via telehealth) by the physician or another physician of the same specialty and group practice within the last 3 years. Generally, other qualified health care professionals (QHPs) are considered to be working in the same specialty as the physicians with whom they work. Refer to Chapter 6, Evaluation and Management Documentation Guidelines, for more information about *new* versus *established* patients.

> ~ **More From the AAP** ~
>
> See "History in the Preventive Service" in the June 2015 *AAP Pediatric Coding Newsletter™* at http://coding.aap.org (subscription required).

- Most health plans will limit the benefits for preventive medicine E/M services covered in a year based on the patient's age.
  - Six visits before the first birthday (recommended at 3–5 days and 1, 2, 4, 6, and 9 months)
  - Three visits before the second birthday (recommended at 12, 15, and 18 months)
  - Two visits before the third birthday (recommended at 24 and 30 months)
  - Once per year beginning with the third birthday

Table 9-1. New and Established Preventive Medicine Codes

Code Description	New Patient Code	Established Patient Code
Comprehensive preventive medicine evaluation and management; infant (age <1 year)	99381	99391
early childhood (age 1–4 years)	99382	99392
late childhood (age 5–11 years)	99383	99393
adolescent (age 12–17 years)	99384	99394
age 18–39 years	99385	99395

- Preventive medicine services include counseling, anticipatory guidance, and risk-factor reduction interventions. No average or typical times are assigned to these services, unlike the times found in many other E/M codes.
- Immunizations, laboratory tests, and other special procedures or screening tests (eg, vision, hearing, developmental screening) that have their own specific *CPT*® codes are reported separately *in addition to* preventive medicine E/M services.
- Most payers will require reporting modifier **25** with the preventive medicine service when immunizations or other services are also performed and reported.
- A comprehensive history and physical examination must reflect an age- and a gender-appropriate history and examination and are *not* synonymous with the "comprehensive" history and examination described in the E/M documentation guidelines from the CMS (see Chapter 6, Evaluation and Management Documentation Guidelines).
- The comprehensive history performed as part of a preventive medicine visit does not require a chief complaint or history of present illness. It does require a comprehensive age-appropriate review of systems (ROS) with an updated past, family, and social history (PFSH). The history should also include a comprehensive assessment or history of age-pertinent risk factors.
  - Generally, the ROS of a preventive medicine service is not a list of systems with pertinent positive and negative responses but, rather, a list of inquiries and patient responses for those areas of risk identified in preventive medicine guidelines as pertinent for patients of that age and gender. However, some payers may require review of all systems regardless of age and gender (eg, required by some Medicaid plans under Early and Periodic Screening, Diagnosis, and Treatment [EPSDT] benefits).
- Routine management of contraception is considered part of the comprehensive preventive medicine E/M service when it is provided during the well-care health supervision visit.
- A comprehensive physical examination is a multisystem examination that may include a routine pelvic and breast examination (when performed in the absence of specific symptoms of a separate problem) depending on the age of the patient and/or sexual history. If the pelvic examination is performed because of a gynecologic problem during a routine preventive medicine service, it may be appropriate to report a problem-oriented E/M service in addition to the preventive medicine service if this required additional physician work and required key components of the E/M code are met.
- State Medicaid programs have requirements for performing, documenting, and reporting certain services in their EPSDT programs. Review your state Medicaid policies for the specific documentation and reporting requirements for services to patients in these programs.
- *ICD-10-CM* well-care diagnosis codes should be linked to the appropriate preventive medicine code (**99381–99395**). *ICD-10-CM* codes for well-child examinations include developmental, hearing, and vision screening.
  - **Z00.110** (health supervision for newborn <8 days)
  - **Z00.111** (health supervision for newborn 8–28 days old)
  - **Z00.121** (routine child health examination [≥29 days] with abnormal findings)
  - **Z00.129** (routine child health examination [≥29 days] without abnormal findings)
  - **Z00.00** (encounter for general adult medical examination without abnormal findings)
  - **Z00.01** (encounter for general adult medical examination with abnormal findings)

* For the purpose of assigning codes from this category, an *abnormal finding* is a newly discovered condition or a known or chronic condition that has increased in severity (eg, uncontrolled, acutely exacerbated). Assign additional codes for any abnormal findings.

* ICD-10-CM does not specify an age at which codes **Z00.00** and **Z00.01** are reported in lieu of codes **Z00.121–Z00.129**. The age of majority varies by state and payers may or may not adopt the Medicare Outpatient Code Editor assignment of age limitations (29 days–17 years) to codes **Z00.121–Z00.129**, as indicated in many *ICD-10-CM* references.

* When an existing problem is addressed at the preventive medicine service but is not a newly discovered condition or a known or chronic condition that has increased in severity, report routine child health examination without abnormal findings and code also the condition addressed.

* Code **Z23** must be reported in addition to the routine health examination codes (eg, **Z00.129**) when immunizations are administered at the preventive medicine encounter. *ICD-10-CM* instructs to code **Z00** first, followed by code **Z23**.

Examples

➤ **A 2-year-old is seen for an established patient preventive medicine service.** The child was seen 1 week ago for acute otitis media of the left ear. Parents report no fever or signs of further illness or pain. On examination, the tympanic membrane is slightly bulging but improved from prior encounter. An age- and a gender-appropriate preventive service is provided and documented. Parents are reassured that the ear infection is resolving as expected and instructed to follow up if new concerns arise. Diagnoses are resolving otitis media of the left ear (**H65.192**) and well-child visit.

ICD-10-CM	CPT®
Z00.129 (routine child health exam without abnormal findings) **H65.192** (other acute nonsuppurative otitis media, left ear)	**99392** (preventive medicine visit; age 1–4)

   Teaching Point: Because the otitis media is not newly identified and not failing to respond adequately to treatment, this is not an abnormal finding. However, it is appropriate to report the code for the otitis media that is still present in addition to code **Z00.129**. In this example, the work of noting the improved otitis media did not equate to a significant, separately identifiable E/M service.

➤ **A 3-year-old was diagnosed 1 week ago with recurrent bilateral otitis media with effusion** (**H65.196**). Antibiotics were prescribed. The child presents today for a previously scheduled preventive service and follow-up visit. On examination, eardrums are still inflamed, and the child complains of intermittent pain. Prescription of a different class of antibiotic is provided and referral to an otolaryngologist is made after discussion with parents about risks and benefits of myringotomy. The age- and gender-appropriate preventive service is also provided and documented. The diagnoses are well-child visit and recurrent bilateral otitis media.

ICD-10-CM	CPT
Z00.121 (routine child health exam with abnormal findings) **H65.196** (other acute nonsuppurative otitis media, recurrent, bilateral)	**99392** (preventive medicine visit; age 1–4) **99213 25**

   Teaching Point: Because the otitis media was inadequately controlled, the routine health examination included an abnormal finding. If the otitis media had resolved, code **Z00.129** (routine child health exam without abnormal findings) would be reported. See more on reporting problem-oriented E/M services in conjunction with a preventive service later in this chapter.

Sports/Camp Physicals

CPT® guidelines recommend that preventive medicine service codes (**99381–99395**) be reported when possible for physicals performed to determine eligibility for participation because they most accurately describe the services performed in that they are preventive and age appropriate in nature and physicians offer counseling on, for example, appropriate levels of exercise or injury prevention. However, the need for these services often arises after the child has had a yearly preventive medicine service, thereby rendering this service non-covered by some health plans, which allow only one preventive service per year. In this case, the parent may be billed if the payer contract allows because the service is non-covered.

> ### ~ More From the AAP ~
> For more information on reporting preparticipation physical evaluations, see the following *AAP Pediatric Coding Newsletter*™ articles at http://coding.aap.org (subscription required): "Preparing for Preparticipation Physical Evaluations" (July 2018) and "Sports and Camp Physicals" (June 2017).

Office visit codes (**99211–99215**) may be used if a problem is discovered during the service. Outpatient consultation codes (**99241–99245**) might be considered if the coach or school nurse requested the physician's opinion of a suspected problem (ie, exercise cough associated with reduced performance in cold weather). The medical record must include documentation of the written or verbal request and a copy of the written report with the physician's opinion or advice sent back to the coach or school nurse. *ICD-10-CM* code **Z02.5** is reported for an encounter for examination for participation in sports. If the preparticipation physical evaluation is incorporated into the annual well visit, use code **Z00.121** or **Z00.129** in lieu of **Z02.5**. Any problems or conditions that are addressed during the course of the visit would also be reported.

When reporting sports or camp physicals for patients with Medicare or Medicaid managed care plans, check the plan's policy on payment for these services and instructions for coding and billing. These physicals may be covered even when the child has already had an annual preventive medicine service under some Medicaid plans.

Immunizations

Vaccine services are reported using 2 families of *CPT* codes—one for the vaccine serum (the product) and one for the services associated with the administration of the vaccine.

Vaccines and Toxoids

Codes **90476–90748** are used to report the vaccine or toxoid product only. They do not include the administration of a vaccine.

- The AAP Commonly Administered Pediatric Vaccines table (see Appendix II) provides a quick reference to codes, descriptors, and the number of vaccine components for each vaccine linked to the brand and manufacturer for each.
- The exact vaccine product administered needs to be reported to meet the requirements of immunization registries, vaccine distribution programs, and reporting systems (eg, Vaccine Adverse Event Reporting System), as well as for payment.
- Codes may be specific to the product manufacturer and brand, schedule (number of doses or timing), chemical formulation, dosage, appropriate age guidelines, and/or route of administration.
- Codes for combination vaccines (eg, **90707**, measles, mumps, rubella, and varicella [MMRV] virus vaccine) are available, as are separate codes for single-component vaccines (eg, **90716**, varicella virus vaccine).
- It is not appropriate to code each component of a combination vaccine separately using separate vaccine product codes when a combination vaccine is administered. However, if a combination vaccine is commercially available but a physician elects to administer the component vaccines due to unavailability or other clinical reason, each vaccine product administered would be separately reported. See Appendix II, Vaccine Products: Commonly Administered Pediatric Vaccines, for a list of vaccine product codes.

> ### ⁞⁞⁞ Coding Pearl ⁞⁞⁞
> The administration of immune globulins (including palivizumab [Synagis]) is not reported using the immunization administration codes. See codes **96365–96368, 96372, 96374,** and **96375**.

New Vaccines/Toxoids

The *CPT®* Editorial Panel, in recognition of the public health interest in vaccine products, has chosen to publish new vaccine product codes prior to US Food and Drug Administration (FDA) approval. The American Medical Association (AMA) uses its *CPT* site (https://www.ama-assn.org/practice-management/category-i-vaccine-codes) to provide updates of *CPT* Editorial Panel actions on new vaccine products. Once approved by the *CPT* Editorial Panel, vaccine/toxoid product codes are typically made available for release on a semiannual basis (July 1 and January 1). As part of the electronic distribution, there is a 6-month implementation period from the initial release date (ie, codes released on January 1 are eligible for use on July 1; codes released on July 1 are eligible for use on January 1). These codes are indicated with a lightning bolt symbol (⚡) and will be tracked by the AMA to monitor FDA approval status. The lightning bolt symbol will be removed once the FDA status changes to "approved." Refer to the AMA *CPT* site indicated earlier for the most up-to-date information on codes with this symbol. More rapid code release and implementation may occur when a government agency has identified the need for a vaccine as urgent to address an emergent health issue and the FDA has granted an expedited review process for the vaccine. In such cases, codes may be approved and released on an immediate (outside the normal code consideration schedule) or rapid (within the normal code consideration schedule but released shortly after approval with an implementation date within 3 months of release) basis.

Before administering any new vaccine product or an existing vaccine product with new recommendations, make certain the CDC, in the *Morbidity and Mortality Weekly Report,* or the AAP, in *Pediatrics,* has endorsed the use or recommendations of the vaccine. You may also want to verify with your carriers if the vaccine will be covered.

If a vaccine enters the market this year and is FDA approved, recommendations for use are published by the CDC or AAP, and no code exists for the specific vaccine, use code **90749** (unlisted vaccine/toxoid) and list the specific vaccine given.

> ||||||||| **Coding Pearl** |||||||||
>
> The word *component* refers to an antigen in a vaccine that prevents disease(s) caused by one organism.

National Drug Code

Many payers, specifically Medicare, Medicaid, and other government payers (eg, Tricare) and other private payers, require the use of the National Drug Code (NDC) when reporting vaccine product codes. The NDCs are universal product identifiers for medications, including vaccines. NDCs are found on outer packaging, product labels, and/or product inserts. This is discussed more fully in Chapter 1, The Basics of Coding.

The NDCs are 10-digit, 3-segment numbers that identify the product, labeler, and trade package size. The Health Insurance Portability and Accountability Act of 1996 standards require an 11-digit code. Table 9-2 shows how the 10-digit codes are converted to the 11-digit format for reporting.

> **~ More From the AAP ~**
>
> For more information on reporting National Drug Codes, see Chapter 1, The Basics of Coding, as well as "National Drug Code Unit Errors Prompt Refund Requests" in the December 2017 *AAP Pediatric Coding Newsletter*™ at http://coding.aap.org (subscription required).

Table 9-2. National Drug Code Format Examples

Product	10-digit NDCs	11-digit NDCs (Added zero [0] is underscored.)
RotaTeq 2-mL single-dose tube, package of 20	0006-4047-20 (4-4-2 format)	00006-4047-20
Fluzone Quadrivalent 0.25-mL prefilled single-dose syringe, package of 10	49281-517-25 (5-3-2 format)	49281-0517-25
Synagis 0.5-mL in 1 vial, single dose	60574-4114-1 (5-4-1 format)	60574-4114-01

Abbreviation: NDC, National Drug Code.

If you are not currently reporting vaccines with NDCs, be sure to coordinate the requirements with your billing software company. For more information on NDCs, visit www.fda.gov/Drugs/InformationOnDrugs/ucm142438.htm or link through www.aap.org/cfp.

Immunization Administration

CPT® codes **90460** and **90461** *or* **90471–90474** are reported *in addition to* vaccine/toxoid code(s) **90476–90749**. If a significant, separately identifiable E/M service (eg, office or other outpatient services, preventive medicine services) is performed, the appropriate E/M service code appended with modifier **25** should be reported in addition to the vaccine and toxoid administration codes. If vaccines are given during the course of a preventive medicine service and another E/M service, both E/M services will need modifier **25** if required by the payer.

Codes **90460** and **90461**

90460   Immunization administration through 18 years of age via any route of administration, with counseling by physician or other qualified health care professional; first or only component of each vaccine or toxoid administered

+90461   each additional vaccine or toxoid component administered
            (List separately in addition to code for primary procedure.)

When reporting codes **90460** and **90461**

* Physicians or other QHPs must provide *face-to-face* counseling to the patient and/or family (patient aged ≤18 years) at the time of the encounter for the administration of a vaccine. (See the Codes **90471–90474** section later in this chapter for immunization administration [IA] without physician counseling or to patients older than 18 years.)
* CPT defines a physician or other QHP as follows:
  A "physician or other qualified health care professional" is an individual who by education, training, licensure/regulation, facility credentialing (when applicable), and facility privileging (when applicable) performs a professional service within his/her scope of practice and independently reports that professional service. These professionals are distinct from "clinical staff." A clinical staff member is a person who works under the supervision of a physician or other qualified health care professional and who is allowed by law, regulation, and facility policy to perform or assist in the performance of a specified professional service, but who does not individually report that professional service. Other policies may also affect who may report specific services.
  ❖ Therefore, although nurses may be allowed by state scope of practice laws to explain risks and benefits of vaccines, their counseling does not fall under the description of code **90460** or **90461**, and codes **90471–90474** must be reported for immunization administration without counseling by a physician or QHP.
* When a private payer contract does not allow QHPs to report services under their own name and National Provider Identifier (NPI), check with the payer to determine eligibility of these professionals to report immunization counseling (**90460**, **90461**) and report under the name and number of the supervising physician.
* Documentation of immunization counseling should include a listing of all vaccine components with notation that counseling was provided for all listed components with authentication (electronic or written signature and date) by the physician or other QHP. Supply of the Vaccine Information Statement (VIS) without discussion of risks and benefits does not constitute counseling. Some payers require documentation of parent or caregiver questions or concerns that were addressed during counseling.
* Code **90460** is reported for the *first (or only) component of each vaccine administered* (whether single or combination) on a day of service and includes the related vaccine counseling.
* Code **90461** is only reported in conjunction with **90460** and is used to report the work of counseling for *each additional component(s) beyond the first* in a given combination vaccine. (See Vaccines for Children Program section later in this chapter for reporting administration of vaccines containing multiple components to this program.)

❋ Combination vaccines are those vaccines that contain multiple vaccine components. Refer to Appendix II, Vaccine Products: Commonly Administered Pediatric Vaccines, for the number of components in the most commonly reported pediatric vaccines.

❋ The IA codes include the physician or other QHP's work of discussing risks and benefits of the vaccines, providing parents with a copy of the appropriate CDC VIS for each vaccine given, the cost of clinical staff time to record each vaccine component administered in the medical record and statewide vaccine registry, giving the vaccine, observing and addressing reactions or side effects, and cost of supplies (eg, syringe, needle, bandages).

For each individual vaccine administered, report code **90460** because every vaccine will have, at minimum, one vaccine component. Depending on the specific vaccine, code **90461** is additionally reported for counseling on each additional component of each combination vaccine. No modifier is typically required for reporting multiple units of the IA codes. Most payers advise reporting multiple units of the same service on a single line of the claim. However, individual payer guidance may vary.

Examples

➤ **A 15-year-old patient receives the 9-valent HPV (9vHPV) vaccine from his physician.** The ordering physician discusses risks of the vaccine and the disease for which it provides protection. The parent/guardian is given the CDC VIS. The parent/guardian consents; the nurse provides the VIS and prepares the vaccine. The nurse administers the vaccine by a single injection, charts the required information, and accesses and enters vaccine data into the statewide immunization registry. The patient is discharged home after the nurse confirms that there are no serious immediate reactions.

ICD-10-CM	CPT®
Z23 (encounter for immunization)	**90651** (9vHPV) **90460**

Teaching Point: Because the physician personally performed the counseling, code **90460** is reported for this single-component vaccine. No other services are reported because the purpose of the visit was for administration of the vaccine only.

➤ **An 11-year-old girl (new patient) presents to a pediatrician for a preventive medicine service.** In addition to the preventive E/M service with no abnormal findings, the physician discusses risks of the HPV vaccine and the disease for which it provides protection. The parent/guardian is given the CDC VIS. The parent/guardian consents; the nurse prepares to administer the vaccine. However, the patient then refuses to receive the immunization, and counseling by the nurse does not change her decision. The physician returns to the examination room and provides additional counseling, but the patient becomes tearful and continues to refuse the vaccine. The patient's mother wishes to discuss with the child's father and return on a later date. A follow-up appointment is scheduled.

ICD-10-CM	CPT
Z00.129 **Z28.21** (immunization not carried out because of patient refusal)	**99383**

Teaching Point: Because the vaccine was not administered, no charge for the product or the administration would be reported. When the patient returns for follow-up, the codes reported will depend on the outcome of the encounter. If the vaccine is administered after additional physician counseling at the same encounter, code **90460** would be reported in addition to the appropriate vaccine product code. If the patient returns for administration by a nurse without additional counseling by a physician, code **90471** would be reported in lieu of **90460**. Additional counseling at the follow-up visit that does not result in immunization may be reported with a preventive medicine counseling code (**99401–99404**) based on the physician's face-to-face time with the patient.

Chapter 9: Preventive Services

➤ **You administer measles, mumps, rubella (MMR) vaccine and a varicella vaccine at the same encounter.**

Report code **90460** with 2 units (1 unit for the first component of each vaccine given) and code **90461** with 2 units for counseling related to additional components of the combination vaccine. Link the vaccine and administration *CPT®* codes to *ICD-10-CM* code **Z23** on health insurance claims.

➤ **A patient receives the diphtheria, tetanus toxoids, acellular pertussis; inactivated poliovirus; and** *Haemophilus influenzae* **type b (DTaP-IPV/Hib) vaccine as a combination vaccine and an influenza vaccine.**

Report **90460** for each vaccine administered (2 units) and **90461** with 4 units for counseling related to additional components of the combination vaccine (DTaP-IPV/Hib). The DTaP-IPV/Hib vaccine product is reported with code **90698**. *Note:* While not as common, some physicians provide single-component vaccines versus combinations. Therefore, for this example, **90460** would be reported with 4 units for the first components of the 4 vaccine products and **90461** with 2 units for the additional components of the DTaP vaccine. Link the vaccine and administration *CPT* codes to *ICD-10-CM* code **Z23** on health insurance claims.

➤ **A 4-month-old established patient receives the DTaP-IPV/Hib combination vaccine, rotavirus vaccine (RV5), and pneumococcal conjugate vaccine (PCV13) from her physician at the time of her preventive medicine visit.** The ordering physician discusses the risks of each vaccine component (eg, tetanus, pertussis) and the diseases for which each vaccine component provides protection. The parent/guardian is given the CDC VIS for all vaccine components and consents for each of the additional vaccine components. The nurse charts the required information and enters data into the statewide immunization registry for each vaccine component.

ICD-10-CM	*CPT*
Z00.129 (routine infant or child check without abnormal findings) **Z23** (encounter for immunization)	**99391 25** (preventive medicine visit; younger than 1 year)
Z00.129 (routine infant or child check without abnormal findings) **Z23** (encounter for immunization)	**90698** (DTaP-IPV/Hib) **90680** (RV5) **90670** (PCV13) **90460** × 3 units for counseling for first component of each of 3 vaccines **90461** × 4 units for counseling for additional components (eg, tetanus, pertussis, IPV, Hib)

Teaching Point: Code **90460** is reported for each vaccine administered and includes the work of counseling for the first component of each vaccine administered (diphtheria, rotavirus, and pneumococcus). Code **90461** is reported in conjunction with **90460** for each additional component that is part of the combination vaccine DTaP-IPV/Hib. Payers who have adopted the Medicare National Correct Coding Initiative (NCCI) edits will require that modifier **25** be appended to code **99391** to signify that it was significant and separately identifiable. (For more information on NCCI edits, see Chapter 2, Modifiers and Coding Edits.) *ICD-10-CM* code **Z00.129** is reported first, followed by code **Z23**.

> **~ More From the AAP ~**
>
> The American Academy of Pediatrics *Quick Reference Guide to Coding Pediatric Vaccines 2019* may be purchased from shopAAP at https://shop.aap.org/quick-reference-guide-to-coding-pediatric-vaccines-2019.

➤ **A 12-year-old established patient is seen for his preventive medicine visit by the certified pediatric nurse practitioner (CPNP), who bills under her own NPI.** The patient complains of an increasingly severe itchy rash on his hands, arms, and legs for 3 days. A problem-focused history related to the complaint is performed. He is diagnosed and treated for a moderately severe case of poison ivy, requiring a prescription for a topical steroid. He has not yet received his tetanus, diphtheria, and acellular pertussis (Tdap), meningococcal (MenACWY, intramuscular), or human papillomavirus (9vHPV) vaccines. The CPNP counsels the parents on the risks and protection from each of the diseases. The CDC VISs are given to the parents and the nurse administers the vaccines.

ICD-10-CM	CPT®
Z00.121 (well-child check with abnormal findings) **L23.7** (allergic contact dermatitis due to plants, except food)	**99394 25** (preventive medicine visit, established patient, age 12 through 17 years)
Z00.121 **Z23**	**90715** (Tdap, 7 years or older, intramuscular) **90734** (MenACWY) **90651** (9vHPV) **90460** × 3 units (for first component of 3 vaccines) **90461** × 2 units (for 2 additional components)
L23.7 (allergic contact dermatitis due to plants, except food)	**99212 25** (office/outpatient E/M, established patient)

Teaching Point: Medical record documentation supports that a significant, separately identifiable E/M service was provided and is reported in addition to the preventive medicine service. Modifier **25** is appended to code **99212** to signify that it is significant and separately identifiable from the preventive medicine service. Modifier **25** is also appended to code **99394** to signify it is significant and separately identifiable from IA. Because the child is younger than 18 years and vaccine counseling was performed by the CPNP with her own NPI, codes **90460** and **90461** may be reported as appropriate.

When assigning an *ICD-10-CM* code for "with abnormal findings," additional code(s) should be assigned to identify the specific abnormal finding(s). The code for the abnormal finding is linked to the claim lines for the preventive and problem-oriented E/M services.

Coding Conundrum: Vaccine Counseling on Day Different From Administration

Current Procedural Terminology® states that codes **90460** and **90461** are reported when the physician or other qualified health care professional (QHP) provides face-to-face counseling of the patient and family during the administration of a vaccine. However, there are situations in which vaccine counseling is performed on a day different from the actual administration. For example, the physician or QHP might provide vaccine counseling during an encounter, but because the child is ill, the vaccines are deferred to a later date. Or the physician or QHP may counsel the patient and parent on all vaccines needed during the annual preventive medicine service visit, but the parent refuses multiple vaccines on the same day, and some of the vaccines are given over a series of encounters for vaccine administration only. How would a physician then report immunization administration (IA)?

Because these circumstances split the actual administration from vaccine counseling, codes **90460** and **90461** cannot be reported. In these situations, IA is reported using codes **90471–90474** on the day the vaccines are administered without physician counseling on the same date.

Codes 90471–90474

90471	Immunization administration (includes percutaneous, intradermal, subcutaneous, or intramuscular injections); one vaccine (single or combination vaccine/toxoid)
+90472	each additional vaccine (single or combination vaccine/toxoid)

(List separately in addition to code for primary procedure.) (Use code **90472** in conjunction with **90460**, **90471**, or **90473**.)

90473	Immunization administration by intranasal or oral route; one vaccine (single or combination vaccine/toxoid)
+90474	each additional vaccine (single or combination vaccine/toxoid)

(List separately in addition to code for primary procedure.) (Use code **90474** in conjunction with **90460**, **90471**, or **90473**.)

Codes **90471–90474** will be reported when criteria for reporting the 2 pediatric IA codes (**90460** and **90461**) have not been met (ie, physician or QHP does not counsel patient/family or does not document that the counseling was personally performed, or when the patient is ≥19 years).

The CMS has assigned 0.58 RVUs to codes **90460**, **90471**, and **90473** and 0.36 RVUs to codes **90461**, **90472**, and **90474**. Appropriate reporting of codes **90460** and **90461** in lieu of codes **90471–90474** should result in higher payment based on reporting of multiple units of code **90461** for *each additional vaccine component* versus reporting of codes **90472** and **90474** for *each additional vaccine product*. Individual payers may or may not assign payment values based on the RVUs published by the CMS. (Administration of vaccines provided through the Vaccines for Children [VFC] program is paid differently. See more about the VFC program later in this chapter.)

When reporting codes **90471–90474**

- Codes **90471–90474** are reported for each vaccine administered, whether single or combination vaccines.
- *Only one* "first" IA code (**90460**, **90471**, or **90473**) may be reported on a calendar day.

    The "first" IA code can be reported from either family or either route of administration (eg, when a patient receives an immunization via injection and a second one via intranasal route, IA services can be reported with codes **90471** and **90474** or with codes **90473** and **90472**).

- The Medicare NCCI edits pair code **90460** with codes **90471** and **90473**, not allowing codes from both sets to be reported on the same day of service by the same physician or physician of the same group and specialty. If a physician personally performs counseling on one vaccine but not on another when given during the same encounter, IA will be reported using codes **90460** (and **90461** if appropriate) and either **90472** (IA, each additional vaccine via injection) or **90474** (each additional vaccine via intranasal or oral route).

For more information on vaccine administration, please see the following examples and Appendix II, Vaccine Products: Commonly Administered Pediatric Vaccines.

Examples

➤ **A 4-year-old patient is seen by a nurse per physician's order to follow up on impetigo and clearance to return to preschool.** The father also requests that his daughter receive influenza vaccination. The nurse performs an interval history and very brief examination and finds the impetigo has resolved. After assessing the patient and verifying she is in good health, the nurse confirms there are no contraindications to the immunization per CDC guidelines. Next, the nurse reviews the VIS with the father and the antipyretic dosage for weight and obtains the father's consent for the immunization. The nurse then administers the influenza vaccine and observes for immediate reactions.

ICD-10-CM	CPT®
Z09 (encounter for follow-up examination after completed treatment for conditions other than malignant neoplasm) Z87.2 (personal history of diseases of the skin and subcutaneous tissue)	99211 25 (E/M service)
Z23 (encounter for immunization)	90686 (influenza vaccine [IIV4], preservative free, 0.5 mL, intramuscular) 90471 (IA, first injection)

Teaching Point: If the payer follows NCCI edits, CPT code 99211 will never be paid for separately from vaccine administration (eg, 90471), even with modifier 25. See Coding Conundrum: Reporting Evaluation and Management Services With Immunization Administration later in this chapter for more information on reporting code 99211 with IA.

➤ A 5-year-old established patient presented 2 weeks ago for her 5-year check and vaccines. At that appointment, her physician provided counseling for each recommended vaccine component and corresponding VISs. The patient's mother asked that the vaccines be split, so only the DTaP and IPV vaccines were given at that encounter. The patient returns today for an immunization-only visit to get the MMR and varicella vaccines.

ICD-10-CM	CPT
Z23 (encounter for immunization)	90707 (MMR, live) 90471 (IA, first injection) 90716 (varicella vaccine) 90472 (IA, subsequent injection)

Teaching Point: Counseling for all vaccines occurred at the last encounter and all VISs were handed out, so only administration occurred today. CPT® codes 90460 and 90461 would be reported with the appropriate codes for DTaP and IPV vaccines that were administered during the previous encounter. However, services on this date did not include physician counseling. (See Coding Conundrum: Vaccine Counseling on Day Different From Administration earlier in this chapter.) Only report codes 90460 and 90461 when physician counseling is provided on the date of vaccine administration.

➤ A 19-year-old established patient presents for college entrance examination. In addition to providing a preventive medicine service, the physician counsels the patient on the need for meningococcal serogroup B (MenB-4C) immunization. The vaccine is administered, and a medical history and physical form provided by the college are completed.

ICD-10-CM	CPT
Z02.0 (encounter for examination for admission to educational institution)	99395 25 (preventive medicine service, established patient, 18–39 years old)
Z23 (encounter for immunization)	90620 (MenB-4C) 90471 (IA, first injection)

Teaching Point: Because the patient is older than 18 years, code 90460 cannot be reported even though the physician provided counseling for the vaccine provided. Code Z00.00 (encounter for general adult medical examination without abnormal findings) is not reported because ICD-10-CM excludes reporting of code Z00.00 in conjunction with codes in category Z02. Code Z02.0 is appropriate as the reason the patient presented for the encounter.

Coding Conundrum: Reporting Evaluation and Management Services With Immunization Administration

Evaluation and management (E/M) services most often reported with the vaccine product and immunization administration (IA) include new and established patient preventive medicine visits (*Current Procedural Terminology* [*CPT®*] codes **99381–99395**), problem-oriented visits (**99201–99215**), and preventive medicine counseling services (**99401–99404**).

The E/M service must be medically indicated, significant, and separately identifiable from the IA.

Payers may require modifier **25** (significant, separately identifiable E/M service by the same physician on the same day of the procedure or other service) to be appended to the E/M code to distinguish it from the administration of the vaccine.

If a patient is seen for the administration of a vaccine only, it is not appropriate to report an E/M visit if it is not medically necessary, significant, and separately identifiable.

CPT code **99211** (established patient E/M, minimal level, not requiring physician presence) *should not* be reported when the patient encounter is for vaccination only because Medicare Resource-Based Relative Value Scale (RBRVS) relative values for IA codes include administrative and clinical services (ie, greeting the patient, routine vital signs, obtaining a vaccine history, presenting the VIS and responding to routine vaccine questions, preparation and administration of the vaccine, and documentation and observation of the patient following administration of the vaccine). However, if the service is medically necessary, significant, and separately identifiable, it may be reported with modifier **25** appended to the E/M code (**99211**). The medical record must clearly state the reason for the visit, brief history, physical examination, assessment and plan, and any other counseling or discussion items. The progress note must be signed with the physician's countersignature. For more information and clinical vignettes on the appropriate use of E/M services during IA, visit www.aap.org/cfp, access code AAPCFP24. Payers who do not follow the Medicare RBRVS may allow payment of code **99211** with IA. Know your payer guidelines, and if payment is allowed, make certain the guidelines are in writing and maintained in your office. Be aware that a co-payment will be required when the "nurse" visit is reported.

The same guidelines apply to physician visits (**99201–99215**).

See FAQ: Immunization Administration online at www.aap.org/cfp, access code AAPCFP24, for further discussion of coding for immunization administration.

Vaccines for Children Program

The VFC program makes vaccines available to children up to 19 years of age who meet any of the following criteria: are enrolled in the Medicaid program (depending on the state Managed Medicaid), do not have health insurance, have no coverage of immunizations under their health plan, or are American Indians or Alaska Natives. Vaccines are provided at no cost to the participating physician or patient, and payment is made only for administration of the vaccine.

If reporting the VFC vaccine with administration codes and not the product code, data for the vaccine products administered must be captured for registry and quality initiatives. This can be accomplished by entering the vaccine codes with a $0 charge (if your billing system allows) and appending modifier **SL** (state-supplied vaccine) to the vaccine code. However, follow individual payer rules for reporting.

Providers are encouraged to use code **90460** for administration of a vaccine under the VFC program unless otherwise directed by a state program. If code **90461** is used for a vaccine with multiple antigens or components, it should be given a $0 value for a child covered under the VFC program. This applies to Medicaid-enrolled VFC-entitled children as well as non–Medicaid-enrolled VFC-entitled children (ie, uninsured, underinsured, and American Indian or Alaska Native children not enrolled in Medicaid). Please be aware that some state Medicaid programs do have reporting rules that differ from VFC. *Be sure to get this policy in writing from your state Medicaid program* and follow it to avoid denied payment. The AAP continues to advocate to the CMS to allow for recognition and payment for component-based vaccine counseling and administration (ie, code **90461**). Under the current statute, administration can only be paid "per vaccine" and not component.

Chapter 9: Preventive Services

Participants in the VFC program should be aware of program-specific guidance, including storage of VFC vaccine separate from privately purchased vaccines. For more information on the VFC program, visit www.cdc.gov/vaccines/programs/vfc/index.html.

Screening Tests and Procedures

Recommendations for age-appropriate screening services are outlined in the AAP "Recommendations for Preventive Pediatric Health Care" (www.aap.org/periodicityschedule) or in your state's EPSDT plan.

Hearing Screening

92551	Screening test, pure tone, air only
92552	Pure tone audiometry (threshold); air only (full assessment)
#92558	Evoked otoacoustic emissions, screening (qualitative measurement of distortion product or transient evoked otoacoustic emissions), automated analysis
92583	Select picture audiometry
92567	Tympanometry (impedance testing)
92568	Acoustic reflex testing, threshold portion

Audiometric tests require the use of calibrated electronic equipment, recording of results, and a written report with interpretation. Services include testing of both ears. If the test is applied to one ear only, modifier 52 (reduced services) must be appended to the code.

- Code **92551** (screening test, pure tone, air only) is used when earphones are placed on the patient and the patient is asked to respond to tones of different pitches and intensities. This is a limited study.

- Code **92552** (full pure tone audiometric assessment; air only) is used when earphones are placed on the patient and the patient is asked to respond to tones of different pitches and intensities. The threshold, which is the lowest intensity of the tone that the patient can hear 50% of the time, is recorded for a number of frequencies.

- Code **92558** (evoked otoacoustic emissions [OAEs] screening) is used when a probe tip is placed in the ear canal to screen for normal hearing function. The probe tip emits a repeated clicking sound (transient evoked emissions) or 2 tones at 2 frequencies (distortion product emissions). The sounds pass through the tympanic membrane and middle ear to the inner ear. In the inner ear, the sound is picked up by the hair cells in the cochlea, which, in turn, bounce the sound back in low-intensity sound waves (OAEs). These OAEs are recorded and analyzed by computerized equipment and the results are automated.

- Code **92583** (select picture audiometry) is typically used for younger children. The patient is asked to identify different pictures with the instructions given at different sound intensity levels.

- Other commonly performed procedures include codes **92567** (tympanometry [impedance testing]) and **92568** (acoustic reflex testing, threshold portion). However, both codes may have limited coverage; check with payers.

- Automated audiometry testing is reported with Category III codes **0208T–0212T**.

> ‖|‖|‖‖‖ *Coding Pearl* ‖|‖|‖‖‖
>
> *International Classification of Diseases, 10th Revision, Clinical Modification* codes for well-child examinations include developmental, hearing, and vision screening.

> ‖|‖|‖‖‖ *Coding Pearl* ‖|‖|‖‖‖
>
> In *Current Procedural Terminology®* references, code **92558** is preceded by the number sign or pound symbol (#) to indicate that this code is not listed in numerical order. Code **92558** is listed between codes **92586** and **92587**.

> ‖|‖|‖‖‖ *Coding Pearl* ‖|‖|‖‖‖
>
> When hearing screening is performed in the physician office because of a failed screening in another setting (eg, school), report *International Classification of Diseases, 10th Revision, Clinical Modification* codes from category **Z01.11-**. Code **Z01.110** is reported for a normal screening result following a failed screening. Code **Z01.118** indicates a failed repeat screening. An additional code is reported to identify the abnormality found following the failed repeat screening.

Chapter 9: Preventive Services

0208T	Pure tone audiometry (threshold), automated; air only
0209T	air and bone
0210T	Speech audiometry threshold, automated
0211T	with speech recognition
0212T	Comprehensive audiometry threshold evaluation and speech recognition (0209T, 0211T combined), automated

Examples

➤ **George is a 16-year-old established patient presenting for a preventive service and clearance to participate in school sports.** A complete preventive E/M service (99394) is provided. George has not received a hearing screening since he was 13 years old, so pure tone, air-only screening audiometry is performed (92551). No abnormalities are found, and George receives clearance to participate in sports. The *ICD-10-CM* code reported for each of the services is Z00.129 (encounter for routine child health examination without abnormal findings).

➤ **Sally is a 6-year-old who failed a hearing screening at school and is referred to her pediatrician for additional evaluation.** Sally's parents indicate no prior concerns about her hearing, and risk factor assessment is negative. The pediatrician chooses to perform screening audiometry (92551), which produces typical results. The *ICD-10-CM* code reported is Z01.110 (encounter for examination of ears and hearing without abnormal findings). If the key components (history, examination, and medical decision-making [MDM]) support a separate office or other outpatient E/M service, this is separately reported (eg, 99212).

➤ **Sally, who failed a hearing screening at her pediatrician's office, is seen by an audiologist for a hearing evaluation.** The audiologist conducts a pure tone, air-only audiometry test with positive findings. Bone conduction testing (92553) and speech audiometry with speech recognition (92556) are additionally performed. Code 92557 (comprehensive audiometry threshold evaluation and speech recognition [92553 and 92556 combined]) is reported in conjunction with the appropriate *ICD-10-CM* code for the hearing abnormality identified.

Vision Screening

99173	Screening test of visual acuity, quantitative, bilateral
99174	Instrument-based ocular screening (eg, photoscreening, automated-refraction), bilateral; with remote analysis and report
99177	with on-site analysis
0333T	Visual evoked potential, screening of visual acuity, automated, with report
0469T	Retinal polarization scan, ocular screening with on-site automated results, bilateral

◦ Screening test of visual acuity (99173) must use graduated visual stimuli that allow a quantitative estimate of visual acuity (eg, Snellen chart).

  ❖ Medical record documentation must include a measurement of acuity for both eyes, not just a pass or fail score.

  ❖ Code 99173 is only reported when vision screening is performed in association with a preventive medicine visit. It is not reported when it is performed as part of an evaluation for an eye problem or condition (eg, examination to rule out vision problems in a patient presenting with problems with schoolwork) because the assessment of visual acuity is considered an integral part of the eye examination.

◦ Instrument-based ocular screening (99174, 99177) is used to report screening for a variety of conditions, including esotropia, exotropia, isometropia, cataracts, ptosis, hyperopia, myopia, and others, that affect or have the potential to affect vision. These tests are especially useful for screening infants, preschool patients, and those older patients whose ability to participate in traditional acuity screening is limited or very time intensive.

Chapter 9: Preventive Services

Chapter 9: Preventive Services

* Code **99177** specifies screening using an instrument that provides an on-site (ie, in-office) pass or fail result.
* Code **99174** specifies the use of a screening instrument that incorporates remote analysis and report.
* These screenings cannot be reported in conjunction with codes **92002–92700** (general ophthalmologic services), **99172** (visual function screening), or **99173** (screening test of visual acuity, quantitative) because ocular screening is inherent to these services. An AAP policy statement on instrument-based pediatric vision screening is available at http://pediatrics.aappublications.org/content/130/5/983.full.
* Vision screening performed using an automated visual evoked potential system is reported with code **0333T**. This code applies to automated screening using an instrument-based algorithm with a pass or fail result. Code **0333T** was revised to indicate that a report of the result must be documented. Report code **95930** only for comprehensive visual evoked potential testing with physician interpretation and report.
* Retinal polarization scanning (**0469T**) is used to detect amblyopia due to strabismus and defocus. Similar to code **99177**, results of each scan are generated on-site.

Developmental Screening and Health Assessment

Standardized (ie, validated) screening instruments are used for screening and assessment purposes as reported by codes **96110** and **96127**. Examples of assessment and screening tools by code are available in Appendix I, Sample Assessment/Testing Tools. Health risk assessments that are patient focused (**96160**) are differentiated from those such as maternal depression screening that are caregiver focused (**96161**) for the benefit of the patient.

Developmental Screening

96110   Developmental screening with scoring and documentation, per standardized instrument

Structured screening for developmental delay is a universal recommendation of the "Recommendations for Preventive Pediatric Health Care" at 18-month and 2-year visits for autism spectrum disorder (ASD)–specific screening (eg, Modified Checklist for Autism in Toddlers [M-CHAT]) and at 9-month, 18-month, and 2- or 2½-year visits for other developmental screening (eg, Ages & Stages Questionnaire [ASQ]). When reporting these screenings, code **96110** represents developmental screening with scoring and documentation per standardized instrument. (Note that screening results should be included in the patient medical record.)

> 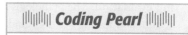 **Coding Pearl** |||||||
>
> *International Classification of Diseases, 10th Revision, Clinical Modification* code **Z13.42**, encounter for screening for global developmental delays (milestones), is not reported for routine developmental testing of an infant or child at the time of a preventive service. An *Excludes1* note directs to codes in subcategory **Z00.1-**.

Code **96110**
* Is reported for standardized developmental screening instruments. It is not reported when the pediatrician conducts an informal survey or surveillance of development as part of a comprehensive preventive medicine service (which is considered part of the history and is not separately billed).
* May be reported for each standardized developmental screening instrument administered.
* Includes standardized screening tools, such as ASQ, Australian Scale for Asperger's Syndrome, M-CHAT, or Parents' Evaluation of Developmental Status (PEDS). Other tools are also used for developmental screening.
* In *CPT 2019*, the introductory text for neuropsychological testing makes clear those codes that include interpretation and report. Code **96110** (developmental screening) does not require interpretation and report (ie, includes scoring and documentation only).
* Is not reported for brief emotional or behavioral assessment; see code **96127**.

Example

➤ **A 20-month-old girl presents to her primary physician with a complaint of pulling at her ears and nasal congestion.** She missed her 18-month well-child checkup. A preventive visit is offered, but mother prefers to come back when she has scheduled more time off work. The mother is given the PEDS and M-CHAT (a standardized screening instrument for ASD in children 16–30 months of age) by the nursing assistant, who explains why the instruments are given and how they should be completed. After the child's mother completes both forms, the nursing assistant scores and attaches them to the child's medical chart. The physician evaluates the patient's upper respiratory symptoms and diagnoses viral upper respiratory infection. The physician also interprets and records the normal results of the PEDS and M-CHAT in the medical record and requests that the mother schedule a full preventive service for the child within the next month.

Code 96110 is reported with 2 units of service (see Claim Form Example 1 for Multiple Units of Service), or 96110 and 96110 59 are reported (see Claim Form Example 2 for Multiple Units of Service), depending on payer requirements. *ICD-10-CM* codes Z13.40–Z13.49 (eg, Z13.42, screening for global developmental delays [milestones]) may be reported to indicate screening for developmental disability in children when the screening is not performed in conjunction with a well-child visit.

Claim Form Example 1 for Multiple Units of Service

21. Diagnosis or nature of illness or injury (Relate A–L to service line below 24E)   ICD Ind. 0

A. J06.9   B. Z13.42   C.   D.

24. A. Dates of service	B. Place of service	C. EMG	D. Procedures, services zor supplies CPT/HCPCS	Modifier	E. Diagnosis Pointer	F. Charges	G. Days or units	H. EPSDT	I. ID Qual	J. Rendering Provider #
1/2/2019–1/2/2019	11		99213	25	A	$$$	1		NPI	123456789
1/2/2019–1/2/2019	11		96110		B	$$$	2		NPI	123456789

Abbreviations: CPT, Current Procedural Terminology; EMG, emergency; EPSDT, Early and Periodic Screening, Diagnosis, and Treatment; HCPCS, Healthcare Common Procedure Coding System; ICD, International Classification of Diseases; NPI, National Provider Identifier.

Claim Form Example 2 for Multiple Units of Service

21. Diagnosis or nature of illness or injury (Relate A–L to service line below 24E)   ICD Ind. 0

A. J06.9   B. Z13.41   C. Z13.42   D.

24. A. Dates of service	B. Place of service	C. EMG	D. Procedures, services or supplies CPT/HCPCS	Modifier	E. Diagnosis Pointer	F. Charges	G. Days or units	H. EPSDT	I. ID Qual	J. Rendering Provider #
1/2/2019–1/2/2019	11		99213	25	A	$$$	1		NPI	123456789
1/1/2019–1/2/2019	11		96110		B	$$$	1		NPI	123456789
1/1/2019–1/2/2019	11		96110	59	C	$$$	1		NPI	123456789

Abbreviations: CPT, Current Procedural Terminology; EMG, emergency; EPSDT, Early and Periodic Screening, Diagnosis, and Treatment; HCPCS, Healthcare Common Procedure Coding System; ICD, International Classification of Diseases; NPI, National Provider Identifier.

Teaching Point: There is a Medically Unlikely Edit (MUE) on code 96110. The MUE is 2; therefore, if the payer follows MUEs, you cannot report more than two 96110 codes per line on the claim form. (See Chapter 2, Modifiers and Coding Edits, for more details.) *ICD-10-CM* codes Z13.41 (autism screening) and Z13.42 (screening for delayed milestones) also help identify the reason for 2 units of service. Proactive recommendations and delivery of preventive services support quality initiatives.

Chapter 9: Preventive Services

Emotional/Behavioral Assessment

96127   Brief emotional/behavioral assessment (eg, depression inventory, ADHD scale), with scoring and documentation, per standardized instrument

Code **96127**

❖ Is reported for standardized emotional/behavioral assessment instruments.

❖ Represents the practice expense of administering, scoring, and documenting each standardized instrument. No physician work value is included. Physician interpretation is included in a related E/M service.

❖ Is not reported in conjunction with preventive medicine counseling/risk-factor reduction intervention (**99401–99404**) or psychiatric or neurologic testing (**96130–96139**), or **96146**.

❖ Can involve 2 or more separately reported completions of the same form (eg, attention-deficit/hyperactivity disorder [ADHD] rating scales by teacher and by parent). Note that MUEs limit reporting to 2 units per claim line. When reporting to payers adopting MUEs, additional units beyond the first 2 must be reported on a separate claim line with an NCCI modifier (eg, **59**, distinct procedural service). As always, documentation should support the appropriateness of the additional units of service.

❖ Can be reported for standardized depression instruments that are required under US Preventive Services Task Force (USPSTF) and Bright Futures recommendations (see AAP/Bright Futures "Recommendations for Preventive Pediatric Health Care" [Periodicity Schedule] insert).

Examples of assessment and screening tools by code are available in Appendix I, Sample Assessment/Testing Tools, or online at www.aap.org/cfp, access code AAPCFP24.

Example

➤ **A 12-year-old boy is seen for an established patient well-child health supervision and sports physical encounter.** In addition to the preventive medicine service, the physician's staff administers and scores a recommended depression screening instrument (eg, Patient Health Questionnaire-9). The physician reviews the score, documents that the screening result is negative for symptoms of depression, and completes the preventive medicine service. Clearance is given to participate in sports.

The preventive medicine service code (**99394**) would be reported in addition to code **96127**. The diagnosis code reported is **Z00.129** (encounter for routine child health examination without abnormal findings). Link **Z00.129** to the claim service line for code **96127**. Remember that *ICD-10-CM* guidelines state to link routine screening services to the well-child/adolescent code. A code for the sports physical (**Z02.5**) is not reported because *ICD-10-CM* excludes reporting of codes in category **Z02** in conjunction with codes in category **Z00**.

When screening results are positive and the physician performs further evaluation, leading to a diagnosis of depression, code the preventive service with abnormal findings (**Z00.121**) followed by the appropriate code for the diagnosed depression (eg, **F32.0**, major depressive disorder, single episode, mild). When appropriate, a significant and separately identifiable E/M service to evaluate and manage depression may be reported by appending modifier **25** to an office or other outpatient E/M code (eg, **99213**). Documentation should clearly support the key components of the separate service or, if billing based on time spent in counseling and/or coordination of care, the time and a summary of the service provided (eg, education on the condition, questions answered, patient and/or caregiver concerns, management options discussed, plan of care).

Health Risk Assessment

96160   Administration of patient-focused health risk assessment (eg, health hazard appraisal) with scoring and documentation, per standardized instrument

96161   Administration of caregiver-focused health risk assessment (eg, depression inventory) for the benefit of the patient, with scoring and documentation, per standardized instrument

Code **96160** is reported for a patient-focused health risk assessment. This is differentiated from code **96161**, which is used to report a health risk assessment focused on a caregiver for the benefit of the patient.

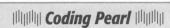

- Code **96160** is reported for administration (with scoring and documentation) of a standardized patient-focused health risk assessment instrument (eg, health hazard appraisal). Code **96160** cannot be used in conjunction with assessment and brief intervention for alcohol/substance abuse (**99408** and **99409**). Check individual payer guidance to determine if and for what purposes code **96160** is included as a covered and payable service under the payer's policies (eg, some Medicaid plans pay for adolescent health questionnaires, such as HEADSSS [*h*ome, *e*ducation (ie, school), *a*ctivities/employment, *d*rugs, *s*afety, *s*exuality, and *s*uicidality/depression], reported with **96160**).

- Code **96161** is reported for administration of a health risk assessment to a patient's caregiver. Examples are a postpartum depression inventory administered to the mother of a newborn and administration of a validated caregiver strain instrument to parents of a seriously injured or ill child.

- Report 1 unit of **96160** or **96161** for each standardized instrument administered. Payer edits may limit the number of times codes **96160** and **96161** may be reported for an individual patient and/or on the same date of service.

- Sparse coverage for codes **96160** and specifically **96161** has been noted by the AAP, and advocacy efforts are being made.

> |||||||| *Coding Pearl* ||||||||
>
> Report only one structured screening instrument for both the Patient Health Questionnaire (PHQ)-2 and PHQ-9. The PHQ-2 consists of the first 2 questions of the PHQ-9. If the PHQ-2 screening result is positive for depression, the remaining portion of the PHQ-9 is often used to confirm the positive screening result.

Example

> ➤ **As part of a health supervision visit for a 2-month-old established patient, the physician directs clinical staff to administer a screening for postpartum depression.** Clinical staff explain the purpose of the instrument to the infant's mother. After the mother has completed the screening instrument, clinical staff score and document the result in the patient record. The physician completes the preventive medicine service. Included is anticipatory guidance advising the mother that her screening indicates no current signs of postpartum depression and of symptoms that should prompt a call to her physician.

ICD-10-CM	CPT®
Z00.129 (encounter for routine child health examination without abnormal findings)	**99391** (preventive medicine visit) **96161** (administration of caregiver-focused health risk assessment [eg, depression inventory] for the benefit of the patient, with scoring and documentation, per standardized instrument)

Teaching Point: The screening for postpartum depression is caregiver focused (sign/symptoms of depression in mother) but performed in this setting for the benefit of the infant. This service is reported as a service provided to the infant with code **96161**. Check payer policy on adoption of code **96161** versus a requirement to report as a service to the mother (ie, to mother's health plan) with code **96127** (brief emotional/behavioral assessment [eg, depression inventory, ADHD scale], with scoring and documentation, per standardized instrument). Many Medicaid plans provide separate payment for maternal depression screening at well-child visits, but specific reporting instructions may apply. Also, never report the new *ICD-10-CM* code **Z13.32** (encounter for maternal depression screen) on the baby's chart/bill.

Chapter 9: Preventive Services

Prevention of Dental Caries

Application of Fluoride Varnish

99188   Application of topical fluoride varnish by a physician or other qualified health care professional

☀ Topical fluoride application by primary care physicians is a recommended preventive service for children from birth through 5 years of age (Grade B rating by the USPSTF). This service may be covered when provided alone or in conjunction with other services. Coverage is usually limited to once every 6 months.

☀ ICD-10-CM code Z29.3 is reported to identify encounter for prophylactic fluoride administration. When applicable, diagnosis of dental caries may be reported as a secondary diagnosis with codes in category K02. Encounter for prophylactic fluoride administration is reported separately from the encounter for routine child health examination (Z00.121 or Z00.129) when both services are provided at the same encounter.

☀ Although code 99188 specifies application by a physician or QHP, payers may allow billing of services by trained clinical staff under direct physician supervision (incident to). Some Medicaid plans require training of clinical staff through specific programs. It is important to identify the requirements of individual payers prior to providing this service.

☀ Code on Dental Procedures and Nomenclature (CDT®) codes also exist for topical application of fluoride varnish and fluoride. In addition, CDT codes exist for nutrition counseling to prevent dental disease, oral hygiene instruction, and oral evaluations. However, acceptance of these codes by health plans may be limited to state Medicaid plans.

> ## |||||||| Coding Pearl ||||||||
>
> National Correct Coding Initiative (NCCI) edits bundle codes 96160 and 96161 with code 96110 and with immunization administration (90460–90474) services, but a modifier is allowed when each code represents a distinct service and is clinically appropriate. Append modifier 59 to the bundled code (second column of NCCI edits) when these services are reported on the same date to a payer that has adopted NCCI edits.

Counseling to Prevent Dental Caries

Some payers will provide coverage for oral evaluation and health risk assessment or other dental preventive services when provided on the same day as a preventive medicine visit; other payers will allow services only when they are provided at an encounter separate from a preventive medicine visit. Know payer requirements for reporting.

☀ Preventive counseling for oral health may be included as part of the preventive medicine service (99381–99395) or, if performed at a separate encounter, reported under the individual preventive medicine counseling service codes (99401–99404) or with an office or outpatient E/M service code (99201–99215). ICD-10-CM code Z13.84 may be reported for an encounter for screening for dental disorders.

☀ For those carriers (particularly state Medicaid plans under EPSDT) that cover oral health care, some will require a modifier. These modifiers are payer specific and should only be used as directed by your state Medicaid agency or other private payer.

SC Medically necessary service or supply

EP Services provided as part of Medicaid EPSDT program

U5 Medicaid Level of Care 5, as defined by each state

> ## ~ More From the AAP ~
>
> An oral health coding fact sheet is available at https://www.aap.org/en-us/Documents/coding_factsheet_oral_health.pdf.

> ## ~ More From the AAP ~
>
> The American Academy of Pediatrics Section on Oral Health also has state-specific information; see https://www.aap.org/en-us/about-the-aap/Committees-Councils-Sections/Oral-Health/Map/Pages/State-Information-and-Resources-Map.aspx.

Chapter 9: Preventive Services

Screening Laboratory Tests

◦ A test performed in the office laboratory should be billed using the appropriate laboratory code and, if performed, the appropriate blood collection code (36400–36416).

◦ Codes 36415 (collection of venous blood by venipuncture) and 36416 (collection of capillary blood specimen [eg, finger, heel, ear stick]) are used for any age child when the physician is not needed to perform the procedure.

◦ When a physician's skill is required to perform venipuncture (eg, access is too difficult for other staff to attain) on a child younger than 3 years, codes 36400–36406 are reported based on the anatomic site of the venipuncture. Report code 36400 when performed on a femoral or jugular vein, code 36405 when on the scalp vein, or code 36406 when another vein is accessed.

◦ When a physician's skill is required to perform venipuncture on a child 3 years or older, code 36410 (venipuncture, age 3 years and older, necessitating physician's skill, for diagnostic or therapeutic purposes [not to be used for routine venipuncture]) is reported.

◦ If the physician performs the venipuncture as a convenience or because staff is not trained in the procedure, code 36415 is reported because the physician's skill was not required.

◦ Although typically not required, some payers will require that modifier 25 be appended to the E/M code if a separate and significant E/M service is reported on the same day of service.

◦ Laboratories and physician offices performing waived tests may need to append modifier QW to the *CPT*® code for Clinical Laboratory Improvement Amendments (CLIA)–waived procedures. The use of modifier QW is payer specific. To review the list of CLIA-waived procedures, go to http://cms.hhs.gov/Regulations-and-Guidance/Legislation/CLIA/Categorization_of_Tests.html.

◦ *ICD-10-CM* allows separate reporting of special screening examinations (codes in categories Z11–Z13) in addition to the codes for routine child health examinations when these codes provide additional information. A screening code is not necessary if the screening is inherent to a routine examination. Payer guidelines for reporting screening examinations may vary. When specific *ICD-10-CM* codes are required to support payment for a screening service, be sure to link the appropriate *ICD-10-CM* code to the claim line for the screening service.

Anemia

85018 QW Blood count; hemoglobin

Screening for anemia is reported with *ICD-10-CM* code Z13.0, encounter for screening for diseases of the blood and blood-forming organs and certain disorders involving the immune mechanism.

Lead Testing

83655 QW Lead, quantitative analysis

◦ This test does not specify the specimen source or method of testing. Alternative tests sometimes (though now rarely) used for lead screening are 82135 (aminolevulinic acid, delta), 84202 (protoporphyrin, red blood cell count, quantitative), and 84203 (protoporphyrin, red blood cell count, screen).

◦ Some states provide lead testing at no cost to patients covered under the Medicaid EPSDT program. Check your state Medicaid requirements for reporting this service.

◦ Report *ICD-10-CM* code Z13.88 (encounter for screening for disorder due to exposure to contaminants) when performing lead screening. Some payers require Z77.011, contact with and (suspected) exposure to lead, in lieu of Z13.88.

Tuberculosis Skin Test (Mantoux)

86580   Tuberculosis, intradermal (includes administration)

❋ The tuberculosis (TB) skin test (Mantoux) using intradermal administration of purified protein derivative (PPD) is the recommended diagnostic skin test for TB. (This is not the BCG TB vaccine.)

❋ Code **99211** is the appropriate code to report when the patient returns for the reading of a PPD test. In the case of a positive test result, when the physician sees the patient and forms a further diagnostic or treatment plan, the complexity may lead to a higher-level code (ie, **99212–99215**). The appropriate *ICD-10-CM* code is **Z11.1** (encounter for screening for respiratory TB).

❋ There is not a separate administration code reported when the TB test is performed.

> ### ~ More From the AAP ~
>
> Not all payers and health care organizations agree with reporting code **99211** when a patient returns for evaluation of a tuberculosis (TB) skin test. However, this is supported by the American Medical Association *CPT Assistant* (July 2006). A template letter for responding to payers that deny code **99211** for evaluation of a TB skin test is available in the Coding Resources at https://coding.aap.org (subscription required).

Dyslipidemia

80061 QW   Lipid panel (must include total serum cholesterol, lipoprotein by direct measurement high-density cholesterol [HDL], and triglycerides) *or*

82465 QW   Cholesterol, serum, total

83718 QW   Lipoprotein, direct measurement, high-density cholesterol (HDL cholesterol)

84478 QW   Triglycerides

The appropriate *ICD-10-CM* code for dyslipidemia screening is **Z13.220** (encounter for screening for lipoid disorders).

Sexually Transmitted Infection

86701 QW   Antibody; HIV-1

G0433 QW   Infectious agent antibody detection by enzyme-linked immunosorbent assay (ELISA) technique, HIV-1 and/or HIV-2, screening

❋ Screening laboratory tests for chlamydia, gonorrhea, and syphilis require more than waived testing laboratory certification. These include

86631   Antibody; chlamydia

86632   Antibody; chlamydia, IgM

86703   Antibody; HIV-1 and HIV-2; single assay

87081   Culture, presumptive, pathogenic organisms, screening only

87110   Culture, chlamydia, any source

87205   Smear, primary source with interpretation; Gram or Giemsa stain for bacteria, fungi, or cell types

❋ *ICD-10-CM* codes supporting screening laboratory tests are **Z11.8**, encounter for screening for other infectious and parasitic diseases (eg, chlamydia); **Z11.3**, encounter for screening for infections with a predominantly sexual mode of transmission (eg, syphilis and gonorrhea); and **Z11.4**, encounter for screening for HIV. Codes in category **Z72**, problems related to lifestyle, may also be required to support screening of a sexually active adolescent.

Preventive Care Provided Outside the Preventive Visit

Counseling and/or Risk-Factor Reduction

Codes **99401–99404**, **99411**, and **99412** are used to report risk-factor reduction services provided for the purpose of promoting health and preventing illness or injury in persons without a specific illness.

Table 9-3 lists the codes for counseling individuals and groups.

Table 9-3. Preventive Medicine Counseling and/or Risk-Factor Reduction	
Code	**Description**
99401	Preventive medicine counseling and/or risk-factor reduction intervention(s) provided to an individual (separate procedure); approximately 15 minutes
99402	approximately 30 minutes
99403	approximately 45 minutes
99404	approximately 60 minutes
99411	Preventive medicine counseling and/or risk-factor reduction intervention(s) provided to individuals in a group setting; approximately 30 minutes
99412	approximately 60 minutes

- Services will vary with age and address issues such as diet, exercise, sexual activity, dental health, injury prevention, safe travel, and family problems.
- Services are reported based on time. The midpoint rule applies (ie, time is met when the midpoint is passed).
- Counseling, anticipatory guidance, and risk-factor reduction interventions provided at the time of an initial or periodic comprehensive preventive medicine examination are components of the periodic service and not separately reported.
- Risk-factor reduction may be reported separately with other E/M services.
  - ❖ Evaluation and management services (other than preventive medicine E/M services) reported on the same day must be separate and distinct.
  - ❖ Time spent in the provision of risk-factor reduction may not be used as a basis for the selection of the other E/M code.
- When reporting a distinct E/M service, append modifier 25 to the code for the distinct E/M service.

> |||||||| **Coding Pearl** ||||||||
>
> Codes **99401–99404, 99411,** and **99412** are time-based codes. Once the midpoint is passed, you may report the code with the closet time. To report code **99401**, the midpoint to pass is 8 minutes.

However, preventive medicine service codes (99381–99395) include counseling, anticipatory guidance, and/or risk-factor reduction interventions that are provided at the time of the periodic comprehensive preventive medicine examination. *CPT* states to "refer to codes 99401, 99402, 99403, 99404, and 99411–99412 for reporting those counseling/anticipatory guidance/risk-factor reduction interventions that are provided at an encounter separate from the preventive medicine examination." Therefore, according to *CPT*, do not report 99401–99404, 99411, or 99412 in addition to 99381–99397.

Preventive Medicine, Individual Counseling Codes

Table 9-4. Time Ranges for Codes 99401–99404	
99401	8–22 min
99402	23–38 min
99403	39–52 min
99404	≥53 min

Report codes 99401–99404
- Based on a physician or other QHP's face-to-face time spent providing counseling.
- For a new or an established patient.
- When the medical record includes documentation of the total counseling time and a summary of the issues discussed. Time is met when the midpoint is passed (eg, 8 minutes of service required to report a 15-minute service). **Table 9-4** contains time ranges for each code.

See the Expectant Parent Counseling and Risk Reduction Intervention box later in this chapter for a discussion of counseling and risk-factor reduction intervention with expectant parents.

Examples

➤ **A physician provides counseling to parents of a child who may be a stem cell donor to an ill sibling.** Discussion includes addressing the parents' questions about risks to the healthy child as a donor and the typical course of care. The physician documents 20 minutes of face-to-face time spent with the parents. Code **99401** (preventive medicine counseling and/or risk factor reduction intervention[s] provided to an individual [separate procedure]; approximately 15 minutes) is reported.

   Teaching Point: If the time of service had been 23 minutes or more, the midpoint between codes **99401** and **99402** (preventive medicine counseling approximately 30 minutes) would be exceeded and code **99402** would be reported.

➤ **Parents of a 2-month-old patient come to their physician's office to discuss immunizations.** To date, they have refused to have their child immunized. Although the physician has discussed the need for vaccines during the child's previous visits, the parents indicate they have further questions. The physician spends 25 minutes counseling the parents about current recommendations, safety and efficacy of vaccines, and their importance in preventing disease.

ICD-10-CM	CPT
Z71.89 (other specified counseling) **Z28.3** (personal history of under-immunization status) **Z28.82** (vaccination not carried out because of caregiver refusal)	**99402** (risk-factor reduction counseling)

➤ **A 3-year-old unvaccinated new patient comes to the pediatrician with a fever.** The physician performs an appropriate history and physical examination and diagnoses the child with left acute otitis media. Documentation supports code **99203**. A discussion about the importance of vaccinations is initiated at the physician's discretion for 10 minutes. The child's parents remain opposed to immunization. Total time of the face-to-face encounter is 20 minutes.

ICD-10-CM	CPT
H66.92 (otitis media, unspecified, left ear)	**99203 25**
Z71.89 (other specified counseling) **Z28.3** (personal history of under-immunization status) **Z28.82** (vaccination not carried out because of caregiver refusal)	**99401** (risk-factor reduction counseling)

   Teaching Point: If the physician documented that more than 50% of the total face-to-face time of service were spent in counseling and/or coordination of care (could include counseling about management of otitis media in addition to immunization counseling), a single office and other outpatient E/M code could be selected based on time rather than reporting separate codes for the E/M of otitis media and risk-factor reduction counseling. It is preferable to obtain parent/caregiver consent prior to the risk-factor reduction service that may increase the cost of an encounter.

Preventive Medicine, Group Counseling Codes

99411   Preventive medicine counseling and/or risk factor reduction intervention(s) provided to individuals in a group setting (separate procedure); approximately 30 minutes

99412   approximately 60 minutes

Example

➤ **A group of 4 overweight patients attend a 30-minute session in the physician's office to discuss diet and exercise.** The physician conducts the counseling session.

ICD-10-CM	CPT
Z71.3 (dietary counseling and surveillance)	**99411** (risk-factor reduction counseling, group)
E66.3 (overweight)	
Use additional code from category **Z68** to identify BMI.	
Z71.82 (exercise counseling)	

Teaching Point: Services are documented in each patient's medical record and are reported for each child. Services provided to a group of patients may not be reported as individual office E/M visits (**99201–99215**) because only face-to-face time spent counseling the individual patient may be reported based on time spent counseling and/or coordinating care when reporting office or other outpatient E/M visits. See **Table 9-5** for more information on BMI codes in category **Z68**.

Table 9-5. Diagnosis Codes for Body Mass Index Percentile[a]

BMI	ICD-10-CM Code
BMI <5th percentile	**Z68.51**
BMI 5th–<85th percentile	**Z68.52**
BMI 85th–95th percentile	**Z68.53**
BMI ≥95th percentile	**Z68.54**

Abbreviations: BMI, body mass index; ICD-10-CM, International Classification of Diseases, 10th Revision, Clinical Modification.

[a] Codes for BMI are reported only in conjunction with diagnosis of a related condition (eg, underweight, overweight, obesity).

Expectant Parent Counseling and Risk Reduction Intervention

Current Procedural Terminology (*CPT*®) codes **99401–99404** may be reported if a parent or family is seen by the physician to discuss a risk reduction intervention (ie, seeking advice to avoid a future problem or complication). If a family is referred by its obstetrician for an existing problem, the outpatient consultation should be reported using office-based consultation codes (**99241–99245**) or other appropriate evaluation and management (E/M) codes as directed by payer policy. (See Chapter 7, Evaluation and Management Services in the Office and Outpatient Clinics, and Chapter 16, Noncritical Hospital Evaluation and Management Services.)

International Classification of Diseases, 10th Revision, Clinical Modification (*ICD-10-CM*) code **Z76.81** (expectant parent[s] pre-birth pediatrician visit) would be reported for pre-birth counseling visits in addition to other relevant *ICD-10-CM* codes as applicable. Family history codes may also be relevant for reporting the reason for pre-birth and/or preconception counseling (eg, **Z82.79**, family history of other congenital malformations, deformations, and chromosomal abnormalities).

When counseling and risk reduction interventions are provided to a mother or her fetus prior to delivery, report them under the mother's insurance. Verification of the payer's benefit policy for these services is recommended prior to service; if non-covered, an advance beneficiary notice should be signed by the patient. An advance beneficiary notice or waiver is a written notice to the patient of noncoverage or potential out-of-pocket costs provided prior to delivery of a service. Verify payer requirements and applicable state regulations prior to using waivers in your practice. A copy of the signed notice should be kept on file with the practice's billing records.

An encounter for a meet and greet is not considered a medically necessary service and will most likely not be covered. Check health plan contracts to determine if charging direct to the patient's caregiver is allowed and whether advance notification of noncoverage is required.

Behavior Change Intervention

Behavior change interventions are for persons who have a behavior that is often considered an illness itself, such as tobacco use and addiction or substance abuse or misuse. Behavior change services may be reported when performed as part of the treatment of conditions related to or potentially exacerbated by the behavior or when performed to change the harmful behavior that has not yet resulted in illness.

Table 9-6 lists behavior change intervention codes.

Table 9-6. Behavior Change Intervention	
99406	Smoking and tobacco use cessation counseling visit; intermediate, >3 minutes up to 10 minutes
99407	intensive, >10 minutes
99408	Alcohol and/or substance (other than tobacco) abuse structured screening (eg, AUDIT, DAST), and brief intervention services; 15–30 minutes
99409	>30 minutes

Abbreviations: AUDIT, Alcohol Use Disorders Identification Test; DAST, Drug Abuse Screening Test.

- Behavior change intervention codes **99406–99409** are reported when
  - Services are provided by a physician or QHP for patients who have a behavior that is often considered an illness (eg, tobacco use and addiction, substance abuse or misuse).
  - Services involve specific validated interventions, including assessing readiness for and barriers to change, advising change in behavior, providing specific suggested actions and motivational counseling, and arranging for services and follow-up care.
- Codes **99406–99409** include specific time requirements that must be met (eg, at least 15 minutes must be spent in counseling to support reporting of code **99408**).
- Medical record documentation supports the total time spent in the performance of the service, and a detail of the behavior change intervention is provided.
- Behavior change intervention services cannot be performed on a parent or guardian of a patient and reported under the patient's name.
- Behavior change interventions may be reported separately with preventive medicine or other E/M services.
  - Evaluation and management services reported on the same day must be separate and distinct.
  - Time spent in the provision of behavior change intervention may not be used as a basis for the selection of the other E/M code.
- When reporting a distinct E/M service, append modifier **25** to the code for the distinct E/M service (eg, **99213 25**).
- Code **99078** is reported when a physician counsels groups of patients with symptoms or an established illness. This service is reported for each participating child. (See the Physician Group Education Services section in Chapter 11, Common Testing and Therapeutic Services in Office Settings, for an example of how code **99078** is used.)

Examples

➤ **During an office visit for a 14-year-old new patient for an unrelated problem, it is learned that he has been smoking for 2 years.** After counseling him about the dangers and potential health problems associated with smoking, he and his mother express interest in assistance to help him stop using tobacco. The physician spends 10 minutes discussing specific methods to overcome barriers, pharmacological options, behavioral techniques, and nicotine replacement. The patient is referred to a community support group and a follow-up visit is scheduled in 2 weeks to provide additional encouragement and counseling as needed. Diagnosis is tobacco use.

ICD-10-CM	CPT®
Use diagnosis code appropriate for problem addressed.	99201–99205 25 (based on service performed and documented)
Z72.0 (tobacco use) Z71.6 (tobacco abuse counseling)	99406

Teaching Point: If only general advice and encouragement to stop smoking had been provided, it would be considered part of the new patient office visit. Counseling time must be documented.

➤ **During a preventive medicine service for a 14-year-old established patient, it is learned that he drinks beer at a friend's house.** The physician uses a structured screening tool to interview the patient about substance use. The result is positive, and the physician spends a total of 20 minutes interviewing the patient about substance use history and counseling the patient about risks associated with alcohol and drug use, not driving or riding with someone under the influence, and seeking an agreement to avoid future use.

||||||| *Coding Pearl* |||||||

International Classification of Diseases, 10th Revision, Clinical Modification guidelines state that substance use codes should only be assigned when the use is associated with a mental or behavioral disorder and such a relationship is documented by the provider.

ICD-10-CM	CPT
Z00.129 (routine child health examination without abnormal findings)	99394 25 (preventive medicine visit)
Z71.89 (other specified counseling)	99408

Preventive Medicine Services Modifier

33   Preventive services

Modifier 33 is used to differentiate services provided as recommended preventive care when the service might also be provided for diagnostic indications. Some payers provide a listing of services for which modifier 33 is required when provided as a preventive service.

- The appropriate use of modifier 33 will reduce claim adjustments related to preventive services and corresponding payments to members.
- Modifier 33 should only be appended to codes represented in one or more of the following 4 categories:
  - Services rated A or B by the USPSTF
  - Immunizations for routine use in children, adolescents, and adults as recommended by ACIP
  - Preventive care and screenings for children as recommended by Bright Futures (AAP) and newborn testing (American College of Medical Genetics and Genomics)
  - Preventive care and screenings provided for women supported by HRSA
- **DO *NOT* USE MODIFIER 33**
  - **When the CPT code(s) is identified as inherently preventive (eg, preventive medicine counseling)**
  - **When the service(s) is not indicated in the categories noted previously**
  - **With an insurance plan that continues to implement the cost-sharing policy on preventive medicine services (grandfathered health plan)**
- Check with your payers before fully implementing the use of modifier 33 to verify any variations in reporting requirements. Modifier 33 *is not used for benefit determination by some payers* and may be required by others only for services that may be either diagnostic/therapeutic or preventive.

Chapter 9: Preventive Services

Examples

> **A 9-month-old patient presents for her age-appropriate preventive medicine service.** The physician completes the age-appropriate history and physical examination and provides anticipatory guidance. While reviewing immunization history, the physician notes the patient is behind on her Hib vaccine because of a recent shortage from the manufacturer. The physician counsels the mother on the vaccine (ActHIB) and orders it. The physician also reviews the periodicity schedule and notes the patient is due for a developmental screening as part of the Bright Futures recommendations. The nurse administers the screening to the mother and scores it. The physician reviews the unremarkable results with the mother and the next routine visit is scheduled for 12 months.

ICD-10-CM	CPT®
Z00.129 Z23	99391 96110 33 (developmental screen) 90648 33 (Hib) 90460 33

   Teaching Point: Append modifier **33** to those services that fall within the 4 listed categories previously discussed. In this case, the developmental screening falls under Bright Futures recommendations for a 9-month-old and the vaccine product and administration fall under routine immunizations recommended by ACIP. Note that the modifier does not have to be appended to code **99391** because that service is inherently preventive.

> **An 11-year-old is seen for an established patient office visit on Monday for a rash.** The physician provides an E/M service with a problem-focused history and physical examination and straightforward MDM. The physician notes the patient is scheduled for a preventive medicine service one afternoon next week and has not been screened for dyslipidemia. The physician orders a fasting lipid panel to be performed prior to the preventive service. The patient returns the next morning and the in-office laboratory performs the lipid panel test. The results are reported to the physician.

ICD-10-CM	CPT
Monday: **R21** (rash)	Monday: **99212**
Tuesday: **Z13.220** (encounter for screening for lipoid disorders)	Tuesday: **80061 QW 33**

   Teaching Point: Append modifier **33** to code **80061** to indicate the test was performed as a preventive service, even though it is ordered and performed on a date when no preventive medicine service was provided. Modifier **QW** is also appended when required by the payer to indicate the test is CLIA waived.

Other Preventive Medicine Services

99429   Unlisted preventive medicine service

   Code **99429** may be reported if these options are not suitable. If the unlisted code is used, most payers will require a copy of the progress notes filed with the claim.

||||||||| Coding Pearl |||||||||

Although a separate evaluation and management service is not reported when a minor problem or chronic condition requires less than significant additional work, the diagnosis code for the problem or chronic condition may be reported in addition to code **Z00.121** (routine child health examination with abnormal findings).

Reporting a Preventive Medicine Visit With a Problem-Oriented Visit

When a problem or abnormality is addressed *and requires significant additional work* (eg, symptomatic atopic dermatitis, exercise-induced asthma, migraine headache, poor academic performance in a patient with ADHD) to perform the required key components and is medically necessary, it may be reported using the office or other outpatient services codes (99201–99215) in addition to the preventive medicine services code.

When reporting both E/M services

- The levels of history and examination performed and documented relative to the problem or abnormality may be limited by the work already included in the preventive medicine service (ie, elements that are included in the preventive service cannot be counted toward the level of service for the problem-oriented service). Because of this, typically, the level of E/M service reported will be one level lower than if the patient presented solely for the problem, unless coding is based on time.
  - An age- and a gender-appropriate examination is included in the preventive medicine service, but an extended examination of the affected body area(s) and other symptomatic or related organ system(s) would be separately considered in determining the level of E/M service provided to address the problem.
  - Because *CPT*® states that the comprehensive history of a preventive medicine service includes a comprehensive or interval PFSH, the level of problem-oriented history on the same date may be limited to expanded problem focused unless you can show that elements of the PFSH were obtained only in relation to the problem being addressed.
  - Payers may require MDM as 1 of the 2 key components met (ie, history and MDM or examination and MDM) to support an established patient visit.
- Documentation for each service should be maintained in the medical record. That documentation may be on a separate progress note (preferred) or, if included on the same progress note, must clearly reflect the additional work performed. If the problem-oriented visit is reported based on time, documentation must clearly reflect the total time spent in the face-to-face encounter addressing the issue(s) or problem(s), the total time spent in counseling and/or coordination of care, and a summary of the issues discussed.
- *ICD-10-CM* well-care diagnosis codes (see code list on page 203) should be linked to the appropriate preventive medicine service code (99381–99395) and the sick care diagnosis code linked to the problem-oriented service code (99201–99215).
- It is important to make parents aware of any additional charges that may occur at the preventive medicine encounter. This includes, but is not limited to, a significant, separately identifiable E/M service. The AAP has developed a template letter that can be used to outline what may not be covered under the no-cost-sharing preventive medicine services (www.aap.org/en-us/professional-resources/practice-transformation/getting-paid/Coding-at-the-AAP/Pages/Evaluation-and-Management.aspx).

> **Coding Pearl**
>
> **Some payers have adopted policy that problem-oriented evaluation and management (E/M) services provided on the same date as a preventive medicine E/M service will be paid at 50% of the contractual amount agreed on under the health plan contract. When reporting to these payers, be sure to include all work related to the problem-oriented encounter in determining the level of service provided. Physicians should not reduce the level of service reported.**

In the following claim form example, a patient received an established patient preventive service (99392) and a problem-oriented E/M service (99213) to address recurrent bilateral otitis media on the same date. Claim Form Example 3 shows diagnosis codes Z00.121 and H65.196 (recurrent bilateral otitis media) listed in fields 21A and 21B. The A and B are diagnosis pointers used in column 24E to link the appropriate diagnosis codes to the procedure codes included on each service line. Note that diagnosis code H65.196 (diagnosis pointer B) is linked to the preventive and problem-oriented services in column 24E. Modifier 25 is appended to code 99213 (field 24D under "Modifier") to indicate the significant, separately identifiable E/M service was provided in addition to the preventive medicine service (99392).

Coding Conundrum: Reporting 2 New Patient Codes on the Same Day

When a preventive medicine visit and problem-oriented evaluation and management service are performed on the same day to a new patient, both codes may be reported with the appropriate new patient codes (eg, **99381** and **99203 25**).

Before reporting 2 new patient codes on the same patient on the same day of service, consider

- A new patient office or outpatient visit requires that all 3 key components (history, physical examination, and medical decision-making) or typical time (if more than 50% of the total face-to-face encounter is spent in counseling and/or coordination of care) be met.
- If only 2 of the 3 required key components are met (eg, the physical examination was part of the comprehensive preventive medicine service), the code selection would have to be based on an established patient code (**99212–99215**).
- The physical examination can be counted as a key component only in situations in which the examination component of the problem-oriented visit would be considered as distinct or in addition to what is normally performed during the preventive medicine examination.

Claim Form Example 3: Preventive and Problem-Oriented Services

21. Diagnosis or nature of illness or injury (Relate A–L to service line below 24E) A. Z00.121 B. H65.196 C. D.					ICD Ind. 0				

24. A. Dates of service B. Place of service	C. EMG	D. Procedures, services or supplies CPT/HCPCS	Modifier	E. Diagnosis Pointer	F. Charges	G. Days or units	H. EPSDT	I. ID Qual	J. Rendering Provider #
1/2/2019–1/2/2019	11		99392		A, B	$$$	1		NPI	123456789
1/2/2019–1/2/2019	11		99213	25	B	$$$	1		NPI	123456789

Abbreviations: CPT, Current Procedural Terminology; *EMG, emergency; EPSDT, Early and Periodic Screening, Diagnosis, and Treatment; HCPCS, Healthcare Common Procedure Coding System;* ICD, International Classification of Diseases; *NPI, National Provider Identifier.*

- The presence of a chronic condition(s) in and of itself does not change a preventive medicine visit to a problem-oriented visit; nor does it unilaterally support a separate problem-oriented E/M service (**99201–99215**) with the well visit, unless it is significant and has been separately addressed.
- An insignificant problem or condition (eg, minor diaper rash, stable chronic problem, renewal of prescription medications) that does not require additional work to perform the required key components cannot be reported as a separate E/M service.
- Modifier **25** (significant, separately identifiable E/M service by the same physician on the same day of the procedure or other service) should be appended to the problem-oriented service code (eg, **99212**). If vaccines are given at the same encounter, append modifier **25** to the problem-oriented E/M service code and the preventive medicine service code to avoid payer bundling edits that may allow payment only for the immunization administration.
- Some patients will be required to provide a co-payment for the non–preventive medicine visit code under the terms of their plan benefit even when there is no co-payment required for the preventive medicine visit. Legally, this co-payment cannot routinely be written off. The AAP has developed a letter addressing this issue that can be found at www.aap.org/cfp (access code AAPCFP24).
- The AAP has developed forms that promote good documentation of preventive medicine services. Examples can be ordered from the AAP by calling 888/227-1770 or visiting https://shop.aap.org/product-list/?q=documentation%20forms. Additionally, some state Medicaid programs have developed documentation templates for preventive services delivered in their EPSDT program.

Chapter 9: Preventive Services

Examples

➤ **A 3-year-old presents for a well-child visit.** The patient has history of removal of Wilms tumor 2 years ago followed by 8 months of chemotherapy. The patient is under care of a geneticist for arginosuccinate lyase deficiency. He has a port-a-cath in the right axilla, hearing aids, and ankle orthotics; is on the liver transplant list; and receives occupational, speech, and physical therapy. The parents are concerned that the child has little association with other children due to risk of infection that could delay transplant opportunity. In addition to the preventive medicine examination with no new abnormal findings or exacerbated problems, the physician spends 15 minutes discussing the need to avoid acquiring infection through preschool attendance and other high-risk community settings. The pediatrician also discusses a care plan for signs of illness in the child and continuation of current protein-restricted diet (managed by the geneticist) and therapies.

Preventive medicine visit	**ICD-10-CM** **Z00.129** (well-child check without abnormal findings) **Z71.3** (dietary counseling and surveillance) **E72.29** (other disorders of urea cycle metabolism)
	CPT® **99392**
Problem-oriented visit *MDM:* Low complexity *History:* Expanded problem focused *Physical examination:* Problem focused	**ICD-10-CM** **E72.29** (other disorders of urea cycle metabolism) **Z76.82** (awaiting organ transplant status) **Z85.52** (personal history of other malignant neoplasm of kidney) **Z92.21** (personal history of antineoplastic chemotherapy)
	CPT® **99213 25**

Teaching Point: This child with complex chronic illness required problem-oriented counseling in addition to the provision of the anticipatory counseling inherent to the preventive medicine service. Documentation should clearly support the separate time of the problem-oriented E/M service and portion of that time spent in counseling/coordination of care, discussion topics, and plan of care for the problems addressed.

Codes for preventive counseling and risk-factor reduction intervention (eg, **99401**) are not appropriate for this example. Risk-factor reduction services are used for persons without a specific illness for which the counseling might otherwise be used as part of treatment. This patient has specific illness that prompts the counseling.

➤ **A 14-year-old established patient presents for a preventive medicine service.** The patient's mother also notes increased signs of depression and anxiety (previously diagnosed). Patient-completed Beck Depression Inventory-II and Screen for Child Anxiety Related Disorders (SCARED) instruments indicate severe depression and anxiety. The patient has not followed through with previous recommendations for counseling except short-term counseling at school because she doesn't like to talk about her problems. In addition to providing the preventive medicine service, the physician documents 25 minutes spent in discussion of depression and anxiety and developing a plan of care including prescription medication, precautions related to adverse effects of medication, and weekly follow-up visits for at least 4 weeks.

Preventive medicine visit	**ICD-10-CM** **Z00.121** (well-child check with abnormal findings) **F32.9** (major depressive disorder, single episode, unspecified) **F41.9** (anxiety disorder, unspecified)
	CPT® **99394**

Chapter 9: Preventive Services

Chapter 9: Preventive Services

Problem-oriented visit 25 minutes spent counseling	**ICD-10-CM** **F32.9** (major depressive disorder, single episode, unspecified) **F41.9** (anxiety disorder, unspecified)
	CPT® **99214 25** **96127** x 2 (brief emotional/behavioral assessment [eg, depression inventory, ADHD scale], with scoring and documentation, per standardized instrument)

Teaching Point: The level of service for the problem-oriented E/M service was selected based on time spent counseling and/or coordinating care. Physician documentation must clearly support the time spent in providing the problem-oriented service versus time spent in anticipatory counseling as part of the preventive service. Code **96127** may be reported for the completion and scoring of the Beck Depression Inventory-II and SCARED instruments. Additional codes may be reported for dietary (**Z71.3**) and exercise counseling (**Z71.82**) and/or documentation of BMI (**3008F**) when applicable.

➤ **A 12-month-old girl is seen for a new patient visit for painful urination.** Mother states that the girl has been crying when voiding for 2 days and her urine "smells bad." Review of systems reveals that she had a fever of 100.4°F (38°C) last night, is voiding more frequently, and is irritable. A history of present illness and comprehensive physical examination are performed. Urinalysis (**81003**) is consistent with a urinary tract infection (UTI). A urine culture is ordered. The result of a complete blood cell count with differential is normal. Blood culture is obtained and pending. A full preventive medicine service is completed, including age-appropriate counseling and anticipatory guidance, and vaccines are deferred. She is placed on antibiotics for 10 days. Mother is advised to follow up in 2 days.

Preventive medicine visit	**ICD-10-CM** **Z00.121** (well-child check with abnormal findings) **Z28.01** (immunization not carried out because of acute illness of patient) **N39.0** (UTI)
	CPT® **99382**
Problem-oriented visit *MDM:* Moderate complexity *History:* Expanded problem focused *Physical examination:* Included in preventive medicine visit	**ICD-10-CM** **N39.0** (UTI)
	CPT® **99213 25** **36415** (venipuncture) **85025** (blood count; complete [CBC], automated [Hgb, Hct, RBC, WBC and platelet count] and automated differential WBC count) **81003** (urinalysis, by dip stick or tablet reagent for bilirubin, glucose, hemoglobin, ketones, leukocytes, nitrite, pH, protein, specific gravity, urobilinogen, any number of these constituents; automated, without microscopy)

Teaching Point: Examination of external genitalia and back does not constitute examination beyond the comprehensive examination included in the preventive service. Because the physical examination was included as part of the preventive medicine visit, only 2 of the required 3 components needed to select the code for a new patient office or outpatient visit were provided and considered in the selection of the problem-oriented service. Therefore, the problem-oriented service is reported using the established patient visit code **99213**. By including code **Z28.01**, the practice indicates delay in immunization due to an acute illness and may use the diagnosis code as part of a recall system to follow up with patients who miss appointments for immunization.

> **A 2-year-old boy with history of macrocephaly is seen for a preventive medicine visit.** He is referred to an ophthalmologist because of strabismus noted by photoscreening with remote analysis.

Preventive medicine visit Photoscreening	*ICD-10-CM* **Z00.121** (well-child check with abnormal findings) **H50.9** (strabismus, unspecified) **Q75.3** (macrocephaly)
	CPT **New Patient Established Patient** **99382 99392** **99174** (instrument-based ocular screening, bilateral, with remote analysis and report)

Teaching Point: Because this scenario includes no additional workup of the strabismus, only the preventive medicine and photoscreening services are reported. The diagnosis code for strabismus discovered during the preventive medicine service is reported as an additional diagnosis to the code for the well-child check. If more work is needed or required, a separate E/M service could be reported based on documentation.

See the following Coding Continuum Model: Problem-Oriented and Preventive Evaluation and Management on the Same Date section and **Table 9-7** for additional illustration of coding for problem-oriented E/M services provided on the same date as preventive E/M services.

Coding Continuum Model: Problem-Oriented and Preventive Evaluation and Management on the Same Date

Table 9-7. Continuum Model for Problem-Oriented and Preventive Evaluation and Management on the Same Date			
CPT® Code Vignette (Appropriate preventive E/M service codes are also reported.)	**Medical Decision-making**	**History**	**Physical Examination**
99211 Nursing visit (not typically allowed in conjunction with a preventive medicine E/M service, as this would not represent a significant, separately identifiable E/M service)			
99212 A 4-year-old presents today for a previously scheduled preventive service and follow-up visit for recurrent bilateral otitis media with effusion (**H65.196**) diagnosed 1 week ago.	Straightforward 1. Established problem—resolving. 2. No data reviewed. 3. Continue antibiotics and return in 1 week.	Problem focused 1. Chief complaint—otitis media 2. Modifying factor—resolving with first-line antibiotics	Problem focused 1. ENMT

~ More From the AAP ~

The American Academy of Pediatrics *Quick Reference Guide to Coding Pediatric Preventive Services 2019* may be purchased from https://shop.aap.org/quick-reference-guide-to-coding-pediatric-preventive-services.

Table 9-7. Continuum Model for Problem-Oriented and Preventive Evaluation and Management on the Same Date (*continued*)

CPT® Code Vignette (Appropriate preventive E/M service codes are also reported.)	Medical Decision-making	History	Physical Examination

99213
A 4-year-old presents today for a previously scheduled preventive service and follow-up visit for recurrent bilateral otitis media with effusion (H65.196) diagnosed 1 week ago. On examination, eardrums are still inflamed, and the child complains of intermittent pain.
	Low complexity
	1. Established problem, not resolving; option of referral to otolaryngologist discussed
	2. No data reviewed
	3. Prescription of second-line antibiotic
		Expanded problem focused
		1. Chief complaint—otitis media
		2. Brief HPI plus pertinent ROS
		  a. Symptoms
		  b. Duration of illness
		  c. Compliance with first-line antibiotic
		  d. Additional symptoms from ROS
			Expanded problem focused
			1. Constitutional (overall appearance, hydration status)
			2. Eyes (conjunctiva)
			3. ENMT

99214
Infant presents for preventive service with fever and cough. Patient is found to have third episode of otitis media within the past 2–3 months. Children at child care have been diagnosed with strep pharyngitis.
	Moderate complexity
	1. Established problem; worsening.
	2. Treatment including antibiotics and supportive care.
	2. Consider/discuss tympanocentesis (**69420** or **69421**).
	3. Hearing evaluation planned.
	4. Discuss possible referral to an allergist or otolaryngologist for tympanostomy.
	5. Discuss contributing environmental factors and supportive treatment.
		Detailed
		1. Chief complaint
		2. Detailed HPI plus pertinent ROS and pertinent social history
		  a. Symptoms of illness
		  b. Fever, other signs
		  c. Any other medications
		  d. Allergies
		  e. Frequency of similar infection in past and response to treatment
		  f. Environmental factors (eg, tobacco exposure, child care)
		  g. Immunization status
		  h. Feeding history
			Detailed
			1. Constitutional (overall appearance, hydration status)
			2. Eyes
			3. ENMT
			4. Cardiovascular
			5. Respiratory
			6. Skin

99215 A 16-year-old patient presents for a preventive medicine service. He completes a depression screening instrument with a positive score necessitating E/M.	40 minutes or more beyond the time of the preventive medicine service is spent face-to-face with the patient obtaining additional information on the patient's symptoms of depression and familial, social, and environmental factors; discussing the diagnosis of depression and management options; and developing and obtaining agreement to a plan of care. (Documentation should specifically state time is separate from that spent providing the preventive medicine service and include details of the counseling and/or coordination of care provided.)		
Note regarding **99214** or **99215**: In many cases, a problem that requires these higher levels of E/M service may warrant delay of the preventive E/M service. Time-based E/M: Time is the key factor when counseling and/or coordination of care are more than 50% of the face-to-face time with the patient. For **99214**, the total visit time would be 25 minutes; for **99215**, the total time is 40 minutes. Time spent on counseling and/or coordination of care and the areas discussed must be documented. Do not include the time of the preventive E/M service (eg, anticipatory counseling) in the time attributed to the problem-oriented E/M service.			

Abbreviations: CPT, Current Procedural Terminology; E/M, evaluation and management; ENMT, ears, nose, mouth, throat; HPI, history of present illness; PFSH, past, family, and social history; ROS, review of systems.

CHAPTER 10

Surgery, Infusion, and Sedation in the Outpatient Setting

Contents

Surgical Package Rules

Current Procedural Terminology (*CPT®*) surgical codes (**10004–69990**) are packaged or global codes. To understand documentation and coding of procedural services, it is necessary to know what is included in each service from a coding and payment perspective. *CPT* directs that each procedure code represents a "surgical package" of service components. These include

- Evaluation and management (E/M) services subsequent to the decision for surgery on the day before and/or day of surgery (including the history and physical examination)
- Local or topical anesthesia, including metacarpal, metatarsal, and/or digital block
- Immediate postoperative care
- Writing orders
- Evaluation of the patient in the recovery area
- Typical postoperative follow-up care

Using the *CPT* definition of the surgical package, relative value units (RVUs) are assigned to each procedure based on the typical preoperative, intraoperative, and postoperative physician work; practice expense (eg, procedure room, instruments, supplies, support staff); and professional liability. Payers that use RVUs to calculate payments will typically not pay separately for any components of the surgical package.

> 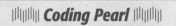 **Coding Pearl** |||||||
>
> The relative value units assigned to procedures include the supplies typically used. When applicable, see the Supplies section later in this chapter.

Medicare Surgical Package Definition

The Medicare definition of the surgical package differs from that of *CPT*. Most state Medicaid programs follow the Medicare definition.

- Medicare defines procedures as minor (procedures assigned a 0- or 10-day global period or endoscopies) or major (procedures assigned a 90-day global period). (See **Table 10-1** for information on global periods for common pediatric procedures.) The day of surgery is day 0 (zero); the postoperative period begins the next day.
- For "minor" procedures, the E/M visit on the date of the procedure is considered a routine part of the procedure *regardless of whether it is prior or subsequent to the decision for surgery.* In these cases, modifier **57** (decision for surgery) is not recognized.
- Medicare states an E/M code may be reported on the same day as a minor surgical procedure only when a significant, separately identifiable E/M service is performed with modifier **25** appended to the E/M code. *CPT* does not specifically include the initial E/M service prior to a minor procedure when the decision for surgery occurs at the visit.
- *CPT* also does not include care related to surgical complications in the surgical package. Medicare considers care related to complications following surgery to be included in the surgical package unless a return to the operating room is necessary.
- Global periods and minor or major surgery are not defined in *CPT*. Global periods are defined in the Medicare Physician Fee Schedule (MPFS). Although other payers can assign different global periods, most follow the MPFS.
    - ❖ The RVUs and global period assigned to each service can be found in the current MPFS at https://www.cms.gov/medicare/medicare-fee-for-service-payment/physicianfeesched.

Most office and outpatient clinic procedures will have 0- or 10-day global periods. Exceptions are certain services such as care of fractures (discussed later in this chapter).

> 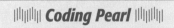 **Coding Pearl** |||||||
>
> Most state Medicaid programs follow the Medicare surgical package guidelines.

Table 10-1. The Medicare Surgical Package

Global Periods	0-Day Global Surgeries	10-Day Global Surgeries	90-Day Global Surgeries
Services before the date of surgery	Not included	Not included	All related services 1 day before surgery if after decision for surgery
Services on the date of procedure	E/M services typically included regardless of when decision for surgery is made	E/M services typically included regardless of when decision for surgery is made	All related services except E/M services at which decision for surgery is made
Postoperative services	Typical postoperative care on the same date	All related care on date of service and 10 days following	All related care on date of service and 90 days following, including care for complications that does not require a return to the OR

Abbreviations: E/M, evaluation and management; OR, operating room.

Significant Evaluation and Management Service and Procedure

Often, a single encounter involves both an E/M service to diagnose and recommend a plan of care for a patient's presenting problem and a related procedural service (eg, incision with removal of foreign body). However, an E/M service is only separately reported on the same date as a procedure when it is significant and separately identifiable from the preservice and post-service work of the procedural service.

The Medicare Resource-Based Relative Value Scale (RBRVS) is used by most private payers and Medicaid plans to determine RVUs and global periods for services. (Learn more about the RBRVS in Chapter 4, The Business of Medicine: Working with Current and Emerging Payment Systems.) Under this payment methodology, procedural services include some preservice and post-service E/M by the performing physician. Payer edits, such as the National Correct Coding Initiative (NCCI) edits used by Medicare, Medicaid, and many other payers, also bundle E/M services with certain procedures.

For minor procedures, separate payment for a significant, separately identifiable E/M service is allowed when modifier **25** is appended to the E/M code. However, care should be taken to use modifier **25** only when documentation supports a significant and separately identifiable E/M service.

For major procedures (typically 90-day global period), modifier **57** may be appended when the decision for surgery or procedure is made during the E/M service on the same date as the procedure. Documentation should clearly show E/M of the problem resulting in the initial decision to perform the related procedure.

Coding Conundrum: Procedure, or Evaluation and Management and Procedure?

The differences in the Centers for Medicare & Medicaid Services (CMS) and *Current Procedural Terminology* (*CPT*®) surgical package guidelines are somewhat open to interpretation, often leading to confusion. Try to answer the following questions when determining if you should report a procedure alone or a procedure with an evaluation and management (E/M) service:

- Did you address a problem or condition prior to making a decision to perform the procedure (above and beyond the usual preoperative care associated with the procedure) or a significant and separately identifiable problem? If yes, report an E/M service and procedure.
- Does the medical record documentation clearly support the performance of a medically necessary E/M service (required key components), the procedure (procedure note), the medical necessity for both, and the decision to perform the surgery? If yes, report an E/M service and procedure.
- Was the purpose of the visit for the procedure only? If yes, do *not* report an E/M service.
- Does the payer follow the *CPT* or CMS guidelines with regard to reporting surgical procedures? If the focus of an E/M service is related to the procedure, the history and physical examination are part of preoperative service and only the surgical procedure should be reported.

Examples

➤ **A physician sees a patient who complains of fullness in his ears and decreased hearing.** On examination, the physician notes cerumen impaction in both ears. The physician documents removal of the impacted cerumen in each canal using an otoscope, lavage (unsuccessful), and wax curettes. Documentation also includes notation of patient/caregiver consent, patient tolerance, outcome, and postprocedural examination findings (brief hearing assessment is included in the procedure). The patient's symptoms are relieved, and no further E/M is necessary.

International Classification of Diseases, 10th Revision, Clinical Modification (ICD-10-CM)	*CPT*
H61.23 (impacted cerumen, bilateral)	69210 50

Teaching Point: No significant and separately identifiable E/M service beyond the preservice/post-service work of the procedure was provided. Code 69210 (removal of impacted cerumen requiring instrumentation, unilateral) is reported with modifier 50 (bilateral). (Payer instructions for reporting bilateral procedures may vary. Not all payers will make additional payment for this procedure when performed bilaterally versus unilaterally.)

➤ **A physician sees an established 10-year-old patient with complaint of fever, cough, and runny nose.** On examination, the right ear canal is found to be blocked by impacted cerumen. The physician documents removal of the impacted cerumen in the right ear canal using an otoscope, lavage (unsuccessful), and wax curettes. The physician documents an E/M service with an expanded problem-focused history and examination and low-complexity medical decision-making (MDM). The diagnoses are upper respiratory infection and cerumen impaction, right ear.

ICD-10-CM	*CPT*
J06.9 (upper respiratory infection)	99213 25
H61.21 (impacted cerumen, right)	69210

Teaching Point: Modifier 25 indicates that the physician provided an E/M service to diagnose the patient's problem that was significant and separately identifiable in the medical record.

Reporting Postoperative Care

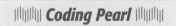

> ||||||||| **Coding Pearl** |||||||||
>
> Payers may reduce payment of a surgical procedure if the physician does not report code 99024.

- ◉ Report *CPT*® code 99024 (postoperative follow-up visit) for follow-up care provided during the global surgery period.
  - ❖ Reporting code 99024 allows a practice to track the number of visits performed during the postoperative period of specific procedures, calculate office overhead expenses (eg, supplies, staff, physician time) associated with the procedure, and potentially use the data to negotiate higher payment rates.
  - ❖ Payers track the postoperative care provided. If a physician is not providing or reporting the postoperative care typically performed for a procedure, payers may reduce payment for the surgical service because payment includes postoperative care as part of the procedure.
- ◉ When the physician who performed the procedure provides an unrelated E/M service during the postoperative period, modifier 24 (unrelated E/M service by the same physician during a postoperative period) should be appended to the E/M service code.
- ◉ When a physician *other than the surgeon* provides unrelated services to a patient during the postoperative period, the services are reported without a modifier. Despite the use of different National Provider Identifiers and diagnosis codes, some payers with assigned follow-up surgical periods will deny the service. The claim should be appealed for payment with a letter advising the payer that the service was unrelated to any surgery.

Chapter 10: Surgery, Infusion, and Sedation in the Outpatient Setting

Example

➤ **A 4-year-old patient returns within 8 days of removal of a foreign body from his right foot (10120 RT) with fever, sore throat, and right ear pain of 2 days' duration.** The child's temperature is slightly elevated, and he appears ill. A rapid strep test is negative. A detailed history and examination is documented. The patient is diagnosed with acute suppurative otitis media of the right ear with pharyngitis and prescribed antibiotics for the otitis media. The physician also rechecks the wound on the right foot that is healing as expected.

ICD-10-CM	CPT
H66.001 (acute suppurative otitis media, right ear) J02.9 (acute pharyngitis, unspecified) S90.851D (superficial foreign body, right foot, subsequent encounter)	99214 24 87880 (rapid strep test)

Teaching Point: Modifier 24 is reported to identity that the service provided was unrelated to the prior procedure. The evaluation of the healing wound during the postoperative period is not included in determining the level of service for the encounter because it is included in postoperative care when provided during the 10-day global period. Code 87880 is reported for testing by infectious agent antigen detection by immunoassay with direct optical observation; *Streptococcus*, group A.

Supplies and Materials

99070   Supplies and materials provided by the physician over and above those usually included with the office visit or other services rendered

❈ Items such as elastic wraps, clavicle splints, or circumcision and suturing trays may be reported with this code. Remember that some supplies (eg, suturing trays, circumcision trays) may be included with the surgical procedure if the payer uses RVUs as its basis for payment.

❈ Only the supplies purchased in an office-based practice may be reported.

❈ Some payers will require the use of Healthcare Common Procedure Coding System (HCPCS) codes. More specific HCPCS codes are available for a number of supplies (eg, codes Q4001–Q4051 for cast and splint supplies). Use HCPCS codes when they are more specific. For more information on HCPCS codes, please see Chapter 1, The Basics of Coding.

> ||||||| **Coding Pearl** |||||||
> If reporting code 99070, identify the supplies or materials on the claim form and be prepared to submit an invoice.

Reporting Terminated Procedures

When a procedure is started but cannot be completed due to extenuating circumstances, physicians should consider the individual situation, including the reason for termination of the procedure and the amount of work that was performed, when determining how to report the service rendered.

When a procedure was performed but not entirely successful (eg, portion of foreign body removed), it may be appropriate to report the procedure code that represents the work performed without modification. Only report reduced services (modifier 52) or discontinued procedure (modifier 53) when the service was significantly reduced from the typical service. (See Chapter 2, Modifiers and Coding Edits, for more information on modifiers.) If the work performed prior to discontinuation was insignificant, it may be appropriate to not report the procedure. When not reporting the procedure, consider whether the level of a related E/M service was increased due to the complexity of MDM associated with the attempted procedure, any complicating factors, and the revised management or treatment plan.

> ~ **More From the AAP** ~
> For more information on reporting discontinued or incomplete procedures, see "Reporting Terminated Procedural Services" in the November 2014 *AAP Pediatric Coding Newsletter* at http://coding.aap.org (subscription required).

> ||||||| **Coding Pearl** |||||||
> Payers may reduce payment of a surgical procedure if the physician does not report code 99024.

Common Pediatric Procedures

Table 10-2 details the number of global days for each of the commonly reported office procedures. Remember that when reporting any procedures containing 0, 10, or 90 global days, modifier 25 or 57 is required on any separately identifiable E/M service done on the same day (or, in some instances, the previous day prior to a planned major surgery). Also, those E/M services that are unrelated to the procedure that take place within the code's 10- or 90-day global period will require modifier 24.

Table 10-2. Common Office Procedures and Global Days		
CPT® Code	**Description[a]**	**Global Period (d)**
10060, 10061	Drainage of skin abscess	10
10120, 10121	FB removal, SQ	10
11200	Removal of skin tags	10
11760	Repair of nail bed	10
12001–12018	Laceration repair, simple	0
12031–12057	Laceration repair, intermediate	10
13100–13153	Laceration repair, complex	10
16000–16030	Burn care	0
17110, 17111	Destruction benign lesions (eg, warts)	10
17250	Chemical cautery	0
23500	Treatment of clavicle fracture	90
24640	Treatment of elbow dislocation (nursemaid elbow)	10
28190	FB removal, foot	10
28192	FB removal, foot, complex	90
28490	Treatment big toe fracture (closed)	90
30300	Removal intranasal FB, office	10
30310	Removal intranasal FB w/general anesthesia	10
30901	Nosebleed cautery/packing	0
40650	Repair of vermilion border of lip	90
41010	Incision in lingual frenulum	10
41250–41252	Laceration repairs of tongue	10
45915	Removal, fecal impaction or anal FB w/general anesthesia	10
51701, 51702	Bladder catheterization	0
54150	Circumcision	0
69090	Ear piercing	N/A[b]

Abbreviations: CPT, Current Procedural Terminology; FB, foreign body; N/A, not applicable; SQ, subcutaneous; w/, with; w/o, without.

[a] Descriptors are abbreviated. Please see your 2019 coding reference for full descriptors and code selection.

[b] Ear piercing (69090) is not valued in the Medicare Physician Fee Schedule, so no global days are assigned. Payers typically do not cover this or other services that are not medically necessary.

Minor Procedures That Do Not Have a Code

Some minor procedures are considered inherent to an E/M code or do not have separate *CPT*® codes. However, any supplies used may be reported. The following procedures are included in an E/M service:

- Insertion or removal of an ear wick.
- Removal of nonimpacted cerumen from the ear.
- Nasal aspiration.
- Nasogastric tube insertion without fluoroscopic guidance.
- Removal of an umbilical clamp.
- Removal of foreign bodies from skin that do not require an incision.
- Puncture of abscess without aspiration.
- Wound closure with Steri-Strips only.
- The use of fluorescein dye and a Wood lamp to examine for a corneal abrasion or foreign body of the eye is included in the E/M service and is not reported separately. However, the work of a detailed eye examination and history may allow the reporting of a higher-level E/M code.

For other procedural services, verify separate reporting through your procedural coding reference. There is value in capturing the procedural services that are distinct from E/M services, as shown in **Table 10-3**.

Table 10-3. Comparing Relative Value Units: 2018 Medicare Resource-Based Relative Value Scale[a]

Code	Description	Total Non-facility RVUs
99201	Level 1 office visit, new patient	1.26
99202	Level 2 office visit, new patient	2.12
99203	Level 3 office visit, new patient	3.05
99212	Level 2 office visit, established patient	1.24
99213	Level 3 office visit, established patient	2.06
99214	Level 4 office visit, established patient	3.04
30300	Foreign body removal from nose	5.02
10120	Foreign body removal from subcutaneous tissue	4.38

Abbreviations: RBRVS, Resource-Based Relative Value Scale; RVU, relative value unit.

[a] The 2019 Medicare RBRVS was not available at the time this manual was printed. For an online copy of the pediatric-specific 2018 Medicare RBRVS, go to www.aap.org/cfp, access code AAPCFP24.

Integumentary Procedures

Incision and Drainage

10060   Incision and drainage of abscess (eg, carbuncle, suppurative hidradenitis, cutaneous or subcutaneous abscess, cyst, furuncle, or paronychia); simple or single

10061   complicated or multiple

- The global period for codes **10060** and **10061** is 10 days.
- *CPT*® does not provide differentiation between simple and complicated incision and drainage (I&D) and leaves code selection to the physician's judgment.
- The simple I&D procedure typically involves local anesthesia, an incision, expression of purulent drainage, obtaining a culture, irrigation, completely opening the cavity, and packing/dressing the wound.
- Complex I&D often typically involves a deeper incision, breakdown of multiple loculations, placement of a drain, and/or debridement of the cavity.
- The difference in RVUs for **10060** (3.33 total non-facility) and **10061** (5.86 total non-facility) indicates the significant additional work and practice expense associated with complicated or multiple I&D procedures.

Example

➤ **A 7-year-old presents with an abscess on his right lower leg.** The decision is made to perform I&D. The physician documents administration of local anesthetic, incision of skin above the abscess, and expression of purulent material. The wound was irrigated and packed. The patient will return in 3 days for reevaluation.

Code **10060** is reported for the procedure. All related visits (eg, follow-up visit to recheck the wound) within the 10 days following the date of surgery may be reported with code **99024** and no charge.

Removal of Skin Tags and Congenital Accessory Digits

11200   Removal of skin tags, multiple fibrocutaneous tags, any area; up to and including 15 lesions

Code **11200** is used to report the removal of a sixth digit from a newborn. It is equivalent to a skin tag and would not fall under the coding of an actual digit removal. The *ICD-10-CM* codes for accessory digits would be **Q69.0**, accessory fingers; **Q69.1**, accessory thumb; **Q69.2**, accessory toes; or **Q69.9**, unspecified. A 10-day global period applies under the MPFS.

Destruction of Benign Lesions (eg, Warts)

17110   Destruction (eg, laser surgery, electrosurgery, cryosurgery, chemosurgery, surgical curettement) of benign lesions other than skin tags or cutaneous vascular proliferative lesions; up to 14 lesions

17111   15 or more lesions

Report destruction of common or plantar warts, flat warts, or molluscum contagiosum with code **17110** or **17111** (with 1 unit of service), depending on the number of lesions removed. Do not report both **17110** and **17111** because they are mutually exclusive. Report *ICD-10-CM* using code **B08.1** for molluscum contagiosum, **B07.8** for common warts, or **B07.0** for plantar warts. A 10-day global period applies to both **17110** and **17111**.

Chemical Cauterization of Granulation Tissue

17250   Chemical cauterization of granulation tissue (ie, proud flesh)

Code **17250** is appropriately reported for cauterization of an umbilical granuloma. Do not report **17250** with removal or excision codes for the same lesion, for achieving wound hemostasis, or in conjunction with active wound care management. A 0-day global period applies.

Example

➤ **A 2-week-old presents for her well-baby check.** On examination, a moderate-sized umbilical granuloma is noted. The physician takes a very brief history and decides to cauterize. The routine well-baby check is completed.

ICD-10-CM	CPT
Z00.121 (encounter for routine child health examination with abnormal findings)	99391 25
P83.81 (umbilical granuloma)	17250

Teaching Point: Preservice work includes explanation of the procedure, obtaining informed consent, positioning and draping, preparing the site, and scrubbing in. Post-service work includes discussing follow-up care with parents/caregivers. Supplies and equipment, such as silver nitrate and an applicator, are included in the value assigned to the code when reporting to payers using RVUs. This service has a 0-day global period.

Laceration Repairs

12001–12018	Simple repair
12031–12057	Intermediate repair
13100–13160	Complex repair

- Categories of difficulty of wound repairs are described as
  - *Simple:* Superficial wound and/or subcutaneous wound requiring a simple single-layer closure or tissue adhesives
  - *Intermediate:* Wound requiring layered closure of one or more of the deeper layers of subcutaneous tissue and non-muscle fascia in addition to skin closure or contaminated wound that requires extensive cleaning or removal of particulate matter
  - *Complex:* Wounds requiring reconstructive surgery, complicated closure, or grafting
- Codes **12001–13160** are used to report wound closure using sutures, staples, or tissue adhesives (eg, Dermabond), singly or in combination with adhesive strips.
- Wound closure using adhesive strips (eg, Steri-Strips, butterfly bandages) only is considered inherent to the E/M service. However, the supplies (eg, Steri-Strips, butterfly bandages) may be reported separately using code **99070** (supplies and materials) or **A4450** (tape, non-waterproof, per 18 sq in). There is not a specific HCPCS code for Steri-Strips or butterfly bandages.
- Some payers may accept HCPCS code **G0168** (wound closure using tissue adhesive[s]) in lieu of simple repair codes (eg, **12001**, **12011**).
- Codes are reported based on the difficulty of the repair, measured length of the wound, and the location. To report wound repair, measure the length of the repaired wound(s) in centimeters.
  - If multiple wounds belong to the same category of difficulty and location, add the lengths and report with a single code.
  - If multiple wounds do not belong in the same category, report each repair separately with the more complicated repair reported as the primary procedure and the less complicated repair reported as the secondary procedure. Modifier **51** (multiple procedures) should be appended to the secondary code(s).
- Simple ligation of vessels is considered as part of the wound closure.
- Wound debridement and/or cleaning and the provision of topical or injected local anesthesia are considered to be included in the wound repair code. Debridement is considered a separate procedure only when gross contamination requires prolonged cleaning, excessive amounts of devitalized tissue are removed, or debridement is performed without immediate primary closure. To report extensive tissue debridement, see codes **11042–11047** for selective debridement of subcutaneous, muscle, fascial tissues, and/or bone (includes debridement of dermis and epidermis when performed) or **97597** and **97598** for debridement of skin, epidermis, and/or dermis.

> 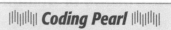 **Coding Pearl** |ו|ון|ון|
>
> *International Classification of Diseases, 10th Revision, Clinical Modification* code **Z48.02** (encounter for removal of sutures) is not reported for removal of sutures placed to repair an injury. For aftercare of an injury, assign the acute injury code with the seventh character **D** (subsequent encounter).

Examples

➤ A 10-year-old sustained a 1.5-cm laceration on his left knee requiring an intermediate (layered) repair after a fall from playground equipment.

ICD-10-CM	CPT®
S81.012A (laceration without foreign body left knee, initial encounter) **W09.8XXA** (fall on or from other playground equipment, initial encounter) **Y92.838** (other recreation area)	**12031** (repair, intermediate, wounds of scalp, axillae, trunk, and/or extremities; 2.5 cm or less)

Teaching Point: External cause codes (eg, **W09.8XXA**) are assigned for each encounter for treatment with a seventh character indicating initial (**A**), subsequent (**D**), or sequela (**S**). Place of occurrence (eg, **Y92.838**) is reported only for the initial encounter for an injury and requires no seventh character. Reporting the place of occurrence of an injury may aid in claims adjudication (ie, indicate that no other party is liable for the claim).

➤ **A 10-year-old fell from playground equipment and sustained a 1.5-cm laceration on his left knee and a 1.5-cm laceration on his left forearm, with each laceration requiring an intermediate repair.**

ICD-10-CM	*CPT*
S81.012A (laceration without foreign body left knee, initial encounter) **S51.812A** (laceration of left forearm without foreign body, initial encounter) **W09.8XXA** **Y92.838**	**12032** (intermediate repair, extremities, 2.6–7.5 cm)

Teaching Point: The measurement of both wounds (3 cm) is between 2.6 and 7.5 cm, both wounds are in the same family of anatomic sites, and both require the same level of repair. If the patient returns for wound follow-up within the 10 days following the date of repair, code **99024** (postoperative follow-up visit) is reported for the encounter because intermediate repair has a 10-day global period. There is no separate charge for care within the global period.

➤ **An 8-year-old sustained a 0.5-cm laceration on her forehead.** The wound on her face requires a simple repair. She is seen in follow-up 7 days later. The wound is clean, and sutures are removed.

ICD-10-CM	*CPT*
S01.81XA (laceration without foreign body of other part of head, initial encounter)	**Initial visit** **12011** (simple repair of the facial laceration 2.5 cm or less)
S01.81XD (laceration without foreign body of other part of head, subsequent encounter)	**Follow-up visit** **99212** (problem-focused E/M visit, office or outpatient)

Teaching Point: The seventh character **D** (ie, **S01.81XD**) is reported for encounters after the patient has received active treatment of the condition and is receiving routine care for the condition during the healing or recovery phase. Simple laceration repair has a 0-day global period, so any medically necessary follow-up care is separately reported.

➤ **A 3-year-old with 5 sutures placed in the emergency department presents at her pediatrician's office for suture removal.** The child is uncooperative, and 2 clinical staff members are required to assist the pediatrician in removing the sutures.

ICD-10-CM	*CPT*
Appropriate code for injury with seventh character **D** (eg, **S51.812D**, laceration of left forearm without foreign body, subsequent encounter)	**S0630** (removal of sutures by a physician other than the physician who originally closed the wound) or Appropriate E/M code (eg, **99212**) based on key components necessary for evaluation of the injury

Teaching Point: Although the suture removal required extended time, this service cannot be reported based on time. See "You Code It! Removal of Sutures" in the March 2018 *AAP Pediatric Coding Newsletter*™ (https://coding.aap.org; subscription required) for more information on reporting removal of sutures placed by another physician.

Coding Conundrum: Suture Removal

Suture removal can be coded in a variety of ways depending on the circumstances involved.

Sutures Placed by a Different Physician

When sutures are removed by another physician with a different tax identification number, an evaluation and management (E/M) office visit code may be reported for the suture removal. Some payers may allow reporting of Healthcare Common Procedure Coding System (HCPCS) code **S0630**. Code **S0630** is for removal of sutures by a physician other than the physician who originally closed the wound. **S** codes are HCPCS Level II codes, designated by the Centers for Medicare & Medicaid Services and recognized by national Blue Cross and Blue Shield payers, but coverage is on a payer-by-payer basis.

Sutures Placed by Same Physician or Physician of the Same Specialty in the Same Group (Same Tax Identification Number)

Simple Repair

The Medicare global surgery period for *Current Procedural Terminology*® codes **12001–12018** (simple repair of superficial wound) is 0 days, meaning payment includes the procedure or service plus any associated care provided on the same day of service. Therefore, practices may report a separate E/M service for removal of sutures placed in the office.

Intermediate or Complex Repair

The Medicare global surgery period for intermediate (**12031–12057**) and complex (**13100–13153**) wound repairs is 10 days. Payment includes the procedure or service plus any associated follow-up care for a period of 10 days. Therefore, the charge for the procedure already includes suture removal by the same physician or physician of the same group and specialty as part of the global surgical package.

Other Repairs

Code **11760** (repair of nail bed) is reported when part or all of the nail plate is lifted and a laceration of the nail bed is repaired.

Report code **40650** (repair of vermilion border of the lip) when a laceration of the full thickness of the lip and vermilion is repaired.

Laceration repairs of the tongue (**41250–41252**) are reported based on size and location (eg, repair of laceration 2.5 cm or less, anterior two-thirds of the tongue is reported using code **41250**).

Burn Care

CPT code **16000** (initial treatment, first-degree burn, where no more than local treatment is required) is reported when initial treatment is performed for the symptomatic relief of a first-degree burn that is characterized by erythema and tenderness.

16020   Dressings and/or debridement of partial-thickness burns, initial or subsequent; small or less than 5% total body (eg, finger)

Code **16020**

* Is used to report treatment of burns with dressings and/or debridement of small partial-thickness burns (second degree), whether initial or subsequent.

* An E/M visit with modifier **25** appended may be reported if a significant, separately identifiable E/M service is medically indicated, performed, and documented in addition to the burn care.

* See full discussion of burn care in Chapter 19, Common Surgical Procedures and Sedation in Facility Settings, for coding of larger partial-thickness or full-thickness burns.

Examples

➤ **A 9-year-old is seen by the physician complaining of sunburn on her shoulders.** There is redness and tenderness but no blistering. Topical treatment is applied and an over-the-counter treatment for the first-degree burn is ordered.

ICD-10-CM	CPT®
L55.0 (first-degree sunburn)	16000 (first-degree burn requiring local treatment)

➤ **A 4-year-old is seen in the office after sustaining a burn on the first finger of her right hand from touching a hot pan.** The area is red and blistered. Following examination by the physician, the finger is treated with a topical cream and bandaged.

ICD-10-CM	CPT
T23.221A (second-degree burn of single finger, initial encounter) X15.3XXA (contact with other heat and hot saucepan or skillet, initial encounter)	16020

Teaching Point: External cause of injury codes like **X15.3XXA** are used to report the source, place, and/or intent of a burn injury. These codes are only required when state regulations mandate reporting of cause of injury (typically applies to emergency department services). However, it is appropriate to report external cause of injury codes when cause is known.

97605 Negative pressure wound therapy (eg, vacuum assisted drainage collection), utilizing durable medical equipment (DME), including topical application(s), wound assessment, and instruction(s) for ongoing care, per session; total wound(s) surface area less than or equal to 50 square centimeters
97606 total wound(s) surface area greater than 50 square centimeters
97607 Negative pressure wound therapy, (eg, vacuum assisted drainage collection), utilizing disposable, non-durable medical equipment including provision of exudate management collection system, topical application(s), wound assessment, and instructions for ongoing care, per session; total wound(s) surface area less than or equal to 50 square centimeters
97608 total wound(s) surface area greater than 50 square centimeters

It has become common in recent years for physicians to include use of negative pressure wound therapy (NPWT) or vacuum-assisted closure in the management of traumatic and surgical wounds. Codes **97605** and **97606** represent NPWT provided via a system that includes a *non-disposable* suction pump and drainage collection device. Codes **97607** and **97608** are used for NPWT that uses a *disposable* suction pump and collection system. Codes **97607** and **97608** are not reported in conjunction with codes **97605** and **97606**. Payer policies may limit coverage to care of specific types of wounds that require NPWT to improve granulation tissue formation and to certain types of NPWT equipment. Be sure to verify the coverage policy of the patient's health plan prior to provision of services.

Negative pressure wound therapy
* Requires direct (one-on-one) physician or other qualified health care professional (QHP) contact with the patient.
* May be initiated in a hospital or surgical center setting and continued in the home setting after discharge.
* Includes application of dressings.
* Is reported once for each session, which includes wound assessment and measurement and application of NPWT dressings and equipment.
* Is separately reported when performed in conjunction with surgical debridement (**11042–11047**).
* Documentation should include current wound assessment, including quantitative measurements of wound characteristics (eg, site, surface area and depth), any previous treatment regimens, debridement (when performed), prescribed length of treatment, dressing types and frequency of changes, and other concerns that affect healing. Encounters for ongoing NPWT may include documentation of progress of healing and changes in the wound, including measurement, amount of exudate, and presence of granulation or necrotic tissue.

* Supplies, including dressings, are reportable with HCPCS codes (eg, **A6550**, wound care set, for NPWT electrical pump, includes all supplies and accessories). Supplies for a disposable system are reported with code **A9272**, which also includes all dressings and accessories.

Removal of Foreign Bodies

CPT® includes codes for reporting removal of foreign bodies from many different body sites. **Table 10-4** summarizes foreign body removal services from other than skin or muscle. Removal of a foreign body from within the subcutaneous tissues above the fascia is reported with a code from the integumentary system regardless of the site (eg, hand, foot). Musculoskeletal codes are reported when a foreign body is removed from *within the fascia, subfascial, or muscle.* Always check the *CPT* index to direct you to the most accurate code.

* Code **10120** (removal of a foreign body from subcutaneous tissue via simple incision) includes the removal of splinters or ticks when the physician has to "break open" or incise the skin to retrieve the splinter.
* Code **10121** is used to report the complicated removal of a foreign body by incision.

The physician determines whether the procedure is simple or complex, but the significant difference in physician work RVUs for the procedures may be used as an indicator of the difference—1.22 for **10120** versus 2.74 for **10121**. Clearly, a procedure described by code **10121** would involve double the time and effort of the simple procedure. *CPT* offers no examples of simple versus complicated. A complicated removal may require extended exploration and removal of multiple foreign bodies (eg, pieces of glass), use of imaging to help locate the foreign body, or removal that is complicated by the anatomic site of the foreign body (eg, area that is not easily seen) and will have a greater intensity of physician work.

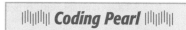

Coding Pearl

Do not report code **10120** or **10121** when a foreign body is removed using forceps alone with no incision. Report instead an evaluation and management service.

The removal of an embedded earring requiring an incision would be reported with code **10120** or **10121**, depending on the complexity of the procedure required to remove it. If the earring is removed by wiggling it out or another method that does not require incision, this work is included in the E/M service.

Table 10-4. Codes for Removal of Foreign Bodies Other Than From Skin or Muscle

Site	Code(s)
Anal foreign body or fecal impaction	Use appropriate E/M code or **45999** (unlisted procedure, rectum) unless removed under anesthesia (**45915**, more than local anesthesia).
External auditory canal (For removal of impacted cerumen, see discussion later in this chapter.)	**69200** (removal foreign body from external auditory canal; without general anesthesia)
Eye	**65205** (removal of foreign body, external eye; conjunctival superficial) **65220** (removal of foreign body, external eye; corneal, without slit lamp)
Nose	**30300** (removal of intranasal foreign bodies when performed in the office) **30310** (removal of intranasal foreign bodies under general anesthesia)
Vagina	Use appropriate E/M code or **58999** (unlisted procedure, female genital system) unless removed under anesthesia (**57415**, more than local anesthesia).

Abbreviation: E/M, evaluation and management.

- *Musculoskeletal foreign body:* Codes in the musculoskeletal system are not reported for removal of foreign bodies within the skin and subcutaneous fat. Examples of codes for removal of foreign bodies within the musculoskeletal system are
  - ❖ *Foot:* For foreign body removal *from within the fascia, subfascial, or muscle,* code **28190** is used to report the removal of a subcutaneous foreign body from the foot; code **28192** is used to report removal of a foreign body from the deep tissue of the foot.
  - ❖ *Upper arm or elbow:* Report removal of foreign bodies from subcutaneous tissues within the fascia (**24200**) or deep, below the fascia or in the muscle (**24201**) of the upper arm or elbow area.

Fracture and/or Dislocation Care

Casts/Strapping/Splints

- Codes for the application of casts, splints, or strapping (**29000–29590**) cannot be reported for the initial (first) application when fracture or dislocation care is reported because they are included as part of the global surgery package.
- May be reported when they are replacements for the initial application or performed as part of the initial E/M visit and fracture care is not reported.

  The following codes are commonly used when treating a fracture or dislocation:
- Application of splints
  - ❖ Short arm splint (forearm to hand): static (**29125**); dynamic (**29126**)
  - ❖ Finger splint: static (**29130**); dynamic (**29131**)
  - ❖ Short leg splint (calf to foot): **29515**
- Strapping
  - ❖ Shoulder: **29240**
  - ❖ Elbow or wrist: **29260**

Example

➤ **An established patient presents to an urgent care practice with an injury to the left wrist.** The patient states he tripped and fell while playing soccer with friends at a soccer field. After examination, a 3-view radiograph of the wrist is ordered and performed in the office. The physician interprets the radiograph, determines that the patient has a fracture of the left proximal scaphoid, and applies a short arm splint pending consultation with an orthopedist in 2 days.

ICD-10-CM	CPT®
S62.035A (nondisplaced fracture of proximal third of navicular [scaphoid] bone of left wrist, initial encounter for closed fracture) **W01.0XXA** (fall on same level from slipping, tripping and stumbling without subsequent striking against object, initial encounter) **Y92.322** (soccer field as the place of occurrence of the external cause) **Y93.66** (activity, soccer) **Y99.8** (recreation or sport not for income or while a student)	**99212–99215 25**
	29125 (application of short arm splint [forearm to hand]; static) **73110** (radiologic examination, wrist; complete, minimum of three views)

Teaching Point: The physician reports splinting of the fracture because only the initial care and referral to an orthopedist were provided in lieu of restorative fracture care. An E/M service for evaluation of the extent of injury would be reported with modifier **25** appended to the E/M code. Payers must have accident information to determine if another party (eg, school, automobile, homeowner's insurance) is liable for a claim. Inclusion of codes for external cause of injury, though not required, may provide information that facilitates timely payment.

Supplies

* Supplies associated with fracture care may be billed with every application, including the initial casting, splinting, or strapping performed in association with the global surgery procedure code when the service is performed in the private office setting.

* HCPCS codes **A4580**, **A4590**, and **Q4001–Q4051** may be reported for cast supplies; codes **E1800–E1841** may be reported for splints. Check with your major payers and/or review their payment policies for reporting these supplies.

* HCPCS codes are accepted by many Medicaid and commercial payers and are very specific to the age of the patient and type of supply and/or material.

* A description of supplies may be required when reporting special supplies code **99070**.

* The following codes are commonly used:

99070	Supplies and materials (except spectacles)
A4565	Slings
A4570	Splint
L3650–L3678	Clavicle splints
Q4001–Q4051	Cast and splint supplies
S8450–S8452	Splint, prefabricated for finger, wrist, ankle, or elbow

> ||||||| **Coding Pearl** |||||||
>
> When reporting codes for radiographs, documentation should include a report that includes the indication for the test, number of views, findings, and, when applicable, comparison to previous radiographs. Do not report a charge for interpretation and report when reviewing images that have been previously interpreted (eg, by a radiologist). The independent review of previously interpreted images is included in an evaluation and management service.

Fracture and Dislocation Care Codes

Codes for fracture/dislocation care

* Are listed by anatomic location.

* Are provided (in most cases) for closed or open treatment, with or without manipulation, and with or without internal fixation.

* Most include a 90-day period of follow-up care under the Medicare global package.

* Include the initial casting, splinting, or strapping.

* Do not include radiographs or E/M to determine the extent of injury and treatment options.

* Fractures most commonly seen in a primary care pediatric practice include closed fractures (ie, skin is intact on presentation), and treatment is typically closed (ie, fracture site is not surgically opened) without manipulation (an exception is treatment of nursemaid elbow).

* Clavicular fracture: Report closed treatment without manipulation with code **23500**.

* Nursemaid elbow: Report closed treatment of radial head subluxation (nursemaid elbow) with manipulation with code **24640**. (This code has a 10-day global period.)

* Radial fracture: Report code **25500** for closed treatment of radial shaft fracture without manipulation and **25600** for closed treatment of distal radius fracture without manipulation.

* Phalanx fracture: Closed treatment of a proximal or middle phalanx, finger, or thumb (each) without manipulation is reported with code **26720**. Closed treatment of a distal phalangeal fracture (each) without manipulation is reported with code **26750**.

* Great toe fracture: Code **28490** is reported for the closed treatment of a fracture of the great toe, phalanx, or phalanges without manipulation.

* Metatarsal fracture: Report code **28470** for closed treatment of a metatarsal fracture without manipulation.

* Lesser toe fracture: Closed treatment of fracture, phalanx, or phalanges, other than great toe without manipulation, is coded with **28510**.

* When a patient presents for follow-up care after initial fracture care is provided in another setting (eg, emergency department, urgent care), it is necessary to determine if the provider of initial fracture care reported a code for fracture care with modifier **54** (surgical care only) or reported only casting/strapping for the initial care. If initial fracture care has been reported with modifier **54**, the physician providing continued fracture care reports the fracture care code with modifier **55** (postoperative care only) appended.

Coding Conundrum: Reporting Fracture Care

If a payer follows Medicare payment policy, the physician has the option of using the appropriate evaluation and management (E/M) codes and reporting each service separately in lieu of using procedure codes. The decision to use the global fracture code rather than E/M service codes requires an analysis of payment by payers for these codes.

Current Procedural Terminology® code **25600** (closed treatment of distal radial fracture, without manipulation) includes all associated preoperative care, application of the splint, and follow-up care for 90 days. If there was a significant, separately identifiable E/M service provided on the day of the fracture care (eg, child sustained sprain to other arm), an E/M service could also be reported with modifier **25** appended to the E/M service. Radiology services (eg, **73100**, radiologic exam, wrist, two views) are separately reported. Follow-up visits would be reported with code **99024** (postoperative follow-up visit included in surgical package). If a physician chooses not to bill fracture care, an E/M visit would be reported with code **29075** (application of short arm cast). You could also report code **Q4012** (cast supplies, short arm cast, pediatric, fiberglass). Any diagnostic procedures, such as radiographs, would be reported in either situation.

Before you decide how to bill the service, consider your total payments for the care associated with this fracture.

Reporting Fracture Care Codes		Reporting E/M and Follow-up	
Code	**2018 Medicare Non-facility RBRVS[a]**	**Code**	**2018 Medicare Non-facility RBRVS[a]**
25600	9.42	99213	2.06
73100	0.89	73100	0.89
		29075	2.49
Q4012[b]	—	Q4012[b]	—
99024	0.00	99212	1.24
Total	10.31		6.68

Abbreviations: E/M, evaluation and management; RBRVS, Resource-Based Relative Value Scale.

[a] The 2019 Medicare RBRVS was not available at the time this manual was printed. For an online copy of the pediatric-specific 2018 Medicare RBRVS, go to www.aap.org/cfp, access code AAPCFP24.

[b] Supplies are not valued on the RBRVS.

Ideally, documentation to support fracture care will include interpretation and report of radiographic findings, that appropriate stabilization or immobilization without neurovascular compromise was achieved, precautions, and instructions to return for follow-up care.

Tip: Unrelated services that are provided during the global surgery period by the same physician (or physician of the same group and specialty) may be reported. Modifier **24** would be appended to the unrelated E/M service. Refer to Chapter 2, Modifiers and Coding Edits, for instructions for reporting modifiers.

Examples

➤ An urgent care physician performs and documents a comprehensive evaluation on a child with multiple injuries, including a fracture of the shaft of the left clavicle and abrasions on the left upper arm and cheek, after a fall from the monkey bars.

ICD-10-CM	CPT®
S40.812A (abrasion upper arm, initial encounter) **S00.81XA** (abrasion face, initial encounter) **W09.8XXA** (fall from playground equipment, initial encounter)	99201–99205 57
S42.022A (displaced fracture shaft of clavicle, closed, initial encounter) **W09.8XXA**	**23500** (closed treatment clavicle fracture without manipulation)

Teaching Point: Fractures not specified as displaced or non-displaced are reported with an *ICD-10-CM* code for a displaced fracture. Fractures not specified as open or closed are reported with a code for a closed fracture. Because code **23500** is assigned a 90-day global period in the MPFS and is placed in the surgery section of *CPT*, many payers may require modifier **57** (decision for surgery) appended to the E/M code. Individual payers may have different policies.

➤ **A physician evaluates a 16-month-old girl whose parents report that she will not move her left arm.** The child was playing in the yard when another child tried to pull her up the ladder of a playhouse. Mother thinks child fell, hitting her head and left side. Mother noted no bump or bruises but soon noticed she was not using her left arm. The fall was from no more than 3 feet off the ground. The patient is otherwise in good health, with no past hospitalizations or surgeries and no allergies or medications. Immunizations are up-to-date. The patient lives with her parents and 2 older siblings. Review of systems is negative for headache, vomiting, dizziness, or changes in behavior other than protection of left arm. On examination, the child is alert but apprehensive. She has no hematoma or skull defect, her face is symmetric, pupils are equal and responsive to light and accommodation, and her neck is supple. The child holds her left arm in front of her body with her right hand supporting her left forearm. Left upper extremity shows no visible signs of deformity or swelling, and skin is intact. Pain is elicited at the head of the radius. Subluxation of the radial head is reduced by manipulation. Reassessment after 10 minutes shows the child uses both arms now when presented with a balloon. The parents are counseled about potential for recurrent injury and avoidance. A follow-up with previously scheduled 18-month visit is arranged unless otherwise indicated.

ICD-10-CM	CPT
S53.032A (nursemaid's elbow, left, initial encounter) **W11.XXXA** (fall on and from ladder)	**99214 25** **24640** (closed treatment of radial head subluxation in child, nursemaid elbow, with manipulation)

Teaching Point: The physician provided a significant and separately identifiable E/M service to evaluate extent of injury in addition to treatment of nursemaid elbow. Although not specifically stated, the patient is established, as she is to return for an already scheduled 18-month preventive service. The history and examination are detailed, and the MDM is of moderate complexity. Modifier **25** is required by most payers to indicate the E/M service was significant and separately identifiable from the preservice work of the minor procedure performed on the same date of service.

➤ **A 9-year-old established patient is seen with complaints of left and right arm pain following a fall while snowboarding.** An expanded problem-focused history and physical examination are performed. The radiograph demonstrates a left Colles fracture (distal radius with dorsal [posterior] displacement of the wrist and hand). A fiberglass cast is applied, and the patient is advised to return for follow-up.

The physician can elect to report the fracture care (closed treatment without manipulation, **25600**, or with manipulation, **25605**) or the E/M services provided over the course of the global surgery period (see the Coding Conundrum: Reporting Fracture Care box earlier in this chapter).

Ear, Nose, and Throat Procedures

Control of Nasal Hemorrhage

30901   Control nasal hemorrhage, anterior, simple (cautery or packing)

30903   Control nasal hemorrhage, anterior, complex (extensive cautery and/or packing) any method

⚙ If performing cautery or packing on both sides, report **30901** with modifier **50**.

⚙ If bleeding is controlled with manual pressure or placement of a nasal clamp (clip), only the appropriate level of E/M service is reported.

Example

➤ **A 7-year old established patient presents with a facial injury.** He was walking with his class on the school sidewalk to the cafeteria when he tripped and fell. He did try to catch himself, but his face partially hit the pavement, and he had mild bruising on his nose and a significant nosebleed. Review of systems revealed no headache, vomiting, or loss of consciousness. Medical history was negative for a bleeding disorder, and family history was negative for a bleeding disorder within the family.

On examination, there was minimal abrasion and ecchymosis on the tip of the nose, with no pain on palpation over the bridge of the nose and cheeks. Septum was not deviated, and no hematoma was present. There was a moderate amount of crusted blood from left nare, and the physician could visually see a small bleed medially of left nare. The remainder of the examination was normal. The decision was made to cauterize with silver nitrate.

ICD-10-CM	CPT®
R04.0 (epistaxis) **S00.31XA** (abrasion of nose) **W01.0XXA** (fall on same level from slipping, tripping and stumbling without subsequent striking against object, initial encounter) **Y92.480** (sidewalk as the place of occurrence of the external cause) **Y93.01** (activity walking, marching, and hiking)	**99214 25** (established patient office E/M: a detailed history; a detailed examination; MDM of moderate complexity) **30901**

Removal of Impacted Cerumen

69209   Removal of impacted cerumen using irrigation/lavage, unilateral
69210   Removal of impacted cerumen requiring instrumentation, unilateral

For cerumen removal that is not impacted, report the appropriate E/M service code.

Modifier **25** should be appended to the significant, separately identifiable E/M service (eg, **99213**) provided on the same date as removal of impacted cerumen based on NCCI edits. Payers that incorporate NCCI edits may deny the service when submitted without modifier **25**. For more information on NCCI edits, see Chapter 2, Modifiers and Coding Edits.

Code **69209** is used to report removal of impacted cerumen by ear wash without direct visualization and instrumentation. *Do not report* **69209** for removal of cerumen that is not impacted. This code is intended to capture the practice expense associated with the service and is not valued to include physician work. Separately report any significant and separately identifiable E/M service provided by a physician or other QHP on the same date (modifier **25** may be appended to the E/M code when required by payers).

> |||||||| **Coding Pearl** ||||||||
> Removal of cerumen that is not impacted is included in an evaluation and management code regardless of how it is removed.

⁕ For bilateral procedure, report **69209** with modifier **50**.
⁕ Do not report **69209** in conjunction with **69210** when performed on the same ear (modifiers **LT** and **RT** may be used to identify contralateral procedures).

Code **69210** is *only* reported when the physician, under direct visualization, removes impacted cerumen using, at a minimum, an otoscope and instruments such as wax curettes or by using an operating microscope and suction plus specific ear instruments (eg, cup forceps, right angles).

⁕ Medical record documentation must support that the cerumen was impacted and removed by the physician and include a description of what equipment and method were used to perform the procedure.
⁕ Report code **69210** with modifier **50** when bilateral procedures are performed.
⁕ Removal of cerumen that is not impacted is included in an E/M code regardless of how it is removed.

Coding Conundrum: Unsuccessful Removal of Impacted Cerumen

If a physician or other qualified health care professional attempts to remove impacted cerumen but finds the impaction too hard for safe removal, what code is reported for the attempt? The answer depends on the individual situation, including the amount of work that was performed and whether another procedure was successful.

If the portion of the procedure completed required insignificant work and practice expense (eg, staff time), report only the services completed on that date (eg, evaluation and management).

If the patient is instructed to use softening drops and return later for removal, consider whether the effort and practice expense were sufficient to justify reporting the removal with reduced services modifier 52.

If the procedure was discontinued after significant effort and practice expense due to extenuating circumstances or concerns that the procedure may threaten the patient's well-being, report the procedure code with modifier 53 (discontinued procedure).

If, after attempted removal by a physician is discontinued, softening drops are administered in the office and clinical staff perform removal of the impaction by lavage (69209), report only the completed procedure.

Note: Medicare does not recognize modifier 50 when reported with code 69210 (impacted cerumen removal); therefore, those payers that follow Medicare payment policy will not recognize it and may deny the claim outright. Check with your payers.

Examples

➤ **A physician orders removal of impacted cerumen from the right ear by lavage.** Clinical staff perform the lavage, removing the impacted cerumen. Because the child is uncooperative, the procedure takes 10 minutes.

ICD-10-CM	CPT®
H92.01 (otalgia, right ear) H61.21 (impacted cerumen, right ear)	99201–99215 25 Report if appropriate and use modifier 25 if required by payer.
H61.21	69209 RT (RT indicates right ear)

Teaching Point: This procedure was unilateral. If it were bilateral, modifier 50 would be appended to code 69209. The anatomic modifier RT (right) is informational and typically does not affect payment. The extended time of service alone is not sufficient to support reporting increased procedural service (ie, modifier 22).

➤ **Physician documents, "Impacted cerumen removed from both ears using an otoscope and curette," in patient with complaint of decreased hearing.** Following the procedure, the patient's hearing is assessed as normal.

ICD-10-CM	CPT
H61.23 (impacted cerumen, bilateral)	99201–99215 25 Report if appropriate and use modifier 25 if required by payer.
	69210 50

Digestive System Procedures

Incision Lingual Frenulum

41010   Incision in the lingual frenum to free the tongue

☀ Note that code **41115** (excision of lingual frenum) is not appropriate when an incisional release of tongue-tie is performed rather than excision of the frenum.

Example

➤ **A 14-day-old is seen for feeding difficulty caused by ankyloglossia.** The physician documents the obtaining of informed consent, positioning and restraining of the neonate, and gentle lifting of the tongue with a sterile, grooved retractor to expose the frenulum. The frenulum, adjacent to the ventral aspect of the tongue, is divided by 2 to 3 mm using sterile scissors. Afterward, the newborn is immediately returned to his mother for comfort and feeding. The latch appears improved. After feeding, the neonate is reevaluated prior to discharge with no evidence of complications. Code **41010** is reported for the procedure.

ICD-10-CM	CPT®
Q38.1 (congenital ankyloglossia)	**41010**

Teaching Point: If a significant and separately identifiable E/M service was provided in addition to the preservice work of the procedure, modifier **25** would be appended to the appropriate E/M code. Any related visit within the 10 days following the procedure may be reported (with no charge) with code **99024**.

Gastrostomy Tube Replacement

●**43762**   Replacement of gastrostomy tube, percutaneous, includes removal, when performed, without imaging or endoscopic guidance; not requiring revision of gastrostomy tract

●**43763**   requiring revision of gastrostomy tract

Code **43760** is deleted in 2019. To report gastrostomy tube change without imaging or endoscopic guidance, see codes **43762** and **43763**. See codes **49450** and **43246** for placement with imaging or endoscopic guidance. A significant, separately identifiable E/M service on the same date may be reported with modifier **25** appended to the E/M code (eg, **99213 25**). An E/M service should not be reported when the encounter is solely for replacement of the gastrostomy tube. Codes **43762** and **43763** include the gastrostomy tube kit.

Genitourinary System Procedures

Urinary Catheterization

51701   Urinary catheterization, straight

Report code **51701** when you insert a urinary catheter to collect a clean-catch urine specimen, after which the catheter is removed.

51702   Urinary catheterization, temporary

Code **51701** is reported when a non-indwelling bladder catheter (straight catheterization) is inserted (eg, for residual urine, for a urine culture collection). Code **51702** is reported when a temporary indwelling bladder catheter is inserted (ie, Foley).

256 ||||||||| PART 2: PRIMARILY FOR THE OFFICE AND OTHER OUTPATIENT SETTINGS

Lysis/Excision of Labial or Penile Adhesions

54450 Foreskin manipulation including lysis of preputial adhesions and stretching
54162 Lysis or excision of penile post-circumcision adhesions
56441 Lysis of labial adhesions

If lysis of labial or penile adhesions is performed by the application of manual pressure without the use of an instrument to cut the adhesions, it would be considered part of the E/M visit and not reported separately.

Code **54450** does not require general anesthesia. It has an RVU of 2.00 when performed in a non-facility setting (eg, office). Medicare has assigned it a 0-day global surgery period. This procedure is performed on the uncircumcised foreskin and the head of the penis. Adhesions are broken by stretching the foreskin back over the head of the penis onto the shaft or by inserting a clamp between the foreskin and the head of the penis and spreading the jaws of the clamp.

Code **54162** is only reported when lysis is performed under general anesthesia or regional block, with an instrument, and under sterile conditions. This code has an RVU of 7.31 when performed in a non-facility setting (eg, office) and a Medicare 10-day global surgery period, which payers may or may not use. If post-circumcision adhesions are manually broken during the postoperative period by the physician or physician of the same group and specialty who performed the procedure, it would be considered part of the global surgical package. Report the service with *ICD-10-CM* code **N47.0**, adherent prepuce in a newborn, or **N47.5**, adhesions of prepuce and glans penis (patients older than 28 days).

Code **56441** is performed by using a blunt instrument or scissors under general or local anesthesia. The total RVUs for this procedure in a non-facility setting are 4.09. This procedure also includes a Medicare 10-day global surgery period, which may or may not be used by payers. *ICD-10-CM* code **Q52.5** (fusion of labia) would be reported with *CPT* code **56441**. When provided without anesthesia, modifier **52** may be appended to indicate reduced services. Payer guidance may vary with regard to use of modifier **52**.

Newborn Circumcision

54150 Circumcision, using clamp or other device with regional dorsal penile or ring block
- If the circumcision using a clamp or other device is performed without dorsal penile or ring block, append modifier **52** (reduced services) to **54150**.
- Medicare has a global period of 0 (zero) assigned to code **54150**. When an E/M service (eg, well-baby visit) is provided on the same date, append modifier **25** to the E/M code. Link the appropriate *ICD-10-CM* code (eg, **Z00.110**, health check for newborn under 8 days old) to the E/M service and link *ICD-10-CM* code **Z41.2** (encounter for routine and ritual male circumcision) to the circumcision code.
54160 Circumcision, surgical excision other than clamp, device, or dorsal slit; neonate (28 days of age or less)
54161 older than 28 days

Unlike code **54150**, Medicare has a global period of 10 days assigned to codes **54160** and **54161**. When circumcisions are performed in the office
- If a payer does not base payment on a global surgical package, a supply code for the surgical tray can be reported with code **99070**. The description of the supply (circumcision tray) would need to be included on the claim form.
- Anesthetic creams (eutectic mixture of local anesthetics) are included in the circumcision code itself and should not be reported unless a third-party payer pays separately for topical anesthetic agents. In that case, they would be reported with code **99070**.

Hydration, Injections, and Infusions

Services included as inherent to an infusion or injection are the use of local anesthesia, starting the intravenous (IV) line, access to indwelling IV lines or a subcutaneous catheter or port, flushing lines at the conclusion of an infusion or between infusions, standard tubing, syringes and supplies, and preparation of chemotherapy agents.

These codes are intended for reporting by the physician or other QHP in an office setting. They are not reported by a physician or other QHP when performed in a facility setting because the physician work associated with these procedures involves only affirmation of the treatment plan and direct supervision of the staff performing the services. If a significant, separately identifiable E/M service is performed, the appropriate code may be reported with modifier **25** appended. The diagnosis may be the same for the E/M service and codes **96360–96379**.

Therapeutic, Prophylactic, and Diagnostic Injections

96372   Therapeutic, prophylactic, or diagnostic injection (specify substance or drug); subcutaneous or intramuscular

96373   intra-arterial

96374   intravenous push, single or initial substance/drug

+96375   each additional sequential intravenous push of a new substance/drug (List separately in addition to **96365**, **96374**, **96409**, or **96413**)

❋ Report code **96372** for the administration of a diagnostic, prophylactic, or therapeutic (eg, antibiotic) subcutaneous or intramuscular (IM) injection. Do not report for the administration of a purified protein derivative test. For administration of immunizations, see discussion of codes **90460**, **90461**, and **90471–90474** in Chapter 9, Preventive Services.

Examples

➤ **A 2-year-old established patient presents with moderate symptoms of croup that began last evening and worsened during the night.** After obtaining a detailed history and performing a detailed examination, the physician recommends injection of dexamethasone sodium phosphate. Seven milligrams of dexamethasone sodium phosphate is administered by IM injection. The child is observed for reaction and released to home with instructions and precautions.

ICD-10-CM	CPT®
J05.0 (acute obstructive laryngitis [croup])	99214 25 (established patient level IV E/M) 96372 (IM injection) J1100 x 7 units (injection, dexamethasone sodium phosphate per 1 mg)

Teaching Point: The medication is reported with HCPCS code **J1100**, which indicates the unit of measure for reporting is 1 mg. Because 7 mg were administered, 7 units of service are reported. Report also the appropriate National Drug Code (NDC) and units. (See Chapter 1, The Basics of Coding, for more information on NDCs.)

The E/M service is described as including detailed history and examination, which supports code **99214**. (The MDM also likely supports **99214** with moderate complexity based on a new problem and injection of a prescription medication.) Modifier **25** must be appended to the E/M service code to indicate the significant, separately identifiable E/M service on the date of the injection for payers that use NCCI edits.

➤ **A 2-year-old girl presents with a fever (39.4°C [103.0°F]), and mom states the girl has been tugging at her right ear for 2 days.** An expanded problem-focused history and examination are completed. When the doctor examines the ears, he notices that the right middle ear is very inflamed (pus is present) and the child is extremely uncomfortable. The child's mother states that it is very difficult to get her daughter to swallow medicine rather than spit it out. The doctor decides to administer a single injection of ceftriaxone sodium 600 mg to the child. The final diagnosis is right acute suppurative otitis media without rupture of eardrum. Medical decision-making is moderate.

ICD-10-CM	CPT®
H66.001 (acute suppurative otitis media without spontaneous rupture of ear drum, right ear)	99213 25 (established patient level E/M) 96372 (IM injection) J0696 × 3 units (injection, ceftriaxone sodium, per 250 mg)

Teaching Point: The medication is reported with HCPCS code J0696, which indicates the unit of measure for reporting is 250 mg. Because 600 mg was administered, 3 units are reported for each date of service. However, if the payer accepts actual dosage, 2.4 units (2 units for the first two 250 mg of the medication and 0.4 units for the last 100 mg) would be reported rather than 3 units. Report also the appropriate NDC.

Modifier 25 must be appended to the E/M service code (99213) to indicate the significant, separately identifiable E/M service on the date of the injection for payers that use NCCI edits.

➤ **A 2-year-old (12-kg) patient with a history of multiple ear infections who has been on multiple antibiotics in the past 3 months presents for left ear pain and fever for 2 days.** History and physical examination support a diagnosis of acute recurrent suppurative otitis media of the left ear. Due to history of multiple courses of antibiotics in the past few months, the physician recommends a 3-day course of ceftriaxone 50 mg/kg by IM injection. The first dose of 600 mg is given at the time of the visit, and the patient returns in 24 hours and in 48 hours with clinical staff administering the next 2 doses. The E/M service provided includes detailed history and examination and moderate MDM.

ICD-10-CM	CPT®
H66.005 (acute suppurative otitis media without spontaneous rupture of ear drum, recurrent, left ear)	**Day 1** 99214 25 (established patient level E/M) 96372 (IM injection) J0696 × 3 units (injection, ceftriaxone sodium, per 250 mg) **Days 2 and 3** (report on each date) 96372 J0696 × 3 units

Teaching Point: The medication and administration code are reported for each of the 3 dates of service.

Modifier 25 must be appended to the E/M service code (99214) to indicate the significant, separately identifiable E/M service on the date of the injection for payers that use NCCI edits.

❋ Report code 96373 for an initial intra-arterial injection and 96374 for an initial injection administered by IV push. Sequential IV push of a new substance or drug is reported with add-on code 96375. Code 96375 may be reported in addition to codes for IV infusion (96365), initial IV push (96374), or chemotherapy administration (96409, 96413).

❋ Additional sequential IV push of the same substance or drug (96376) is not reported for services provided in the physician office (ie, is reported only by a facility).

❋ Each drug administered is reported separately with the appropriate infusion code.

> |||||||| **Coding Pearl** ||||||||
>
> Short infusions of less than 15 minutes should be reported with code 96374.

Codes **96374** and **96375** are only used when the health care professional administering the substance or drug is in constant attendance during the administration *and* must observe the patient. The IV push must be less than 15 minutes. Short infusions of less than 15 minutes are reported as a push (eg, **96374**).

Hydration and Infusions

Hydration and infusion codes are reported based on the time (time medication administration begins to end of administration). Time must be documented.

When reporting multiple infusions on the same date, physicians select an initial service based on the service that is the primary reason for infusion services on that date. For example, a patient receives infusion of a medication and a separate infusion of hydration fluid. The physician determines whether the primary service was the therapeutic infusion or the hydration and selects the appropriate initial service code. The other service is reported with a code for sequential or subsequent administration.

Table 10-5 lists primary and additional IV infusion and IV push codes. See the table notes for additional instructions on reporting multiple services.

Hydration

Codes **96360** (IV infusion, hydration; initial, 31 minutes to 1 hour) and **96361** (each additional hour)

- Are intended to report IV hydration infusion using prepackaged fluid and/or electrolyte solutions (eg, physiologic [normal] saline solution, D_5-0.45% physiologic saline solution with potassium).
- Typically require direct physician supervision for purposes of consent, safety oversight, or supervision of staff with little special handling for preparation or disposal of materials.
- Do not typically require advanced training of staff because there usually is little risk involved with little patient monitoring required.
- Are reported based on the actual time over which the infusion is administered and do not include the time spent starting the IV and monitoring the patient after infusion. Medical record documentation must support the service reported.
- Code **96360** may be reported for hydration infusion lasting more than 31 minutes and up to 1 hour. Code **96361** is reported for each additional hour of hydration infusion and for a final interval of greater than 30 minutes beyond the last hour reported.
- Are not reported when IV infusions are 30 minutes or less.
- Are not used to report infusion of drugs or other substances; nor are they reported when it is incidental to non-chemotherapeutic/diagnostic or chemotherapeutic services.
- Code **96361** is reported if an IV hydration infusion is provided secondary or subsequent to a therapeutic, prophylactic, or diagnostic infusion and administered through the same IV access.

Therapeutic, Prophylactic, and Diagnostic Infusions

96365 Intravenous infusion, for therapy, prophylaxis, or diagnosis (specify substance or drug); initial, up to 1 hour

+96366 each additional hour (List separately in addition to **96365** or **96367**.)

+96367 additional sequential infusion of a new drug/substance, up to 1 hour (List separately in addition to **96365, 96374, 96409, 96413**.)

+96368 concurrent infusion (List separately in addition to **96365, 96366, 96413, 96415**, or **96416**.)

Codes **96365–96368**

- Are for infusions for the purpose of administering drugs or substances.
- Typically require direct physician supervision and special attention to prepare, calculate dose, and dispose of materials.
- If fluid infusions are used to administer the drug(s), they are considered incidental hydration and are not reported.
- Each drug administered is reported separately with the appropriate infusion code.
- Short infusions of less than 15 minutes are reported as a push (eg, **96374**).

* Only one initial service code (eg, **96365**) should be reported unless the protocol or patient condition requires that 2 separate IV sites must be used. A second IV site access is also reported using the initial service code with modifier **59** appended (eg, **96365, 96365 59**).

* Subcutaneous infusion is reported with codes **96369–96371** (see **Table 10-5** for descriptions).

Table 10-5. Primary and Additional Intravenous Infusion Codes[a]

For all services, you must specify the substance or drug administered.

Service (Select the primary reason for encounter irrespective of order of infusion services.)[b]	IV infusion, for therapy, prophylaxis, or diagnosis	Subcutaneous infusion for therapy or prophylaxis [b]	Therapeutic, prophylactic, or diagnostic injection IV push
Initial service, up to 1 h	**96365** (16 min–1 h)	**96369** (16 min–1 h)	**96374** IV push or infusion ≤15 min
Each additional hour (>30 min) of *same substance or drug*	**+96366**[c] (List separately in addition to **96365, 96367**)	**+96370** (Use **96370** in conjunction with **96369**)	
Additional sequential infusion of *new substance or drug*	**+96367**[c]	**+96371** Additional pump set-up with establishment of new subcutaneous infusion site(s)	**+96367**
Sequential IV push of a *new substance/drug*	**+96375**		**+96375**
Concurrent infusion (Report only once per date of service)	**+96368**		

Abbreviation: IV, intravenous.

[a] If IV infusion for hydration of >30 minutes is provided in addition to a therapeutic infusion service (**96360, 96365, 96374**) through the same IV access, report **+96361** in addition to **96365** or **96374**.

[b] Includes pump set-up and establishment of infusion site(s). Use **96369** and **96371** only once per encounter.

[c] Report **96367** only once per sequential infusion of same infusate mix. Report **96366** for each additional hour (includes final time unit of 31 minutes or more) beyond the first hour of the service reported with **96367**.

Example

➤ A 3-year-old established patient is seen with a complaint of vomiting and fever for the past 24 hours. She has refused all food and liquids and last voided 12 hours prior to the visit. A detailed history and physical examination with moderate-level MDM are performed. Her diagnosis is bilateral acute suppurative otitis media and dehydration. Intravenous fluids are initiated with physiologic (normal) saline solution, and IV ceftriaxone (750 mg) is infused over 30 minutes for her otitis media. After 1 hour and 45 minutes of IV hydration, she urinates, begins tolerating liquids, and is released to home.

ICD-10-CM	CPT®
E86.0 (dehydration) **H66.003** (acute suppurative otitis media without spontaneous rupture of ear drum, bilateral)	**99214 25** (established patient office E/M) **96365** (IV infusion, for therapy) **96361** (IV infusion, hydration, each additional hour) **J0696** × 3 units (ceftriaxone sodium, per 250 mg) **J7030** (infusion, normal saline solution, 1,000 cc)

Teaching Point: Link the appropriate diagnosis code to each procedure (eg, code **H66.003** is linked to code **J0696**). The medication and infusion solution may need to be reported with the NDC if required by the payer. The fluid used to administer ceftriaxone is not reported because it is considered incidental hydration.

Coding Conundrum: Multiple and Concurrent Infusions or Injections

When administering multiple infusions, injections, or combinations, only one "initial" service code should be reported for a given date, unless protocol requires that 2 separate intravenous (IV) sites must be used. Do not report a second initial service on the same date due to an IV line requiring a restart, an IV rate not being able to be reached without 2 lines, or a need to access a port of a multi-lumen catheter. If an injection or infusion is of a subsequent or concurrent nature, even if it is the first such service within that group of services, a subsequent or concurrent code from the appropriate section should be reported. For example, the first IV push given subsequent to an initial 1-hour infusion is reported using a subsequent IV push code.

When services are performed in the physician's office, report as follows:

Initial Infusion

Physician reporting: Report the code that best describes the *key* or *primary* reason for the service regardless of the order in which the infusions or injections occur. Only one initial service code (eg, **96365**) should be reported unless the protocol or patient condition requires using 2 separate IV sites. The difference in time and effort in providing this second IV site access is also reported using the *initial* service code with modifier **59**, distinct procedural service, appended (eg, **96365, 96365 59**).

Facility reporting: An initial infusion is based on the hierarchy. Only one initial service code (eg, **96365**) should be reported unless the protocol or patient condition requires using 2 separate IV sites. The difference in time and effort in providing this second IV site access is also reported using the *initial* service code with modifier **59**, distinct procedural service, appended (eg, **96365, 96365 59**).

Sequential Infusion

This is an infusion or IV push of a new substance or drug following a primary or initial service. For example, if an IV push was performed through the same IV access subsequent to an IV infusion for therapy, the appropriate codes to report would be **96365** and **96375**. If an IV push was performed through a different IV access route, the services would be reported using codes **96365** and **96374**. Sequential infusions are reported only one time for the same infusate. However, if additional hours were required for the infusion, the appropriate "each additional hour" add-on code would be reported. Different infusates can be reported using the same code as the original sequential code. Hydration may not be reported concurrently with any other service. All sequential services require that there be a new substance or drug, except that facilities may report a sequential IV push of the same drug using **96376**.

Concurrent Infusion

This is an infusion of a new substance or drug infused at the same time as another drug or substance. This is not time-based and is only reported once per day regardless of whether a new drug or substance is administered concurrently. Hydration may not be reported concurrently with any other service. A separate subsequent concurrent administration of another new drug or substance (the third substance or drug) is not reported.

If IV hydration (**96360, 96361**) is given from 11:00 pm to 2:00 am, code **96360** would be reported once with **96361** with 2 units of service. However, if instead of a continuous infusion, a medication were given by IV push at 10:00 pm and 2:00 am, both administrations would be reported as initial (**96374**) because the services are not continuous. For continuous services that last beyond midnight, use the date in which the service began and report the total units of time provided continuously. Although in conflict with *Current Procedural Terminology*® guidelines, some payers may require that the primary infusion code be reported for each day of service.

Other Injection and Infusion Services

96523   Irrigation of implanted venous access device for drug delivery systems

Code **96523** is used to report irrigation required for implanted venous access devices for drug delivery systems when services are provided on a separate day from the injection or infusion service. Do not report **96523** in conjunction with other services.

Chemotherapy and Other Highly Complex Drug/Biologic Agent Administration

Codes **96401–96549** are reported for chemotherapy administration. *CPT*® defines chemotherapy administration as parenteral administration of non-radionuclide antineoplastic drugs, antineoplastic agents provided for treatment of non-cancer diagnoses and to substances such as certain monoclonal antibody agents, and other biologic response modifiers.

Example

➤ **A patient with severe persistent asthma is receiving injections of omalizumab 225 mg every 2 weeks.** The patient presents for administration of the medication. The medication is divided and injected at 2 different sites, as only 150 mg may be injected to a single site. The diagnosis code reported is **J45.50** (severe persistent asthma). Omalizumab injection is reported as a chemotherapy administration of monoclonal antibody (**96401**) with only 1 unit of service *unless prohibited by payer policy.* Omalizumab is provided in 150-mg single-use vials with an NDC of 50242-040-62. HCPCS code **J2357** (injection, omalizumab, 5 mg) is used to report the medication supplied by the physician practice. The sample claim form illustrates reporting for this example.

21. Diagnosis or nature of illness or injury (Relate A–L to service line below 24E)				ICD Ind. 0					
A. J45.50	B.	C.	D.						
24. A. Dates of service	B. Place of service	C. EMG	D. Procedures, services or supplies CPT/HCPCS	Modifier	E. Diagnosis Pointer	F. Charges	G. Days or units	H. EPSDT	I. ID Qual	J. Rendering Provider #
1/1/2019–1/1/2019	11		96401		A	$$$	1		NPI	0123456789
N450242004062 UN2										
1/1/2019–1/1/2019	11		J2357		A	$$$	45		NPI	0123456789

Abbreviations: CPT, Current Procedural Terminology; *EMG, emergency; EPSDT, Early and Periodic Screening, Diagnosis, and Treatment; HCPCS, Healthcare Common Procedure Coding System; ICD, International Classification of Diseases; NPI, National Provider Identifier.*

Teaching Point: Check payer policies before reporting administration of omalizumab and other highly complex drug/biologic agents. *CPT* instructs that administration of certain monoclonal antibody agents may be reported with code **96401**. However, not all payers accept code **96401** for administration of omalizumab. Some payers limit reporting to code **96372** (subcutaneous or IM injection) and/or allow only one administration code despite requirements to administer by 2 or more separate injections.

The HCPCS codes and NDCs for the omalizumab are included on the claim with units based on the HCPCS code descriptor (per 5 mg) and NDC quantity (payers may require NDC units per vial—2 units or per gram—**GR0.225**) to identify the substance administered. Some payers allow reporting of the full amount of single-dose vials when only a portion of the medication is provided to a patient to account for drug waste. Report units for the full single-dose vial only as instructed by payer policy.

Moderate Sedation

Moderate sedation codes **99151–99153** and **99155–99157** are used for reporting moderate sedation when intraservice time is 10 minutes or more. **Table 10-6** contains sedation codes and descriptors.

Moderate sedation is a drug-induced depression of consciousness. No interventions are required to maintain cardiovascular functions or a patent airway, and spontaneous ventilation is adequate. Moderate sedation codes are not used to report administration of medications for pain control, minimal sedation (anxiolysis), deep sedation, or monitored anesthesia care (**00100–01999**).

Moderate sedation provided and reported by the same physician or QHP who is performing the diagnostic or therapeutic service requires the presence of an independent trained observer. An *independent trained observer* is an individual qualified to monitor the patient during the procedure but who has no other duties (eg, assisting at surgery) during the procedure. Alternatively, a physician or QHP other than the person performing the diagnostic or therapeutic service may provide and report moderate sedation services.

Table 10-6. Moderate Sedation		
Moderate Sedation and Procedure by the Same Physician or QHP	**First 10–22 min of Intraservice Time**	**Each Additional 15 min of Intra-service Time**
Moderate sedation services provided by the same physician or other QHP performing the diagnostic or therapeutic service that the sedation supports, requiring the presence of an independent trained observer to assist in the monitoring of the patient's level of consciousness and physiological status; initial 15 minutes of intra-service time, patient younger than 5 years of age	99151	+99153
5 years or older	99152	+99153
Moderate Sedation and Procedure by 2 Different Physicians/QHPs		
Moderate sedation services (other than those services described by codes 00100–01999) provided by a physician other than the health care professional performing the diagnostic or therapeutic service that the sedation supports; younger than 5 years	99155	+99157
5 years or older	99156	+99157

Abbreviation: QHP, qualified health care professional.

Codes 99151, 99152, and 99153 are reported when

* The administration of moderate sedation is provided by the physician who is simultaneously performing a procedure (eg, fracture reduction, vessel cutdown, central line placement, wound repair).
* An independent trained observer is present to assist the physician in the monitoring of the patient during the procedure or diagnostic service.

Codes 99155, 99156, and 99157 are reported when

* A second physician or QHP other than the health care professional performing the diagnostic or therapeutic services provides moderate sedation.
* Codes 99153 and 99157 are reported for each additional 15 minutes of intraservice time. The midpoint between the end of the previous 15-minute period must be passed to report an additional unit of intraservice time (ie, intraservice time must continue for at least 8 minutes beyond the last full 15 minutes of intraservice time).

Note: Documentation must include the description of the procedure, name and dosage(s) of the sedation agent(s), route of administration of the sedation agent(s), and who administered the agent (physician or independent observer); the ongoing assessment of the child's level of consciousness and physiological status (eg, heart rate, oxygen saturation levels) during and after the procedure; and the presence, name, and title of the independent observer and total time from administration of the sedation agent(s) (start time) until the physician's face-to-face service is no longer required (end time).

* Codes are selected based on intraservice time. Intraservice time
  ❖ Begins with the administration of the sedating agent(s)
  ❖ Ends when the procedure is completed, the patient is stable for recovery status, and the physician or other QHP providing the sedation ends personal continuous face-to-face time with the patient
  ❖ Includes ordering and/or administering the initial and subsequent doses of sedating agents
  ❖ Requires continuous face-to-face attendance of the physician or other QHP
  ❖ Requires monitoring patient response to the sedating agents, including
    — Periodic assessment of the patient
    — Further administration of agent(s) as needed to maintain sedation
    — Monitoring of oxygen saturation, heart rate, and blood pressure
* Moderate sedation service of less than 10 minutes of intraservice time is not separately reported.

⊛ Preservice work of moderate sedation services *is not separately reported* and is not included in intraservice time. Preservice work includes

❖ Assessment of the patient's past medical and surgical history with particular emphasis on cardiovascular, pulmonary, airway, or neurologic conditions

❖ Review of the patient's previous experiences with anesthesia and/or sedation

❖ Family history of sedation complications

❖ Summary of the patient's present medication list

❖ Drug allergy and intolerance history

❖ Focused physical examination of the patient, with emphasis on

— Mouth, jaw, oropharynx, neck, and airway for Mallampati score assessment

— Chest and lungs

— Heart and circulation

— Vital signs, including heart rate, respiratory rate, blood pressure, and oxygenation, with end-tidal carbon dioxide when indicated

❖ Review of any pre-sedation diagnostic tests

❖ Completion of a pre-sedation assessment form (with American Society of Anesthesiologists physical status classification)

❖ Patient informed consent

❖ Immediate pre-sedation assessment prior to first sedating doses

❖ Initiation of IV access and fluids to maintain patency

⊛ Do not separately report or include the time of post-service work in the intraservice time. Post-service work of moderate sedation includes

❖ Assessment of the patient's vital signs, level of consciousness, neurologic, cardiovascular, and pulmonary stability in the post-sedation recovery period

❖ Assessment of patient's readiness for discharge following the procedure

❖ Preparation of documentation for sedation service

❖ Communication with family or caregiver about sedation service

⊛ Oxygen saturation (94760–94762) cannot be reported separately.

⊛ Codes 99151–99157 are distinguished by service provider, patient age, and time spent (see **Table 10-6**).

> |||||||| **Coding Pearl** ||||||||
>
> Do not report a separate evaluation and management service for preservice or post-service work associated with moderate sedation.

Examples

➤ **A 24-month-old requires a layered closure of a 2.5-cm laceration of the right knee in an urgent care setting.** Moderate sedation is required and is performed by the Pediatric Advanced Life Support–trained physician with an independent trained observer who has been trained in pediatric basic life support. The physician supervises the administration of the sedating agent and assesses the child until an effective, safe level of sedation is achieved and continues to assess the child's level of consciousness and physiological status while also performing the laceration repair. The procedure, from the time of administration of the agent until the physician completes the repair and determines the child is stable and face-to-face physician time is no longer required, takes a total of 28 minutes.

ICD-10-CM	CPT®
S81.011A (laceration without foreign body, right knee, initial encounter) Codes for external cause, activity, and place of injury are reported when documented.	12031 (intermediate repair of wound of extremities, 2.5 cm or less) 99151 (moderate [conscious] sedation, patient younger than 5 years, first 15 minutes) +99153 (moderate [conscious] sedation, each additional 15 minutes of intraservice time)

Teaching Point: If a medically necessary, significant, and separately identifiable E/M service had also been performed, an E/M visit with modifier **25** appended could be reported. The agent itself should also be reported.

➤ **Same patient as previous example, except moderate sedation is performed by the Pediatric Advanced Life Support–trained physician while another physician performs the repair.** The procedure, from the time of administration of the agent until the repair is complete and the child is stable and no longer requires face-to-face physician time, takes a total of 28 minutes.

ICD-10-CM	*CPT®*
S81.011A (laceration without foreign body, right knee, initial encounter) Codes for external cause, activity, and place of injury are reported when documented.	*The physician repairing the wound reports* **12031** (intermediate repair of wound of extremities, 2.5 cm or less)
	The physician performing moderate sedation reports **99155** (moderate [conscious] sedation, patient younger than 5 years, first 15 minutes) **+99157** (moderate [conscious] sedation, each additional 15 minutes of intraservice time)

Teaching Point: Each physician reports the service provided. The time of moderate sedation used in code selection is only the intraservice time.

CHAPTER 11

Common Testing and Therapeutic Services in Office Settings

Contents

Chapter 11: Common Testing and Therapeutic Services in Office Settings

This chapter includes discussion of codes for some of the common tests and therapeutic services performed in physician offices and outpatient clinics. See Chapter 9, Preventive Services, for discussion of recommended preventive screenings. See also Chapter 14, Mental and Behavioral and Mental Health Services, for discussion of central nervous system assessments and tests and behavior identification assessments.

Professional and Technical Components

26   Professional component: When the physician or other qualified health care professional is reporting only the professional component of a service, append modifier **26** to the procedure code.

TC   Technical component: When reporting only the technical component of a service, append modifier **TC** to the procedure code.

Certain procedures (eg, electrocardiograms [ECGs], radiographs, surgical diagnostic tests, laboratory tests) include a professional and technical component. The professional component includes the physician work (eg, interpretation of the test, written report). The technical component includes the costs associated with providing the service (eg, equipment, salaries of technical personnel, supplies, facility expense). Some codes were developed to distinguish between the technical and professional components (eg, routine ECG codes **93000–93010**); however, many are not. If a physician is performing a service or procedure with equipment owned by a facility or another entity and the codes are written as a global service, services are reported with modifier **26** (professional component). *Current Procedural Terminology* (*CPT®*) does not include a modifier for reporting the technical component. However, most payers recognize Healthcare Common Procedure Coding System (HCPCS) modifier **TC**. Facilities or an office providing use of its equipment only would report the same service using modifier **TC**.

> ### ~ More From the AAP ~
>
> For more information on reporting professional and technical components of service, see "Professional Component Services: More Than Codes" in the July 2014 *AAP Pediatric Coding Newsletter*™ at http://coding.aap.org (subscription required).

When the physician owns the equipment and is performing the technical and professional services, a modifier should not be appended to the code.

No modifier is appended when the code descriptor for the service identifies whether the professional, technical, or global service is being reported.

Examples

➤ **A pediatrician orders a 2-view chest radiograph on a child.** The child is sent to a neighboring physician's office (or outpatient department) for the radiograph. The films are then brought back to the office and the pediatrician interprets them and creates a report of the findings.

     Pediatrician: **71046 26** (radiologic examination, chest; 2 views)

     Other office or outpatient department: **71046 TC**

➤ **A pediatrician orders a 12-lead ECG on an adolescent patient.** The patient is sent to another office with the ECG machine to perform the ECG. The tracings are taken back to the pediatrician for review and written interpretation and report.

     Pediatrician: **93010** (routine ECG with at least 12 leads; interpretation and report only)

     Other office: **93005** (routine ECG with at least 12 leads; tracing only, without interpretation and report)

Do not separately report review of another physician's interpretation and report or personal review of the tracing that has been interpreted by another physician. These activities contribute to the medical decision-making for any related evaluation and management (E/M) service.

When interpreting an ECG at a location remote from the site of the tracing, follow payer guidelines for reporting. The place of service for remote interpretation and report is typically the site where the technical component of the test was performed (eg, outpatient hospital). Payer guidelines may vary.

Chapter 11: Common Testing and Therapeutic Services in Office Settings

Supplies and Medications

The relative value units (RVUs) assigned to testing services include the value of supplies (eg, masks, tubing, gauze, needles) that are typically required for each service. Supplies should be separately reported when a payer does not use a payment methodology based on the RVUs assigned to each code under the Medicare Physician Fee Schedule (MPFS). However, most payers today use a payment method based on RVUs and do not provide separate payment for supplies.

When a payer pays separately for supplies, report HCPCS codes (eg, A7003, administration set, with small volume nonfiltered pneumatic nebulizer, disposable).

Medications used in testing or treatment (eg, albuterol) are not included in the value of service and are separately reported using HCPCS codes (eg, J7613, albuterol, inhalation solution, US Food and Drug Administration [FDA]-approved final product, noncompounded, administered through durable medical equipment [DME], unit dose, 1 mg). **Table 11-1** lists HCPCS codes for some medications commonly administered in pediatric practices.

Table 11-1. Common Healthcare Common Procedure Coding System J Codes			
Inhalation Solution	**Brand Name(s)[a]**	**J Code**	**Administration**
Albuterol, inhalation solution, FDA-approved final product, noncompounded, administered through DME, concentrated form, 1 mg	Proventil, Ventolin	J7611	**94640** or **94644** (for first hour)
Levalbuterol, inhalation solution, FDA-approved final product, noncompounded, administered through DME, concentrated form, 0.5 mg	Xopenex	J7612	**94640** or **94644** (for first hour)
Albuterol, inhalation solution, FDA-approved final product, noncompounded, administered through DME, unit dose, 1 mg	AccuNeb, Proventil, Ventolin	J7613	**94640** or **94644** (for first hour)
Levalbuterol, inhalation solution, FDA-approved final product, noncompounded, administered through DME, unit dose, 0.5 mg	Xopenex	J7614	**94640** or **94644** (for first hour)
Levalbuterol, inhalation solution, compounded, administered through DME, unit dose, 0.5 mg	Levalbuterol hydrochloride	J7615	**94640** or **94644** (for first hour)
Albuterol, up to 2.5 mg, and ipratropium bromide, up to 0.5 mg, FDA-approved final product, noncompounded, administered through DME	Albuterol, DuoNeb, ipratropium bromide	J7620	**94640** or **94644** (for first hour)
Budesonide, inhalation solution, FDA-approved final product, noncompounded, administered through DME, unit dose form, up to 0.5 mg	Pulmicort	J7626	**94640** or **94644** (for first hour)
Budesonide, inhalation solution, compounded product, administered through DME, unit dose form, up to 0.5 mg	Pulmicort Respules	J7627	**94640** or **94644** (for first hour)
Injection	**Brand Name(s)[a]**	**J Code**	**Administration**
Epinephrine, 0.1 mg	Adrenalin chloride, Sus-Phrine	J0171	**96372**
Ampicillin, 500 mg	Omnipen-N, Totacillin-N	J0290	**96372** (IM) (IV)[b]
Atropine sulfate, 0.01 mg	Atropen	J0461	**96372**
Penicillin G benzathine and penicillin G procaine, 100,000 units	Bicillin CR	J0558	**96372**
Penicillin G benzathine, 100,000 units	Bicillin L-A	J0561	**96372**

Table 11-1. Common Healthcare Common Procedure Coding System J Codes (*continued*)

Injection (*continued*)	Brand Name(s)[a]	J Code	Administration
Ceftriaxone, per 250 mg	Rocephin	J0696	96372 (IM) (IV)[b]
Cefotaxime, per gram	Claforan	J0698	96372 (IM) (IV)[b]
Betamethasone acetate, 3 mg, and betamethasone sodium phosphate, 3 mg	Celestone Soluspan	J0702	96372
Dexamethasone acetate, 1 mg	Decadron LA	J1094	96372
Dexamethasone sodium phosphate, 1 mg	Decadron	J1100	96372 (IM) (IV)[b]
Phenytoin sodium, per 50 mg	Dilantin	J1165	96374
Diphenhydramine hydrochloride, up to 50 mg	Benadryl	J1200	96372
Gamma globulin, IM, 1 cc Gamma globulin, IM, more than 10 cc	Gammar Gamastan	J1460 J1560	96372
Immunoglobulin, 500 mg	Gammar-IV	J1566	96374
Gentamicin, up to 80 mg	Garamycin	J1580	96372 (IM) (IV)[b]
Glucagon, per 1 mg	GlucaGen	J1610	96374
Heparin sodium (heparin lock flush), per 10 units	Hep-Lock	J1642	96374
Hydrocortisone sodium succinate, up to 100 mg	Solu-Cortef	J1720	96374
Promethazine hydrochloride, up to 50 mg	Phenergan	J2550	96372
Other	**Brand Name(s)[a]**	**J Code**	**Administration**
Prednisolone, oral, 5 mg	Delta-Cortef	J7510	None
Prednisone, immediate release or delayed release, oral, 1 mg	Rayos	J7512	None
Antiemetic drug, rectal/suppository, not otherwise specified	Phenergan	J8498	None
Dexamethasone, oral, 0.25 mg	Decadron	J8540	None

Abbreviations: DME, durable medical equipment; FDA, US Food and Drug Administration; IM, intramuscular; IV, intravenous.

[a] Brand names are furnished for identification purposes only. No endorsement of the manufacturers or products is implied.

[b] For IV administration codes, see **Table 10-5**.

The 2019 Healthcare Common Procedure Coding System codes were released subsequent to the publication of this book. Refer to www.aap.org/cfp for updates.

Blood Sampling for Diagnostic Study

Collection of blood samples for testing (eg, venipuncture) in a physician practice is reported regardless of whether the laboratory test is performed in the office or at an outside facility.

Venipuncture

36400	Venipuncture, younger than age 3 years, necessitating the skill of a physician or other qualified health care professional, not to be used for routine venipuncture; femoral or jugular vein
36405	scalp vein
36406	other vein

36410   Venipuncture, age 3 years or older, necessitating the skill of a physician or other qualified health care professional (separate procedure), for diagnostic or therapeutic purposes (not to be used for routine venipuncture)

36415   Collection of venous blood by venipuncture

36416   Collection of capillary blood specimen (eg, finger, heel, ear stick)

36591   Collection of blood specimen from a completely implantable venous access device

Codes **36415** and **36416** are used for any age child when the physician is not needed to perform the procedure. Code **36416** is considered bundled under the MPFS and, therefore, not separately payable. Some payers may follow this bundling practice.

- When a physician's skill is required to perform venipuncture (eg, access is too difficult for other staff to attain) on a child younger than 3 years, codes **36400–36406** are reported based on the anatomic site of the venipuncture. Report code **36400** when performed on the femoral or jugular vein, code **36405** when performed on the scalp vein, or code **36406** when another vein is accessed.

- When a physician's skill is required to perform venipuncture on a child 3 years and older, code **36410** is reported.
    - ❖ If the physician performs the venipuncture as a convenience or because staff is not trained in the procedure, code **36415** is reported because the physician's skill was not required.
    - ❖ Although typically not required, some payers will require that modifier **25** be appended to the E/M code if an E/M service is reported on the same day of service.

- It is not appropriate to report *CPT®* code **99211** along with code **36415** if the nurse only collects the blood specimen and no medically necessary and separately identified E/M service is provided.

- Code **36591** (collection of blood specimen from a completely implantable venous access device) is reported only when in conjunction with a laboratory service.

> |||||||| **Coding Pearl** ||||||||
>
> Report code **36415** when the physician performs a venipuncture as a convenience.

Arterial Puncture

36600   Arterial puncture, withdrawal of blood for diagnosis

Arterial puncture (eg, radial artery) with withdrawal of blood for diagnosis is reported with code **36600**. See Chapter 19, Common Surgical Procedures and Sedation in Facility Settings, for discussion of arterial catheterization.

Pathology and Laboratory Procedures

CPT® laboratory codes may be generic for a particular analyte that is independent of testing method or else have a specific *CPT* code, depending on the method used for the particular analysis.

- A test performed in the office's laboratory should be billed using the appropriate laboratory code and, if performed, the appropriate blood collection code (**36400–36416**).

- If the specimen (eg, blood, urine, stool, cerebrospinal fluid) is collected in the office and sent to an outside laboratory, the office visit (if applicable) plus any specimen acquisition procedure code (eg, venipuncture, capillary blood collection, spinal tap) and a handling fee (**99000**) should be billed.

- If the laboratory bills the pediatrician for the test, bill the patient using the appropriate laboratory analysis code with modifier **90** to indicate the procedure was performed in an outside laboratory.

- Link the appropriate diagnosis code to the laboratory procedure and/or venipuncture and handling fee. The diagnosis must support the medical necessity or reason for the test or service.

- If the *only service* provided is a urinalysis or obtaining a blood specimen, only the laboratory test and/or venipuncture or capillary stick is reported. It is not appropriate to report a nurse visit (**99211**) in these cases. If a medically necessary nursing E/M service is performed in compliance with payer guidelines (eg, incident to a physician's service) on the same date as venipuncture, append modifier **25** to code **99211**.

- Do not report any laboratory test that is *not performed* in the office (eg, thyroid, laboratory panels, phenylketonuria). Instead, report the appropriate blood-drawing code (36415 or 36416). For example, the physician orders a lead test and the nurse obtains the blood via venipuncture. The specimen is sent to an outside laboratory for processing. Only the venipuncture (36415) and handling fee (99000) would be reported in addition to the E/M service and other procedures performed on that day.

Clinical Laboratory Improvement Amendments–Waived Tests

The Clinical Laboratory Improvement Amendments (CLIA) establish quality standards for all laboratory testing to ensure the accuracy, reliability, and timeliness of patient test results regardless of where the test was performed.

A *laboratory* is defined as any facility that performs laboratory testing on specimens derived from humans for the purpose of providing information for the diagnosis, prevention, and treatment of disease or impairment or assessment of health.

- The term *CLIA waived* refers to simple laboratory examinations and procedures that have an insignificant risk of an erroneous result. One typical test in the *CPT* 80000 series that is CLIA waived is urinalysis without microscopy (81002). Other tests require higher levels of CLIA certification (eg, provider-performed microscopy).
  - Payers may require a practice's CLIA certificate number on claims.
  - Some codes represent both CLIA-waived and higher complexity test systems. Refer to the FDA Web site at www.accessdata.fda.gov/scripts/cdrh/cfdocs/cfClia/analyteswaived.cfm for the currently waived test systems and analytes.
- Laboratories and physician offices performing waived tests may need to append modifier QW to the *CPT* code for CLIA-waived procedures. Some of the CLIA-waived tests are exempt from the use of modifier QW (eg, 81002, 82272). The use of modifier QW is payer specific. To review the list of CLIA-waived procedures, go to www.cms.hhs.gov/CLIA.

Laboratory Panel Coding

All laboratory test panels in *CPT®* were specifically developed for coding purposes only and should not be interpreted as clinical parameters. (See codes 80047–80076 for a component listing of these panels.) For example, the lipid panel (80061) includes total cholesterol (82465), high-density lipoprotein cholesterol (83718), and triglycerides (84478). Any additional tests performed can be coded separately from the panel code. Do not unbundle individual laboratory tests if a laboratory panel code is available.

Direct Optical Observation

Direct optical observation is a testing platform that provides a result (eg, positive or negative) by producing a signal on the reaction chamber (eg, test strip with colored bands) that can be interpreted visually (eg, point-of-care influenza testing). When reporting tests using direct optical observation, the number of results (eg, 2 results—positive for influenza A and negative for influenza B) determines the units of service reported. (See codes 87804 [influenza], 87807 [respiratory syncytial virus], 87880 [group A streptococcus], and 87802 [group B streptococcus].)

Cultures

- Use code 87086 (culture, bacterial; quantitative colony count, urine) once per encounter for urine culture to determine the approximate number of bacteria present per milliliter of urine. Use of a commercial kit with defined media to identify isolates in a positive urine culture is reported with 87088 (culture, bacterial; quantitative colony count, urine with isolation and presumptive identification of each isolate).
- Code 81007 (urinalysis; bacteriuria screen, except by culture or dipstick) (CLIA waived) can be used for a bacteriuria screen by non-culture technique using a commercial kit. The type of commercial kit must be specified.

- Code **87070** (culture, bacterial; any other source except urine, blood, or stool) is reported for throat cultures.
- Use code **87045** to report culture, bacteria of the stool, aerobic, with isolation and preliminary examination (eg, Kligler [triple sugar] iron agar, lysine iron agar) for *Salmonella* and *Shigella* species. Additional pathogens are reported with code **87046** with 1 unit per plate.
- Culture, presumptive pathogenic organisms, screening only (**87081**) is reported for testing for a specific organism (eg, *Streptococcus*).
- Report services with the symptoms (eg, microscopic hematuria) or the confirmed diagnosis (eg, urinary tract infection).

Laboratory Tests Frequently Performed in the Office

Urinalysis

81000	Urinalysis, by dipstick or tablet reagent for bilirubin, glucose, hemoglobin, ketones, leukocytes, nitrite, pH, protein, specific gravity, urobilinogen, any number of these constituents; nonautomated, with microscopy
81001	as per **81000** with microscopy, but automated
81002	as per **81000** but without microscopy (CLIA waived)
81003	as per **81000** but without microscopy, automated (CLIA waived)

It is important to report the correct code for the urinalysis test performed. Code **81000** is reported when the results are shown as color changes for multiple analytes (eg, ketones, specific gravity) that are compared against a standardized chart (nonautomated) and when microscopy (in a second step, the urine is centrifuged and examined under microscope) is performed. Code **81002** is reported if the test results are obtained by the same method but a microscopic examination is not performed. Codes **81001** and **81003** are reported for urinalysis performed by a processor that reads the results (automated).

For urinalysis, infectious agent detection, semiquantitative analysis of volatile compounds, use code **81099**.

Urine Pregnancy Test

81025	Urine pregnancy test, by visual color comparison method (CLIA waived)

Report code **81025** with *International Classification of Diseases, 10th Revision, Clinical Modification* (*ICD-10-CM*) codes **Z32.00–Z32.02**, depending on the findings of the test (ie, unconfirmed result, positive result, or negative result).

Glucose Tests

82947	Glucose, quantitative, blood (without a reagent strip) (CLIA waived)
82948	blood, reagent strip
82951	Glucose tolerance test (GTT), 3 specimens (CLIA waived)
82952	each additional beyond 3 specimens (CLIA waived)
82962	Glucose, blood by glucose monitoring device(s) cleared by the FDA specifically for home use (CLIA waived)
83036	Hemoglobin; glycosylated (A_{1c}) (CLIA waived)
83037	Hemoglobin; glycosylated (A_{1c}) by device cleared by FDA for home use (CLIA waived)

Report code **83037** for in-office hemoglobin A_{1c} measurement using a device that is cleared by the FDA for home use. This test is not limited to use in a patient's home.

Code **82962** describes the method when whole blood is obtained (usually by finger-stick device) and assayed by glucose oxidase, hexokinase, or electrochemical methods and spectrophotometry using a small portable device designed for home blood glucose monitoring. The devices are also used in physician offices, during home visits, or in clinics.

Continuous glucose monitoring is reported with codes **95249–95251** (see discussion later in this chapter).

Hematology

85013	Spun microhematocrit (CLIA waived)
85018	Hemoglobin (CLIA waived)
85025–85027	Complete blood cell count, automated (85025 is CLIA waived.)
88738	Hemoglobin (Hgb), quantitative, transcutaneous

If using a complete blood cell count (CBC) machine to perform only a hemoglobin test, follow these guidelines.

* If the CBC result is normal, only the hemoglobin may be reported because that was the medically necessary test ordered.
* If the CBC reveals an abnormality and it is addressed during the course of the visit, the CBC result may be reported. The abnormality would be linked to the procedure, and the medical record would need to include documentation for the ordering of the test and to support the medical necessity of the procedure.

Influenza—Point-of-Care Testing

87804	Infectious agent antigen detection by immunoassay with direct optical observation; influenza (CLIA waived)

If tests performed separately detect the influenza A and B antigen, providing 2 distinct results, report code 87804 twice with modifier 59 appended to the second service. This applies whether the test kit uses 1 or 2 analytic chambers to deliver 2 distinct results. Check with your payers because some do not recognize modifier 59 and may require reporting with 2 units of service and no modifier.

Lead Testing

83655	Lead, quantitative analysis (CLIA waived)

* This test does not specify the specimen source or the method of testing. Alternative tests sometimes (though rarely) used for lead screening are 82135 (aminolevulinic acid, delta), 84202 (protoporphyrin, red blood cell count, quantitative), and 84203 (protoporphyrin, red blood cell count, screen).
* Some states provide lead testing at no cost to patients covered under the Medicaid Early and Periodic Screening, Diagnosis, and Treatment program. Check your state Medicaid requirements for reporting this service.
* Report *ICD-10-CM* code Z13.88 (encounter for screening for disorder due to exposure to contaminants) when performing lead screening. Some payers require Z77.011, contact with and (suspected) exposure to lead, in lieu of Z13.88.

Mononucleosis—Heterophile Antibodies Screening

86308	Heterophile antibodies; screening (CLIA waived)

This code may be appropriate for rapid mononucleosis screening.

Papanicolaou Tests

* The laboratory performing the cytology and interpretation reports Papanicolaou (Pap) tests with codes 88141–88155, 88164–88167, or 88174 and 88175.
* Obtaining a Pap test specimen is inherent to the physical examination performed during a preventive medicine visit or a problem-oriented office visit.
* Medicare does require reporting HCPCS code Q0091 (screening Papanicolaou, obtaining, preparing, and conveyance of cervical and vaginal smear to laboratory) in addition to the E/M service for preventive medicine and problem-oriented office visits.
  * Some state Medicaid programs and commercial payers may also recognize obtaining a Pap test as a separate service.

- ❖ Code **Q0091** cannot be reported when a patient must return for a repeat Pap test due to inadequate initial sampling.
- ❖ If not reporting **Q0091**, a handling fee (**99000**) can be reported in addition to an E/M service if the Pap test was obtained.
- ☀ The appropriate *ICD-10-CM* code to link to the E/M code or code **Q0091** is either **Z01.411** (encounter for gynecological examination [general] [routine] with abnormal findings) or **Z01.419** (encounter for gyneco-logical examination [general] [routine] without abnormal findings). For screening cervical Pap test not part of a gynecologic examination, report *ICD-10-CM* code **Z12.4** (encounter for screening for malignant neo-plasm of cervix). For high-risk patients, you may also use code **Z92.89** or **Z77.9**. These diagnosis codes may be used as secondary when linked with a routine preventive medicine code or problem-oriented sick visit.

Presumptive Drug Tests

#80305	Drug test(s), presumptive, any number of drug classes, any number of devices or procedures; capable of being read by direct optical observation only (eg, utilizing immunoassay [eg, dipsticks, cups, cards, or cartridges]); includes sample validation when performed, per date of service (CLIA waived)
#80306	read by instrument assisted direct optical observation (eg, utilizing immunoassay [eg, dip-sticks, cups, cards, or cartridges]); includes sample validation when performed, per date of service
#80307	by instrument chemistry analyzers (eg, utilizing immunoassay [eg, EIA, ELISA, EMIT, FPIA, IA, KIMS, RIA]), chromatography (eg, GC, HPLC), and mass spectrometry either with or without chromatography (eg, DART, DESI, GC-MS, GC-MS/MS, LC-MS, LC-MS/MS, LDTD, MALDI, TOF); includes sample validation when performed, per date of service

- ☀ Presumptive drug class screening includes all drugs and drug classes performed by the respective methodology (eg, dipstick kit with direct optical observation) on a single date of service. Sample validation is included in presumptive drug screening service. Venipuncture to obtain samples for drug testing may be separately reportable with code **36415** (collection of venous blood by venipuncture).
- ☀ When testing is performed with a method using direct optical observation to determine the result, code **80305** is reported. Tests that have a waived status under CLIA may be reported with modifier **QW** (waived test).
- ☀ When a reader is used to determine the result of testing (eg, a dipstick is inserted into a machine that determines the final reading), code **80306** is reported.
- ☀ Testing that uses a chemistry analyzer or more effort than tests represented by codes **80305** and **80306** is reported with code **80307**.

See Chapter 14, Mental and Behavioral Health Services, for more information.

Respiratory Syncytial Virus Test

| 87807 | Infectious agent antigen detection by immunoassay with direct optical observation; respiratory syncytial virus (CLIA waived) |
| 87634 | Infectious agent detection by nucleic acid (DNA or RNA); respiratory syncytial virus, amplified probe technique |

For assays that include respiratory syncytial virus with additional respiratory viruses, see **87631–87633**. Tests reported with codes **87631** and **87633** are CLIA waived. Append modifier **QW** if required.

Serum and Transcutaneous Bilirubin Testing

82247	Total bilirubin (CLIA waived)
82248	Direct bilirubin
88720	Transcutaneous total bilirubin

Streptococcal Test

87802	Infectious agent antigen detection by immunoassay with direct optical observation; streptococcus group B
87880	Infectious agent antigen detection by immunoassay with direct optical observation; streptococcus group A (CLIA waived)
87651	Infectious agent detection by nucleic acid (DNA or RNA); streptococcus, group A, amplified probe technique (CLIA waived)
87081	Culture, presumptive pathogenic organisms, screening only
87430	Enzyme immunoassay, qualitative, streptococcus group A

☀ Report the code based on the test method rather than on the site of specimen collection.

☀ Culture plates using sheep blood agar with bacitracin disks should be coded with 87081.

Testing Stool for Occult Blood

82272	Blood, occult, by peroxidase activity (eg, guaiac), qualitative, feces, 1–3 simultaneous determinations, performed for other than colorectal neoplasm screening (CLIA waived)

Code 82272 is reported when a single sample is obtained from a digital rectal examination or a multi-test card is returned from the patient and is tested for blood. Report 82272 with 1 unit when up to 3 cards are returned.

Tuberculosis Skin Test (Mantoux)

86580	Tuberculosis, intradermal

☀ This test is exempt from CLIA requirements.

☀ The tuberculosis (TB) skin test (Mantoux) using the intradermal administration of purified protein derivative (PPD) is the recommended diagnostic skin test for TB. This is not the BCG TB vaccine. The American Academy of Pediatrics supports the use of the Mantoux test (TB, intradermal) for TB screening when appropriate
A separate administration code *is not reported* when the PPD is placed.

☀ Code 99211 is the appropriate code to report the reading of a PPD test when that is the only reason for the encounter. The appropriate *ICD-10-CM* code is Z11.1 (encounter for screening for respiratory TB). In the case of a positive test result when the physician sees the patient, the complexity may lead to a higher-level code.

☀ Because risk-based testing is recommended for pediatric patients, an E/M service to evaluate the need for testing may be indicated when testing is requested by a third party (eg, school, employer). If TB testing by cell-mediated immunity antigen response measurement, gamma interferon (86480) is ordered, and a specimen obtained, venipuncture (36415) may be separately reported.

Zika Virus Testing

86794	Zika virus, IgM
87662	Zika virus, amplified probe technique

☀ The IgM test described by code 87662 is used when suspected patient exposure to the Zika virus was less than 2 weeks before testing.

☀ The amplified probe technique (86794) is used when potential exposure occurred 2 weeks or more prior to testing.

Respiratory Tests and Treatments

Pulmonary Function Tests

National Correct Coding Initiative (NCCI) edits exist between office-based E/M services and all pulmonology services (**94010–94799**). Append modifier **25** to the E/M service as appropriate when also reporting a pulmonology service on the same claim. Refer to Chapter 2, Modifiers and Coding Edits, for more information on coding edits.

There is no code for peak flow analysis. It is considered part of the E/M service and/or a component of pulmonary function testing.

* Codes include laboratory procedure(s) and interpretation of test results. If a separately identifiable E/M service is performed, the appropriate E/M service code may also be reported.
* When spirometry is performed before and after administration of a bronchodilator, report code **94060** (bronchodilation responsiveness, spirometry as in **94010**, pre- and post-bronchodilator administration) only. Code **94640** (nebulizer treatment) is inherent to (ie, included as part of) code **94060**. Report codes for supplies if the payer does not use an RVU payment methodology. Relative value units assigned to codes include typical supplies (eg, masks, tubing). Medication is separately reported with the appropriate HCPCS code (eg, **J7613**, albuterol, inhalation solution, FDA-approved final product, noncompounded, administered through DME, unit dose, 1 mg).
* Measurement of vital capacity (**94150**) is a component of spirometry and is only reported when performed alone.
* Measurement of spirometric forced expiratory flows in an infant or child through 2 years of age is reported with code **94011**.
* Code **94012** is used to report measurement of bronchodilation spirometric forced expiratory flows (before and after bronchodilator) in an infant or child.
* Code **94013** is used to report measurement of lung volumes (eg, functional residual capacity, expiratory reserve volume, forced vital capacity) in an infant or child through 2 years of age.
* Report pulse oximetry (**94760** [noninvasive ear or pulse oximetry for oxygen saturation; single determination] and **94761** [multiple determinations]) because *CPT®* guidelines allow reporting the services, services may be paid if they are the only service received (according to the NCCI), some payers do allow payment, and a practice needs to be aware of all services that are performed and monitor associated costs. See Chapter 2, Modifiers and Coding Edits, for a detailed explanation of NCCI edits.

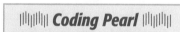

> ||||||||| **Coding Pearl** |||||||||
>
> *Current Procedural Terminology®* code **94060** includes spirometry and pre- and post-bronchodilation. Do not report code **94060** with **94010** or **94640** when they are a component of code **94060**.

* Pulmonary stress testing (**94618**) includes measurement of heart rate, oximetry, and oxygen titration, when performed. If spirometry is performed prior to and following a pulmonary stress test, separately report 2 units of spirometry (**94010**).

Inhalation

94640   Pressurized or nonpressurized inhalation treatment for acute airway obstruction for therapeutic purposes and/or for diagnostic purposes such as sputum induction with an aerosol generator, nebulizer, metered dose inhaler (MDI) or intermittent positive pressure breathing (IPPB) device

94644   Continuous inhalation treatment with aerosol medication for acute airway obstruction; first hour
(For services of less than 1 hour, use **94640**)

+94645   each additional hour (List separately in addition to code for primary procedure)

Report **94640**

* When treatment such as aerosol generator, nebulizer, metered-dose inhaler (MDI), or intermittent positive pressure breathing (IPPB) device is administered.

- With modifier **76** (repeat procedure) with the number of units when more than one treatment is given on a date of service. Some payers require reporting with the number of units only and no modifier. Follow payer guidelines for reporting these services.
- When any treatment of less than 30 minutes is performed.

At the time of publication, NCCI edit policy does not allow for code **94640** to be reported more than once per patient encounter. The American Academy of Pediatrics is working with NCCI edit staff to change this policy.

Report codes **94644** and **94645** when

- A treatment lasts 31 minutes or longer.
- The total time spent in the provision of continuous inhalation treatments is documented in the medical record.

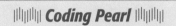

> **Coding Pearl**
>
> Peak flow analysis is included in an evaluation and management service.

Codes **94644** and **94645** are not reported by physicians when services are provided in a facility setting because no physician work value is assigned to these codes.

Report code **94664** (demonstration and/or evaluation of patient utilization of an aerosol generator, nebulizer, MDI, or IPPB device) when an initial or subsequent demonstration and/or evaluation is performed and documented. This code is intended to be reported only once per day. No physician work is attributed to code **94664**. Physicians providing nebulizer instruction in conjunction with an E/M service may include the time of nebulizer instruction in the time of counseling and/or coordination of care.

Note that peak flow analysis and administration of oxygen do not have *CPT*® codes. They are inherent to E/M services.

Examples

> **A 6-year-old established patient with asthma arrives to the office in acute exacerbation.** Pulse oximetry is performed and indicative of moderate asthma exacerbation. One nebulizer treatment is given via a small-volume nebulizer. Physical examination after first treatment shows decreased wheezing and work of breathing. Pulse oximetry is remeasured and normal. An asthma control test is completed, scored, and documented. An order is written for continuing treatments at home, evaluation and education in use of MDI, and return to the office as needed. The nurse documents her evaluation of use and education for home use of the MDI. Later the same day, the patient returns, again in acute exacerbation. A second nebulizer treatment is given by a small-volume nebulizer. Physical examination after the second treatment shows no improvement and the patient is borderline hypoxic on second pulse oxygen measurement. He is sent to the hospital to be admitted to observation by the hospitalist. Diagnosis is acute exacerbation of mild persistent asthma with hypoxemia.

ICD-10-CM	CPT
J45.31 (mild persistent asthma with acute exacerbation) **R09.02** (hypoxemia)	**99212–99215 25** (office/outpatient E/M, established patient) **94640 76** × 2 units or **94640** × 2 (nebulizer treatments × 2) **96160** (administration of patient-focused health risk assessment instrument [eg, health hazard appraisal] with scoring and documentation, per standardized instrument) **94664 59** (MDI demonstration) Medication (See HCPCS codes listed in **Table 11-1**.) **94761** (pulse oximetry, multiple determinations)

Teaching Point: Modifier **59** appended to **94664** indicates the MDI demonstration is reported in addition to nebulizer treatments provided via a different device. See the Coding Conundrum: Reporting **94664** With **94640** box for more information. Physicians should also report any medications provided at the expense of the practice. HCPCS codes describe medications such as albuterol. (See HCPCS codes listed in **Table 11-1**.)

➤ **A 12-year-old with severe exacerbation of mild persistent asthma is seen in the physician's office.** Pulse oxygen indicates hypoxemia. The patient is placed on continuous bronchodilator therapy for an hour and a half. The patient is monitored closely during the procedure. Multiple pulse oxygen measurements are obtained and indicate continued hypoxemia following treatment. Medical record documentation supports the total time of the treatment and frequent assessments. The patient is transferred to the emergency department by ambulance. Diagnosis is mild persistent asthma with status asthmaticus.

ICD-10-CM	CPT
J45.32	**99212–99215 25** (office/outpatient E/M, established patient) **94644** (continuous inhalation treatment with aerosol medication for acute airway obstruction; first hour) **94645** (each additional hour) **94761** (pulse oximetry, multiple determinations) Medication (See HCPCS codes listed in **Table 11-1**.)

Teaching Point: Payers that use the MPFS as a basis for payment may bundle pulse oximetry with any other service on the same date.

Coding Conundrum: Reporting 94664 With 94640

When the physician or nurse (of the same group and specialty) performs demonstration and/or evaluation of patient use of a nebulizer (**94664**) on the same day as a nebulizer treatment (**94640**), modifier **59** (distinct procedural service) should be appended to code **94664** to indicate to the payer that the services were separate and distinct and that both were clinically indicated. Per the 2018 Medicaid National Correct Coding Initiative (NCCI) manual, the demonstration and/or evaluation described by code **94664** is included in code **94640** if it uses the same device (eg, aerosol generator) that is used in the performance of *Current Procedural Terminology®* code **94640**. The NCCI edits pair code **94664** with **94640** but allow an override of the edit with modifier **59** when the services are indicated. However, as currently written, some payers may not allow the use of modifier **59** in this instance because the 2 services did not occur at separate encounters. Check with your Medicaid payers.

Modifier **25** should be appended to the evaluation and management service to signify a separately identifiable service. All services must be documented in the medical record as significant, separately identifiable, and medically necessary.

Car Seat/Bed Testing

▲**94780**   Car seat/bed testing for airway integrity, for infants through 12 months of age, with continual clinical staff observation and continuous recording of pulse oximetry, heart rate and respiratory rate, with interpretation and report; 60 minutes

+▲**94781**   each additional full 30 minutes (List separately in addition to **94780**.)

To report codes **94780** and **94781**, the following conditions must be met:

❉ The patient must be an infant (12 months or younger). Reassessment after the patient is 29 days or older may be necessary.

❉ Continual clinical staff observation with continuous recording of pulse oximetry, heart rate, and respiratory rate is required.

❉ Inpatient or office-based services may be reported separately on the same date (eg, discharge day management [**99238**] or a significant, separately identifiable office or other outpatient E/M service [eg, **99213 25**]).

❉ Vital signs and observations must be reviewed and interpreted and a written report generated by the physician.

❉ Codes are reported based on the total observation time spent and documented.

- If less than 60 minutes is spent in the procedure, code 94780 may not be reported.
- Each additional full 30 minutes (ie, not less than 90 minutes) is reported with code 94781.

Example

➤ **A male neonate born at 34 weeks' gestation was released from the hospital 2 weeks ago with instructions to the parents to use only a car bed when transporting him until the pediatrician retests and determines that the neonate can safely ride in a car seat.** The newborn is seen in the outpatient clinic for a preventive medicine visit, and car seat testing is conducted for a period of 1 hour and 45 minutes. The physician reviews and interprets the nurse's records of pulse oximetry, heart and respiratory rates, and observations during the testing period. The interpretation is documented in a formal report and plan of care clearing the neonate to begin use of a rear-facing car seat. The plan of care is discussed with the parents, who also receive further instruction on appropriate use of the car seat.

ICD-10-CM	CPT
Codes for conditions of the newborn **P07.37** (preterm newborn, gestational age 34 completed weeks)	**94780** (car seat/bed testing; first 60 minutes) **94781** (each additional full 30 minutes)

Teaching Point: In this scenario, a total of 105 minutes of testing was conducted. This would be reported with 1 unit of code 94780 for the initial 60 minutes of testing and 1 unit of code 94781 for the last 45 minutes (only one full period of 30 minutes beyond the first 60 minutes was performed). The 15 minutes beyond the last full 30-minute period are not separately reported.

Pediatric Home Apnea Monitoring

94774   Pediatric home apnea monitoring event recording including respiratory rate, pattern and heart rate per 30-day period of time; includes monitor attachment, download of data, review, interpretation, and preparation of a report by a physician or other qualified health care professional

94777   review, interpretation and preparation of report only by a physician or other qualified health care professional

- Codes 94774–94777 are reported once per 30-day period.
- Codes 94774 and 94777 are reported by the physician.
  - ❖ Code 94774 is reported by the physician when he or she orders home monitoring, chooses the monitor limits, and arranges for a home health care provider to teach the parents. It includes reviewing and interpreting data and preparation of the report.
  - ❖ Code 94777 is reported when the physician receives the downloaded information on disc or hard copy, reviews the patterns and periods of abnormal respiratory or heart rate, and summarizes, in a written report, the findings and recommendations for continuation or discontinuation of monitoring. This information is provided to the primary care physician and/or the family.
- Codes 94775 and 94776 are reported by the home health agency because there is no physician work involved.

Please see Chapter 20, Digital Medicine Services: Technology-Enhanced Care Delivery, for more information on pediatric home apnea monitoring and codes 94774–94777.

Home Ventilator Management

94005   Home ventilator management care plan oversight of a patient (patient not present) in home, domiciliary or rest home (eg, assisted living) requiring review of status, review of laboratories and other studies and revision of orders and respiratory care plan (as appropriate), within a calendar month, 30 minutes or more

◉ Services include determining ventilator settings, establishing a plan of care, and providing ongoing monitoring.

◉ Ventilator management includes all the E/M services (physical examination, review of the medical record or diagnostic tests performed, counseling the patient and/or parents, coordinating care with other health care professionals, and documenting the medical record) performed by the physician responsible for providing the ventilation management.

◉ Code **94005** is used to report home ventilator management care plan oversight. It may only be reported when 30 or more minutes of care plan oversight is provided within a calendar month.

◉ See Chapter 20, Digital Medicine Services: Technology-Enhanced Care Delivery, for more information on reporting ventilation assist and management.

Allergy and Clinical Immunology

Allergy Testing

95004	Percutaneous tests (scratch, puncture, prick) with allergenic extracts, immediate type reaction, including test interpretation and report, specify number of tests
95017	Allergy testing, any combination of percutaneous (scratch, puncture, prick) and intracutaneous (intradermal), sequential and incremental, with venoms, immediate type reaction, including test interpretation and report, specify number of tests
95018	Allergy testing, any combination of percutaneous (scratch, puncture, prick) and intracutaneous (intradermal), sequential and incremental, with drugs or biologicals, immediate type reaction, including test interpretation and report, specify number of tests
95024	Intracutaneous (intradermal) tests with allergenic extracts, immediate type reaction, including test interpretation and report, specify number of tests
95027	Intracutaneous (intradermal) tests, sequential and incremental, with allergenic extracts for airborne allergens, immediate type reaction, including test interpretation and report, specify number of tests
95028	Intracutaneous (intradermal) tests with allergenic extracts, delayed type reaction, including reading, specify number of tests

◉ *CPT®* codes for allergy testing are reported by type of test.
  ❖ Percutaneous, immediate type reaction (**95004**)
  ❖ Intracutaneous (intradermal) with immediate (**95024**, **95027**) or delayed type reaction (**95028**)
  ❖ Any combination of percutaneous and intracutaneous, sequential and incremental tests with venoms (**95017**) or with drugs or biologicals (**95018**)

◉ Specification of the number of tests applied is required for accurate reporting of the units of service provided. Medicaid NCCI edits do not allow inclusion of positive or negative controls in the number of tests reported.

◉ Codes **95004**, **95017**, **95018**, **95024**, and **95027** include test interpretation and report. Code **95028** includes reading.
  ❖ An E/M service should not be reported for interpretation and report. However, if a significant, separately identifiable E/M service is performed and documented, it may be reported with modifier **25** appended to the appropriate E/M code.

Example

➤ **A patient with seasonal allergies undergoes percutaneous testing with 24 allergenic extracts.** A clinician administers the extracts as per physician's order and monitors the patient for signs of reaction. For each extract administered, the reaction (eg, size of wheal) or lack of reaction is noted. The physician interprets the test and creates a report of the findings.

The physician reports code 95004 with 24 units of service. If a significant E/M service is provided on the same date and is separately identifiable in the documentation from the preservice and post-service work of the testing (eg, interpretation and report), append modifier 25 to the code for the E/M service provided.

- Patch and photo patch testing are reported with code 95044–95056.
- Specific challenge testing (95060–95079) is coded according to target organ (eg, ophthalmic mucous membrane, nasal, inhalation bronchial challenges without pulmonary function testing, ingestion).
- Nasal cytology, a test for allergy-type cells (eosinophils) or infection-type cells (neutrophils) on a nasal scraping, is reported with code 89190.
- Nitric oxide expired gas determination is reported with code 95012. Nitric oxide determination by spectroscopy should be reported with code 94799.

Allergen Immunotherapy

Table 11-2 includes codes for reporting allergen immunotherapy based on the service provided: preparation and provision of allergen extract only; administration only; or provision and administration.

Table 11-2. Allergen Immunotherapy Services

Service	Codes	
Extract prepared and provided (not administered)	95144	Professional services for the supervision of preparation and provision of antigens for allergen immunotherapy, single-dose vials(s) (specify number of vials)
	95145	Professional services for the supervision of the preparation and provision of antigens for allergy immunotherapy (specify number of doses); single stinging insect venom
	95146	2 stinging insect venoms
	95147	3 stinging insect venoms
	95148	4 stinging insect venoms
	95149	5 stinging insect venoms
	95165	Professional services for the supervision of preparation and provision of antigens for allergen immunotherapy; single or multiple antigens (specify number of doses)
	95170	Professional services for the supervision of preparation and provision of antigens for allergen immunotherapy; whole body extract of biting insect or other arthropod (specify number of doses)
Extract administered (not prepared/provided)	95115	Professional services for allergen immunotherapy not including provision of allergenic extracts; single injection
	95117	2 or more injections
Provision and administration	95120	Professional services for allergen immunotherapy in the office or institution of the prescribing physician or other qualified health care professional, including provision of allergenic extract; single injection
	95125	2 or more injections
	95130	Professional services for allergen immunotherapy in the office or institution of the prescribing physician or other qualified health care professional, including provision of allergenic extract; single stinging insect venom
	95131	2 stinging insect venoms
	95132	3 stinging insect venoms
	95133	4 stinging insect venoms
	95134	5 stinging insect venoms

- An appropriate office or outpatient code may be reported with allergen immunotherapy codes. Modifier 25 is appended to the E/M service when it is performed and documented.

Coding Conundrum: National Correct Coding Initiative Immunotherapy Edits

The Medicaid National Correct Coding Initiative (NCCI) manual instructs that for purposes of reporting units of service (UOS) for antigen preparation (ie, *Current Procedural Terminology*® codes **95145–95170**), the physician reports "number of doses." The NCCI program defines a dose for reporting purposes as 1 mL. Thus, if a physician prepares a 10-mL vial of antigen, the physician may only report a maximum of 10 UOS for that vial even if the number of actual administered doses is greater than 10. Verify payer policies on units of service before reporting.

Preparation and Provision of Extract Only

- Codes **95144–95170** are used to report preparation and provision of antigens for allergen immunotherapy without administration of the allergenic extract.
    - Codes **95144–95170** describe the preparation of the antigen, the antigen extract itself, the physician's assessment and determination of the concentration and volume to use based on the patient's history and results of previous skin testing, and the prospective planned schedule of administration of the extract.
    - The number vials must be specified when reporting code **95144**. Codes **95145–95170** are reported based on the *number of doses* (eg, preparation of 2 vials that will provide 20 doses of extract containing 4 insect venoms is reported with code **95148** and 20 units of service). See the Coding Conundrum: National Correct Coding Initiative Immunotherapy Edits box for information on reporting to Medicaid and payers that use the Medicaid NCCI edits.
    - Services may be reported at the time the allergenic extract is prepared because injections occur on later dates (prospectively planned) or may not occur at all.
    - Administration of the allergenic extract is not included.
- Codes **95146–95149** are reported for preparation of extracts containing more than one single stinging venom (eg, code **95146** is reported for 2, **95147** for 3).

Administration of Extract Only

Codes **95115** and **95117** are used to report administration of the allergenic extract only. Code **95115** or **95117** (not both) is reported when another health care professional (eg, the patient's allergist) prepares and supplies the allergenic extract or when a physician (usually an allergist) administers the prospectively prepared extract (ie, prepared with the intent to administer on a planned schedule).

Same Encounter Provision of Allergenic Extract With Administration

- Codes **95120–95134** are reported when the entire service of preparing, providing, and administering (injection) allergenic extract is performed at one patient encounter.
- Codes **95131–95134** are reported for extracts containing more than one single stinging insect venom.
- Codes **95115** and **95117** *cannot* be reported with codes **95120–95134**.
- *CPT*® recommends codes **95120–95134** be reported only when specifically required by the payer.
- Codes **95120** and **95125** are reported based on the number of injections administered (ie, a single injection or ≥2 injections). Codes **95130–95134** are reported per injection. Therefore, if 2 separate injections of 2 stinging insect venoms (eg, wasp and bee) are provided, code **95131** would be reported 2 times.
- For rapid desensitization per hour, see code **95180**.

Examples

➤ An allergist prepares a 10-dose vial of allergen extract and administers 1 dose at the time of the visit (allergenic extract was prepared with the intent to administer on a planned schedule).

The allergist will report code **95165** with 10 units of service and **95115** with 1 unit of service and the specific diagnosis code. Allergic rhinitis due to pollen would be reported with *ICD-10-CM* code **J30.1** or, if due to food, code **J30.5**.

➤ **The patient has a reaction to the allergenic extract.** The physician injects epinephrine using an auto-injector device (eg, EpiPen Jr).

The injection using an auto-injection device would be reported as an intramuscular injection with code **96372**. Although code **J0171** is used to report provision of epinephrine, the auto-injector is not described by this code. Prior to claim submission, it is advisable to verify payer policy addressing submission of code **J0171** (epinephrine 0.01 mg) versus **J3490** (unspecified drug) with the product National Drug Code (NDC) to specify the exact product provided. (The NDCs are universal product identifiers for prescription drugs and insulin products. Codes are 10-digit, 3-segment numbers that identify the product, labeler, and trade package size. The Health Insurance Portability and Accountability Act of 1996 standards require an 11-digit code. If you are not currently reporting injectables with NDCs, be sure to coordinate the requirements with your billing software company. See Chapter 1, The Basics of Coding, for more information on NDCs.)

➤ **The pediatrician administers 3 injections of allergen extract for a patient with allergic rhinitis due to pollen.** The extract was prepared and supplied by the allergist.

The pediatrician will report code **95117** with *ICD-10-CM* code **J30.1**.

Coding Conundrum: Centers for Medicare & Medicaid Services Allergen Immunotherapy Guidelines

The Centers for Medicare & Medicaid Services (CMS) Medicare program will only accept codes **95115**, **95117**, and **95144–95170** and will not allow payment for codes **95120–95134**. State Medicaid and commercial payers may follow the CMS Medicare guidelines or may have their own established guidelines. Therefore, before reporting these services, research the reporting policies of your major payers.

EpiPen Administration

Administration of epinephrine via an EpiPen in the office or other outpatient setting is reported with code **96372** (therapeutic, prophylactic, or diagnostic injection [specify substance or drug]; subcutaneous or intramuscular). Follow payer guidance for reporting an EpiPen kit furnished by the practice. Many payers require submission of code **J0171** (injection, adrenalin, epinephrine, 0.1 mg) with 1 unit for 1 injection. Other payers may require code **J3490** (unclassified drugs). Inclusion of the NDC provides additional information on the exact product. See Chapter 1, The Basics of Coding, for more information on reporting NDCs.

Immunoglobulins

When reporting codes **90281–90399**, remember that they are only for the cost of the immunoglobulin and the appropriate separate administration code should also be reported (eg, **96372**, **96374**). A significant, separately identifiable E/M service performed during the same visit may also be billed if indicated. *ICD-10-CM* diagnosis codes to support immunoglobulin services include codes from categories **D80–D84** for certain disorders involving the immune mechanism or codes for specific conditions, such as mucocutaneous lymph node syndrome (**M30.3**).

Note: This information does not apply to immunization services. Immunization services and vaccines are discussed in length in Chapter 9, Preventive Services.

> ||||||| **Coding Pearl** |||||||
>
> When reporting administration of immunoglobulin, report the diagnosis code for the condition for which immunoglobulin administration is performed (eg, pulmonary hypertension, exposure to disease).

Example

➤ An infant with moderate pulmonary hypertension is seen for administration of the second of 5 monthly doses of palivizumab. A nurse administers the immunoglobulin under direct physician supervision.

Code **96372** (intramuscular injection) is reported in addition to code **90378** (respiratory syncytial virus, monoclonal antibody, recombinant, for intramuscular use, 50 mg, each). The appropriate number of units reported for the dose given is 1 unit per 50 mg. The NDC for each vial should be included on claims for most payers. (See Chapter 1, The Basics of Coding, for more on reporting NDCs.)

Hearing Screening and Other Audiological Function Testing Codes

*(For central auditory function evaluation, see **92620**, **92621**.)*

Audiometric tests require the use of calibrated electronic equipment, recording of results, and a written report with interpretation. Services include testing of both ears. If the test is applied to one ear only, modifier **52** (reduced services) must be appended to the code.

|||||||| **Coding Pearl** ||||||||

Report hearing tests conducted following a failed hearing screening with *International Classification of Diseases, 10th Revision, Clinical Modification* code **Z01.110** if results are typical. If findings are atypical, report code **Z01.118** and a code to identify the abnormality.

- ☀ Code **92551** (screening test, pure tone, air only) is used when earphones are placed on the patient and the patient is asked to respond to tones of different pitches and intensities. This is a limited study to identify the presence or absence of a potential hearing problem. Code **92551** is not used to report hearing screenings performed on newborns and infants.

- ☀ Code **92552** (full pure tone audiometric assessment) is used when earphones are placed on the patient and the patient is asked to respond to tones of different pitches and intensities. The threshold, which is the lowest intensity of the tone that the patient can hear 50% of the time, is recorded for a number of frequencies. Bone thresholds are obtained in a similar manner. Air and bone thresholds (**92553**) may be obtained and compared to differentiate among conductive, sensorineural, or mixed hearing losses.

- ☀ Code **92558** is reported for evoked otoacoustic emissions, screening (qualitative measurement of distortion product or transient evoked otoacoustic emissions), automated analysis. This is used when the results are obtained automatically. Coverage for this is typically limited to newborn screening, including follow-up newborn screening from a failed screen in the hospital and screening on younger children. Check with your payers, however.

- ☀ Code **92583** (select picture audiometry) is typically used for younger children. The patient is asked to identify different pictures with the instructions given at different intensity levels.

- ☀ Auditory evoked potentials for evoked response audiometry and/or testing of the central nervous system, comprehensive, is reported with code **92585**. A limited study is reported with code **92586**.

- ☀ Distortion product evoked otoacoustic emissions codes are reported based on the number of frequencies used. Code **92587** is used to report testing for confirmation of the presence or absence of a hearing disorder, 3 to 6 frequencies. Code **92588** is reported when a comprehensive (quantitative analysis of outer hair cell function by cochlear mapping) diagnostic evaluation with a minimum of 12 frequencies is performed. A written interpretation and report are required. Do not report these codes for automated analysis.

|||||||| **Coding Pearl** ||||||||

Automated audiometry testing is reported with Category III codes **0208T–0212T**.

- ☀ Other commonly performed procedures include codes **92567** (tympanometry [impedance testing]) and **92568** (acoustic reflex testing, threshold portion). Code **92550** is reported when tympanometry and reflex threshold measurements are performed.

- Optical coherence tomography of the middle ear with interpretation and report is reported with Category III codes based on whether the service was unilateral (0485T) or bilateral (0486T). Be sure to verify payer policy prior to provision of services.

- Most audiological procedures are bundled with impacted cerumen removal services (69209, 69210) and, therefore, will not be separately payable. Report only the audiology test to payers that bundle impacted cerumen removal services.

Example

➤ **A 3-year-old with bilateral acute recurrent otitis media undergoes optical coherence tomography of the middle ears to evaluate the presence and purulence of effusion in the middle ears.** After sufficient images are collected and areas of interest identified, a printout of selected data is obtained and reviewed by the physician or other qualified health care professional (QHP), who creates a report of the findings. Diagnosis is bilateral acute recurrent otitis media with effusion.

ICD-10-CM	CPT®
H66.006 (acute suppurative otitis media without spontaneous rupture of ear drum, recurrent, bilateral)	0486T (optical coherence tomography [OCT] of middle ear, with interpretation and report; bilateral)

Teaching Point: If a unilateral procedure were performed, code 0485T would be reported in lieu of 0486T. Note that the printout produced in testing is not the physician or QHP interpretation and report but provides information for the interpretation and report.

Endocrinology Services

95250   Ambulatory continuous glucose monitoring of interstitial tissue fluid via a subcutaneous sensor for a minimum of 72 hours; physician or other qualified health care professional (office) provided equipment, sensor placement, hook-up, calibration of monitor, patient training, removal of sensor, and printout of record

#95249   patient-provided equipment, sensor placement, hookup, calibration of monitor, patient training, and printout of recording

95251   Ambulatory continuous glucose monitoring of interstitial tissue fluid via a subcutaneous sensor for a minimum of 72 hours; analysis, interpretation and report

- When ambulatory glucose monitoring using monitoring equipment is initiated and data are captured for a minimum of 72 hours, report either 95249 or 95250 based on the supplier of the equipment (patient or physician office).

- Physicians report code 95249 only if the patient brings the data receiver in to the physician's or other QHP's office with the entire initial data collection procedure conducted in the office.

- Report code 95249 only once for the entire duration of time that a patient has a receiver even if the patient receives a new sensor and/or transmitter. If a patient receives a new or different model of receiver, code 95249 may be reported again when the entire initial data collection procedure is conducted in the office.

- Analysis, interpretation, and report (95251) may be performed without a face-to-face encounter on the same date of service. This service is reported only once per month.

Emotional/Behavioral Assessment

Please see Chapter 14, Mental and Behavioral Health Services, for discussion of diagnostic testing of the central nervous system. Also, see Chapter 9, Preventive Services, for discussion of developmental screening, brief emotional and/or behavioral assessment, and health risk assessment as preventive services.

96127   Brief emotional/behavioral assessment (eg, depression inventory, attention-deficit/hyperactivity disorder [ADHD] scale), with scoring and documentation, per standardized instrument

Code **96127**

* Represents the practice expense of administering, scoring, and documenting each standardized instrument. No physician work value is included. Physician interpretation is included in a related E/M service.
* May be used for screening but also for assessment in monitoring treatment efficacy and to support clinical decision-making.
* Not reported in conjunction with **96105**, **96125**, and **99483**.
* Two separate completions (eg, by teacher and parent) of the same form may be separately reported (ie, 2 units of service). When reporting multiple units of service, it is advisable to learn if the payer has specific guidance for reporting as a single line item with the total number of units or requires splitting to multiple claim lines. Medically Unlikely Edits may apply. (See Chapter 2, Modifiers and Coding Edits, for more information on Medically Unlikely Edits.)

Example

➤ **The mother of an 8-year-old girl expresses concerns about the child daydreaming and not paying attention at school.** The parent version of a behavior assessment system for children is administered to the mother and scored for the physician's review. The physician recommends that an additional behavioral assessment be completed by the girl's teacher to confirm or rule out predominantly inattentive ADHD.

The appropriate E/M service code (preventive medicine visit, new or established patient office visit, or consultation) would be reported in addition to code **96127**. Because the physician did not diagnose ADHD, assign *ICD-10-CM* code **R41.840** for symptoms of attention and concentration deficit.

Radiology Services

The following general guidelines are for reporting radiology services:

* Report only the service provided. See the Professional and Technical Components section earlier in this chapter for appropriate reporting when the physician does not provide the global service.
* An authenticated (signed) written report of the physician's or QHP's interpretation of imaging is an integral part of the professional component of a radiologic service.
* A reference to *image* in *CPT* may refer to that which is acquired on film or in digital format. Images must contain anatomic information unique to the patient for which the imaging service is provided.
* Certain health plans, including Medicaid plans, may require use of modifier **FX** (x-ray taken using film) when reporting the technical component or global radiology service (ie, combined professional and technical components). Verify health plan requirements, as payment may be reduced for radiographs taken using film.

Several categories of codes for radiology services have been revised in recent years. The following sections highlights some of these changes. Please see your coding reference for a full listing of codes and reporting instructions.

Imaging Guidance

Many procedures include imaging guidance. When a code descriptor for a procedure or *CPT* instruction indicates that the procedure includes imaging guidance, do not separately report a code for supervision and interpretation of imaging (eg, radiography, fluoroscopy, ultrasonography, magnetic resonance imaging, computed tomography, nuclear medicine).

◉ Do not report imaging guidance when a non-imaging guided tracking or localizing system (eg, radar or electromagnetic signals) is used.

Abdominal Radiographs

74018	Radiologic examination, abdomen; 1 view
74019	2 views
74021	3 or more views
74022	complete acute abdomen series, including supine, erect, and/or decubitus views, single view chest

Chest Radiographs

71045	Radiologic examination, chest; single view
71046	2 views
71047	3 views
71048	4 or more views

◉ The types of views (eg, frontal and lateral) obtained no longer affect coding of chest radiographs.

◉ Do not separately report a single-view chest radiograph when obtained in conjunction with an acute abdomen series (74022).

Hip Radiographs

73501	Radiologic examination, hip, unilateral, with pelvis when performed; 1 view
73502	2-3 views
73503	performed minimum of 4 views
73521	Radiologic examination, hips, bilateral, with pelvis when performed; 2 views
73522	3-4 views
73523	minimum of 5 views
73525	Radiologic examination, hip, arthrography, radiological supervision and interpretation
73592	Radiologic examination lower extremity, infant, minimum of 2 views

Codes 73501–73523 include radiograph of the pelvis when performed. Do not separately report a single-view radiograph of the pelvis (72170) when performed in conjunction with a radiograph of the hip.

Total Spine Radiographs

72081	Radiologic examination, spine, entire thoracic and lumbar, including skull, cervical and sacral spine if performed (eg, scoliosis evaluation); one view
72082	2 or 3 views
72083	4 or 5 views
72084	minimum of 6 views

◉ Previously reported with a single code regardless of the number of views, examination of the entire thoracic and lumbar spine is now reported based on the number of views obtained.

◉ Codes 72081–72084 describe imaging of the entire thoracic and lumbar spine and, when performed, the skull, cervical, and sacral spine. Do not separately report codes for views of the individual spinal segments or skull when performed in conjunction with radiologic examination of the spine. Rather, select the code that represents the number of views obtained of the hip and/or pelvis.

Administrative Services and Supplies

Administrative Services

Codes in this section cover some of the administrative aspects of medical practice.

99071 Educational supplies, such as books, tapes, and pamphlets, for the patient's education at cost to physician or other qualified health care professional

99075 Medical testimony

99082 Unusual travel (eg, transportation and escort of patient)

99091 Collection and interpretation of physiological data (eg, ECG, blood pressure, glucose monitoring) digitally stored and/or transmitted by the patient and/or caregiver to the physician or other qualified health care professional, requiring a minimum of 30 minutes of time (Do not report more than once in a 30-day period.)

 Codes 99071–99091 are for administrative services.

- Code 99071 may be reported when the physician incurs costs for educational supplies and provides them to the patient at his or her cost.
- Code 99075 may be reported when a physician presents medical testimony before a court or other administrative body.
- With the exception of code 99091, none of these services are assigned Medicare RVUs.
- HCPCS code S9981 (medical records copying fee, administrative) or S9982 (medical record copying fee, per page) may be reported when it is appropriate to charge for copies of medical records. Commercial payers and some Medicaid programs may accept S codes.
- State medical insurance departments or medical associations determine the amount a practice can charge for copying medical records. Be sure to know the state charge limitations and do not overcharge. The Health Insurance Portability and Accountability Act regulations, where more stringent, will override state regulations. For information on charges to patients for copying health records, see www.hhs.gov/hipaa/for-professionals/privacy/guidance/access/index.html#newlyreleasedfaqs.

Physician Group Education Services

99078 Physician or other qualified health care professional qualified by education, training, licensure/regulation (when applicable), educational services rendered to patients in a group setting (eg, prenatal, obesity, or diabetic instructions)

Code 99078 is used to report physician educational services provided to established patients in group settings (eg, obesity or diabetes classes).

- There are no time requirements.
- Modifier 25 (significant, separately identifiable E/M service) should *not* be appended to the E/M service because 99078 is an adjunct service.
- Documentation in each medical record includes the education and training provided, follow-up for ongoing education, and total time of the education.
- Services are reported on each participating child.
- Payers may require that these services be reported differently.
- For preventive medicine and risk-factor reduction counseling to patients in a group setting, see codes 99411 and 99412.

Supplies and Materials

99070   Supplies and materials provided by the physician over and above those usually included with the office visit or other services rendered

* Items such as elastic wraps, clavicle splints, or circumcision and suturing trays may be reported with this code. Remember that some supplies (eg, suturing trays, circumcision trays) may be included with the surgical procedure if the payer uses the Resource-Based Relative Value Scale as its basis for payment.

* Only the supplies purchased in an office-based practice may be reported.

* Some payers will require the use of HCPCS codes. More specific HCPCS codes are available for a number of supplies (eg, codes **Q4001–Q4051** for cast and splint supplies). Use HCPCS codes when they are more specific.

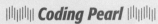

> **||||||||| Coding Pearl |||||||||**
>
> If reporting code **99070**, identify the supplies or materials on the claim form and be prepared to submit an invoice.

Medications

See **Table 11-1** for a list of the most commonly used HCPCS **J** codes.

* The practice must have incurred a cost for the medication reported.

* Most payers do not cover services reported with nonspecific codes.

* Check with payers to determine if they accept these HCPCS codes or if they require reporting with code **99070**.

* Drugs are listed with a base dosage. When the dosage exceeds the amount listed, report additional units for the total dosage administered.

* Some payers require use of the NDC instead of or in addition to **J** codes. The NDC should always be reported in addition to code **99070** or **J3490** (unclassified drug).

For more information on NDCs, see Chapter 1, The Basics of Coding.

Chapter 11: Common Testing and Therapeutic Services in Office Settings

Managing Chronic and Complex Conditions

Contents

Managing Chronic and Complex Conditions

Children with chronic and complex health care needs are patients who require greater levels and amounts of multidisciplinary medical, psychosocial, rehabilitation, and habilitation services than their same-aged peers. The child with special health care needs will require extra services, such as prolonged services, home care visits, and care management, with an increased frequency of evaluation and management (E/M) visits. Patient-centered medical home recognition programs and related quality initiatives have focused on care of children with chronic and episodic health conditions and complex care through planning and coordination, management between face-to-face encounters, and use of electronic technology for population management, increased access to care, and quality measurement. However, physician practices have faced challenges in receiving adequate funding for the infrastructure necessary to effectively coordinate and manage care for patients with multiple and complex conditions. In response, codes have been developed with the aim of capturing the components of care that go beyond those included in preservice, intraservice, and post-service values of the traditional face-to-face visit. Services such as chronic care management (CCM) and transitional care management (TCM) have been defined and valued and are separately reportable services in addition to other face-to-face services.

New in 2019 is a code for CCM services personally performed by a physician or other qualified health care professional (QHP) rather than clinical staff working under supervision of a physician or QHP.

Codes and payment policy for many of these services continue to evolve. Awareness of the codes for these services and the related coding instructions may offer additional opportunities for providing and/or coordinating comprehensive care for all children. Reporting these services and the diagnosis codes representing the patient's chronic and complex conditions can play an important role in demonstrating the higher quality, lower cost care that is a key element of emerging payment methodologies. (See Chapter 4, The Business of Medicine: Working With Current and Emerging Payment Systems, for information on emerging payment methodologies, such as value-based purchasing.) Payers that have adopted value-based or enhanced payment initiatives, such as per-member, per-month payment models, may consider certain care management services bundled into the services for which the enhanced payment is made. However, practices may choose to assign codes for use in internal calculations of the cost to provide enhanced care in comparison to any enhanced payments.

To take advantage of opportunities for providing and reporting services related to management of chronic conditions and complex health care needs, physicians must identify the services that their practice capabilities will support. For instance, provision of TCM services requires timely identification of patients who are discharged from an inpatient or observation stay such that contact may be made with the patient within 2 business days of facility discharge. Payers may also require specific electronic capabilities (eg, having a system that meets specifications required by the Medicaid electronic health record [EHR] incentive programs and/or Merit-based Incentive Payment System [MIPS]).

Identification of patients who may qualify for care management services must be accomplished through a standardized methodology. This may involve developing checklists or processes for identifying characteristics of patients with complex health care needs (eg, patients with chronic or episodic conditions that are expected to last at least 12 months and increase the risk of morbidity and mortality, acute exacerbation or decompensation, or functional decline may require CCM services). Examples of such characteristics (*examples only; not a practice guideline*) include

- Number of chronic conditions
- Number of visits for nonroutine care in the past year
- Number of days the child did not attend school due to health condition
- Emergency department (ED) visits or hospitalizations in the past 6 months
- Number of current medications or medications prescribed or revised in the last 6 months
- Number of physicians and other providers (eg, home health care provider, nutritionist)
- Lack of resources (eg, housing, health plan coverage, access to care in community)
- Assistance required for activities of daily living
- Other psychosocial considerations (eg, language barriers, multiple family members with complex care needs)

Electronic systems may be used to identify patients whose records include specific diagnoses and/or services that may indicate the need for care management. However, standardized procedures for identifying the need for services and documenting orders for and delivery of services are necessary to support billing and payment.

Chapter 12: Managing Chronic and Complex Conditions

For more information on preparing your practice to provide care to patients with complex health care needs, see the American Academy of Pediatrics (AAP) policy statement, "Patient- and Family-Centered Care Coordination: A Framework for Integrating Care for Children and Youth Across Multiple Systems" (http://pediatrics.aappublications.org/content/early/2014/04/22/peds.2014-0318). This policy statement, coauthored by the AAP Council on Children With Disabilities and the Medical Home Implementation Project Advisory Committee, specifically outlines the essential partnerships that are critical to this framework. To further augment and facilitate application of the recommendations within this policy statement, the freely accessible Boston Children's Hospital Care Coordination Curriculum (https://www.pcpcc.org/resource/care-coordination-curriculum) provides content that can be adapted to the needs of any entity (eg, a single practice, a network of practices, parent and family organizations, a statewide organization). By design, most of the content is universally relevant, but the curriculum is optimally used when it is adapted and customized to reflect local needs, assets, and cultures.

Physicians may also choose to incorporate other health care professional services (eg, medical nutrition therapist, psychologist, behavioral health care manager) into their medical practice to meet the needs of patients with complex health care needs. See Chapter 13, Allied Health and Clinical Staff Services, and Chapter 14, Mental and Behavioral Health Services, for information on reporting services by nonphysician providers (NPPs).

Provider Terminology

Of particular importance to correct reporting of services that include clinical staff and other NPPs is identifying the providers included when terms such as "physician or other qualified health care professional" or "qualified, nonphysician health care professional" are used in *Current Procedural Terminology* (*CPT*®) and/or payer instruction.

Current Procedural Terminology® Provider Definitions

Current Procedural Terminology provides definitions of *providers* as follows:
- **Physician or other qualified health care professional:** an individual who is qualified by education, training, licensure/regulation (when applicable), and facility privileging (when applicable) who performs a professional service within his or her scope of practice and independently reports that professional service
- **Clinical staff member:** a person who works under the supervision of a physician or other qualified health care professional and who is allowed by law, regulation, and facility policy to perform or assist in the performance of a specific professional service but does not individually report that professional service

Throughout the *CPT* code set, the use of terms such as "physician," "qualified health care professional," or "individual" is not intended to indicate that other entities may not report the service. In selected instances, specific instructions may define a service as limited to professionals or to other entities (eg, hospital, home health agency).

Clinical staff member is used in *CPT* mostly in the context of staff who provide components of physician or QHP services, such as TCM and CCM, and services that are always billed by a supervising physician or QHP.

The *CPT* definition of *physician or other QHP* creates a broad category of providers (eg, advanced practice providers, therapists, social workers). The definition of physician or other QHP is used in relation to services such as E/M services (**99201–99499**) and immunization administration with physician counseling (**90460, 90461**) and to codes *not reported* by physicians, such as genetic counseling (**96040**).

However, this definition may be confusing, as payer policies commonly differentiate QHPs such as advanced practice providers, who may perform and prescribe services much like a physician, from those who provide specialized services under the supervision and order of a physician or advanced practice provider. Payers may offer direct reporting by certain QHPs (eg, advanced practice provider, psychologist) while requiring others to report services in the name of the supervising physician or advanced practice QHP. To aid in differentiating how services are typically reported by these subcategories of QHPs, the following definitions will apply in discussions and examples in this chapter:
- **Physician:** Signifies an individual licensed under state law to practice medicine or osteopathy (Medicare also includes individuals licensed to provide dental, podiatric, optometric, and chiropractic services in the definition of physician.)

- **Qualified health care professional**: Signifies advanced practice providers, such as advanced practice nurses and physician assistants, whose scope of practice includes E/M services beyond minimal services incident to a physician (ie, **99211**) and who can individually report their professional services within their scope of practice
- **Clinical staff member** (as defined by *CPT®* in differentiating from a physician or QHP): A health care team member (eg, registered nurse, licensed practical nurse, medical assistant) who works under the supervision of a physician or other QHP and who is allowed by law, regulation, and facility policy to perform or assist in the performance of a specific professional service but does not individually report that professional service
- **Allied health professional** (AHP): Represents a broad category of health care professionals (eg, social workers, nutritionists) who typically would not independently prescribe and manage, whose professional services are typically performed under the order and supervision of a physician or QHP (eg, nutritional counseling, occupational therapy), and whose scope of practice does not include E/M services beyond **99211**

Note: CPT does not include any requirements for licensure but, rather, advises physicians to follow state regulations and the related scopes of practice defined by regulations (eg, regulations defining services that require a nursing license).

Coding for Management of Complex Medical Conditions

Coordination and delivery of complex care may include use of technology such as access to the medical home through telephone and online medical evaluations and subspecialty care through telemedicine or interprofessional consultation. In addition, medical team conferences may be performed on occasion to coordinate or manage care and services or to present findings and recommendations that are used to develop or revise a plan of care that includes coordination across multiple disciplines. Several different types of non–face-to-face E/M services may be performed within the same calendar month, so practices must be cognizant of *CPT* coding guidelines.

Many inclusion and exclusion rules are applied to the services included in this chapter. These rules often bundle certain niche services (eg, management of end-stage renal disease [ESRD]) in addition to prohibiting separate reporting of services that may be considered components of care management during a period when more comprehensive care management is reported. Tables are provided to summarize the patient population, work, and potentially bundled services for each type of service.

Tracking Time of Periodic Services

Documentation and tracking of time for services that are reported on a periodic basis, such as per calendar month, require establishment of routine processes that prevent lost revenue due to failure to capture all billable services. Some practices use manual systems, such as spreadsheets, while others have adapted their EHR with flow sheets to capture each activity and the related time throughout a period of service and provide a report of time per patient within each period of service.

The following example illustrates one manual method of using pseudocodes that are set to never bill out on claims but provide a basis for tracking time-based services. Practice and system capabilities vary.

> ||||||||| **Coding Pearl** |||||||||
>
> Transitional care management services (**99495, 99496**) are reported for a 30-day period beginning with the date of discharge from a facility setting. All chronic care management, care plan oversight, psychiatric collaborative care management, and care management for behavioral health conditions are reported per calendar month of service.

Example

➤ **Dr Joe at ABC Pediatric Clinic is the primary care pediatrician for 18-month-old Izzy, who has cystic fibrosis with exocrine pancreatic insufficiency and failure to thrive.** Dr Joe's clinical coordinator, Jill, works with Izzy's mother to coordinate care by her occupational therapist, nutritionist, gastroenterologist, and pulmonologist in addition to primary care and early intervention services. Jill also consults with the practice's social worker and various community agencies to find assistance for Izzy and her family as needed. Izzy recently underwent insertion of a feeding tube. During the calendar month, a substantial change is made to Izzy's care plan to include commencement of tube feeding.

Chapter 12: Managing Chronic and Complex Conditions

All times and activities are documented in the EHR via free text note entries, with the cumulative time captured through use of internally created pseudocodes selected for each activity during the calendar month (eg, code COORD is attached to a note to capture time spent coordinating with other care providers, with 1 unit assigned for each documented minute of time spent in the activity). At the end of the calendar month the care coordinator reviews a report of all pseudocodes entered for each patient who received care management services during the month and determines what codes are supported by the documentation. Jill determines that between herself and Dr Joe, a total of 80 minutes was spent in care management activities for Izzy in December.

Time of 80 minutes of care management activities along with substantial revision of the patient's care plan support reporting of complex CCM.	**_CPT®_** **99487** (complex chronic care management services, with the following required elements: ⚬ multiple [two or more] chronic conditions expected to last at least 12 months, or until the death of the patient, ⚬ chronic conditions place the patient at significant risk of death, acute exacerbation/decompensation, or functional decline, ⚬ establishment or substantial revision of a comprehensive care plan, ⚬ moderate or high complexity medical decision making; ⚬ 60 minutes of clinical staff time directed by a physician or other qualified health care professional, per calendar month)
	International Classification of Diseases, 10th Revision, Clinical Modification (ICD-10-CM) **E84.8** (cystic fibrosis with other manifestations) **K86** (exocrine pancreatic insufficiency) **R62.51** (failure to thrive) Codes for any other conditions addressed in the calendar month

Collaboration with system vendors, professional colleagues, and practice management consultants may be invaluable to successful delivery, documentation, and reporting of time-based services.

Care Management Services

Chronic Care Management (CCM) Services

New in 2019 for Chronic Care Management

⚬ **99491** is added for reporting chronic care management (CCM) personally performed by a physician or other qualified health care professional (QHP).
⚬ Changes to the guidelines for CCM services allow reporting of time spent by clinical staff performing CCM activities on the same date as a physician's or QHP's evaluation and management service to the same patient except on the day of an initiating visit (changed in _CPT® 2018_ via errata).
⚬ Site of service (ie, inpatient or observation) no longer affects reporting of time spent in CCM activities.

Chronic care management services are management and support services that are provided by physicians or QHPs or by clinical staff under the direction of a physician or other QHP to individuals with 2 or more chronic conditions who reside at home or in a domiciliary, rest home, or assisted living facility. Care management includes provision or oversight of the management and/or coordination of services, as needed, for all the patient's medical conditions, psychosocial needs, and activities of daily living. A comprehensive care plan for all the patient's health problems is created, implemented, monitored, and revised as needed.

Chronic care management includes 2 levels of care management. Codes 99487 and 99489 require additional elements of service and greater clinical staff time than codes 99490 and 99491.

Tables 12-1 and 12-2 provide CCM code descriptions and services not separately reported with CCM (99490, 99491) and complex CCM (99487, 99489) services.

The appropriate CCM code is reported once per calendar month by only one physician or other QHP who has assumed this management role for the patient's care. Face-to-face E/M services may be separately reported by the same physician or QHP during the same calendar month. See Appendix III for an example of a worksheet for tracking CCM services (or see it online at www.aap.org/cfp, access code AAPCFP24).

> ||||||| **Coding Pearl** |||||||
>
> The midpoint rule commonly applied for coding based on time does not apply to chronic care management or complex chronic care management services (99487–99491).

Guidelines Applicable to All CCM Services

* Time, activities (eg, patient education, communication with other health care providers), and identification of the individual conducting each activity must be documented.
* Only one CCM service is reported per calendar month (eg, 99490 and 99491 are not reported for the same month).
* Creation or revision of a care plan must be documented. Plans created by other entities (eg, home health agencies) do not substitute for a care plan established by the individual reporting CCM services.
* Cannot be reported if performed within the postoperative portion of the global period of a surgery or procedure reported by the same physician or other physician of the same specialty and same group practice.
* Cannot be reported for any post-discharge CCM services for any days within 30 days of discharge, if reporting code 99495 or 99496 (TCM services).
  * When care management resumes after a discharge in a new month, start a new period or report TCM services (99495, 99496) as appropriate.
  * If discharge occurs in the same month, continue the reporting period or report TCM services.

Table 12-1. Chronic Care Management Services

99490 Chronic care management services by clinical staff
Patient Population
Patients have multiple (2 or more) chronic or episodic conditions expected to last at least 12 months, or until the death of the patient, that place the patient at significant risk of death, acute exacerbation/decompensation, or functional decline.
Work Required
* Comprehensive care plan established, implemented, revised, or monitored
* At least 20 minutes of clinical staff activity directed by a physician or other QHP, per calendar month

#●99491 Chronic care management services by physician
Patient Population
Patients have multiple (2 or more) chronic or episodic conditions expected to last at least 12 months, or until the death of the patient, that place the patient at significant risk of death, acute exacerbation/decompensation, or functional decline.
Work Required
* Comprehensive care plan established, implemented, revised, or monitored
* At least 30 minutes of time personally spent by a physician or other QHP, per calendar month

99487, +99489 Complex chronic care management services by clinical staff/physician/QHP
Patient Population
Patients have multiple (2 or more) chronic or episodic conditions expected to last at least 12 months, or until the death of the patient, that place the patient at significant risk of death, acute exacerbation/decompensation, or functional decline.
Work Required
* Establishment or substantial revision of a comprehensive care plan
* Moderate- or high-complexity medical decision-making
* At least 60 minutes of clinical staff activity directed by a physician or other QHP, per calendar month

Abbreviation: QHP, qualified health care professional.

Chapter 12: Managing Chronic and Complex Conditions

Table 12-2. Services Not Separately Reported in Same Calendar Month as Chronic Care Management or Complex Chronic Care Management Services

Code	Description
90951–90970	End-stage renal disease performed in an outpatient setting
93792, 93793	Home INR management
98960–98962	Education and training for patient self-management by AHP
98966–98968	Telephone A/M service provided by AHP
98969	Online A/M service provided by AHP
99071	Educational supplies
99078	Physician or other QHP educational services to a group
99080	Special reports such as insurance forms
#▲99091	Collection and interpretation of physiologic data
99339, 99340	Care plan oversight in home, domiciliary, or rest home
99358, 99359	Prolonged E/M service before and/or after direct patient care
99366–99368	Medical team conferences
99374, 99375	Supervision of patient under care of home health agency in home, domiciliary, or equivalent environment
99377, 99378	Supervision of hospice patient
99379, 99380	Supervision of a nursing facility patient
99441–99443	Telephone E/M service by a physician or other QHP
99444	Online E/M service by a physician or other QHP
99490	Chronic care management services
99495, 99496	Transitional care management services
99605–99607	Medication therapy management by a pharmacist

Abbreviations: AHP, allied health professional; A/M, assessment and management; E/M, evaluation and management; INR, international normalized ratio; QHP, qualified health care professional.

Chronic Care Management Required Practice Capabilities

- Use an electronic health record system that allows care providers timely access to clinical information.
- Use a medical record form and format that are standardized within the practice.
- Identify patients who require care management using a standardized methodology.
- Adopt an internal care management process to provide care management services in a timely manner following identification of need for these services.
- Provide access to care providers or clinical staff 24 hours a day, 7 days a week, including providing patients and caregivers with a means to make contact with health care professionals in the practice to address urgent needs, regardless of the time of day or day of the week.
- Provide continuity of care through scheduling of the patient's successive routine appointments with a designated member of the care team.
- Provide timely access and management for necessary follow-up when a patient is discharged from the emergency department or hospital.
- Engage and educate patients and caregivers.
- Coordinate care among all service providers, as appropriate for each patient.

- Do not count any time of the clinical staff on the day of an initiating visit (eg, the creation of the care plan, initial explanation to patient and/or caregiver, obtaining consent). However, previous instruction ("Do not count any clinical staff time on a day when the physician or qualified health care professional reports an E/M service...") was deleted in 2018.
- When provided during the same calendar month, behavioral or psychiatric collaborative care management (PCCM) services (99484, 99492–99494) may be separately reported. Do not count the same period toward CCM and behavioral or PCCM services.

Chronic Care Management Clinical Staff Activities

- Face-to-face and non–face-to-face time spent communicating with and engaging the patient and/or family, caregivers, other professionals, community services, and agencies
- Developing, revising, documenting, communicating, and implementing a comprehensive care plan
- Collecting health outcomes data and registry documentation
- Teaching patient and/or family/caregiver patient self-management, independent living, and activities of daily living
- Identifying community and health resources
- Facilitating access to care and other services needed by the patient and/or family
- Management of care transitions not reported as part of transitional care management (99495, 99496)
- Ongoing review of patient status, including review of laboratory and other studies not reported as part of an evaluation and management service
- Assessment and support for adherence to the care plan

Guidelines Specific to CCM Services Based on Clinical Staff Time

Codes 99487, 99489, and 99490 are reported only once per calendar month.

- These codes are reported in any calendar month when the clinical staff time requirements are met. Only time spent by clinical staff employed directly by or under contract with the reporting professional's practice is included. If multiple clinical staff members meet about one patient, count the time for only one staff member.
  - More than one clinical staff member may spend time in CCM activities on a single date. Count all time that is not overlapping, but do not count the same period more than once.
- Services include all face-to-face and non–face-to-face clinical staff time spent in CCM activities. Time spent in other reported clinical staff services (eg, time of prolonged clinical staff service [99415, 99416]) may not be included to meet requirements for reporting CCM.
- If the physician personally performs clinical staff activities, his or her time may be counted toward the required clinical staff time to meet the elements of the code. If a physician or QHP personally performs at least 30 minutes of CCM services, see the CCM by a Physician or Other Qualified Health Care Professional (99491) section later in this chapter.

CCM

99490   Chronic care management services, at least 20 minutes of clinical staff time directed by a physician or other qualified health care professional, per calendar month, with the following required elements:
- multiple (two or more) chronic conditions expected to last at least 12 months, or until the death of the patient,
- chronic conditions place the patient at significant risk of death, acute exacerbation/decompensation, or functional decline,
- comprehensive care plan established, implemented, revised, or monitored

Chronic care management code 99490 was developed to align with the Centers for Medicare & Medicaid Services (CMS) benefit specifications for Medicare coverage of CCM. The CMS has outlined specific coverage criteria that may be adopted by Medicaid and private health plans, including 2 points of consideration for physicians who wish to provide CCM services.

1. Practices providing CCM services must have certain capabilities, including use of an EHR. Health plans may adopt the CMS requirement for use of an EHR that meets certification requirements of the Medicaid EHR incentive programs and/or MIPS in place on December 31 of the prior year.
2. Chronic care management activities are provided by clinical staff under the supervision of the physician or QHP reporting CCM services. Check with payers for the level of supervision required. The CMS has allowed an exception to the requirement for direct supervision (ie, physician presence in the office suite when staff perform activities) for CCM services provided to Medicare patients. This exception allows

staff to perform CCM activities under the physician's or QHP's general supervision (ie, supervising provider is available as needed by phone) as long as all other incident-to requirements are met. See Chapter 13, Allied Health and Clinical Staff Services, for information on incident-to requirements.

To report code **99490**, physicians must meet the required practice capabilities and supervise clinical staff activities of CCM. At least 20 minutes of clinical staff time spent in CCM activities must be documented. Time spent in activities personally performed by a physician may be counted toward CCM when provided on a date when no face-to-face service was provided. Chronic care management may be reported even if no substantial revision is made to the care plan.

Example

➤ **A 12-year-old has severe atopic disease and moderate persistent asthma, which has led to multiple ED visits, hospital admissions, lost school days, and behavioral adjustment reactions.** Clinical staff spend 30 minutes in the calendar month providing education; care plan creation, implementation, monitoring, and/or revision, including documentation; and facilitating access to community services.

Code **99490** is reported. *ICD-10-CM* codes reported are **J45.4-** (moderate persistent asthma [see *ICD-10-CM* reference for required fifth character]), **Z91.09** (other allergy status, other than to drugs and biological substances) or appropriate code for more specific atopic condition, **R43.2-** (adjustment disorders [fifth character required; see *ICD-10-CM* reference for specified disorder]), and codes for other acute or episodic conditions that affected CCM activities.

Complex CCM

99487   Complex chronic care management (CCM) services, with the following required elements:
- multiple (two or more) chronic conditions expected to last at least 12 months, or until the death of the patient,
- chronic conditions place the patient at significant risk of death, acute exacerbation/decompensation, or functional decline,
- establishment or substantial revision of a comprehensive care plan,
- moderate or high complexity medical decision-making;
- 60 minutes of clinical staff time directed by a physician or other qualified health care professional, per calendar month

+99489   each additional 30 minutes of clinical staff time directed by a physician or other qualified health care professional, per calendar month (List separately in addition to **99487**.)

> ### ~ More From the AAP ~
>
> For more examples of reporting complex chronic care management, see articles in the April 2017 *AAP Pediatric Coding Newsletter*™ at http://coding.aap.org (subscription required).

Complex CCM services (**99487** and **99489**) require additional physician work and clinical staff time. Medical decision-making (MDM) for the reporting period must be of moderate or high complexity. Code **99487** is reported when at least 60 and up to 89 minutes of clinical staff time is spent in care management activities. Code **99489** is reported in addition to **99487** when at least 90 minutes are spent in complex CCM and for each additional full 30 minutes of clinical staff time spent in care management activities during the calendar month. Do not report **99489** for care management services of less than 30 minutes beyond the first 60 minutes or last full 30 minutes of complex CCM services during a calendar month.

The reporting physician or other QHP must develop or substantially revise the plan of care for all health problems. (See the *CPT*® manual for a description of a typical care plan.) Complex CCM is not reported when the care plan is unchanged or requires minimal change (eg, medication change, adjustment of a treatment modality).

In contrast, substantial revision of the care plan is not required for CCM (**99490**, **99491**).

The significant difference in work and practice expense required for delivery of complex CCM services is reflected in the 2018 total non-facility relative value units (RVUs) assigned to codes **99487** (2.63), **99489** (1.31), and **99490** (1.19). For more information on how RVUs affect payment, see Chapter 5, Preventing Fraud and Abuse: Compliance, Audits, and Paybacks.

Example

➤ **A 6-year-old has spastic quadriplegia, gastrostomy, gastroesophageal reflux with recurrent bouts of aspiration pneumonia and mild persistent asthma, myoclonic epilepsy, failure to thrive, and expressive language disorder.** He receives home occupational, physical, and speech therapy services. During the course of a calendar month, the care plan is substantially revised to address changes in nutritional requirements, side effects of treatment, and need for additional home health services to address activities of daily living that the primary caregivers can no longer handle on their own. Significant time is spent assisting with development of an individual education plan for the patient. A referral and prior authorization for neurology consultation is necessary due to changes to the patient's preferred provider network. Clinical staff confirm that the patient's medical records are received by the consulting neurologist prior to the child's appointment and assist with arranging transportation services to the appointment. Clinical staff time of CCM services is 110 minutes.

   Codes **99487** and **99489** (1 unit) are reported. *ICD-10-CM* codes reported are **G80.0** (spastic quadriplegic cerebral palsy), **K21.9** (gastroesophageal reflux disease without esophagitis), **G40.409** (other generalized epilepsy and epileptic syndromes, not intractable, without status epilepticus), **R62.51** (failure to thrive [child]), and **F80.1** (expressive language disorder). If applicable during the reporting period, report **J69.0** (pneumonitis due to inhalation of food and vomit), **J45.3-** (mild persistent asthma [see *ICD-10-CM* reference for required fifth character]), and codes for other acute or episodic conditions that affected CCM activities.

CCM by a Physician or Other Qualified Health Care Professional

#●99491   Chronic care management services, provided personally by a physician or other qualified health care professional, at least 30 minutes of physician or other qualified health care professional time, per calendar month, with the following required elements: multiple (two or more) chronic conditions expected to last at least 12 months, or until the death of the patient, chronic conditions place the patient at significant risk of death, acute exacerbation/decompensation, or functional decline; comprehensive care plan established, implemented, revised, or monitored

   Code **99491** is reported when a physician or QHP *personally* performs care management services for 30 minutes or more within a calendar month. Codes for CCM reported based on time spent by clinical staff (**99487–99489** or **99490**) are not reported for the same calendar month as **99491**.

⦿ For **99491**, only count the time personally performed by the physician. Time spent by clinical staff is not counted toward the time to support **99491**.

⦿ Do not report **99491** for time of less than 30 minutes.

   This service includes all the same elements and practice specifications as that described by code **99490**, but *only the physician or QHP's time* of personally performed service (30 minutes or more) is counted toward the time of care management. No time spent by clinical staff may be counted toward the time for code **99491**. The list of services not reported in conjunction with CCM services provided under the general guidelines for reporting CCM are not reported in the same calendar month as **99491**.

Example

➤ **A 12-year-old has severe atopic disease and moderate persistent asthma, which has led to multiple ED visits, hospital admissions, lost school days, and behavioral adjustment reactions.** A physician or QHP spends 30 minutes in the calendar month providing counseling; care plan creation, implementation, monitoring, and/or revision, including documentation; and coordinating with other providers of care, including the school nurse. The physician or QHP reports code **99491** with *ICD-10-CM* codes, as in the example previously provided for code **99490**.

Coding Conundrum: Chronic Care Management or Care Plan Oversight?

Chronic care management (CCM) personally performed by a physician or other qualified health care professional (QHP) (99491) is similar to care plan oversight for patients in their home setting, under care of home health or hospice, or residing in a nursing facility (99339, 99340; 99374, 99375; 99377–99380). Which should be reported for a physician's or QHP's services?

There are differences that may determine the appropriate code to report, as shown in the table at the end of this box. For instance, CCM is reported by a physician whose practice has certain qualifications (eg, provides access to care providers or clinical staff 24 hours a day, 7 days a week, including providing patients and caregivers with a means to make contact with health care professionals in the practice to address urgent needs, regardless of the time of day or day of the week). Care plan oversight (CPO) does not require specific practice capabilities.

At the time of publication, the relative value units have not been assigned to code 99491, so a comparison of potential revenue is not included here.

	CPO (99339, 99340; 99374, 99375; 99377–99380)	CCM Personally Performed by the Physician or QHP (99491)
Time (minute)/month	At least 15	At least 30 (CCM)
Level of physician/QHP involvement	Required to personally perform	Required to personally perform services
Patient setting/type	Home, domiciliary, rest home, assisted living facility, or nursing facility	Home or domiciliary, rest home, or assisted living facility
Number of chronic conditions	At least 1	At least 2
Care plan work	Regular development and/or revision	Comprehensive care plan established, implemented, revised, or monitored

Abbreviations: CCM, chronic care management; CPO, care plan oversight.

Transitional Care Management Services

99495   Transitional care management services with the following required elements:
- ⦿ Communication (direct contact, telephone, electronic) with the patient and/or caregiver within 2 business days of discharge
- ⦿ Medical decision-making of at least moderate complexity during the service period
- ⦿ Face-to-face visit, within 14 calendar days of discharge

99496   Transitional care management services with the following required elements:
- ⦿ Communication (direct contact, telephone, electronic) with the patient and/or caregiver within 2 business days of discharge
- ⦿ Medical decision-making of high complexity during the service period
- ⦿ Face-to-face visit, within 7 calendar days of discharge

Transitional care management includes services provided to a new or an established patient whose medical and/or psychosocial problems require moderate- or high-complexity MDM during the transition from an inpatient hospital setting, observation care setting, or skilled nursing facility to the patient's home, domiciliary, rest home, or assisted living facility. Because moderate to high MDM is a requirement for TCM, follow-up care that includes low-intensity services such as relaying findings of test results,

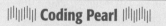
‖|‖|‖ Coding Pearl ‖|‖|‖

To provide direct patient contact within 2 days of discharge and to schedule appointments within 7 or 14 days, practices must have a process for receiving notification of observation and inpatient hospital discharges. Failure to make contact within 2 business days of discharge or to provide a face-to-face visit within 14 days of discharge eliminates the possibility of reporting transitional care management services.

which require only straightforward or low MDM (discussion of improving or normal laboratory results), are not reported with codes for TCM.

Transitional care management services were valued at 4.64 non-facility RVUs for code 99495 and 6.57 RVUs for code 99496 in the 2018 Medicare Physician Fee Schedule (MPFS). This equates to $167.04 and $236.52, respectively, for providing TCM services over a 30-day period.

- Transitional care management services are not limited to the attending provider of the related facility stay (eg, hospitalist) or any specific specialty. However, the individual reporting TCM services provides or oversees the management and/or coordination of services necessary *for all* the patient's medical conditions, psychosocial needs, and activities of daily living.
- Only one physician or other QHP may report these services and only once per patient within 30 days of discharge.
- The TCM services begin on the date of discharge and continue for the next 29 days.
- One face-to-face visit is included in addition to non–face-to-face services performed by the physician or other QHP and/or licensed clinical staff under the direction of the physician or other QHP.
- Non–face-to-face services provided by the physician or other QHP may include obtaining and reviewing the discharge information; reviewing, ordering, or following up on pending diagnostic tests and treatments; communication or interaction with or education provided to family, caregivers, or other QHPs; scheduling assistance for necessary follow-up services; and arranging referrals and community resources as necessary.
- Licensed clinical staff time (under the direction of the physician or other QHP) may include
  - Face-to-face and non–face-to-face time spent communicating with the patient and/or family, caregivers, other professionals, and agencies
  - Revising, documenting, and implementing the care plan
  - Collecting health outcomes data and registry documentation
  - Teaching patient and/or family/caregiver patient self-management
  - Assessment and support for adherence to treatment plan and medication management
  - Facilitating access to care and other services needed by the patient and/or family, including identification of community and health resources

Codes 99495 and 99496
- Require a face-to-face visit, initial patient contact, and medication reconciliation within specified time frames.
- *Medication reconciliation* refers to the process of avoiding inadvertent inconsistencies across transitions in care by reviewing the patient's complete medication regimen at the time of admission, transfer, and discharge and comparing it with the regimen being considered for the new setting of care.
- Medication management must occur *no later than* the date of the face-to-face visit.
- Code selection is based on the level of MDM and the date of the first face-to-face visit, as shown in **Table 12-3**. Note that all 3 components (communication within 2 business days, type of MDM, and timing of face-to-face visit) must be met to report TCM services, although only the MDM and time of the face-to-face visit differentiate code selection.

Table 12-3. Levels of Transitional Care Management

Type of Medical Decision-making	Face-to-face Visit Within 7 Days	Face-to-face Visit Within 8 to 14 Days
Moderate complexity	99495	99495
High complexity	99496	99495

- The first face-to-face visit is included in the TCM service and is not reported separately.
- Additional face-to-face E/M services during the 30-day TCM period but provided on dates subsequent to that of the first face-to-face visit may be separately reported.
- Another TCM service may not be reported by the same provider (or provider of the same group) for any subsequent discharge(s) within the 30 days.

- Hospital or observation discharge services (**99238**, **99239**, or **99217**) can be reported by the same physician reporting TCM services. Discharge services do not qualify as the required face-to-face visit for TCM.
- The TCM services cannot be reported when provided during a postoperative portion of the global period of a service reported by the same physician or other physician of the same specialty and same group practice.
- Services include care plan oversight (CPO) services (**99339**, **99340**, **99374–99380**), prolonged services without direct patient contact (**99358**, **99359**), home international normalized ratio monitoring (**93792**, **93793**), medical team conferences (**99366–99368**), education and training (**98960–98962**, **99071**, **99078**), telephone services (**98966–98968**, **99441–99443**), ESRD services (**90951–90970**), online medical evaluation services (**98969**, **99444**), preparation of special reports (**99080**), analysis of data (**99091**), CCM services (**99487–99490**), or medication therapy management services (**99605–99607**). These services may not be separately reported by the same physician or physicians of the same group practice during a period of TCM.
- Medical decision-making is defined by the E/M service guidelines. Medical decision-making over the service period reported is used to define the MDM of TCM. Documentation includes the timing of the initial post-discharge communication with the patient or caregivers, date of the face-to-face visit, and complexity of MDM.
- Only one individual may report these services and only once per patient within 30 days of discharge. Another TCM service may not be reported by the same individual or group for any subsequent discharge(s) within the 30 days.
- Follow payer guidelines for reporting. The CMS allows reporting of TCM services once the included face-to-face visit has been completed (ie, prior to the end of the service period). Other payers may not allow billing until the complete service period has elapsed.

Table 12-4 provides an overview of the patient population, work, and services not separately reported with TCM services.

Examples

➤ **A child with cystic fibrosis is discharged from the hospital after an admission for recurrent *Pseudomonas aeruginosa* infection.** Two days after discharge, the physician speaks with the mother. Clinical staff assesses adherence with the treatment plan and educates the parents on management of the child. The child is seen by the physician in follow-up 10 days after discharge. Medical decision-making is highly complex.

Code **99495** is reported. This service did not meet the requirements for code **99496** because the face-to-face visit did not occur within 7 days of discharge. Diagnosis codes may include **E84.0** (cystic fibrosis with pulmonary manifestations), **B96.5** (*Pseudomonas* as the cause of diseases classified elsewhere), and, if pneumonia persists, **J15.1** (pneumonia due to *Pseudomonas*).

➤ **A 6-month-old born at 25 weeks' gestation with a diagnosis of bronchopulmonary dysplasia resulting in chronic lung disease requiring home oxygen, diuretics, bronchodilators, and high-caloric formula is discharged from the hospital after an admission for respiratory failure.** The physician speaks with the mother the day after discharge. Clinical staff assesses adherence with the treatment plan and educates the parents on management of the child. The child is seen by the physician in follow-up in 5 days. Medical decision-making is highly complex.

Code **99496** is reported. Diagnosis is **P27.1** (bronchopulmonary dysplasia originating in the perinatal period) and **P07.24** (extreme immaturity of newborn, gestational age 25 completed weeks).

Table 12-4. Transitional Care Management Services

Service	Services Not Separately Reported in Same Calendar Month
99495,99496 Transitional care management services **Patient Population** ◉ Patients are new or established and have medical and/or psychosocial problems that require moderate- or high-complexity medical decision-making. ◉ Patients are transitioning from care in an inpatient hospital setting, partial hospital, observation status in a hospital, or skilled nursing facility/nursing facility to the patient's community setting.	**90951–90970** End-stage renal disease performed in an outpatient setting **98960–98962** Education and training for patient self-management by AHP **98966–98968** Telephone A/M service provided by AHP **98969** Online A/M service provided by AHP **99071** Educational supplies **99078** Physician or QHP educational services to a group **99080** Special reports such as insurance forms **99091** Collection and interpretation of physiologic data **99339,99340** Care plan oversight in home, domiciliary, or rest home **99358,99359** Prolonged E/M service before and/or after direct patient care **93792,93793** Home INR management **99366–99368** Medical team conferences **99374,99375** Supervision of patient under care of home health agency in home, domiciliary, or equivalent environment **99377,99378** Supervision of hospice patient **99379,99380** Supervision of a nursing facility patient **99441–99443** Telephone E/M service by a physician or other QHP **99444** Online E/M service by a physician or other QHP **99487–99491** Care management services **99605–99607** Medication therapy management by a pharmacist
Work Required ◉ Communication (direct contact, telephone, electronic) with the patient and/or caregiver within 2 business days of discharge. ◉ Medication reconciliation and management (ie, updating and reviewing medications and dosages) must occur no later than the date of the face-to-face visit. ◉ Face-to-face visit within 7 or 14 calendar days of discharge. ◉ Medical decision-making of moderate or high complexity during the service period.	

Abbreviations: AHP, allied health professional; A/M, assessment and management; E/M, evaluation and management; INR, international normalized ratio; QHP, qualified health care professional.

Medical Team Conferences

99366   Medical team conference with interdisciplinary team of health care professionals, face-to-face with patient and/or family, 30 minutes or more; participation by nonphysician qualified health care professional

99367   Medical team conference with interdisciplinary team of health care professionals, patient and/or family not present, 30 minutes or more; participation by physician

99368   Medical team conference with interdisciplinary team of health care professionals, patient and/or family not present, 30 minutes or more; participation by nonphysician qualified health care professional

Medical team conference codes are used to report participation by a minimum of 3 physicians and/or QHPs or NPPs of different specialties in conferences to coordinate or manage care and services for established patients with chronic or multiple health conditions (eg, child who is ventilator dependent with developmental delays, seizures, and gastrostomy tube for nutrition).

* Codes differentiate provider (physician vs other QHP or AHP) and between face-to-face and non–face-to-face (patient and/or family is not present) patient team conference services.

* *CPT*® code descriptors for medical team conferences do not differentiate between NPPs who do not independently report E/M services and QHPs who may do so when state licensing and scope of practice allow. However, *CPT* instructs that physicians or other QHPs who may report E/M services should report their time spent in a team conference with the patient and/or family present using E/M codes (and time as the key controlling factor for code selection when counseling and/or coordination of care dominates the service).

* If licensed QHPs (including clinical nurse specialists and clinical nurse practitioners) participated in a conference without direct physician supervision, they may report the service (**99367**) if it is within the state's scope of practice and they use their own National Provider Identifier. State Medicaid and commercial payers may follow these Medicare requirements or have their own specific rules.

* Medical team conferences may not be reported if the facility or organization is contractually obligated to provide the service, they are informal meetings or simple conversations between physicians and other QHPs and NPPs, or less than 30 minutes of conference time is spent in the team conferences.

* Code **99367** is the only code that may be reported by a physician, and it can only be reported when the patient and/or family is not present at the team conference.

* When the physician participates in a medical team conference with the patient and/or family present, the appropriate-level E/M code (eg, **99212–99215** if an outpatient setting) will be reported based on the place of service and total face-to-face time spent in counseling and/or coordination of care.

* Medical team conferences may be reported separately from other E/M services provided on the same day of service with modifier **25** appended to the appropriate-level E/M code, with the exception of neonatal and pediatric critical care (**99468–99476**) and intensive care (**99477–99480**). However, the time reported for these conferences may not be used in the determination of time for CPO (**99339**, **99340**; **99374–99380**), CCM services (**99487–99491**), TCM services (**99495** and **99496**), prolonged services (**99354–99359**), psychotherapy (**90832–90853**), or any E/M service.

Table 12-5 provides an overview of the patient population, work, and services not separately reported with medical team conference services.

Table 12-5. Medical Team Conference Services

Service	Services Not Separately Reported in Same Calendar Month
99366–99368 Medical team conference with interdisciplinary team of health care professionals (Physicians report other evaluation and management codes when patient or caregivers attend conference.) **Patient Population** Established patients with chronic and multiple health conditions or with congenital anomalies (eg, cleft lip and palate, craniofacial abnormalities) **Work Required** At least 30 minutes of face-to-face services from different specialties or disciplines Performed face-to-face evaluations or treatments of the patient, independent of any team conference, within the previous 60 days Presentation of findings and recommendations Formulation of a care plan and subsequent review/proofing of the plan	**99487–99491** Care management services **99495, 99496** Transitional care management services

Medical team conferences require

◉ Face-to-face participation by a minimum of 3 physicians and/or QHPs or NPPs from different subspecialties or disciplines (eg, speech-language pathologists, dietitians, social workers), with or without the presence of the patient, family member(s), community agencies, surrogate decision-maker(s) (eg, legal guardian), and/or caregiver(s).

◉ Active involvement in the development, revision, coordination, and implementation of health care services needed by the patient by each participant.

◉ Face-to-face evaluations and/or treatments by the participant that are separate from any team conference within the previous 60 days.

◉ Only one individual from the same specialty may report codes **99366–99368** for the same encounter. However, physicians of different specialties may each report their participation in a team conference.

◉ Medical record documentation supporting the participation of the physician or other QHP, the time spent from the beginning of the review of an individual patient until the conclusion of the review, and the contributed information and subsequent treatment recommendations.

Examples

➤ **A 14-year-old boy is under the care of a pediatrician, psychologist, and school counselor for injuries incurred during an explosive rage at school.** Over the past 3 months, the patient has shown increased anger with destructive behavior at home and school. *Without the patient or family present,* the pediatrician participates in a medical team conference with the psychologist and school psychologist. The psychologist discusses a change in diagnosis from bipolar disorder to disruptive mood dysregulation disorder and recommends changes to the patient's care plan. The patient's parents are unable to attend the conference but have expressed desire for new treatment options for their child. Each of the health care professionals participates in discussion and planning including changes to behavioral therapy and medication, potential side effects of treatment, and accommodations necessary at home and at school. The conference lasts 60 minutes.

Each participating physician (if they are different specialties and/or from different practices [ie, separate tax identification numbers])	*ICD-10-CM* **F34.81** (disruptive mood dysregulation disorder) The pediatrician may include codes for injuries if these conditions affected the plan of care. ***CPT*®** **99367**
Each nonphysician AHP (eg, respiratory therapist, occupational therapist)	*CPT* **99368**

The physician reports code **99367** because the patient and family were not present. If the patient and/or parents were present during the conference, the physician would report an applicable E/M service based on the time of counseling and/or coordination of care. Verify payer policies for non–face-to-face participation in a medical team conference (eg, by telephone or Internet). Participation in team conferences via real-time audiovisual technology *has not yet been added* to the lists of services reported with modifier **95** or the Medicare list of services approved for provision via telehealth.

➤ **A patient with mixed cerebral palsy requires coordination with multiple health care professionals (eg, physical and occupational therapists, neurologist, pediatrician).** Each participant in the conference has completed his or her evaluation of the patient within 60 days prior to the conference, and a team conference of 40 minutes is held to assess the current plan of care and therapy. The patient's family is present at this conference.

Because the patient's family is present, the participating physicians must report an appropriate E/M service rather than team conference services. The appropriate E/M code for the site of service (eg, **99215**), based on typical time, would be reported by each participating physician if they are different specialties and/or from different practices (ie, separate tax identification numbers). Code **99368** would be reported by the physical and occupational therapists. *ICD-10-CM* code **G80.8** (other cerebral palsy) is reported. Additional codes would be reported for any diagnoses addressed that are not integral to mixed cerebral palsy.

Care Plan Oversight Services

> ### ~ More From the AAP ~
>
> For more information on reporting transitional care management (**99495, 99496**), see "Transitional Care Management: Revisiting the Basics" in the July 2017 *AAP Pediatric Coding Newsletter*™ at http://coding. aap.org (subscription required).

99339   Individual physician supervision of a patient (patient not present) in home, domiciliary, or rest home (eg, assisted living facility) requiring complex and multidisciplinary care modalities involving regular physician development and/or revision of care plans, review of subsequent reports of patient status, review of related laboratory and other studies, communication (including telephone calls) for purposes of assessment or care decisions with health care professional(s), family member(s), surrogate decision-maker(s) (eg, legal guardian), and/or key caregiver(s) involved in patient's care, integration of new information into the medical treatment plan, and/or adjustment of medical therapy, within a calendar month; 15-29 minutes

+99340   ≥30 minutes (Report in addition to **99339**)

99374   Supervision of a patient under care of home health agency (patient not present) in home, domiciliary or equivalent environment (eg, Alzheimer's facility) requiring complex and multidisciplinary care modalities involving regular development and/or revision of care plans by that individual, review of subsequent reports of patient status, review of related laboratory and other studies, communication (including telephone calls) for purposes of assessment or care decisions with health care professional(s), family member(s), surrogate decision-maker(s) (eg, legal guardian) and/or key caregiver(s) involved in patient's care, integration of new information into the medical treatment plan and/or adjustment of medical therapy, within a calendar month; 15-29 minutes

+99375   ≥30 minutes (Report in addition to **99374**)

99377   Supervision of a hospice patient (patient not present) requiring complex and multidisciplinary care modalities involving regular development and/or revision of care plans by that individual, review of subsequent reports of patient status, review of related laboratory and other studies, communication (including telephone calls) for purposes of assessment or care decisions with health care professional(s), family member(s), surrogate decision-maker(s) (eg, legal guardian) and/or key caregiver(s) involved in patient's care, integration of new information into the medical treatment plan and/or adjustment of medical therapy, within a calendar month; 15-29 minutes

+99378   ≥30 minutes (Report in addition to **99377**)

99379   Supervision of a nursing facility patient (patient not present) requiring complex and multidisciplinary care modalities involving regular development and/or revision of care plans by that individual, review of subsequent reports of patient status, review of related laboratory and other studies, communication (including telephone calls) for purposes of assessment or care decisions with health care professional(s), family member(s), surrogate decision-maker(s) (eg, legal guardian) and/or key caregiver(s) involved in patient's care, integration of new information into the medical treatment plan and/or adjustment of medical therapy, within a calendar month; 15-29 minutes

+99380   ≥30 minutes (Report in addition to **99379**)

Care plan oversight is recurrent physician or QHP supervision of a complex patient or a patient who requires multidisciplinary care and ongoing physician or QHP involvement. Chronic care management or TCM services would not be reported in conjunction with CPO services. (See Coding Conundrum: Chronic Care Management or Care Plan Oversight? earlier in this chapter to compare CPO to CCM services.) Care plan oversight services are not face-to-face and reflect the complexity and time required to supervise the care of the patient. The codes are reported separately from E/M office visits.

Medicare requires the use of Level II Healthcare Common Procedure Coding System codes for CPO services provided to patients under the care of a home health agency (G0181) or hospice (G0182). To report these G codes, Medicare requires a minimum of 30 minutes of physician supervision per calendar month. Because some state Medicaid programs may follow suit, check with your payer to learn its requirements for reporting these services.

Table 12-6 provides a comparison of CPO services, including patient population, work included, and services not separately reported. (Work included and services not separately reported are the same for all CPO services).

Care plan oversight services

⊙ Are reported only by the individual (physician/QHP) who has the predominant supervisory role in the care of the patient or is the sole provider of the services. A face-to-face service with the patient must have been provided by the physician prior to assuming CPO.

⊙ Include

❖ Regular development and/or revision of care plans

❖ Review of subsequent reports of the patient's status

❖ Review of related laboratory or other diagnostic studies

❖ Communication (including telephone calls) for purposes of assessment or care decisions with health care professionals, family members, surrogate decision-makers (eg, legal guardians), and/or key caregivers involved in the patient's care

❖ Integration of new information into the medical treatment plan or adjustment of medical therapy

❖ Team conferences

❖ Prolonged E/M service before and/or after direct patient care when the same time is attributed to CPO

Table 12-6. Care Plan Oversight Services

Service—Codes and Patient Population

Note: Patients receiving care plan oversight require complex and multidisciplinary care modalities involving regular physician development and/or revision of care plans.

99339, 99340 Care plan oversight in home, domiciliary, or rest home (eg, assisted living facility) *Patient Population:* Patients in home settings not under the care of a home health or hospice agency	**99374, 99375** Supervision of patient under care of home health agency in home, domiciliary, or equivalent environment *Patient Population:* Patients are under the care of a home health agency.
99377, 99378 Supervision of hospice patient *Patient Population:* Patients are under the care of a hospice agency.	**99379, 99380** Supervision of a nursing facility patient *Patient Population:* Patients reside in nursing facility.

Work Included in Care Plan Oversight Services

⊙ At least 15 minutes by physician in regular development and/or revision of care plans
⊙ Review of subsequent reports of the patient's status
⊙ Review of related laboratory or other diagnostic studies
⊙ Communication for purposes of assessment or care decisions
⊙ Integration of new information into the medical treatment plan or adjustment of medical therapy

Services Not Separately Reported in Same Calendar Month[a]

98966–98968[a] Telephone A/M service provided by AHP
98969[a] Online A/M service provided by AHP
99091 Collection and interpretation of physiologic data
99358, 99359[a] Prolonged E/M service before and/or after direct patient care
99441–99443[a] Telephone E/M service by a physician/QHP
99444[a] Online E/M service by a physician or QHP
99487–99491 Care management services
99495, 99496 Transitional care management services

Abbreviations: AHP, allied health professional; A/M, assessment and management; E/M, evaluation and management; QHP, qualified health care professional.

[a] Telephone and online assessments and prolonged physician service before and/or after direct patient care may be separately reported when the time of each service is distinct and nonoverlapping with time spent in care plan oversight.

- Require recurrent supervision of therapy. Provision of very low-intensity or infrequent supervision services is considered part of the pre- and post-encounter work for home, office/outpatient, hospital, and nursing facility or domiciliary visit codes. For example, a physician monitors test results from follow-up bilirubin testing for a newborn discharged from the hospital with low risk for hyperbilirubinemia. The test results are called in to the physician's office and the physician relays the findings to the mother. These low-intensity services would be included in the post-service work of the hospital services.

- Are reported once per month based on the amount of time spent by the physician during that calendar month.

- Cumulative time begins with the first day of the month and ends with the last day of the month.

- Are reported based on the patient's location or status (eg, home, hospice) and the total time spent by the physician within a calendar month. Less than 15 minutes' cumulative time within a calendar month cannot be reported.

- Are reported separately from other office or outpatient, hospital, home, nursing facility, or domiciliary E/M services.

- Do not require specific practice capabilities as are defined for CCM services.

Time spent on the following activities *may not* be considered CPO:

- Travel time to or from the facility or place of domicile
- Services furnished by clinical staff (ancillary or incident-to staff)
- Very low-intensity or infrequent supervision services included in the pre- and post-encounter work for an E/M service
- Interpretation of laboratory or other diagnostic studies associated with a face-to-face E/M service
- Informal consultations with health professionals not involved in the patient's care
- Routine postoperative care provided during the global surgery period of a procedure
- Time spent on telephone calls or online medical evaluation or in medical team conferences if they are separately reported with codes **99441–99444** or **99367**

> ||||||| **Coding Pearl** |||||||
>
> Unlike nonphysician chronic care management and transitional care management services, time included in care plan oversight is only that of the physician or other qualified health care professional and not that of clinical staff.

A CPO log serves as medical record documentation and as an encounter form for reporting purposes. A template is found in Appendix IV and online at www.aap.org/cfp (access code AAPCFP24). See Care Plan Oversight Encounter Worksheet on the next page for an example of a completed CPO log.

Advance Care Planning

99497   Advance care planning including the explanation and discussion of advance directives such as standard forms (with completion of such forms, when performed), by the physician or other qualified health care professional; first 30 minutes, face-to-face with the patient, family member(s) and/or surrogate

+99498   each additional 30 minutes (List separately in addition to code for primary procedure)

Codes **99497** and **99498** include

- Face-to-face service by a physician or QHP to a patient, family member, or surrogate spent in counseling and discussion of advance directives
- Completion of forms, when applicable (eg, Health Care Proxy, Durable Power of Attorney for Health Care, Living Will, and Medical Orders for Life-Sustaining Treatment)

Active management of problems is not included in advance care planning. Other E/M services provided on the same date as advance care planning may be separately reported with the exceptions of hourly critical care services (**99291**, **99292**), inpatient neonatal and pediatric critical care (**99468**, **99469**; **99471–99476**), and initial and continuing intensive care services (**99477–99480**). Do not report codes **99497** and **99498** in conjunction with codes **99291**, **99292**, **99468**, **99469**, **99471–99476**, or **99477–99480**.

Do not report code **99497** for less than 16 minutes of physician face-to-face time.

Care Plan Oversight Encounter Worksheet

Physician: <u>Dr IM Good, MD</u>   Patient Name: <u>Babe Ruth</u>

Services Provided:

The letter that corresponds with each service provided should be placed in column #2.

A. Regular physician development and/or revision of care plans

B. Review of subsequent reports of patient status

C. Review of related laboratory or other studies

D. Communication (including telephone calls not separately reported with codes 99441–99443) with other health care professionals involved in patient's care

E. Integration of new information into the medical treatment plan and/or adjustment of medical therapy

F. Other (Attach additional explanatory materials on the services provided.)

Date of Service XX/XX/XXXX	Services Provided	Contact Name and Agency	Start Time	End Time	Total Minutes	Monthly Subtotal
08/04/2019	C, D	Consultation with pediatric endocrinologist	12:00 pm	12:06 pm	6	6
08/04/2019	D, A	Phone call to mother, change in medication	12:15 pm	12:21 pm	6	12
08/15/2019	C	Review of individual education plan (IEP)	5:15 pm	5:25 pm	10	22
08/16/2019	D	Phone calls to mother and teacher re: changes in IEP	5:30 pm	5:45 pm	15	37

Explanation for additional services provided:

Date:_____/_____

_____

Date:_____/_____

_____

Date:_____/_____

_____

Physician Signature: IM Good, MD Date 01/31/2018

See www.aap.org/cfp for an online version of this worksheet (access code AAPCFP24).

Advance care planning services may be considered bundled to enhanced payment methodologies and not separately paid. However, *CPT®* requires reporting of the code that is specific to the service provided regardless of payment policy. Advance care planning services should not be reported as another service (eg, office visit) in an effort to avoid denial as a bundled service.

Relative value units assigned for a non-facility site of service are 2.39 for 99497 and 2.11 for 99498 (based on 2018 MPFS), making the allowed amounts $86.02 and $75.94, respectively, when paid at the 2018 Medicare conversion factor of $35.99 per RVU.

Example

➤ **A child and his parents, who have learned at a recent visit that the child's prognosis is poor, return for advance care planning.** The physician spends 50 minutes face-to-face with the patient and parents and assesses their understanding of the diagnosis and confirms and documents the desire to limit lifesaving measures and decisions regarding palliative care. A plan of care is developed and documented, and an appointment with the supportive care team at the hospital is scheduled to provide additional counseling to the family and connection to other supportive services.

Chapter 12: Managing Chronic and Complex Conditions

The physician may report codes **99497** and **99498** with 1 unit for the 50 minutes of face-to-face time spent providing the advance care planning. Because the *CPT®* prefatory language and code descriptors for advance care planning do not include other instruction on the time required for reporting, these services may be reported based on general *CPT* instruction to report when the midpoint is passed (eg, 1 unit of **99498** may be reported for services of 46–75 minutes). Exceptions may apply for payers with policy requiring that the time be met or exceeded.

Teaching Point: In this vignette, the service was aimed at advance planning of what care the patient and parents wish to be provided. This is best described by advanced care planning codes **99497** and **99498**. *CPT* instructs that codes reported should accurately describe the service rendered and physicians should not report a code that merely approximates the service provided, so it would be inappropriate to report another service that may have higher RVUs and payment values. However, when a payer does not recognize these codes or the main reason for an encounter is other than advance care planning, consultation codes **99241–99245** or **99251–99255** or other E/M service codes (eg, **99212–99215**) may be appropriately reported (see Chapter 7, Evaluation and Management Services in the Office and Outpatient Clinics, and Chapter 16, Noncritical Hospital Evaluation and Management Services, for discussion of reporting to payers that do not accept consultation codes).

Psychiatric Collaborative Care Management Services

99492 Initial psychiatric collaborative care management, first 70 minutes in the first calendar month of behavioral health care manager activities, in consultation with a psychiatric consultant, and directed by the treating physician or other qualified health care professional, with the following required elements:

- outreach to and engagement in treatment of a patient directed by the treating physician or other qualified health care professional;
- initial assessment of the patient, including administration of validated rating scales, with the development of an individualized treatment plan;
- review by the psychiatric consultant with modifications of the plan if recommended;
- entering patient in a registry and tracking patient follow-up and progress using the registry, with appropriate documentation, and participation in weekly caseload consultation with the psychiatric consultant; and
- provision of brief interventions using evidence-based techniques such as behavioral activation, motivational interviewing, and other focused treatment strategies.

99493 Subsequent psychiatric collaborative care management, first 60 minutes in a subsequent month of behavioral health care manager activities, in consultation with a psychiatric consultant, and directed by the treating physician or other qualified health care professional, with the following required elements:

- tracking patient follow-up and progress using the registry, with appropriate documentation;
- participation in weekly caseload consultation with the psychiatric consultant;
- ongoing collaboration with and coordination of the patient's mental health care with the treating physician or other qualified health care professional and any other treating mental health providers;
- additional review of progress and recommendations for changes in treatment, as indicated, including medications, based on recommendations provided by the psychiatric consultant;
- provision of brief interventions using evidence-based techniques such as behavioral activation, motivational interviewing, and other focused treatment strategies;
- monitoring of patient outcomes using validated rating scales; and
- relapse prevention planning with patients as they achieve remission of symptoms and/or other treatment goals and are prepared for discharge from active treatment.

+99494   Initial or subsequent psychiatric collaborative care management, each additional 30 minutes in a calendar month of behavioral health care manager activities, in consultation with a psychiatric consultant, and directed by the treating physician or other qualified health care professional (List separately in addition to code for primary procedure)
         (Use **99494** in conjunction with **99492, 99493**)

Psychiatric collaborative care management services are provided to patients who have a new or existing psychiatric disorder that requires a behavioral health assessment; care plan implementation, revision, or monitoring; and provision of brief interventions. Psychiatric collaborative care management services involve the efforts of a team of 3 health care professionals: a treating physician or QHP, a behavioral health care manager, and a psychiatric consultant. The treating physician or QHP reports codes **99492–99494** when all requirements for reporting are met. Evaluation and management and other services may be reported separately by the same physician or QHP during the same calendar month. Please see Chapter 14, Mental and Behavioral Health Services, for more information on PCCM services.

General Behavioral Health Integration Care Management

99484   Care management services for behavioral health conditions, at least 20 minutes of clinical staff time, directed by a physician or other qualified health care professional, per calendar month, with the following required elements:
- Initial assessment or follow-up monitoring, including the use of applicable validated rating scales;
- Behavioral health care planning in relation to behavioral/psychiatric health problems, including revision for patients who are not progressing or whose status changes;
- Facilitating and coordinating treatment such as psychotherapy, pharmacotherapy, counseling and/or psychiatric consultation; and
- Continuity of care with a designated member of the care team

Code **99484** was created to allow for reporting provision of behavioral health integration care management services by other than the PCCM model. The services are performed by clinical staff for a patient with a behavioral health (including substance use) condition that requires care management services (face-to-face or non–face-to-face) of 20 or more minutes in a calendar month. The service must be initiated and supervised by a physician or QHP who may report E/M services (ie, is not reported by NPPs whose scope of practice does not include E/M services under state regulations or when not allowed by payer policy). A documented treatment plan is required as well as all activities specified in the code descriptor. Please see Chapter 14, Mental and Behavioral Health Services, for more information on behavioral health integration care management services.

Prolonged Services Without Direct Patient Contact

99358   Prolonged evaluation and management service before and/or after direct patient care; first hour
+99359   each additional 30 minutes (Use in conjunction with code **99358**)

Guidelines for reporting non-direct prolonged services include
- Reported when a physician or QHP provides prolonged service that does not involve face-to-face care. Does not include time spent by clinical staff.
- Service must be related to another face-to-face physician or other QHP service. The primary service may be an E/M service (with or without an assigned average time), a procedure, or other non–face-to-face service codes. However, prolonged service must relate to a service or patient where direct (face-to-face) patient care has occurred or will occur and to ongoing patient management.
- The place of service does not affect reporting.
- May be reported on a different date than the related primary service. *CPT*® does not specify a time frame (eg, within 1 week of related service) for provision of prolonged service before and/or after direct patient care.

- Cannot be reported for time spent in any of the following:
  - Medical team conferences (**99366–99368**)
  - Care plan oversight services (**99339, 99340; 99374–99380**)
  - Online medical evaluations (**99444**)
  - Transitional care management (**99495, 99496**)
- Do not report prolonged service during the same month with
  - Chronic care management services (**99487–99491**)
  - Care management for behavioral health conditions (**99484**)
  - Psychiatric collaborative care management (**99492–99494**)
- Time is met when the midpoint is passed.
  - Less than 30 minutes' total duration on a given date cannot be reported.
  - Less than 15 minutes beyond the first hour or beyond the final 30 minutes is not reported separately. Code **99359** may also be used to report the final 15 to 30 minutes of prolonged service on a given date. **Table 12-7** breaks down the time requirements.

Table 12-7. Time Requirements for Non–face-to-face Prolonged Services

Total Duration of Prolonged Service Without Direct Face-to-face Contact	Code(s) and Units of Service Reported
<30 min	Not separately reported
30–74 min	**99358** x 1
75–104 min	**99358** x 1 and **99359** x 1
≥105 min	**99358** x 1 and **99359** x 2

See Chapter 7, Evaluation and Management Services in the Office and Outpatient Clinics, and Chapter 16, Noncritical Hospital Evaluation and Management Services, for discussion of *face-to-face* prolonged services.

Example

➤ A physician requested and received medical records from the former physician of a 6-year-old who was born with hypoplastic left heart syndrome. The patient has undergone staged palliative reconstruction, including Fontan procedure with extracardiac conduit. The child has residual supraventricular tachycardic arrhythmia. On a day separate from any face-to-face service, the physician spends 35 minutes reviewing and summarizing the medical records and documents his time in the medical record.

Prolonged physician services without direct patient contact (30–74 minutes)	**ICD-10-CM** **Q23.4** (hypoplastic left heart syndrome) **I49.1** (supraventricular tachycardia) **Z95.818** (presence of other cardiac implants and grafts)
	CPT® **99358**

||ı|ı||ı| **Coding Pearl** ||ı|ı||ı|

Codes **99358** and **99359** must be related to an evaluation and management service, procedure, or other non–face-to-face service with a published maximum time.

||ı|ı||ı| **Coding Pearl** ||ı|ı||ı|

Codes for congenital malformation or deformity may be used throughout the life of the patient. If a congenital malformation or deformity has been *completely repaired*, a personal history code should be used to identify the history of the (corrected) malformation or deformity.

Chapter 12: Managing Chronic and Complex Conditions

Remote Physiologic Monitoring

#●99457   Remote physiologic monitoring treatment management services, 20 minutes or more of clinical staff/physician/other qualified health care professional time in a calendar month requiring interactive communication with the patient/caregiver during the month

Code **99457** is reported for time spent managing care when the results from a monitoring device(s) are used for treatment management services. This code requires 20 or more minutes of time spent using the results of physiologic monitoring to manage a patient under a specific treatment plan. Please see Chapter 20, Digital Medicine Services: Technology-Enhanced Care Delivery, for more information on this and other remote physiologic monitoring services.

Interprofessional Telephone/Internet Consultations

Patients with chronic conditions may often require collaboration between their primary pediatrician and a subspecialist. A consultation request by a patient's attending or primary physician or other QHP soliciting opinion and/or treatment advice *by telephone, Internet, or EHR* from a physician with specialty expertise (consultant) is reported by the consultant with interprofessional consultation codes **99446–99449** or **99451**. This consultation does not require face-to-face contact with the patient by the consultant. Code **99457** may be reported when 16 to 30 minutes is spent by the requesting individual in a service day preparing for the referral and/or communicating with the consultant. Alternatively, prolonged service codes may be reported by the requesting individual when supported by the time of service. Please see Chapter 20, Digital Medicine Services: Technology-Enhanced Care Delivery, for more information on interprofessional consultations.

Telephone Services

99441   Telephone E/M service by a physician or other qualified health care professional who may report evaluation and management services provided to an established patient, parent, or guardian not originating from a related E/M service provided within the previous 7 days nor leading to an E/M service or procedure within the next 24 hours or soonest available appointment; 5–10 minutes of medical discussion

99442   11–20 minutes of medical discussion

99443   21–30 minutes of medical discussion

98966   Telephone assessment and management services provided by a qualified nonphysician health care professional to an established patient, parent, or guardian not originating from a related assessment and management service provided within the previous 7 days nor leading to an assessment and management service or procedure within the next 24 hours or soonest available appointment; 5–10 minutes of medical discussion

98967   11–20 minutes of medical discussion

98968   21–30 minutes of medical discussion

Telephone services (**99441–99443**) are non–face-to-face E/M services provided to a patient using the telephone by a physician or other QHP, who may report E/M services. Codes **98966–98968** are used to report telephone assessment and management services by health care professionals who may not report E/M services.

Guidelines for reporting of telephone assessment and management services are the same as those for physician and QHP telephone E/M services.

Codes 99441–99443 *may* be reported when	Codes 99441–99443 are *not* reported when
The call was initiated by an established patient or guardian of an established patient.	The call results in a face-to-face encounter within 24 hours.
They include physician management of a new problem that does not result in an office visit within 24 hours from the telephone call or at the next available urgent visit appointment.	There was a face-to-face encounter related to the problem in the previous 7 days from the telephone call.
They include physician management of an existing problem for which the patient was not seen in a face-to-face encounter in the previous 7 days from the telephone call (physician requested or unsolicited patient follow-up) or within the postoperative period of a performed and reported procedure.	The call occurs within the postoperative period of a reported procedure.
The physician documentation of telephone calls includes the date of the call, name and telephone number of the patient, name of person and relationship of the caller, type of service provided (eg, provide consultation or medical management, initiate or adjust therapy, report results), and the time spent in the encounter.	The call occurs within 7 days of a previously reported telephone management service.
	Care plan oversight (99339, 99340, or 99374–99380), care management (99487–99490, or transitional care management (99495 and 99496) services are reported and the calls are included as part of these services.
	Non–face-to-face communication is between the physician and other health care professionals. If applicable, the services may be reported using non–face-to-face prolonged physician service codes 99358 and 99359 or as part of care plan oversight or care management services (99339 and 99340, 99374–99380, 99487–99490, 99495 and 99496).
	Performed by a provider who may not report evaluation and management services. (See codes 98966–98968 for services by qualified providers who may not report evaluation and management services.)

Online Medical Services

An online electronic medical evaluation (99444) is a non–face-to-face E/M service by a physician or other QHP who may report E/M services to a patient using Internet resources in response to a patient's online inquiry. This is in contrast with telemedicine services, which represent interactive audio and video telecommunications systems that permit real-time communication between the physician, at the distant site, and the patient, at the originating site. Code 98969 is used by a qualified AHP to report an online assessment and management service. The reporting guidelines for code 98969 are the same as those required for online services provided by the physician or QHP.

Please see Chapter 20, Digital Medicine Services: Technology-Enhanced Care Delivery, for more information on online medical services.

After-hours and Special Services

Codes **99050–99060** are used to report services that are provided after hours or on an emergency basis and are an adjunct to the basic E/M service provided. Refer to Chapter 7, Evaluation and Management Services in the Office and Outpatient Clinics, for more details on after-hours and special services codes.

Reporting a Combination of Non–face-to-face Services

When CCM or TCM services do not apply or a payer does not provide benefits for these services, it may be necessary to report a combination of codes for non–face-to-face services provided to a child with special health care needs. These may include CPO, online or telephone E/M services, prolonged services, and team conference services.

Be sure to review payer guidance on reporting of these services, as National Correct Coding Initiative edits or other payment policy may require appending modifiers to indicate distinct periods were spent in the provision of each service. For instance, prolonged E/M service is bundled to CPO, but a modifier may be appended to indicate distinct services within the same reporting period. Guidance for reporting and coverage may vary.

Example

➤ **On January 3, several days prior to performing a preventive medicine visit on a 4-year-old new patient with cerebral palsy, the physician reviews medical records that were brought in by the mother.** It takes the physician 30 minutes at noon and another 20 minutes after regular office hours to complete the review. The total time spent is documented.

On January 5, the child is seen by the pediatrician in the morning and a preventive medicine visit is performed and documented. During the visit, the mother relates that the child has had wheezing for 1 day and increased gastroesophageal reflux. A detailed history is performed for the wheezing and reflux. Medications are prescribed and reflux precautions are reviewed in detail.

Later that day, the physician spends 40 minutes developing a care plan and an emergency information form to summarize the medical condition(s), medications, and special health care needs that will be used to inform other health care professionals of the child's special health conditions and needs. The nurse (under direction of the physician) spends 35 minutes scheduling appointments with a neurologist, physical therapist, and social worker.

The next day, an additional 12 minutes is spent by the physician on the telephone with the patient's mother to discuss the care plan and coordination of care. All services and the time spent are documented on the CPO log. On January 16, the child's mother calls the physician because she is concerned that the child will have problems adjusting to his new school. The physician spends a total of 15 minutes on the telephone with the mother to discuss how she should handle the issue. The physician documents the time spent on the telephone call, the history, and issues discussed.

On January 24, the pediatrician attends a medical team conference with the child's neurologist, physical therapist, occupational therapist, and social worker to discuss the current plan of care and therapy and make appropriate revisions. The patient and family are not present at this conference. The conference lasts 35 minutes. Each participant documents the total time spent in conference and a summary of the treatment recommendations and plans.

Pediatrician reports		
	ICD-10-CM	**CPT®**
January 3	**G80.9**(infantile cerebral palsy, unspecified)	**99358**(prolonged E/M service before and/or after direct patient care; first hour)
January 5	**Z00.121**(routine child health check with abnormal findings) **K21.9**(gastroesophageal reflux without esophagitis) **R06.2**(wheezing) **G80.9**(infantile cerebral palsy, unspecified)	**99382**(preventive medicine visit, 1–4 years of age, new patient) **99214 25**(detailed history, moderate-level MDM)
January 16	**Z71.89**(other specified counseling)	**99442**(telephone E/M service; 11–20 minutes of medical discussion) Alternatively, the time spent on the telephone call could be included in the CPO time.
January 24	**G80.9**	**99367**(medical team conference)
January 31	**G80.9**	**99340**(care plan oversight, patient at home, ≥30 minutes) Total physician time spent over the course of the calendar month was 52 minutes (does not include time spent providing other reported services).

Teaching Point: In this vignette, the practice is not reporting CCM services (**99490**or **9949**) although the time requirements for each were met. The physician instead reports code **99340**(CPO, patient at home, ≥30 minutes), which does not require the practice capabilities or extensive medical conditions of CCM. Code **99340**is supported by the 40 minutes of the physician's time spent on January 5 and the 12 minutes spent on the physician-initiated call on January 6, which were not included in other reported services. Code **99442** is applicable for the phone call initiated by the patient's mother on January 16, and this time is not included in the time of CPO.

Practices with the capabilities required for reporting CCM services in lieu of CPO may still report the CPO codes when the service provided and nature of the patient presentation support reporting CPO services. CPO code **99340**is assigned 3.07 RVUs in the MPFS. Code **99490**(≥20 minutes CCM by clinical staff) is assigned 1.19 RVUs. The value assigned to code **99491**was unavailable at the time of publication. Physicians must determine the appropriate code selection based on the practice capabilities, services rendered, and nature of the patient presentation.

CHAPTER 13

Allied Health and Clinical Staff Services

Contents

In the context of providing comprehensive and high-quality primary care to their patients, pediatric physicians are including more nonphysician providers (NPPs) in their practices. In addition to advanced practice providers, such as nurse practitioners and physician assistants, physicians are also including other allied health professionals (AHPs) in their practices to provide specialized services, such as nutrition counseling, condition-specific self-management education, and mental and behavioral health services.

This chapter focuses on services that are provided by health care professionals other than physicians. These services may be provided by AHPs within a physician's group practice based on a physician or other qualified health care professional's (QHP) orders.

Terminology

Of particular importance to correct reporting of nonphysician services is identifying the providers included when terms such as "physician or other qualified health care professional" or "qualified, nonphysician health care professional" are used in *Current Procedural Terminology* (CPT®) and/or payer instruction.

Current Procedural Terminology Provider Definitions

Current Procedural Terminology (CPT) provides definitions of providers as follows:
- **Physician or other qualified health care professional:** An individual who is qualified by education, training, licensure/regulation (when applicable), and facility privileging (when applicable) who performs a professional service within his or her scope of practice and independently reports that professional service
- **Clinical staff member:** A person who works under the supervision of a physician or other qualified health care professional and who is allowed by law, regulation, and facility policy to perform or assist in the performance of a specific professional service but does not individually report that professional service

Throughout the *CPT* code set, the use of terms such as "physician," "qualified health care professional," or "individual" is not intended to indicate that other entities may not report the service. In selected instances, specific instructions may define a service as limited to professionals or other entities (eg, hospital, home health agency).

Clinical staff member is used in *CPT* mostly in the context of staff who provide components of physician or QHP services, such as transitional care management (TCM) and chronic care management (CCM), and services that are always billed by a supervising physician or QHP (eg, nurse visit, medication administration), as discussed in the Medicare Incident-to Requirements: Supervision of Nonphysician Health Care Professionals section later in this chapter.

The *CPT* definition of physician or other QHP creates a broad category of providers (eg, advanced practice providers, therapists, social workers). The definition of *physician and other QHP* is used in relation to services such as evaluation and management (E/M) (99201–99499) and immunization administration with physician counseling (90460, 90461) and to codes *not reported* by physicians, such as genetic counseling (96040).

However, this definition may be confusing, as payer policies commonly differentiate QHPs such as advanced practice providers, who may perform and prescribe services much like a physician, from those who provide specialized services under the supervision and order of a physician or advanced practice provider. To aid in differentiating how services are typically reported by these subcategories of QHPs, the following definitions will apply in discussions and examples in this chapter:

- **Qualified health care professional:** Signifies advanced practice providers, such as advanced practice nurses, clinical nurse specialists, and physician assistants, whose scope of practice includes E/M services beyond minimal services incident to a physician (ie, 99211)
- **Clinical staff member** (as defined by *CPT* in differentiating from a physician or QHP): A health care team member who works under the supervision of a physician or other QHP and who is allowed by law, regulation, and facility policy to perform or assist in the performance of a specific professional service but *does not individually report that professional service*. These include, but are not limited to, registered nurses (RNs), licensed practical nurses (LPNs), and medical assistants (MAs). Staff who perform *only administrative functions* such as receptionist, scheduling, billing, dictation, or scribing are not clinical staff for coding purposes.

☀ **Allied health professional:** Represents a broad category of health care professionals who typically would not independently prescribe and manage, whose professional services are typically performed under the order and supervision of a physician or QHP, and whose scope of practice does not include E/M services beyond 99211. Sometimes they are able to bill under their own National Provider Identifier (NPI). This category includes providers such as clinical psychologists, dietitians/nutritionists, and lactation consultants.

Including Nonphysician Providers in Your Practice

Services such as medical nutrition therapy by a registered dietitian or nutritionist or behavioral health assessment by a licensed social worker or licensed psychologist may be provided within a physician group practice and can be an integral part of providing a full scope of care in the medical home. However, billing and coding of these services must align not only with coding guidelines but also state scope of practice (see the Scope of Practice Laws section later in this chapter) and individual payer policies on credentialing, contracting, and billing for services of the specific NPP. *Before including AHPs within your group practice,* it is important to seek expert advice on related state regulations for scope of practice and supervision requirements, enrollment and payment policies of the group's most common payers, and best practices in employment and/or contractual agreements. The number of services that may be provided can be estimated based on current patient diagnoses or history of referral for services. Reports from electronic health records or billing software may be used in this estimation (eg, report of number of unique patient accounts containing a diagnosis indicating mental or behavioral health conditions).

When physicians choose to arrange for services provided within their practice by AHPs who are not employed or contracted with their group practice, additional counsel should be obtained to avoid conflict with anti-kickback and/or self-referral regulations.

Payment for AHP services begins with negotiating and contracting with payers for coverage and payment of services as described by *CPT®* and/or Healthcare Common Procedure Coding System (HCPCS) codes. (A list of HCPCS codes that may be used to report nonphysician education services is included in the Healthcare Common Procedure Coding System Codes section later in this chapter.) Payers may pay separately for these services when your practice can demonstrate the overall cost savings (eg, decrease in physician or emergency department visits, decreased hospital care) that may be achieved through expanded care in the physician practice. If payers do not agree to directly compensate for individual services, consider opportunities for shared savings and other revenue that may be realized when AHP services support quality improvement initiatives (eg, per-member, per-month compensation for meeting certain quality measures) and redirection of physician and QHP time to services that are restricted to or best delivered within their scope of practice. (For more on quality and performance measurement, see Chapter 3, Coding to Demonstrate Quality and Value.)

Physicians should be especially aware of each payer's policy addressing use of E/M codes for services provided by AHPs or clinical staff. Medicare and payers that adopt Medicare policy do not allow reporting of E/M services provided by AHPs or clinical staff other than 99211 (E/M visit not requiring physician face-to-face service).

Example

CPT describes codes 99401–99404 as representing services provided face-to-face by a physician or other QHP for the purpose of promoting health and preventing illness or injury. However, some payers directly instruct that codes such as 99401 may be reported for specific services by specific AHPs, such as medical nutritionists or certified lactation consultants. See the Lactation Services section later in this chapter for an example of payer policy that includes reporting of codes 99401–99404 for lactation counseling by an RN.

Always keep a printed or electronic copy of payer guidance that is in conflict with *CPT* or standard billing practices.

Scope of Practice Laws

Scope of practice is terminology that is used by state licensing boards for various professions to define the procedures, actions, and processes that are permitted for a licensed individual.

The level of medical responsibility or health services (boundaries within which a health care professional may practice) or range of activities that a practitioner is legally authorized to perform is based on his or her specific education and experience.

Physicians, RNs, clinical nurse practitioners, physician assistants, LPNs, physical therapists, and nutritionists are among some of the professions for which scope of practice laws are defined. However, it can vary by state. Some states limit the autonomous practice of advanced practice professionals and require these QHPs to have written collaboration agreements and either general or direct supervision by a physician. Prescribing authority may also be limited.

Every state has laws and regulations that describe the requirements of education and training for health care professionals. However, some states do not have different scope of practice laws for every level of professional (eg, LPN).

Sources of information on scope of practice laws include each state's licensing authorities, boards of nursing, and medical societies. National organizations representing specific practitioners also provide information on state scope of practice and regulatory bodies.

Scope of practice should be taken into consideration when delegating directly or through standing orders (eg, physician writes order that recommended screening instruments will be completed for all patients presenting for well-baby/well-child examinations).

National Provider Identifier

The NPI is a unique identification number for covered health care providers. The NPI is required on administrative and financial transactions under the Health Insurance Portability and Accountability Act (HIPAA) Administrative Simplification provisions. Anyone who directly provides health care services (eg, physical therapist, nutritionist, audiologist) can apply for and receive an NPI. However, usually only those who will bill for services and/or order services or prescription drugs will need an NPI. The NPI is included on medical claims to indicate who ordered, provided, or supervised the provision of services.

Selecting Codes for Services of Allied Health Professionals

Certain codes are limited to reporting services performed by NPPs who cannot report E/M services under their own NPI. Thus, it is important to differentiate the QHP who may independently report E/M services from the AHP who reports other specific procedure codes rather than E/M services. The examples in **Table 13-1** illustrate the differences in reporting 30 minutes of asthma education by a certified asthma educator using a standardized curriculum based on the provider's scope of practice. Where payer policy directs to report differently, practices should maintain documentation of the payer's instruction and report codes accordingly.

As shown in **Table 13-1**, reporting the appropriate code may result in significantly different payment. This also indicates the value of allowing each provider to work within the full scope of practice as allowed by state regulations and for which he or she is trained. While payment to a QHP who may provide and independently report E/M services is higher, so also is the salary of these providers. Practices should consider the cost to benefit ratio for services by provider type when expanding services offered within the practice.

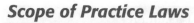

Table 13-1. Asthma Education Service Coding Examples	
QHP (eg, Nurse Practitioner, Physician Assistant) Providing 30 Minutes of Asthma Education Using Standardized Curriculum	**AHP[a] (billed incident to a physician or QHP) Providing 30 Minutes of Asthma Education Using Standardized Curriculum**
CPT 99214 (25 min typical time) Service may include additional elements of E/M service.	*CPT* 98960 Education and training for patient self-management by a qualified, nonphysician health care professional using a standardized curriculum, face-to-face with the patient (could include caregiver/family), each 30 minutes; individual patient
Payment Example Total non-facility RVUs: 3.04 Conversion factor: $40 Payment: $121.60	Payment Example Total non-facility RVUs: 0.79 Conversion factor: $40 Payment: $31.60

Abbreviations: AHP, allied health professional; CPT, Current Procedural Terminology; E/M, evaluation and management; QHP, qualified health care professional; RVU, relative value unit.

[a] Examples: Respiratory therapist, registered nurse with asthma education certification.

Medicare Incident-to Requirements: Supervision of Nonphysician Health Care Professionals

Billing for care provided by AHPs requires careful attention to state licensure and local payer requirements. Most state Medicaid programs and commercial payers follow the Medicare incident-to payment rules. Some have their own policies addressing incident-to provisions and certified AHP billing. Examples of incident-to policies that do not align with Medicare policy include

- One major payer bases incident-to billing on whether or not the nonphysician is credentialed with the payer. If the NPP is credentialed, he or she must report under his or her own NPI (ie, incident to does not apply). However, if the provider is not credentialed with the payer, all services are reported by the credentialed supervising physician or provider in accordance with payer guidance. HCPCS codes and/or modifiers may be used to identify the rendering provider.

- Another major payer requires credentialing for all providers who may independently provide services under applicable state law for their commercial plans and provides a list of services that may not be reported under a physician's NPI.

> ||||||||| **Coding Pearl** |||||||||
>
> Incident-to provisions apply only in the office or other outpatient setting.

Because of the variance in how payers treat the credentialing of NPPs (QHPs and AHPs) and the related payment policies, it is important that practice administrators and/or billing managers verify payer policies prior to provision of services.

For those payers that align with Medicare policy, see the Medicare Requirements for Incident-to Services box for detailed requirements. See also Chapter 12, section 30.6, of the *Medicare Claims Processing Manual* and Chapter 15, section 60, of the *Medicare Benefit Policy Manual* at http://cms.gov/manuals for detailed information on incident-to services. Check with your payers and obtain a copy of their specific policies.

- The Centers for Medicare & Medicaid Services (CMS) defines *incident to* as "services incident to the service of a physician or other professional permitted by statute to bill for services incident to their services when those services meet all of the requirements applicable to the benefit."

- Incident-to services are always provided as a continuation of a physician's services and do not address new problems (eg, a nursing visit performed at patient or caregiver request and not based on a physician's recommendation is not an incident-to service). A treatment plan or order must be documented by a physician or QHP prior to provision of services by an AHP or clinical staff provision of services billed incident-to a physician or QHP.

☀ Although certain QHPs and AHPs otherwise may bill for their services under their own NPI when they provide medically necessary services (within their state's scope of practice), the incident-to provision allows for reporting under the name and NPI of a supervising physician when the requirements of incident-to billing are met. Payment for QHPs and AHPs billing under the incident-to provision may be 100% of the physician payment versus 85% when reporting under the QHP's and AHP's individual NPI.

☀ Nonphysician providers without their own NPI must report services incident to a physician and must meet all incident-to requirements, including physician presence in the office suite and continuation of a physician's previously established plan of care. Medicare makes an exception for the physician's presence in the office suite for CCM, TCM, and behavioral health integration activities by clinical staff. Private payers may also allow inclusion of time spent by clinical staff without direct supervision when reporting these services. For more information on CCM and TCM, see Chapter 12, Managing Chronic and Complex Conditions.

Example

➤ **A patient presents for nutritional counseling by an RN.** The nurse provides the counseling based on a physician's documented order for a nutritional counseling visit for this patient, whose body mass index (BMI) is at the 98th percentile. The nurse spends 20 minutes counseling the patient. The physician is in the office suite at the time of service. The nurse instructs the patient to return to the practice for weight checks every other week for the next 2 months as directed by the physician.

The nurse reports code **99211** (established patient E/M not requiring a physician's presence) for this encounter. However, the return visits for weight checks were ordered by the nurse and were not included in the physician's plan of care for the patient. These services would not meet incident-to requirements.

☀ Physicians and QHPs billing under their own NPI may
  ❖ Bill directly for services they have personally performed.
  ❖ Bill for the services that are performed by any employee, leased employee, or contracted employee (eg, nurse practitioners, physician assistants, therapists, nurses, MAs, technicians). Any services performed by an employee who does not have his or her own individual NPI must be reported as incident to (when provided within the incident-to requirements).

For example, an MA, as allowed under state scope of practice laws, administers a nebulizer treatment that was ordered, documented, and directly supervised by the physician. The treatment (**94640**) would be reported under the physician's NPI. If a certified pediatric nurse practitioner had ordered the treatment, the service would be reported under that practitioner's NPI.

Qualified health care professionals may also perform a split/shared E/M service with a physician. A *split/shared* E/M service is one in which a physician and a QHP from the same group practice each personally perform a medically necessary and substantive portion of one or more face-to-face E/M encounters on the same date. A portion of the key components of the service must be provided face-to-face by the physician to report under the physician's NPI. For more on split/shared visits, see Chapter 16, Noncritical Hospital Evaluation and Management Services. A split/shared E/M service involves a physician and a QHP and not AHPs who may not report E/M services beyond **99211**

Documentation Requirements and Tips When Reporting Incident-to Services

☀ Physicians and QHPs must document their order for a service or treatment (eg, injection) that will be performed as incident to or document their plan for a follow-up visit in the treatment plan (eg, follow-up visit in 1 week for weight check).

☀ To demonstrate compliant incident-to billing, AHPs and clinical staff providing services in continuation of a physician's plan of care *should, ideally, reference the date of the physician order for the service.* This may be documented in the chief complaint for the encounter (eg, "Patient is seen today per Dr Green's 1/3/2018 order for dressing change to left arm wound in 10 days").

Medicare Requirements for Incident-to Services[a]

- Services must be related to the physician service and must be of a type commonly furnished in a physician office or clinic (physician owned and independent of a hospital or other facility), commonly performed without charge, or included in the physician/qualified health care professional (QHP) service (eg, vital signs, assistance with dressing change).

- Services performed must be reasonable and medically necessary.

- Services performed must be within the employee's state scope of practice and require direct physician supervision. Direct supervision of auxiliary personnel requires that the physician (ie, any physician in the group practice) be on the premises (eg, in the office or facility) and be immediately available to provide assistance or direction. The supervising physician who is reporting the service (his or her name is on the claim form) must be the one who was providing the direct supervision.

- Services can only be provided to an established patient after the physician has performed the initial visit, established the plan of care, and established the physician–patient relationship. The physician must evaluate and initiate the treatment of new problems. The physician is not required to be involved in each subsequent patient encounter. Subsequent patient encounters and services must be incidental and integral to the initial service. They do not require physician involvement, but the physician must remain actively involved in a patient's treatment and must personally see the patient periodically. Review of the medical record alone does not constitute active management of the patient.

- Time cannot be used as the controlling factor when counseling and/or coordination of care is performed incident to the physician. Therefore, when an evaluation and management (E/M) service is provided as incident to the physician (physician is not involved in the service) and time is the key factor (ie, history, physical examination, and medical decision-making [MDM] requirements are not met), only code 99211 (minimal office/outpatient E/M service) may be reported. Qualified health care professionals who provide an E/M service with most of the face-to-face time spent in counseling and/or coordination of care may report the service based on time when reporting under their own National Provider Identifier.

- Services provided in a home are covered only if there is direct supervision by the physician.

- Inpatient hospital services can be reported only if the physician sees the patient face-to-face. The physician must perform some portion of the required key components (history, physical examination, MDM) to report the encounter under his or her name. If the E/M encounter is reported based on time, only the physician face-to-face time is considered.

- Incident-to services cannot be billed for E/M services performed in the inpatient or outpatient hospital (unless a split/shared service is performed under the requirements of Transmittal 1776 for a nursing facility or home).

- Although diagnostic tests do not fall under incident-to provisions, the Centers for Medicare & Medicaid Services requires certain levels of physician supervision for covered diagnostic tests. The Medicare Physician Fee Schedule database includes an indicator on each *Current Procedural Terminology*® and Healthcare Common Procedure Coding System (HCPCS) code to define the level of supervision required. The 3 levels of physician supervision include general supervision (ie, the procedure is performed under the physician's overall direction and control, but the physician's presence is not required during the performance of the test and the physician is responsible for personnel training and maintenance of the equipment and supplies), direct supervision (ie, the physician must be on the premises and immediately available to provide assistance or direction), or personal supervision (ie, the physician must be in the room while the test is being performed). Medicare regulations do not allow supervision of diagnostic tests by QHPs (eg, QHPs cannot supervise radiology services).

- Some payers may require the use of HCPCS codes and/or modifiers to identify services provided by allied health professionals.

- Medicare provides an exception to the requirement for direct physician supervision for clinical staff activities included in chronic care management, transitional care management, and behavioral health integration services. Clinical staff may perform these activities under general supervision. All other incident-to provisions apply.

[a] *Note that the term* physician *also includes QHPs billing under their own National Provider Identifier.*

❖ Documentation of incident-to services should fully describe the services provided, including date of service, assessment, concerns noted and addressed, details of care provided (eg, wound cleansed and new bandage applied), and education and/or instructions for home care and follow-up. Inclusion of the supervising physician's name also supports that incident-to requirements were met. Medical record documentation must reflect the identity including credentials and legible signature of the person providing the service.

For Medicare purposes, the physician or QHP billing the service is not required to sign documentation prepared by the clinical staff. Other payer and state regulations may require physician authentication. Documentation may be as simple as "service performed/provided under the direct supervision of Dr X." When applicable, the supervising physician's signature must be legible.

Healthcare Common Procedure Coding System Codes

HCPCS Level II codes may be reported when the narrative differs from the *CPT* code for the service. What follows is a small sample of HCPCS codes and modifiers that may be used for services by AHPs. Payer guidance for reporting HCPCS or *CPT* codes may vary.

Note that HCPCS codes may include the term NPP in lieu of AHP or QHP. These codes are only reported when services are provided by NPPs unless otherwise instructed by a payer. It is advisable to retain copies of a payer's written policies and guidance for reporting HCPCS codes.

Code	Description
G0108	Diabetes outpatient self-management training services, individual, per 30 minutes
G0109	Diabetes outpatient self-management training services, group session (2 or more), per 30 minutes
S0315	Disease management program; initial assessment and initiation of the program
S0316	Disease management program, follow-up/reassessment
S0317	Disease management program; per diem
S0320	Telephone calls by a registered nurse to a disease management program member for monitoring purposes; per month
S9441	Asthma education, NPP; per session
S9443	Lactation classes, NPP, per session
S9445	Patient education, not otherwise classified, NPP, individual, per session
S9446	group, per session
S9449	Weight management classes, NPP, per session
S9451	Exercise class, NPP, per session
S9452	Nutrition class, NPP, per session
S9454	Stress management class, NPP, per session
S9455	Diabetic management program, group session
S9460	nurse visit
S9465	dietitian visit
S9470	Nutritional counseling, dietitian visit

Payers may also instruct certain AHPs to report services by appending a HCPCS modifier to the *CPT* or HCPCS code for services provided.

Modifier	Description
AE	Registered dietitian
AH	Clinical psychologist
AJ	Clinical social worker
HA	Child/adolescent program
HN	Bachelor's degree level
HO	Master's degree level
HP	Doctoral level
HQ	Group setting
UN	Two patients served
UP	Three patients served
UQ	Four patients served
UR	Five patients served
US	Six or more patients served

Nonphysician Services

Nonphysician Evaluation and Management Services

Nursing Visit

99211   Office or other outpatient visit for the evaluation and management of an established patient, that may not require the presence of a physician or other qualified health care professional. Usually, the presenting problem(s) are minimal. Typically, 5 minutes are spent performing or supervising these services

When clinical staff and/or AHPs who do not independently report E/M services provide an E/M service that is not described by another procedure code, code 99211 is reported.

Report 99211 when

* Services meet the incident-to requirements of the payer.
* Problems addressed have previously been addressed by ordering physician or QHP and services are a continuation of care.
* The service is provided based on physician orders and within scope of practice and license.
* The service is rendered face-to-face with the patient/caregiver.

Never report 99211 when

* Another procedure code describes the service provided (eg, 36415, venipuncture).
* The physician performs a face-to-face E/M service on the same date.
* The patient is new or the problem has not been addressed by the physician.

Examples

➤ A physician orders counseling about diet and exercise by a nurse in the practice for a 16-year-old patient who has obesity with borderline hypertension (follow-up visit not on same day as physician visit). The follow-up visit is conducted by an RN who documents the patient's weight, BMI, and blood pressure. The nurse spends 10 minutes face-to-face with the patient going over dietary guidelines, demonstrating proper portion sizes, and encouraging him to continue progress made in adopting an exercise routine and healthier diet.

The RN is not a registered dietitian or licensed medical nutritionist who may report medical nutrition therapy. This service was provided in continuation of the physician's plan of care and under direct (in-office) physician supervision. Code 99211 is reported. Most payers will deny code 99211 when reported on the same date as a physician's E/M service (99201–99205, 99212–99215).

➤ A physician orders education and training on proper use of a metered-dose inhaler (MDI) for a patient seen in the emergency department and treated for new-onset asthma. A respiratory therapist who works part-time in the physician's clinic providing asthma education sees the patient. The patient presents with an MDI and spacer. The therapist demonstrates proper use and evaluates the patient's use of the MDI. The patient is instructed to keep a follow-up appointment with the ordering physician in 10 days.

94664 (demonstration and/or evaluation of patient utilization of an aerosol generator, nebulizer, metered dose inhaler or IPPB device)

This service is not reported with code 99211 because code 94664 describes the service performed.

Prolonged Clinical Staff Service

#+99415   Prolonged clinical staff service (the service beyond the typical service time) during an evaluation and management service in the office or outpatient setting, direct patient contact with physician supervision; first hour (List separately in addition to code for outpatient Evaluation and Management service)

#+99416   each additional 30 minutes (List separately in addition to code 99415)

Codes **99415** and **99416** are used to report 45 minutes or more of prolonged clinical staff time spent face-to-face providing care to a patient under the supervision of a physician or other QHP who has provided an office or other outpatient E/M service at the same session. Report only prolonged service by a physician or other QHP (**99354**, **99355**) when provided on the same date as prolonged clinical staff services. The relative value units assigned to codes **99415** (0.25) and **99416** (0.13) represent only the intraservice time spent by clinical staff, as preservice and post-service times are valued in the related E/M service.

The following guidelines apply to reporting of prolonged clinical staff services:

* Prolonged clinical staff services are reported only in conjunction with E/M services in the office or other outpatient setting. Report **99415** and **99416** in addition to office or other outpatient E/M codes **99201–99215**. The related E/M service by the physician may be reported based on key components or time spent in counseling and/or coordinating care.

* Supervision must be provided by a physician or other QHP during the provision of prolonged clinical staff services.

* Prolonged clinical staff services are reported only when the face-to-face time spent by clinical staff is 45 minutes or more beyond the typical time of the related E/M service on the same date. Documentation of the physician's time spent in provision of the E/M service is not required when the level of service is selected based on key components. (See **tables 7-2 and 7-3** for typical times assigned to office and other outpatient services.)

* Do **not** report prolonged service of less than 45 minutes beyond the typical time of the related E/M service.

* The total time of and medical necessity for the service must be documented.

* Time spent providing separately reported services, such as intravenous medication administration or inhalation treatment, is not counted toward the time of prolonged service.

* It is not required that the clinical staff time be continuous, but each episode of face-to-face time should be documented in the encounter note with authentication by the clinical staff for each episode of care.

* Report code **99416** for each additional 30 minutes of clinical staff time beyond the first hour and for the last 15 to 30 minutes of prolonged clinical staff service. Do not report **99416** for less than 15 minutes beyond the first hour or last 30-minute period.

See Chapter 7, Evaluation and Management Services in the Office and Outpatient Clinics, for more information on prolonged clinical staff services.

Example

➤ **A child is seen for diarrhea and concerns of dehydration.** The physician diagnoses moderate dehydration due to viral gastroenteritis. Oral rehydration is ordered. The physician completes his or her documentation and selects code **99214** for service to this established patient based on the level of history, examination, and medical decision-making. The physician remains in the office suite while clinical staff deliver and monitor a time-based oral rehydration plan using an electrolyte solution. The nurse's total direct care time is 2 hours. The first 25 minutes are included in the practice expense of the physician service. The additional 95 minutes following the physician's service are reported as prolonged clinical staff service.

E/M service by physician Prolonged clinical staff time	***International Classification of Diseases, 10th Revision, Clinical Modification (ICD-10-CM)*** **A08.4** (viral intestinal infection, unspecified) **E86.0** (dehydration)
	CPT® **99214** (typical time of 25 minutes) **99415** × 1 (first hour) and **99416** × 1 (final 35-minute period)

Teaching Point: *CPT* instructs that prolonged clinical staff time reporting begins 45 minutes after the typical time of the E/M service provided by the physician. In this scenario, the typical time of the physician service is 25 minutes, so prolonged clinical staff time is not reported until clinical staff have spent at least 70 minutes in face-to-face patient care. Code **99415** is reported for prolonged clinical staff service of 45 to

74 minutes beyond the typical time of the related E/M service. Code **99416** is reported with 1 unit of service for 75 to 104 minutes of service time. When reporting units of service for code **99416**, only time of 15 to 30 minutes beyond the previous period is reported. In this example, the final 5 minutes beyond the first 90 minutes is not separately reported.

Education and Training for Patient Self-management

98960   Education and training for patient self-management by a qualified, nonphysician health care professional using a standardized curriculum, face-to-face with the patient (could include caregiver/family) each 30 minutes; individual patient

98961   2–4 patients

98962   5–8 patients

Report codes **98960–98962** when

❂ The purpose of these services is to teach the patient and caregivers how to self-manage the illness or disease or delay disease comorbidities in conjunction with the patient's professional health care team.

❂ A physician prescribes the services and a standardized curriculum is used. A standardized curriculum is one that is consistent with guidelines or standards established or recognized by a physician or AHP society, association, or other appropriate source (eg, curriculum established or endorsed by the American Academy of Pediatrics).

❂ Qualifications of the AHPs and the content of the program are consistent with guidelines or standards established or recognized by a physician or AHP society, association, or other appropriate source. For example, these codes apply to diabetic self-management training—an important category of patient self-management education and training. Such training can be provided by diabetic nurse educators—nurses who have received special education in addition to certification from accreditation societies or state licensing panels. In such scenarios, these services could be reported by the supervising physician when the services are rendered by the appropriately certified professional and acknowledged by the payer via the payer contract or published guidance.

❂ Education and training services are provided to patients with an established illness or disease. Code **98960** is reported when services are provided to an individual patient; code **98961** is reported when services are provided to 2 to 4 patients; and code **98962** is reported when 5 to 8 patients receive the education and training.

> **||||||| Coding Pearl |||||||**
>
> Qualifications of the allied health professionals (AHPs) and the content of patient self-management education (**98960–98962**) must be consistent with guidelines or standards established or recognized by a physician or AHP society, association, or other appropriate source.

Code selection is based on the general *CPT®* instruction for reporting services based on time. Time is met when the midpoint is passed (ie, report code **98960** for 16 or more minutes of face-to-face time and with units of service for each additional full 30 minutes and the last 16–30 minutes).

Example

➤ **A 7-year-old patient was recently diagnosed with asthma and is referred to the asthma educator for therapy and training under an approved curriculum.** This includes review of protocols for prevention, use of controller medications (eg, inhaler technique, use of holding chamber or spacer, self-monitoring), and handling potential exacerbations. The total documented time of service is 50 minutes.

The content, type, duration, and patient response to the training must be documented in the medical record. Two units of service are reported with code **98960**, one for the first 30 minutes of service and an additional unit for the last 20 minutes (16–30 minutes is reportable). Reporting of services under the name of the asthma educator or supervising physician or QHP will be determined by payer contract. If payer credentials educators, report under the name and NPI of the educator. If payer does not credential educators, follow payer guidance for reporting. HCPCS modifiers and/or codes may be required to indicate the service was provided by an AHP.

Genetic Counseling Services

96040   Medical genetics and genetic counseling services, each 30 minutes face-to-face with patient/family

- Trained genetic counselors provide services that may include obtaining a structured family genetic history, pedigree construction, analysis for genetic risk assessment, and counseling of the patient and family.
- Only face-to-face time with the patient or caregiver is used in determining the units of service reported. Do not report genetic counseling of 15 minutes or less. Report code **96040** with units of service for the first and each additional 30 minutes and the last 16 to 30 minutes.
- Services may be provided during one or more sessions and may include review of medical data and family information, face-to-face interviews, and counseling services.
- For genetic counseling and education on genetic risks by an AHP to a group, see codes **98961** and **98962**
- Genetic counseling by physicians and other QHPs who may report E/M services are reported with the appropriate E/M service code.

Health and Behavior Assessments/Interventions

96150	Health and behavior assessment, each 15 minutes face-to-face with the patient, initial assessment
96151	reassessment
96152	Health and behavior intervention, each 15 minutes, face-to-face; individual
96153	group (2 or more patients)
96154	family (with patient present)
96155	family (without patient present)

Face-to-face health and behavior intervention services are reported per each 15 minutes of time spent. The total time must be documented in the medical record. Time is met when the midpoint is passed unless payer policy directs otherwise.

Codes **96150–96155**

- May be reported by psychologists, clinical social workers, licensed therapists, and other AHPs within their scope of practice who have specialty or subspecialty training in health and behavior assessment or intervention procedures. Check payer guidelines for any required referral or prior authorization for services.
- Physicians and other QHPs who may report E/M services are instructed to report E/M or preventive service codes.
- Are used when assessing or addressing psychosocial factors affecting patients who have an established medical illness or diagnosis and may benefit from assessments and interventions with a focus on the role that psychosocial adaptation may play on the clinical course of that condition (eg, services differ from preventive medicine counseling and risk-factor reduction interventions).
- Are not used in conjunction with a primary diagnosis of mental disorder. (Payers may deny when a diagnosis code indicating mental disorder is included on the claim for these services.) The first-listed diagnosis should be the medical condition for which the patient may benefit from assessment and intervention focused on helping the patient better manage his or her health condition.
- Are used to identify the psychological, behavioral, emotional, cognitive, and/or social factors needed for the prevention, treatment, or management of physical health problems, with a focus on treating the biopsychosocial factors contributing to physical problems.
- Do not require a standardized curriculum.
- Are not reported with psychiatric codes (**90791–90899** and, when applicable, **90785** when provided on the same day. Only the primary service is reported (ie, either **96150–96155** or **90791–90899**)
- Are not reported with an E/M code (eg, **99201–99215** **99401–99412** on the same day.
- Are not reported in conjunction with adaptive behavior treatment (**97153–97158** **0373T** . See Chapter 14, Mental and Behavioral Health Services, for more information on adaptive behavior treatment.
- The initial assessment (**96150** may include a health-focused clinical interview, behavioral observations, psychophysiological monitoring, and completion of health-oriented questionnaires. Completion of health-oriented questionnaires is not separately reported (eg, do not separately report code **96127** [brief emotional/ behavioral assessment]).

❖ Code **96151** is used to report the reassessment of a patient's condition by interview and behavioral health instruments.

Examples

➤ **A 12-year-old girl undergoing treatment for acute lymphoblastic leukemia is referred to a social worker trained in health and behavior assessment or intervention procedures for assessment of pain, behavioral distress, and combativeness associated with repeated procedures and treatment.** The patient is assessed using standardized questionnaires (eg, Pediatric Pain Questionnaire, Coping Strategies Inventory). The child's parents are also interviewed.

Code **96150** would be reported with, for example, *ICD-10-CM* code **C91.00**, acute lymphoblastic leukemia, without remission. One unit of service would be reported for each 15 minutes of face-to-face time with the patient and/or parents. Time must be documented and does not include time spent before or after face-to-face services.

Results from the health and behavior assessment are used to develop a treatment plan. Thirty minutes is spent with the patient discussing the behavior and suggested coping skills. Code **96152** with 2 units of service would be reported with the same diagnosis as used in the initial assessment.

➤ **A 10-year-old boy diagnosed with attention-deficit/hyperactivity disorder 2 years ago has undergone health and behavior assessment after parents noted the boy was afraid to go to school, where he fears being in trouble and failing.** Based on the assessment conducted at a previous encounter, the clinical psychologist works with the boy to develop new coping skills and improve self-management. Parents are urged to meet with the boy's teacher about adherence to an existing behavioral intervention plan and recommended revisions. A total of 55 minutes is spent face-to-face with the boy and his parents.

Code **96154** is reported with 4 units of service (3 full 15-minute periods and 1 unit for the 10 minutes because the midpoint of 8 minutes beyond the last full period was passed).

Home Health Procedures/Services

99500	Home visit for prenatal monitoring and assessment to include fetal heart rate, non-stress test, uterine monitoring, and gestational diabetes monitoring
99501	Home visit for postnatal assessment and follow-up care
99502	Home visit for newborn care and assessment
99503	Home visit for respiratory therapy care (eg, bronchodilator, oxygen therapy, respiratory assessment, apnea evaluation)
99504	Home visit for mechanical ventilation care
99505	Home visit for stoma care and maintenance including colostomy and cystostomy
99506	Home visit for intramuscular injections
99507	Home visit for care and maintenance of catheter(s) (eg, urinary, drainage, and enteral)
99509	Home visit for assistance with activities of daily living and personal care
99510	Home visit for individual, family, or marriage counseling
99511	Home visit for fecal impaction management and enema administration
99512	Home visit for hemodialysis
99600	Unlisted home visit service or procedure

Codes **99500–99600** are

❖ Typically reported for skilled nursing services ordered by a physician or QHP and are medically necessary services provided to a homebound patient. *Exception:* Nursing visit to a mother and newborn may be covered when provided within a specified time following hospital discharge (verify payer policy for coverage).

❖ Used to report services provided in a patient's residence (including assisted living apartments, group homes, nontraditional private homes, custodial care facilities, or schools). Physicians and QHPs providing E/M services in a patient's home report code **99341–99350**.

◦ Not reported if another code more accurately describes the service provided (eg, report home medical nutrition therapy with 97802–97804 rather than 99509).

Coverage of home health procedures or services by QHPs who are authorized to use E/M home visit codes (99341–99350) may also be reported with codes 99500–99600 if both services are performed and the patient's condition requires a significant, separately identifiable service. Modifier 25 would be appended to codes 99341–99350.

Lactation Services

S9443   Lactation classes, nonphysician provider, per session

Although code S9443 is the code most specific to lactation services, it is not paid under many health plan contracts. Lactation consultation services do not have a specific *CPT®* code, and billing is a source of confusion for many providers. Less-specific codes are often used to report these services. Options for reporting services by AHPs may include

S9445   Patient education, not otherwise classified, nonphysician provider, individual, per session

S9446   Patient education, not otherwise classified, nonphysician provider, group, per session

98960   Education and training for patient self-management by a qualified, nonphysician health care professional using a standardized curriculum, face-to-face with the patient (could include caregiver/family) each 30 minutes; individual patient

99401   Preventive medicine counseling and/or risk-factor reduction intervention(s) provided to an individual (separate procedure); approximately 15 minutes

96150   Health and behavior assessment, each 15 minutes face-to-face with the patient, initial assessment

Key considerations for reporting lactation services include

◦ Practices must verify coverage and reporting instructions for each payer prior to service. Examples of coding instructions from payers are included in the Examples of Payment Policies for Lactation Services box later in this chapter.

◦ Unless the newborn or infant has been diagnosed with a feeding problem, the mother is typically the patient and claims are filed to her health benefit plan. Although included as a covered preventive service under the Patient Protection and Affordable Care Act, breastfeeding services are linked to the mother's health coverage and often considered by payers to be included in E/M services provided to the mother by a physician.

◦ Payer policies typically do not allow separate payment for lactation counseling on the same date as an E/M service.

◦ Recently, licensure of lactation consultants has been approved in at least 2 states (Georgia and Rhode Island). In states where licensure is not yet enacted, issues are seen in credentialing and coverage by payers who cover only services provided by licensed health care professionals, although services provided incident to a physician or QHP may be allowed.

◦ When a medical condition (eg, feeding problem, low weight gain) has been previously diagnosed by the physician at an earlier date, an AHP may see the mother and patient to identify the psychological, behavioral, emotional, cognitive, and social factors important to the prevention, treatment, or management of physical health problems. Codes 96150–96155 may be reportable for these services. Again, payer policy drives the provision (who may provide) and payment for these services.

◦ Codes 99401–99404 are described by *CPT* as services provided face-to-face by a physician or other QHP for the purpose of promoting health and preventing illness or injury. When payer policy instructs to report these codes for services by lactation consultants or other AHPs, a written copy of the payer policy should be kept on file.

◦ Lactation counseling provided in conjunction with a physician's or QHP's E/M service, though not separately reported, may reduce the physician's time spent on history taking, counseling, and education. This may also support quality initiatives.

> ### ~ More From the AAP ~
>
> For more information on coding for lactation counseling services, see "Lactation Counseling: Payer Policies Drive Coding" in the April 2018 *AAP Pediatric Coding Newsletter™* at http://coding. aap.org (subscription required).

Examples of Payment Policies for Lactation Services

- Lactation consultations (98960) are separately paid when filed by a licensed MD/DO or advanced practice professional when the lactation consultation is the only service provided and performed by a certified lactation consultant under the general supervision of a licensed MD/DO or mid-level practitioner. Lactation consultations (98960) are considered not separately paid when provided at the same time as any evaluation and management visit.

- Lactation counseling services may be billed directly by International Board Certified Lactation Consultants (IBCLCs) using codes S9445 and S9446. A physician who employs an IBCLC physician assistant or registered nurse may bill for lactation counseling provided by these health care professionals (S9445 and S9446). Physicians providing lactation counseling must append modifier AF (specialty physician) to code S9445 or S9446.

- Up to 6 individual outpatient breastfeeding or lactation counseling sessions (99401–99404), per birth event, may be covered. These counseling sessions are in addition to breastfeeding or lactation counseling that may be provided during an inpatient maternity stay, outpatient obstetrician visit, or well-child visit. However, these additional counseling sessions are only covered and separately paid when all the following conditions are met:
    - ❖ The breastfeeding or lactation counseling is rendered by an authorized individual professional provider (eg, physician, physician assistant, nurse practitioner, nurse midwife, registered nurse), outpatient hospital, or clinic.
    - ❖ The breastfeeding or lactation counseling is billed using one of the preventive counseling *Current Procedural Terminology* (*CPT*®) procedure codes 99401–99404.
    - ❖ Breastfeeding or lactation counseling is the *only service* being provided.

- The following *CPT*/Healthcare Common Procedure Coding System codes are appropriate for lactation support and counseling services provided by an IBCLC: 99211 and 99401–99404; for lactation classes, use codes S9443, 99411, or 99412.

ICD-10-CM code Z39.1 is reported for encounter for care and examination of a lactating mother. When addressing lactation disorders, such as cracked nipple, suppressed lactation, or agalactia, see codes in category O92. It is important to verify benefits and bill for services to the mother separately from services to address a condition of the newborn. Feeding difficulty in the newborn is reported with codes in category P92 (eg, P92.5 neonatal difficulty in feeding at breast). Remember that codes that define or describe maternal conditions cannot be reported for the baby.

Medical Nutrition Assessments

97802	Medical nutrition therapy; initial assessment and intervention, individual, face-to-face with the patient, each 15 minutes
97803	Reassessment and intervention, individual, face-to-face with the patient, each 15 minutes
97804	group (2 or more individuals), each 30 minutes

Medical nutrition therapy is one of the services for which *CPT*® instruction excludes reporting by a physician or QHP who may report E/M services. Many states restrict the provision of medical nutrition therapy to certain AHPs (eg, registered dietitian, licensed medical nutritionist). Practices providing medical nutrition therapy services should be aware of state licensing and scope of practice regulations. Coverage may be limited to patients with certain conditions (eg, diabetes, kidney disease) and a limited number of units of service or visits per year.

Payers that follow Medicare policy on reporting of E/M services will not accept codes 99201–99205, 99212–99215, or 99217–99499 performed by AHPs. (*Note:* 99211 is reportable by AHPs and clinical staff. Payers may adopt Medicare incident-to policy requirements.) Physicians and QHPs who provide counseling regarding nutrition should report the E/M service that best describes the service provided (eg, office visit based on time spent counseling or preventive medicine counseling [99401–99404]).

- Codes are reported when provided by an AHP who may report medical nutrition therapy services under his or her individual state's scope of practice.

❖ When medical nutrition therapy is provided as a preventive service, modifier 33 may be appended to codes 97802–97804 (For more on modifier 33 see Chapter 2, Modifiers and Coding Edits, and Chapter 9, Preventive Services.)

❖ Services are reported based on time. Per *CPT* instruction, a unit of time is met when the midpoint is passed. Certain payers may require that the time in the code descriptor (eg, 15 minutes) be met or exceeded for each unit of service reported. Time must be documented. Report codes 97802 and 97803 with 1 unit for 8 to 22 minutes of service. An additional unit may be reported for each subsequent 15 minutes and the last 8 to 22 minutes of service.

❖ HCPCS codes may be required by certain payers when providing reassessment and subsequent intervention due to a change in diagnosis, medical condition, or treatment.

G0270   Medical nutrition therapy; reassessment and subsequent intervention(s) following second referral in same year for change in diagnosis, medical condition, or treatment regimen (including additional hours needed for renal disease); individual, face-to-face with the patient, each 15 minutes

G0271   group (2 or more individuals), each 30 minutes

❖ Documentation of services should include the physician or QHP order for services, information on the medical need for services, medical nutrition therapy evaluation and plan for intervention, time, correspondence with the referring provider, and date of service, name, credentials, and signature of the provider of medical nutrition therapy.

Examples

➤ **A 14-year-old girl was seen by her physician for a well-child visit 1 week ago.** Her BMI was at the 90th percentile, blood pressure was at upper limit of normal, and results of cholesterol screening indicated hypercholesterolemia. The patient was referred to the practice's registered dietitian for assessment and counseling on a diet to reduce the risk of cardiovascular and endocrine disorders. The dietitian meets with the child and her parents and spends 30 minutes discussing risk factors and developing a plan with goals to decrease weight, cholesterol, and blood pressure.

ICD-10-CM	CPT®
Z71.3 (dietary counseling and surveillance) E78.00 (pure hypercholesterolemia) Z68.53 (BMI pediatric, 85th percentile to less than 95th percentile for age)	If payer allows billing under registered dietitian's NPI 97802 x 2 (medical nutrition therapy, initial assessment and intervention, individual, face-to-face with the patient, each 15 minutes) If payer requires billing under the NPI of the supervising physician 97802 AE x 2 (medical nutrition therapy as above by a registered dietitian)

Teaching Point: Some Medicaid plans and/or private payers may require that medical nutrition therapy in the physician practice be provided under a physician's order and general supervision. Services are reported as if provided by the physician, but modifier AE indicates the service was provided by a registered dietitian.

➤ **A 12-year-old girl has decided to become a vegetarian.** The patient's laboratory test results have shown iron deficiency, and she is referred by her pediatrician to a nurse practitioner in the same practice for consultation on a vegetarian diet that meets the patient's nutritional requirements. The nurse practitioner spends 30 minutes face-to-face with the patient and parents learning the patient's reasons for choosing a vegetarian diet, assessing the patient's current diet, and counseling on the importance of a plant-based diet that is balanced to provide adequate nutrition. A plan is developed to encourage food choices that support adequate nutrition, and a follow-up visit is scheduled in 2 weeks.

ICD-10-CM	CPT®
Z71.3 (dietary counseling and surveillance) **E61.1** (iron deficiency)	**99214** (25 minutes typical time)

Teaching Point: While nutritional counseling is often provided by physicians and QHPs, use of medical nutrition therapy service codes is typically limited to other providers (eg, registered dietitian, certified nutritionist, clinical nutritionist) who are licensed or certified in the state where practicing. Physicians and other QHPs should verify payer policy prior to delivering services. Reporting with an E/M code based on time spent counseling and/or coordinating care is appropriate per *CPT* instruction.

Medical Team Conferences

99366   Medical team conference with interdisciplinary team of health care professionals, face-to-face with patient and/or family, 30 minutes or more; participation by nonphysician qualified health care professional

99368   Medical team conference with interdisciplinary team of health care professionals, patient and/or family not present, 30 minutes or more; participation by nonphysician qualified health care professional

Medical team conference codes are used to report participation by a minimum of 3 health care professionals (includes physicians, QHPs, and AHPs) of different specialties in conferences to coordinate or manage care and services for established patients with chronic or multiple health conditions (eg, child who is ventilator dependent with developmental delays, seizures, and gastrostomy tube for nutrition).

- Codes differentiate provider (physician or QHP vs AHP) and between face-to-face and non–face-to-face (patient and/or family is not present) patient team conference services. Physicians or other QHPs who may report E/M services should report their time spent in a team conference *with the patient and/or family present* using E/M codes (and time as the key controlling factor for code selection when counseling and/or coordination of care dominates the service). Payer policy may vary.

- If QHPs (including clinical nurse specialists and clinical nurse practitioners) participated in the conference without direct physician supervision, they may report team conference participation *without the patient or caregiver present* as if provided by a physician (**99367**) if it is within the state's scope of practice and they use their own NPI. State Medicaid and commercial payers may follow these Medicare requirements or have their own specific rules.

- Medical team conferences may not be reported if the facility or organization is contractually obligated to provide the service, they are informal meetings or simple conversations between physicians and AHPs (eg, therapists), and less than 30 minutes of conference time is spent in the team conferences.

- Medical team conferences are not reported when provided during a month when the patient is receiving CCM or TCM services provided by the same individual. See Chapter 12, Managing Chronic and Complex Conditions, for more information on CCM and TCM services.

- Medicare assigns a bundled (B) status to team conference services in the Medicare Physician Fee Schedule and does not separate payment for participation in medical team conferences. Payment policies may vary among Medicaid and private health plans.

Medical team conferences require

- Face-to-face participation by a minimum of 3 health care professionals (any combination of AHPs, physicians, and/or QHPs) from different subspecialties or disciplines (eg, speech-language pathologists, dietitians, social workers), with or without the presence of the patient, family member(s), community agencies, surrogate decision-maker(s) (eg, legal guardian), and/or caregiver(s).

- Active involvement in the development, revision, coordination, and implementation of health care services needed by the patient by each participant.

- Face-to-face evaluations and/or treatments by the participant that are separate from any team conference within the previous 60 days.

- Only one individual from the same specialty may report codes **99366–99368** for the same encounter.
- Medical record documentation must support the reporting individual's participation, the time spent from the beginning of the review of an individual patient until the conclusion of the review, and the contributed information and subsequent treatment recommendations.

Examples

▶ **A 14-year-old girl with spinal muscular atrophy is wheelchair bound and receives her education at home.** Over the past 6 months, her respiratory compromise has progressed and she has required 2 inpatient admissions for pneumonia. She is on oxygen at night. She receives physical and occupational therapy services at home and twice-weekly visits from a respiratory therapist. She sees a pediatric pulmonologist every 4 months and a pediatric physiatrist every 6 months. You have started discussions with her parents about how aggressive the family wishes to be if she were to require assisted ventilation. The pediatrician, pulmonologist, physiatrist, occupational and physical therapists, respiratory therapist, home care coordinator, home educator, and social worker attend the conference to discuss the child's current medical status, prognosis for the short and long term, and the child's and family's wishes as her condition deteriorates. The conference lasts 60 minutes.

Each participating physician (if they are different specialties and/or from different practices [ie, separate tax identification numbers])	*ICD-10-CM* **G12.1** (other inherited spinal muscular atrophy) ***CPT*®** **99367**
Each AHP (eg, respiratory therapist, occupational therapist)	***CPT*** **99368**

Code selection is, in part, determined by the type of provider reporting participation in a team conference. Allied health professionals report participation using code **99366** when the patient and/or caregivers are present at the conference or **99368** when the patient/caregivers are not present. However, physicians report an E/M code for the appropriate setting when the patient is present or code **99367** for physician participation in team conference when patient or caregivers are not present. *CPT* allows reporting of codes **99366** and **99368** by QHPs. However, reporting an E/M code for participation when the patient or caregivers are present may be beneficial when allowed or required by individual payer policy.

▶ **A patient with cerebral palsy requires coordination with multiple health care professionals (eg, physical and occupational therapists, neurologist, pediatrician).** Each participant in the conference has completed his or her evaluation of the patient within 60 days prior to the conference, and a team conference of 40 minutes is held to assess the current plan of care and therapy. The patient's family is present at this conference.

Code **99366** would be reported by the physical and occupational therapists.

Medication Therapy Management Services

99605   Medication therapy management service(s) provided by a pharmacist, individual, face-to-face with patient, with assessment and intervention if provided; initial 15 minutes, new patient

99606   initial 15 minutes, established patient

+99607   each additional 15 minutes (List separately in addition to **99605** or **99606**)

Medication therapy management service(s)

- Are provided only by a pharmacist face-to-face with the patient or caregiver and usually in relation to complex medication regimens or medication adherence in conditions such as asthma and diabetes.
- Provided on request of the patient or caregiver, prescribing physician, other QHPs, or prescription drug benefit plan (not reported for routine dispensing-related activities).

- Are reported with codes selected based on whether the patient is new or established and by the pharmacist's face-to-face time with the patient.
- Includes review of pertinent patient history (not limited to drug history).
- Include documentation of review of the pertinent patient history, medication profile (prescription and non-prescription), and recommendations for improving health outcomes and treatment compliance.
- New patients are those who have received no face-to-face service from the pharmacist or another pharmacist of the same clinic or pharmacy within 3 years prior to the current date of service.
- Unless otherwise specified by the payer policy, time is met when the midpoint is passed. Report codes 99605 and 99606 for the first 8 to 22 minutes of face-to-face time with the patient. When time exceeds 22 minutes, code 99607 may be reported for subsequent 15-minute periods and the last 8 to 22 minutes.
- Under the Medicare program, pharmacists may also provide services incident to a physician or QHP and report E/M services with code 99211 when allowed under the scope of practice as defined by state licensure.

Online Medical Assessment

98969   Online assessment and management service provided by a qualified nonphysician health care professional to an established patient or guardian not originating from a related assessment and management service provided within the previous 7 days, using the Internet or similar electronic communications network

An online electronic medical evaluation (98969) is a non–face-to-face assessment and management service by an AHP to an established patient using Internet resources in response to a patient's online inquiry. Online assessment and management refers to use of technology such as secure e-mail and other asynchronous digital communication. This is in contrast to telemedicine services, which represent interactive audio and video telecommunications systems that permit real-time communication between the AHP, at the distant site, and the patient, at the originating site. See Chapter 20, Digital Medicine Services: Technology-Enhanced Care Delivery, for more information on telemedicine services.

Code 98969 is used by an AHP to report an online assessment and management service. One unit of service is reported for the sum of communications pertaining to the online encounter during a 7-day period.

The CMS has not assigned relative value units to online medical evaluation codes and considers them non-covered services. As a result, most third-party payers do not pay for them.

Before providing online medical services, understand local and state laws, ensure that communications will be HIPAA compliant, establish written guidelines and procedures, educate payers and negotiate for payment, and educate patients.

Online assessment and management includes
- Timely reply to the patient/caregiver's request for online service
- Permanent record of the service (hard copy or electronic)
- All related communications during a 7-day episode of care (eg, ordering laboratory or other testing, prescriptions, related phone calls)

Online assessment and management services *are not reported* when
- Related to a service provided by the AHP within the past 7 days regardless of whether the online service was planned or prompted by patient or caregiver concern
  - Result in an appointment within the next 24 hours or next available appointment
  - Within a global period of another service
- When provided during a month when the patient is receiving care plan oversight, CCM, or TCM services provided by the same individual (See Chapter 12, Managing Chronic and Complex Conditions, for more information on CCM and TCM services.)

Example

➤ **The parents of a child who has attention-deficit/hyperactivity disorder contact their psychologist by e-mail for recommendations for helping the child cope with increased demands of school (eg, more homework and written work).** The psychologist responds to the request and e-mails are exchanged to further clarify the nature of the problem and provide management options. The child will be seen reevaluated at a regularly scheduled appointment in 3 weeks.

The psychologist reports code **98969** If the patient had been seen within the past 7 days or scheduled for an appointment in the next 24 hours or next available appointment, this service would not be separately reported.

Telephone Calls

98966   Telephone assessment and management services provided by a qualified nonphysician health care professional to an established patient, parent, or guardian not originating from related assessment and management service provided within the previous 7 days nor leading to an assessment and management service or procedure within the next 24 hours or soonest available appointment; 5–10 minutes of medical discussion

98967   11–20 minutes of medical discussion

98968   21–30 minutes of medical discussion

Codes **98966–98968** are used to report telephone assessment and management services by AHPs. Those QHPs who may independently provide and report E/M services report codes **99441–99443** Report codes **98966–98968** when

☀ The patient or caregiver initiates a call that is not in follow-up to a service by the same AHP within the past 7 days.

☀ Five minutes or more is spent in assessment and management services (*time must be documented*).

☀ No decision to see the patient within 24 hours or at the next available appointment is made during the telephone service.

Services Not Reported as Telephone Assessment and Management

Do not report telephone assessment and management services that

☀ Are related to a service provided by the AHP within the past 7 days, regardless of whether this service was planned or prompted by patient or caregiver concern.

☀ Result in an appointment within the next 24 hours or next available appointment. When telephone assessment and management results in scheduling the patient for an appointment within 24 hours or at the next available appointment, the service is considered preservice work to the face-to-face encounter.

☀ Is within a global period of another service.

☀ During a month when the patient is receiving CCM or TCM services provided by the same individual (see Chapter 12, Managing Chronic and Complex Conditions, for more information on CCM and TCM services).

☀ Most telephone services provided by clinical staff (eg, MA relaying physician instructions) are included in the practice expense value assigned to physician services and not separately reported. Telephone services by clinical staff may contribute to time of CCM or TCM when the services meet the description of the clinical staff activities included in CCM or TCM.

Example

➤ **The parents of a patient who has developed mealtime anxiety due to previous allergic reactions to multiple foods contact their child's registered dietitian for advice.** It has been 3 weeks since the dietitian provided education on food allergies and meeting the child's nutritional needs with a limited diet. The dietitian spends 18 minutes on the phone with the parents discussing techniques for encouraging a healthy diet while acknowledging and alleviating the child's anxiety.

The dietitian reports code 98967 based on the time spent addressing the parent's concerns. This service would not be reported if the call were provided within 7 days of a previous service by the same provider or if the call resulted in an appointment within 24 hours or next available face-to-face appointment.

Psychiatric Collaborative Care Management Services

99492   Initial psychiatric collaborative care management, first 70 minutes in the first calendar month of behavioral health care manager activities, in consultation with a psychiatric consultant, and directed by the treating physician or other qualified health care professional, with the following required elements:
- ✷ outreach to and engagement in treatment of a patient directed by the treating physician or other qualified health care professional;
- ✷ initial assessment of the patient, including administration of validated rating scales, with the development of an individualized treatment plan;
- ✷ review by the psychiatric consultant with modifications of the plan if recommended;
- ✷ entering patient in a registry and tracking patient follow-up and progress using the registry, with appropriate documentation, and participation in weekly caseload consultation with the psychiatric consultant; and
- ✷ provision of brief interventions using evidence-based techniques such as behavioral activation, motivational interviewing, and other focused treatment strategies.

99493   Subsequent psychiatric collaborative care management, first 60 minutes in a subsequent month of behavioral health care manager activities, in consultation with a psychiatric consultant, and directed by the treating physician or other qualified health care professional, with the following required elements:
- ✷ tracking patient follow-up and progress using the registry, with appropriate documentation;
- ✷ participation in weekly caseload consultation with the psychiatric consultant;
- ✷ ongoing collaboration with and coordination of the patient's mental health care with the treating physician or other qualified health care professional and any other treating mental health providers;
- ✷ additional review of progress and recommendations for changes in treatment, as indicated, including medications, based on recommendations provided by the psychiatric consultant;
- ✷ provision of brief interventions using evidence-based techniques such as behavioral activation, motivational interviewing, and other focused treatment strategies;
- ✷ monitoring of patient outcomes using validated rating scales; and
- ✷ relapse prevention planning with patients as they achieve remission of symptoms and/or other treatment goals and are prepared for discharge from active treatment.

+99494   Initial or subsequent psychiatric collaborative care management, each additional 30 minutes in a calendar month of behavioral health care manager activities, in consultation with a psychiatric consultant, and directed by the treating physician or other qualified health care professional (List separately in addition to code for primary procedure)
(Use 99494 in conjunction with 99492, 99493)

Psychiatric collaborative care management (PCCM) services are reported by a supervising physician or QHP for services by a behavioral health care manager (BHM) working under the supervision of the reporting physician or QHP. Psychiatric collaborative care management services are provided to patients who have a new or existing psychiatric disorder that requires a behavioral health assessment; care plan implementation, revision, or monitoring; and provision of brief interventions. These services require a team effort of 3 health care professionals: a treating physician or QHP, a BHM, and a psychiatric consultant. The treating physician or QHP reports codes 99492–99494 when all requirements for reporting are met. Evaluation and management and other services may be reported separately by the same physician or QHP during the same calendar month.
- ✷ The BHM is an AHP or clinical staff member with master's or doctoral-level education *or* specialized training in behavioral health who provides behavioral health care management services under the treating physician's

or QHP's supervision and in consultation with a psychiatric consultant. The BHM provides the following services, as needed:

❖ Assessment of needs including the administration of validated rating scales

❖ Development of a care plan

❖ Provision of brief interventions face-to-face and non–face-to-face

❖ Ongoing collaboration with the treating physician or QHP

❖ Consultation with the psychiatric consultant at least weekly (typically non–face-to-face)

❖ Maintenance of a registry

Reporting requirements for PCCM services include

❁ Psychiatric consultant refers to a medical professional, who is trained in psychiatry or behavioral health and qualified to prescribe the full range of medications. Qualified health care professionals with psychiatry or behavioral health training and who are able to prescribe the full range of medications may act as a psychiatric consultant.

❁ Psychiatric collaborative care management services are time-based services that are subject to the *CPT* midpoint rule for reporting time. Time of service is met when the midpoint is passed. Documentation must support provision of PCCM services for

❖ 36 minutes or more to report a 70-minute service (**99492**)

❖ 31 minutes or more to report a 60-minute service (**99493**)

❖ 16 minutes or more beyond the last full service period to report an additional 30 minutes of service (**99494**)

❁ Time spent by the BHM coordinating care with the emergency department may be included in time attributed to PCCM services. However, time spent while the patient is an inpatient or in observation status at a hospital may not be included in time of PCCM services.

❁ Psychiatric collaborative care management services are provided for an episode of care defined as beginning when the treating physician or QHP directs the patient to the BHM and ending when

❖ The attainment of targeted treatment goals, which typically results in the discontinuation of care management services and continuation of usual follow-up with the treating physician or other QHP

❖ Failure to attain targeted treatment goals culminating in referral to a psychiatric care provider for ongoing treatment

❖ Lack of continued engagement with no PCCM services provided over a consecutive 6-month calendar period (break in episode)

❁ A new episode of care starts after a break in episode of 6 calendar months or more.

Please see Chapter 14, Mental and Behavioral Health Services, for full details on reporting PCCM services.

Example

➤ **A pediatrician orders PCCM services for a 15-year-old patient diagnosed with moderate depression, single episode.** A licensed clinical psychologist acting as the BHM meets with the patient to discuss PCCM services and perform an initial assessment. Standardized assessment instruments are used to further assess the patient's health, and a treatment plan including psychotherapy is agreed on. After the meeting, the BHM enters the patient information into a registry, which will be used to track her medication compliance and progress. Later, the BHM has a regularly scheduled conference call with a consulting psychiatrist who reviews the patient's assessment and approves of the treatment plan. The supervising pediatrician is also consulted and approves the treatment plan. The BHM, whose scope of practice includes psychotherapy, provides 3 individual psychotherapy sessions within the calendar month in addition to PCCM services. The BHM psychologist will separately report the psychotherapy services in addition to PCCM. During the calendar month, the BHM documents 60 minutes of time spent in PCCM services.

PCCM 60 minutes in first calendar month of service	**ICD-10-CM**
Psychotherapy without E/M service	F32.1 (major depressive disorder, single episode, moderate)
	CPT 99492 (initial month PCCM service, first 70 minutes) 90832, 90834, or 90837 (psychotherapy based on time of service; 30, 45, or 60 minutes)

Teaching Point: *CPT* instructs that time of service for PCCM services is met when the midpoint is passed. In this example, the 60 minutes spent by the BHM supports reporting of code 99492, which includes the first 70 minutes of PCCM services in the initial month of service. No time spent in provision of psychotherapy may be attributed to the time of PCCM services. If psychotherapy services were not within the scope of practice for the BHM, the patient might be referred to another provider (eg, the consulting psychiatrist), who would report the services rendered.

General Behavioral Health Integration Care Management

99484   Care management services for behavioral health conditions, at least 20 minutes of clinical staff time, directed by a physician or other qualified health care professional, per calendar month, with the following required elements:

- Initial assessment or follow-up monitoring, including the use of applicable validated rating scales;
- Behavioral health care planning in relation to behavioral/psychiatric health problems, including revision for patients who are not progressing or whose status changes;
- Facilitating and coordinating treatment such as psychotherapy, pharmacotherapy, counseling and/or psychiatric consultation; and
- Continuity of care with a designated member of the care team

CPT® does not define the education or credentials of clinical staff who may provide services described by code 99484. Behavioral health care integration clinical staff are not required to have qualifications that would permit them to separately report services (eg, psychotherapy), but, if qualified and they perform such services, they may report such services separately, as long as the time of the service is not used in reporting 99484.

Services must be provided under general physician supervision and in accordance with the licensing and scope of practice requirements of the state where services are provided. The individual supervising and reporting general behavioral health integration care management services must be able to report E/M services.

Use of validated rating scales is required and is not separately reported (ie, do not report code 96127 for rating scales administered during the period of behavioral health care management services).

See Chapter 14, Mental and Behavioral Health Services, for more information on reporting care management for behavioral health conditions.

Psychiatric Evaluation and Psychotherapy Without Evaluation and Management

+90785   Interactive complexity (List separately in addition to the code for primary procedure)
90791   Psychiatric diagnostic evaluation
90832   Psychotherapy, 30 minutes with patient and/or family member
90834   45 minutes with patient and/or family member
90837   60 minutes with patient and/or family member
90839   Psychotherapy for crisis; first 60 minutes
+90840   each additional 30 minutes (List separately in addition to code 90839)
90846   Family psychotherapy (without the patient present)
90847   Family psychotherapy (conjoint psychotherapy) (with patient present)
90849   Multiple-family group psychotherapy

90853   Group psychotherapy (other than of a multiple-family group)

+90863   Pharmacologic management, including prescription and review of medication, when performed with psychotherapy services (List separately in addition to **90832**, **90834**, **90837**.)

Mental and behavioral health services may be covered through a provider network separate from other health care services. The scope of services may also be limited by payer policies allowing specific licensed providers, such as licensed clinical psychologists, to report certain services, while other AHPs (eg, licensed clinical social workers) may report a smaller scope of services. Verify coverage and billing options prior to provision of services.

A payer may apply bundling edits that do not allow separate payment for mental and behavioral health services and E/M services provided in the same practice on the same date. Follow payer instructions for reporting services such as psychotherapy by an AHP under the name and NPI of a supervising physician and E/M services by the physician on the same date. HCPCS modifiers identifying the type of provider (eg, **AJ**, clinical social worker) may be necessary to override edits that bundle E/M and mental or behavioral health services on the same date. See the Healthcare Common Procedure Coding System Codes section earlier in this chapter for HCPCS modifiers or your current HCPCS coding reference for additional modifiers.

> |||||||||| **Coding Pearl** ||||||||||
>
> Healthcare Common Procedure Coding System modifiers identifying the type of provider may be necessary to override edits that bundle evaluation and management and mental or behavioral health services on the same date.

See Chapter 14, Mental and Behavioral Health Services, for information on codes for psychological and neuropsychological testing.

- Psychiatric diagnostic evaluation or reevaluation (**90791**) is reported once per day. Do not report psychotherapy codes (**90832–90839**) on the same date of service as **90791**.
- Psychotherapy times are for face-to-face services with a patient and/or family member. The patient must be present for all or some of the service except when reporting family psychotherapy without the patient present (**90846**). This allows for the participation of others in the psychotherapy session for the patient as long as the patient remains the focus of the intervention. The patient must be present for a significant portion of the session.
- Psychotherapy differs from family psychotherapy (**90846**, **90847**), which uses family psychotherapy techniques to benefit the patient (eg, attempting to improve family communication or alter family interactions that negatively affect the patient; encouraging interactions to improve family functioning). Family psychotherapy includes sessions with the entire family as well as sessions that may not include the patient.
- In reporting, choose the code closest to the actual time (**Table 13-2**). Do not report psychotherapy of less than 16 minutes' duration.

Table 13-2. Reporting Psychotherapy Services

Duration of Psychotherapy	*CPT* Codes
<16 min	Do not report.
16–37 min	90832
38–52 min	90834
53–89 min	90837

Abbreviation: CPT, Current Procedural Terminology.

- Psychiatric services may be reported "with interactive complexity" (**90785**) when at least one of the following conditions is present:
    - The need to manage maladaptive communication (related to, eg, high anxiety, high reactivity, repeated questions, disagreement) among participants that complicates delivery of care
    - Caregiver emotions or behavior that interferes with the caregiver's understanding and ability to assist in the implementation of the treatment plan
    - Evidence or disclosure of a sentinel event and mandated report to third party (eg, abuse or neglect with report to state agency) with initiation of discussion of the sentinel event and/or report with patient and other visit participants

❖ Use of play equipment, other physical devices, interpreter, or translator to communicate with the patient to overcome barriers to therapeutic or diagnostic interaction between the physician or other QHP and a patient who
  — Is not fluent in the same language as the physician or other QHP
  — Has not developed, or has lost, the expressive language communication skills to explain his or her symptoms and response to treatment or the receptive communication skills to understand the physician or other QHP if he or she were to use typical language for communication

☀ Do not report psychotherapy for crisis (**90839**, **90840**) for service of less than 30 minutes or on the same date as other psychiatry services (**90785–90899**).

☀ Code **90863** was created for medication management when provided on the same day as psychotherapy by QHPs who may not report E/M codes (ie, psychologists licensed to prescribe). This code is an add-on code and may only be reported in addition to one of the stand-alone psychotherapy codes (ie, **90832**, **90834**, **90837**). Time spent providing medication management is not included in the time spent in psychotherapy.

☀ Prolonged services in the office or other outpatient setting (**99354**, **99355**) or inpatient or observation setting (**99356**, **99357**) may be reported in addition to the psychotherapy service code **90837** when 90 minutes or longer of face-to-face time with the patient and/or family member is spent performing psychotherapy services, which are not performed with an E/M service.

☀ Do not report psychotherapy codes in conjunction with codes for adaptive behavior assessment or treatment services (**97151–97158**, **0362T**, **0373T**).

Mental and Behavioral Health Services

Contents

Chapter 14: Mental and Behavioral Health Services

Physicians and Other Mental/Behavioral Health Providers

This chapter focuses on services that are provided to diagnose, manage, or treat mental and behavioral health conditions. Mental and behavioral health services may be covered through a provider network separate from other health care services. Physicians providing these services personally and/or through nonphysician staff within their practice must be aware of the coverage and payment policies of local and regional health plans and determine how these policies affect delivery and payment of services.

Services included in this chapter may be provided by

- Physicians and other qualified health care professionals (QHPs), including licensed clinical psychologists and licensed social workers
- Allied health care professionals (AHPs), such as technicians and developmental specialists, who provide services ordered by physicians and QHPs
- Clinical staff working under direct physician supervision

Of particular importance to correct reporting of nonphysician provider (NPP) services is identifying the providers included when terms such as "physician or other qualified health care professional" or "qualified, non-physician health care professional" are used in *Current Procedural Terminology* (*CPT®*) and/or payer instruction.

Current Procedural Terminology Provider Definitions

Current Procedural Terminology (*CPT*) provides definitions of providers as follows:

- **Physician or other qualified health care professional:** An individual who is qualified by education, training, licensure/regulation (when applicable), and facility privileging (when applicable) who performs a professional service within his or her scope of practice and independently reports that professional service
- **Clinical staff member:** A person who works under the supervision of a physician or other qualified health care professional and who is allowed by law, regulation, and facility policy to perform or assist in the performance of a specific professional service but does not individually report that professional service

Throughout the *CPT* code set, the use of terms such as "physician," "qualified health care professional," or "individual" is not intended to indicate that other entities may not report the service. In selected instances, specific instructions may define a service as limited to professionals or other entities (eg, hospital, home health agency).

Clinical staff member is used in *CPT* mostly in the context of staff who provide components of physician or QHP services, such as transitional care management and chronic care management (CCM), and services that are always billed under incident-to guidelines (eg, nurse visit, medication administration).

The *CPT* definition of physician or other QHP creates a broad category of providers (eg, advanced practice providers, therapists, social workers). The definition of *physician and other QHP* is used in relation to services such as evaluation and management (E/M) (**99201–99499**, which are typically within the scope of practice of physicians and advanced practice professionals but not of other QHPs and AHPs, whose scope of practice may be limited to specific specialized services (eg, psychotherapy without E/M).

Including Nonphysician Providers in Your Practice

Services such as behavioral health assessment by a licensed social worker or licensed psychologist may be provided within a general pediatric group practice and can be an integral part of providing a full scope of care in the medical home. However, billing and coding of these services must align not only with coding guidelines but also stanciate scope of practice (see the Scope of Practice Laws section in Chapter 13) and individual payer policies on credentialing, contracting, and billing for services of the specific NPP. See Chapter 13, Allied Health and Clinical Staff Services, for more information on billing and coding for services of NPPs.

Payment Issues for Mental/Behavioral Health Services

When arranging for or providing psychiatric services, it is very important to explore the options available to the patient in terms of health plan policy. Psychiatry services may be covered through a plan and provider network separate from other health care services. Payer policies may allow specific licensed professionals, such as licensed clinical psychologists, to directly provide and report certain services, while other AHPs (eg, licensed clinical social workers) may be limited to providing services under direct supervision and reporting under the name of the participating health care professional (eg, licensed clinical psychologist or psychiatrist). General pediatric physicians and advanced practice professionals may be ineligible to participate in the behavioral health plan network and limited to reporting E/M services to the health plan based on time spent in counseling and/or coordination of care.

Integration of psychiatric and/or developmental/behavioral health care professionals into the primary care practice may also require an understanding of health plan payment policies. Payer edits may not allow separate payment for mental and behavioral health services when E/M services are provided in the same practice on the same date. (Learn more about payer edits in Chapter 2, Modifiers and Coding Edits.) Verify coverage and billing options prior to provision of services. Healthcare Common Procedure Coding System (HCPCS) modifiers identifying the type of health care professional (eg, **AJ**, clinical social worker) may be necessary to override edits that bundle E/M services provided by a physician/QHP and mental/behavioral health services provided by an AHP on the same date.

Relevant HCPCS modifiers include

AH	Clinical psychologist
AJ	Clinical social worker
AM	Physician, team member service
HA	Child/adolescent program
HN	Bachelor's degree level
HO	Master's degree level
HP	Doctoral level
HQ	Group setting
TL	Early intervention/individualized family service plan (IFSP)
UN	Two patients served
UP	Three patients served
UQ	Four patients served
UR	Five patients served
US	Six or more patients served

Diagnosis Coding

Diagnosis of behavioral and mental health conditions is typically based on the criteria set forth in the *Diagnostic and Statistical Manual of Mental Disorders* (*DSM*) classification system, currently *DSM-5*. Often, a simple crosswalk from *DSM-5* diagnosis to *International Classification of Diseases, 10th Revision, Clinical Modification* (*ICD-10-CM*) code supporting the diagnosis can be made. However, the classifications are not equivalent in many cases. *DSM-5* does not differentiate Asperger syndrome from autism spectrum disorder (ASD). *ICD-10-CM* provides a specific code for Asperger syndrome (**F84.5**), in addition to codes for autistic disorder (**F84.0**) and other pervasive developmental disorders (eg, Rett syndrome, **F84.2**). It is important that documentation clearly reflects a diagnostic statement separate from the assignment of an *ICD-10-CM* code as required by official guidance for *ICD-10-CM*. This statement should include the findings (eg, observations made during the appointment, history, standardized rating scale results, pertinent physical examination findings) supporting the

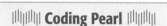

> ||||||||| **Coding Pearl** |||||||||
>
> *International Classification of Diseases, 10th Revision, Clinical Modification* codes for behavioral and emotional disorders with onset usually occurring in childhood and adolescence (**F90–F98**) may be reported for patients of any age. Disorders in this category typically have onset during childhood but may continue throughout life and not be diagnosed until adulthood.

diagnosis. Failure to document the information supporting the diagnostic statement could affect the patient's access to care and the physician's payment for services provided.

ICD-10-CM includes codes for specifying how an accident or injury happened (eg, unintentional or accidental; intentional, such as suicide or assault). Management of patients who have sustained injury or illness (eg, poisoning) due to intentional self-harm are reported with codes signifying the intent (eg, **T52.92ZA**, toxic effect of unspecified organic solvent, intentional self-harm, initial encounter). If the intent of the cause of an injury or other condition is unknown or unspecified, code the intent as accidental intent. All transport accident categories assume accidental intent. External cause codes for events of undetermined intent are only for use if the documentation in the record specifies that the intent cannot be determined (eg, suspected abuse under investigation).

Current Procedural Terminology® Add-on Codes

Many mental and behavioral health services are described by a combination of a base code with add-on codes representing extended services. Add-on codes (marked with a + before the code) are always performed in addition to a primary procedure and are never reported as a stand-alone service. Add-on codes describe additional intraservice work and are not valued to include preservice and post-service work like most other codes.

Central Nervous System Assessments/Tests

The following codes are used to report the services provided during testing of central nervous system (CNS) functions. Central nervous system assessments include, but are not limited to, memory, language, visual/motor responses, and abstract reasoning/problem-solving abilities. The mode of completion can be by a person (eg, paper and pencil) or via automated means. The administration of these tests will generate material that will be interpreted and formulated into a report by a physician or other QHP or an automated result.

Standardized instruments are used in the performance of these services. Standardized instruments are validated tests administered and scored in the consistent or "standard" manner performed during their validation. Informal checklists created by a physician or electronic health record developer are not considered standardized instruments.

Central nervous system assessments/tests are not reported in conjunction with adaptive behavior treatment (**97151–97158, 0362T, 0373T**).

> |||||||| **Coding Pearl** ||||||||
>
> Standardized instruments, used in the performance of central nervous system services, are validated tests administered and scored in the consistent or "standard" manner performed during their validation. Informal checklists created by a physician or electronic health record developer are not considered standardized instruments.

New in 2019

CPT 2019 introduces multiple changes to codes for CNS assessment/tests. Each of the new and revised codes for neuropsychological and psychological testing are discussed later in this section.

- Codes **96101, 96102,** and **96103** (psychological testing) have been deleted. To report psychological testing evaluation and administration and scoring services, see codes **96130, 96131,** and **96136–96146**.
- Code **96111** (developmental testing) has been deleted. To report developmental testing, see codes **96112** and **96113**. Refer to **Table 14-1**.
- Code **96116** now represents *only the first hour* of neurobehavioral status examination by a physician or QHP. Additional hours are reported with code **96121**.
- Codes **96118–96120** (neuropsychological testing) have been deleted. To report neuropsychological testing evaluation and administration and scoring services, see codes **96132–96146**.

Developmental Testing

Table 14-1. Developmental Testing Code Changes	
2018	**2019**
*96111 Developmental testing (includes assessment of motor, language, social, adaptive, and/or cognitive functioning by standardized developmental instruments) with interpretation and report	●96112 Developmental test administration (including assessment of fine and/or gross motor, language, cognitive level, social, memory and/or executive functions by standardized developmental instruments when performed), by physician or other qualified health care professional, with interpretation and report; first hour +●96113 each additional 30 minutes (List separately in addition to code for primary procedure)

Developmental testing services, which include interpretation and report, are now described by codes 96112 and 96113 Developmental testing is used by physicians with a special interest or special training in developmental and behavioral pediatrics.

Codes 96112 and 96113

❀ Allow reporting of developmental testing in which the child is observed doing standardized tasks that are then scored, with interpretation and report.

❀ Include assessment of motor, language, social, and/or cognitive function by standardized developmental instruments, such as the Bayley Scales of Infant and Toddler Development.

❀ Billing time includes both face-to-face time spent in testing and time of interpretation and report. Although not specifically stated in the code descriptor, interpretation and report is included as intraservice work in the assignment of work relative value units for these services. Payer policies may vary on reporting of time spent in interpretation and report. Check the policies of individual health plans when reporting.

❀ These 2 new codes allow billing for more than 76 minutes of testing. Developmental testing time is met when the midpoint is passed. At least 16 minutes of service is necessary to support reporting of a code that includes 30 minutes of service. An hour of service may be reported for 31 minutes or more.

> **||||||| Coding Pearl |||||||**
>
> Developmental screening services are described by **96110**. Developmental screening using a standardized instrument includes scoring and documentation. Interpretation and report as required for developmental test administration is included in the accompanying evaluation and management service.

Examples

➤ **A 5-year-old boy previously diagnosed with ASD but not enrolled in early intervention due to family circumstances presents for extended developmental testing after he could not be successfully assessed for kindergarten entry.** Developmental tests are administered, with total testing time on this date of 75 minutes. The child returns to complete testing 1 week later. Total testing time on the second date is 60 minutes. After the face-to-face encounter, the developmental pediatrician spends another 60 minutes on the same date interpreting the test results and 60 minutes formulating a report of the findings and recommendations. Code 96112 is reported for the 75 minutes of service on the first date. Code 96113 is not reported because the midpoint between 60 and 90 minutes (76 minutes) was not passed. On the second date of service, codes 96112 (for the 60 minutes of developmental testing) and 96113 are reported. 96113 is reported with 4 units of service for the additional 2 hours spent in interpreting the results of the testing and developing the report.

Teaching Point: Payers may require the entire service to be reported on a single claim. For these payers, on the date of the second session, report code 96112 (for the 60 minutes of testing on the first day) and 6 units of 96113 (for the remaining 195 minutes). Remember, the midpoint must be passed for the additional units to be billed. In this case, the remaining time was only 15 minutes.

➤ **A 10-year-old established patient has shown a progressive pattern of academic struggles since the first grade.** He says the fourth-grade work is "too hard." His parents wonder if he is "lazy" or if he may not be "smart enough." His school psychologist says there is no reason for her to do any psychoeducational testing. The physician administers a Kaufman Brief Intelligence Test, 2nd Edition, and a Wide Range Achievement Test 4 to briefly assess overall cognitive level and academic achievement levels. The tests are scored and interpreted. A concise written report is created for the parents to take to the school psychologist. Total time devoted to face-to-face testing, interpretation, and report was 110 minutes.

Code 96112 is reported for the first hour of testing, and code 96113 is reported with 2 units of service for the additional 50 minutes of service (1 unit for the first 30 minutes after the first hour and another unit for the final 20 minutes).

Neuropsychological and Psychological Testing

Neuropsychological and psychological testing evaluation services typically include integration of patient data with other sources of clinical data, interpretation, clinical decision-making, treatment planning, and report. Interactive feedback, conveying the implications of psychological or neuropsychological test findings and diagnostic formulation, is included when performed. Testing by a physician or QHP is separately reportable on the same or a different date as an evaluation service.

Testing codes differentiate tests administered by a physician or other QHP, by a technician, or via an electronic platform. Changes to this code set were approved for 2018. Refer to **Table 14-2**.

Neurobehavioral Status Examination

Table 14-2. Neurobehavioral Status Examination Code Changes	
2018	**2019**
96116 Neurobehavioral status examination (clinical assessment of thinking, reasoning and judgment, eg, acquired knowledge, attention, language, memory, planning and problem solving, and visual spatial abilities), per hour of the psychologist's or physician's time, both face-to-face time with the patient and time interpreting test results and preparing the report	★▲96116 Neurobehavioral status examination (clinical assessment of thinking, reasoning and judgment [eg, acquired knowledge, attention, language, memory, planning and problem solving, and visual spatial abilities]), *by physician or other qualified health care professional*, both face-to-face time with the patient and time interpreting test results and preparing the report; *first hour* +●96121　　　 each additional hour

⦿ Mini-mental status examination performed by a physician would be included as part of the CNS physical examination of an E/M service and not separately reportable.

⦿ Documentation of these services includes scoring, informal observation of behavior during the testing, and interpretation and report. It should include the date and time spent in testing, time of interpretation and report, reason for the test, and titles of all instruments used.

⦿ As specifically noted in the code descriptor for neurobehavioral status examination, time of face-to-face testing and time interpreting test results and preparing a report are included in the time reported for these services. The unit of time is 60 minutes.

Chapter 14: Mental and Behavioral Health Services

Example

➤ An 8-year-old boy, previously diagnosed with attention-deficit/hyperactivity disorder, is being evaluated for gradual problems with remembering directions, organizing his school materials and his room at home, and other behavior concerns. The Woodcock-Johnson Tests of Cognitive Abilities, 4th Edition, is administered, scored, and interpreted in a written report. The results indicate the need for further language, memory, and intelligence testing. The total time for testing, scoring, and report writing is 3½ hours.

This service is reported with codes **96116** (neurobehavioral status examination) and **96121** with 2 units for the additional 2 hours of testing, scoring, and report writing. The diagnosis code would be *ICD-10-CM* code **F90.9** (attention-deficit/hyperactivity disorder, unspecified type). Additional *ICD-10-CM* codes may be assigned for specific developmental disorders diagnosed following testing (eg, **F81.2**, mathematics disorder).

Psychological and Neuropsychological Testing Evaluation Services

Codes for psychological and neuropsychological testing are shown in **Table 14-3**. *Italic font* is added to emphasize key differences between codes.

Table 14-3. 2019 Psychological and Neuropsychological Testing Code Changes

Testing Evaluation Services by a Physician or QHP With Interpretation and Report

●96130 Psychological testing evaluation services by physician or other qualified health care professional, *including integration of patient data, interpretation of standardized test results and clinical data, clinical decision-making, treatment planning and report*, and interactive feedback to the patient, family member(s) or caregiver(s), when performed; first hour

+●96131   each additional hour (List separately in addition to code for primary procedure)

●96132 Neuropsychological testing evaluation services by physician or other qualified health care professional, *including integration of patient data, interpretation of standardized test results and clinical data, clinical decision-making, treatment planning and report*, and interactive feedback to the patient, family member(s) or caregiver(s), when performed; first hour

+●96133   each additional hour (List separately in addition to code for primary procedure)

Physician or QHP Administration and Scoring Only

●96136 Psychological or neuropsychological *test administration and scoring by physician or other qualified health care professional*, two or more tests, any method, first 30 minutes

+●96137   each additional 30 minutes after first 30 minutes (List separately in addition to code for primary procedure)

Administration and Scoring by a Technician

●96138 Psychological or neuropsychological test *administration and scoring by technician*, two or more tests, any method; first 30 minutes

+●96139   each additional 30 minutes (List separately in addition to code for primary procedure)

Automated Test Administration With Automated Result

●96146 Psychological or neuropsychological test administration, with single automated, standardized instrument *via electronic platform, with automated result only*

Abbreviation: QHP, qualified health care professional.

The tests selected, test administration, and method of testing and scoring are the same regardless of whether the testing is performed by a physician, QHP, or technician. Codes differentiate psychological and neuropsychological testing and testing by physicians and QHPs, technicians, and automated system.

Psychological and neuropsychological testing evaluation services by a physician or QHP are described by codes **96130–96133**.

●96130 *Psychological testing* evaluation services by physician or other qualified health care professional, including integration of patient data, interpretation of standardized test results and clinical data, clinical decision making, treatment planning and report, and interactive feedback to the patient, family member(s) or caregiver(s), when performed; first hour

+●96131 each additional hour (List separately in addition to code for primary procedure)

●96132 *Neuropsychological testing* evaluation services by physician or other qualified health care professional, including integration of patient data, interpretation of standardized test results and clinical data, clinical decision making, treatment planning and report, and interactive feedback to the patient, family member(s) or caregiver(s), when performed; first hour

+●96133 each additional hour (List separately in addition to code for primary procedure)

※ These services include integration of patient data, interpretation of test results and clinical data, treatment planning and report, and interactive feedback, when performed.

※ Psychological/neuropsychological testing evaluation services (96130–96133) may be reported with psychological/neuropsychological test administration and scoring services (96136–96139) on the same or different days (ie, each service is separately reported though incorporation of data from test administration, and scoring services performed on the same or a different date may be included in the time attributed to codes 96130–96133).

※ These services follow standard *CPT*® time definitions (ie, a minimum of 31 minutes must be provided to report any per-hour code). The time reported in codes 96130–96133is the face-to-face time with the patient and the time spent integrating and interpreting data.

※ Documentation of these services includes scoring, observation of behavior, and interpretation and report. It should include the date and time spent in testing and the time spent integrating and interpreting data, reason for the testing, and titles of all instruments used.

> **|||||||| Coding Pearl ||||||||**
>
> The time reported in codes **96130–96133** is the face-to-face time with the patient and the time spent integrating and interpreting data. Documentation of the time spent in face-to-face testing and in integration and interpretation of data must be documented to support the time used in code selection.

Example

➤ **An adolescent whose family reports psychotic behavior is referred for psychological testing evaluation.** The patient undergoes physician-administered psychological testing to evaluate emotionality, intellectual abilities, personality, and psychopathology, and to make a mental health diagnosis and treatment recommendations as applicable. The total time of face-to-face testing is 45 minutes. The physician's total time of evaluation and of data integration and interpretation is 75 minutes. Codes 96130and 96136are reported.

Teaching Point: Time of 30 minutes or less would not be reported with codes 96130–96133Time of 91 to 150 minutes would support reporting code 96131with 1 unit of service in addition to 96130 Time of 151 minutes or more would support additional units of service for code 96131(1 unit for each 31 minutes beyond the last full hour).

Testing Administration Services With Scoring

Testing administration services with scoring only (not including data integration or interpretation) performed by a physician or other QHP is reported with codes 96136and 96137

●96136 Psychological or neuropsychological test administration and scoring by physician or other qualified health care professional, two or more tests, any method, first 30 minutes

+●96137 each additional 30 minutes after first 30 minutes (List separately in addition to code for primary procedure)

※ Services include administration of a series of tests, recording of behavioral observations made during testing, scoring, and transcription of scores to a data summary sheet.

※ Codes are selected based on time of testing and scoring. Time is met when the midpoint is passed (ie, a minimum of 16 minutes for 30-minute codes).

※ *Do not include* time spent in integration of patient data or interpretation of test results in the time reported with codes **96136** and **96137**. This time is included with psychological and neuropsychological test evaluation services (**96130–96133**).

※ Psychological or neuropsychological test administration *using a single instrument*, with interpretation and report by physician or QHP, is reported with code **96127** (brief emotional/behavioral assessment [eg, depression inventory, attention-deficit/hyperactivity disorder scale], with scoring and documentation, per standardized instrument).

Example

➤ **An adolescent patient is referred for neuropsychological testing due to chronic physical symptoms without clinical findings and declining academic achievement.** A physician spends 50 minutes administering tests, recording observations, scoring, and transcribing results to a data summary sheet. Codes **96136** and **96137** are reported with 1 unit of service each.

   Teaching Point: Because the time of service exceeded 16 minutes beyond the first 30 minutes, code **96137** is reported in addition to **96136**.

Technician-Administered Testing

Testing and administration services performed by a technician are reported with codes **96138** and **96139**.

●**96138**   Psychological or neuropsychological test administration and scoring by technician, two or more tests, any method; first 30 minutes

+●**96139**   each additional 30 minutes (List separately in addition to code for primary procedure)

※ Codes **96138** and **96139** do not include the work of a physician or QHP. These codes are valued for practice expense and medical liability only.

※ Evaluation services by the physician or QHP are reported with **96133** whether provided on the same or a different date. Do not include time for evaluation services (eg, integration of patient data or interpretation of test results in the time of technician-administered testing).

Example

➤ **An adolescent patient is referred for neuropsychological testing due to chronic physical symptoms without clinical findings and declining academic achievement.** A technician spends 40 minutes administering and scoring tests. The technician also notes any behavioral observations. Code **96138** is reported with 1 unit of service.

   Teaching Point: If a physician or QHP provides evaluation services, including integration and interpretation of data from tests administered by a technician, on the same or different date, see codes **96132** and **96133** for those services.

Automated Testing and Result

When a single test instrument is completed by the patient via an electronic platform without physician, QHP, or technician administration and scoring, report code **96146**.

●**96146**   Psychological or neuropsychological test administration, with single automated, standardized instrument via electronic platform, with automated result only

※ Code **96146** does not include scoring by a health care professional or interpretation and report. Results are generated via the electronic platform.

※ If a test is administered by a physician, QHP, or technician, do not report **96146**. For brief emotional/behavioral assessment, see code **96127**.

Example

➤ **A child who is recovering from a concussion is provided a single computerized test (eg, ImPACT) for post-concussion symptoms.** The patient completes the test and the automated result is included in the patient's medical record.

Code **96146** is reported in addition to the code representing the physician's related E/M service (eg, **99213**).

Adaptive Behavior Assessment and Treatment Services

Adaptive behavior services address
- Deficient adaptive behaviors, such as impaired social, communication, or self-care skills
- Maladaptive behaviors, such as repetitive and stereotype behaviors
- Behaviors that risk physical harm to the patient, others, and/or property

Codes for adaptive behavior services are a combination of Category I and Category III (emerging technology) *CPT*® codes. Adaptive behavior services may be delivered by a physician or QHP, behavioral analyst, and/or licensed psychologist working with assistant behavior analysts or technicians. *It is important to verify health plan policies for coverage and payment of adaptive behavior services, including any required provider qualifications (eg, certification, licensure) prior to provision of services.* Most states mandate coverage of adaptive behavior services for patients diagnosed with ASD. Some states require that behavior analysts providing ASD-related assessment and/or treatment be certified by the Behavior Analyst Certification Board as a Board Certified Behavior Analyst. In the discussion of adaptive behavior services, the QHP includes behavior analysts and licensed psychologists who are able to independently report these services.

Patients who require adaptive behavior assessment and/or treatment may also require combinations of services such as speech/language, physical, or occupational therapy; neurobehavioral status examination; psychiatric examination; or neuropsychological testing. However, these services are not included in or reported as adaptive behavior assessment or treatment. See your procedure coding reference (eg, *CPT*® coding manual) for specific instructions for reporting these services.

Because there are no category-specific instructions on the time of service for adaptive behavior services, the general rule that time is met when the midpoint is passed applies (eg, at least 8 minutes of service is required to support a service specified as 15 minutes).

Until this year, *CPT* codes for adaptive behavior assessment and treatment services were Category III codes, which are not accepted by all payers. Additionally, some payers (eg, Medicaid plans) have required HCPCS codes in lieu of *CPT* codes for certain adaptive behavior assessment and treatment services. Examples of HCPCS codes used in health plan policies for adaptive behavior services include

H2014	Skills training, per 15 minutes
H2019	Therapeutic behavioral services, per 15 minutes
H0025	Behavioral health prevention education service (delivery of services with target population to affect knowledge, attitude and/or behavior)
H0031	Mental health assessment by nonphysician
H0032	Mental health service plan development by nonphysician
H2027	Psychoeducational service, per 15 minutes
S5108	Home care training to home care client, per 15 minutes
S5111	Home care training, family; per session

HCPCS codes are often interpreted and utilized differently by individual health plans. It is important to verify each payer's policy for coverage and payment of adaptive behavior services and to submit codes complying with each payer's policy.

Adaptive Behavior Assessment

Note: This code set is used during evaluations of behaviorally disturbed individuals. Although the term *adaptive behavior assessment* also is used by some publishers of scales of functional status, the services are different, and these codes should not be used to describe the administration and scoring of standardized scales of functional status (eg, Vineland Adaptive Scales, Adaptive Behavior Assessment System).

   CPT codes for behavior identification assessment include

#●97151   Behavior identification assessment, administered by a physician or other qualified health care professional, each 15 minutes of the physician's or other qualified health care professional's time face-to-face with patient and/or guardian(s)/caregiver(s) administering assessments and discussing findings and recommendations, and non-face-to-face analyzing past data, scoring/interpreting the assessment, and preparing the report/treatment plan

#●97152   Behavior identification supporting assessment, administered by one technician under the direction of a physician or other qualified health care professional, face-to-face with the patient, each 15 minutes

▲0362T   Behavior identification supporting assessment, each 15 minutes of technicians' time face-to-face with a patient, requiring the following components:

   ❖ administration by the physician or other qualified health care professional who is on site;

   ❖ with the assistance of two or more technicians;

   ❖ for a patient who exhibits destructive behavior;

   ❖ completion in an environment that is customized to the patient's behavior

---

Current Procedural Terminology Definitions of Functional Behavior Assessment and Functional Analysis

Current Procedural Terminology provides some helpful definitions.

❖ **Functional behavior assessment** comprises descriptive assessment procedures designed to identify environmental events that occur just before and just after occurrences of potential target behaviors and that may influence those behaviors. Information may be gathered by interviewing the patient's caregivers; having caregivers complete checklists, rating scales, or questionnaires; and/or observing and recording occurrences of target behaviors and environmental events in everyday situations.

❖ **Functional analysis** is an assessment procedure for evaluating the separate effects of each of several environmental events on a potential target behavior by systematically presenting and withdrawing each event to a patient multiple times and observing and measuring occurrences of the behavior in response to those events. Graphed data are analyzed visually to determine which events produced relatively high and low occurrences of the behavior.

❖ Behavior identification assessment code 97151 may include analysis of pertinent past data (including medical diagnosis), a detailed behavioral history, patient observation, administration of standardized and/or non-standardized instruments and procedures, functional behavior assessment, functional analysis, and/or guardian/caregiver interview to identify and describe deficient adaptive behaviors, maladaptive behaviors, and other impaired functioning secondary to deficient adaptive or maladaptive behaviors.

❖ If the physician or other QHP personally performs the technician activities, his or her time engaged in these activities should be included as part of the required technician time to meet the components of the code.

❖ Codes 97151, 97152, and 0362T may be repeated on the same or different days until the behavior identification assessment (97151) and, if necessary, supporting assessment(s) (97152, 0362T), are complete.

❖ Code 97152 is reported for assessment by a technician. The reporting physician or QHP is not required to be on site during the assessment. See code 0362T when multiple technicians and a customized assessment environment are required due to destructive behavior(s) of the patient.

⊙ Code **0362T** represents testing of a patient who demonstrates destructive behavior(s), and requires an environment customized to the patient and behavior and multiple technicians. The reporting physician or QHP is required to be on site (immediately available and interruptible to provide assistance and direction throughout the performance of the procedure). The reporting physician or QHP is not required to be in the room during testing.

  ❖ Destructive behavior(s) includes maladaptive behaviors associated with a high risk of medical consequences or property damage (eg, elopement; pica; self-injury requiring medical attention; aggression with injury to others; breaking furniture, walls, windows).

⊙ Only count the time of 1 technician when 2 or more technicians are present. Code **0362T** is reported based on a single technician's face-to-face time with the patient and not the combined time of multiple technicians (eg, 1 hour with 3 technicians equals 1 hour of service) despite the expectation that more than 1 technician will be needed.

Examples

➤ **A 3-year-old boy with symptoms of ASD presents for assessment.** The physician/QHP reviews the patient's medical records, including previous assessments and any previous or current treatment. A structured interview with the parents is conducted to solicit their observations of their child's behaviors and other concerns. The physician/QHP spends 1 hour face-to-face with the patient and/or guardian(s)/caregiver(s) administering assessments and discussing findings and recommendations, and 45 minutes of non–face-to-face time analyzing past data, scoring/interpreting the assessment, and preparing the report/treatment plan. The total time of service is 1 hour, 38 minutes. Code **97151** is reported with 7 units (1 for each full 15 minutes of service and 1 for the last 8 minutes).

  Teaching Point: If fewer than 8 minutes past the last full 15 minutes of service were provided, only the number of 15-minute periods of service would be reported (eg, 1 hour, 37 minutes equals 6 units).

➤ **An additional assessment of the 3-year-old from the previous example is required to assess behavior that interferes with acquisition of adaptive skills.** A technician, under the physician's or QHP's direction, observes and records occurrence of the patient's deficient adaptive and maladaptive behaviors and the surrounding environmental events several times in a variety of situations. The physician/QHP reviews and analyzes data from those observations. The face-to-face time of the technician is 1 hour.

  Code **97152** is reported with 4 units of service.

➤ **An 11-year-old boy with ASD requires evaluation due to increased self-injury and aggression toward others.** A team of technicians conducts the assessment session in a room that is devoid of any objects that might cause injury, under observation by a physician/QHP who is on site and immediately available throughout the session. The technicians implement functional analysis as directed by the physician/QHP and record data. Graphed data are reviewed and analyzed by the physician/QHP to identify the environmental events in whose presence the level of behavior was highest and lowest. The technicians spend a total of 90 minutes face-to-face with the patient during the assessment.

  Code **0362T** is reported with 6 units of service.

Adaptive Behavior Treatment

Adaptive behavior treatment services address specific treatment targets and goals based on results of previous assessments and include ongoing assessment and adjustment of treatment protocols, targets, and goals. Codes describe services to the individual patient, groups of patients, families, and an individual patient who exhibits destructive behavior. See **Table 14-4** for a listing of codes for adaptive behavior treatment.

Table 14-4. 2019 Codes for Adaptive Behavior Treatment

By Protocol

#●97153 Adaptive behavior treatment by protocol, administered by technician under the direction of a physician or other qualified health care professional, face-to-face with one patient; each 15 minutes

#●97154 Group adaptive behavior treatment by protocol, administered by technician under the direction of a physician or other qualified health care professional, face-to-face with two or more patients, each 15 minutes

With Protocol Modification

#●97155 Adaptive behavior treatment with protocol modification administered by physician or other qualified health care professional, which may include simultaneous direction of technician, face-to-face with one patient, each 15 minutes

#●97158 Group adaptive behavior treatment with protocol modification, administered by physician or other qualified health care professional face-to-face with multiple patients, each 15 minutes

▲0373T Adaptive behavior treatment with protocol modification, each 15 minutes of technicians' time face-to-face with a patient, requiring the following components:
- administration by the physician or other qualified health care professional who is on site;
- with the assistance of two or more technicians;
- for a patient who exhibits destructive behavior;
- completion in an environment that is customized to the patient's behavior.

Family

#●97156 Family adaptive behavior treatment guidance, administered by physician or other qualified health care professional (with or without the patient present), face-to-face with guardian(s)/caregiver(s), each 15 minutes

#●97157 Multiple-family group adaptive behavior treatment guidance, administered by physician or other qualified health care professional (without the patient present), face-to-face with multiple sets of guardians/caregivers, each 15 minutes

Codes for adaptive behavior treatment specify services provided by protocol (**97153, 97154**) or with protocol modification (**97155, 97158, 0373T**). Behavior treatment with protocol modification requires adjustments *made in real time* rather than for a subsequent service.

Adaptive Behavior Treatment by Protocol

#●97153 Adaptive behavior treatment by protocol, administered by technician under the direction of a physician or other qualified health care professional, face-to-face with one patient; each 15 minutes

#●97154 Group adaptive behavior treatment by protocol, administered by technician under the direction of a physician or other qualified health care professional, face-to-face with two or more patients, each 15 minutes

- If the physician/QHP personally performs the technician activities, his or her time engaged in these activities should be reported as technician time. The physician is not required to be on site during the provision of these services.
- Adaptive behavior treatment by protocol to a single patient (**97153**) and group adaptive behavior treatment by protocol (**97154**) are administered by a technician under the direction of a physician/QHP, using a treatment protocol *designed in advance* by the physician or other QHP, who may or may not provide direction during the treatment.
  - The service described by code **97153** is face-to-face with one patient only. This code does not include protocol modification.
  - Code **97154** is reported for services face-to-face with 2 or more patients but not more than 8 patients.

Examples

➤ **A 4-year-old girl presents with deficits in language and social skills and emotional outbursts in response to small changes in routines or when preferred items are unavailable.** A QHP directs a technician in the implementation of treatment protocols and data collection procedures. The technician conducts a treatment session in the family home with multiple planned opportunities for the patient to practice target skills. The QHP reviews the technician's recorded and graphed data to assess the child's progress and determine if any treatment protocol needs adjustment. The technician spends 1 hour at the patient's home with face-to-face time of the treatment session of 50 minutes. Code **97153** is reported with 3 units of service.

    Teaching Point: Only the technician's face-to-face time with the patient is used to determine the units of service. This service may also be conducted in a community setting (eg, playground, store).

➤ **Peer social skills training in a small group is recommended for a 7-year-old girl with deficits in social skills.** A technician conducts the group session using treatment protocols and data collection procedures as previously designed by a QHP. The QHP reviews the technician's recorded and graphed data to assess the child's progress and determine if treatment protocols need adjustment. The total face-to-face time of the session is 60 minutes.

    Code **97154** is reported with 4 units.

Adaptive Behavior Treatment With Protocol Modification

#●97155   Adaptive behavior treatment with protocol modification administered by physician or other qualified health care professional, which may include simultaneous direction of technician, face-to-face with one patient, each 15 minutes

#●97158   Group adaptive behavior treatment with protocol modification, administered by physician or other qualified health care professional face-to-face with multiple patients, each 15 minutes

▲0373T   Adaptive behavior treatment with protocol modification, each 15 minutes of technicians' time face-to-face with a patient, requiring the following components:
- administration by the physician or other qualified health care professional who is on site;
- with the assistance of two or more technicians;
- for a patient who exhibits destructive behavior;
- completion in an environment that is customized to the patient's behavior.

- Adaptive behavior treatment with protocol modification (**97155**) is administered by a physician/QHP *face-to-face with a single patient.*
  - ❖ The physician/QHP resolves one or more problems with the protocol and may simultaneously direct a technician in administering the modified protocol *while the patient is present.* Physician/QHP direction to the technician without the patient present is not reported separately.
- Group adaptive behavior treatment with protocol modification (**97158**) is reported for when a physician/QHP provides *face-to-face* protocol modification services with up to 8 patients in a group. The physician/QHP monitors the needs of individual patients and adjusts treatment techniques during the group sessions, as needed.
- Adaptive behavior treatment with protocol modification (**0373T**) is reported for services to a patient who presents with one or more destructive behavior(s). The service time is based on a single technician's face-to-face time with the patient and not the combined time of multiple technicians.
  - ❖ The physician/QHP must be on site and immediately available during the service described by code **0373T.**

Chapter 14: Mental and Behavioral Health Services

Examples

➤ **A 5-year-old boy previously showed steady improvements in language and social skills at home as a result of one-to-one intensive applied behavior analysis intervention, but skill development seems to have reached a plateau recently.** A QHP modifies the written protocols used previously to incorporate procedures designed to build the child's language and social skills into daily home routines (eg, play, dressing, mealtimes). The QHP demonstrates the procedures to the technician and directs the technician to implement the protocols with the child. The QHP then observes and provides feedback as the technician implements the procedures with the child. The technician's face-to-face time with the patient is 45 minutes. Code **97155** is reported with 3 units of service.

> **Teaching Point:** Time spent by the technician and QHP without the patient present is not included in the time of service.

➤ **A 13-year-old girl is reported to be isolated from peers due to poor social skills and odd behavior.** The child attends a group treatment session that focuses on peer social skills. A QHP begins the group session by asking each patient to briefly describe 2 of their recent social encounters with peers, one that went well and one that did not. The information is used to develop a group activity in which each member has the opportunity to practice the skills she or he used in the encounters that went well and to problem-solve the interactions that did not go well. The QHP helps each patient identify social cues that were interpreted correctly and incorrectly and what she or he could have done differently and provides prompts and feedback individualized to each patient's skills. The QHP ends the session by summarizing the discussion. The total time of the session was 70 minutes, including a 10-minute break (ie, 60 minutes of group session). Code **97158** is reported with 4 units of service.

> **Teaching Point:** Only the QHP's face-to-face time providing the service is reported.

➤ **A 16-year-old boy has had 2 surgeries to relieve esophageal blockages due to pica involving repeated ingestion of small metal objects (eg, paper clips, pushpins).** The patient's pica behavior has not responded to previous treatment. The QHP supervising the patient's treatment plan has previously developed written protocols for reducing the patient's pica. A technician carefully inspects the room before the session to make sure there are no potential pica items on the floor. Two technicians are present, with one presenting the patient with a series of trials in which the patient is presented with a food item and a nonhazardous item that resembles a pica item. The second technician prompts the patient to choose the food item and blocks attempts to choose the pica item. The patient's response to each trial is recorded. The QHP is on site and available to assist as needed. The total session lasts 40 minutes. Code **0373T** is reported with 2 units.

> **Teaching Point:** Although 2 technicians were present, time is counted only once.

Family Adaptive Behavior Treatment Guidance

Family adaptive behavior treatment guidance (**97156**) and multiple-family group adaptive behavior treatment guidance (**97157**) are administered by a physician or QHP face-to-face with guardian(s)/caregiver(s) and involve identifying potential treatment targets and training guardian(s)/caregiver(s) to implement treatment protocols designed to address deficient adaptive or maladaptive behaviors.

#●**97156**   Family adaptive behavior treatment guidance, administered by physician or other qualified health care professional (with or without the patient present), face-to-face with guardian(s)/caregiver(s), each 15 minutes

#●**97157**   Multiple-family group adaptive behavior treatment guidance, administered by physician or other qualified health care professional (without the patient present), face-to-face with multiple sets of guardians/caregivers, each 15 minutes

☀ Family adaptive behavior treatment guidance (**97156**) provided to the caregiver(s) of one patient may be performed with or without the patient present.

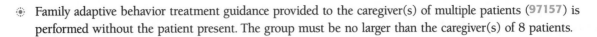

❋ Family adaptive behavior treatment guidance provided to the caregiver(s) of multiple patients (97157) is performed without the patient present. The group must be no larger than the caregiver(s) of 8 patients.

Examples

➤ **Parents of a 6-year-old boy seek training on procedures for helping the child communicate using picture cards (skills he previously developed in adaptive behavior treatment therapy sessions with technicians) during typical family routines.** A physician/QHP trains the parents. The service includes reviewing the written treatment and data collection protocols with the parents, demonstrating how to implement them in role-plays and with the child, and having the parents implement the protocols with the child while the provider observes and provides feedback. The time of service is 1 hour.

  Code 97156 is reported with 4 units of service.

➤ **The parents of a 3-year-old boy who has pervasive hyperactivity and no functional play, social, or communication skills seek training on how to manage his hyperactive and disruptive behavior and help him develop appropriate play, social, and communication skills.** The parents attend a group session (without the patient) lead by a physician who asks each set of parents to identify one skill to be increased or one problem behavior to be decreased in their own child. The physician describes how behavior analytic principles and procedures could be applied to the behavior identified by the parents of this 3-year-old patient. She/he demonstrates a procedure (eg, prompting the child to speak instead of whining when he wants something; not giving him preferred items when he whines). The parents then role-play, implementing that procedure. Other group participants and the physician provide feedback and make constructive suggestions. That process is repeated for skills/behaviors identified by other sets of parents. The group session ends with the physician summarizing the main points, answering questions, and giving each set of parents a homework assignment to practice the skills they worked on during the session. The session lasts 110 minutes. Code 97157 is reported with 7 units.

  Teaching Point: The last 5 minutes are not reported because the midpoint of 8 minutes beyond the last full 15-minute period (105 minutes) was not passed.

Habilitative and Rehabilitative Modifiers

Adaptive behavior services may be either habilitative or rehabilitative. Because the Patient Protection and Affordable Care Act provides that certain health plans must provide equal coverage for habilitative and rehabilitative services and count each type of service separately, it may be necessary to indicate that a service is habilitative or rehabilitative. Modifiers 96 (habilitative services) and 97 (rehabilitative services) are appended to procedure codes to designate the nature of a service. Habilitative services are those provided to help an individual learn skills not yet developed and to keep and/or improve those skills. Rehabilitative services help a patient keep, get back, or improve skills that have been lost or limited due to illness, injury, and/or disability. Modifiers 96 and 97 were added to *CPT®* in 2018 and may not be adopted for use by all payers or may have limited utility. Verify payer policies for these modifiers when providing habilitative and rehabilitative services. See Chapter 2, Modifiers and Coding Edits, for more information on modifiers 96 and 97.

Health and Behavior Assessments/Interventions

96150	Health and behavior assessment, each 15 minutes face-to-face with the patient, initial assessment
96151	reassessment
96152	Health and behavior intervention, each 15 minutes, face-to-face; individual
96153	group (2 or more patients)
96154	family (with patient present)
96155	family (without patient present)

Face-to-face health and behavior intervention services are reported per each 15 minutes of time spent. The total time must be documented in the medical record. Time is met when the midpoint is passed unless payer policy directs otherwise.

Codes 96150–96155

⚬ May be reported by psychologists, clinical social workers, licensed therapists, and other AHPs within their scope of practice who have specialty or subspecialty training in health and behavior assessment or intervention procedures.

⚬ Physicians and other QHPs who may report E/M services are instructed to report E/M or preventive service codes in lieu of 96150–96155.

⚬ Are used when assessing or addressing psychosocial factors affecting patients who have an established medical illness or diagnosis and may benefit from assessments and interventions with a focus on the role that psychosocial adaptation may play on the clinical course of that condition.

⚬ Are not used in conjunction with a primary diagnosis of mental disorder. (Payers may deny when a diagnosis code indicating mental disorder is included on the claim for these services.)

⚬ Are used to identify the psychological, behavioral, emotional, cognitive, and/or social factors needed for the prevention, treatment, or management of physical health problems, with a focus on treating the biopsychosocial factors contributing to physical problems.

⚬ Do not require a standardized curriculum.

⚬ Are not reported with psychiatric codes (90785–90899) when provided on the same day. Only the primary service is reported (ie, either 96150–96155 or 90791–90899).

⚬ Are not reported with an E/M code (eg, 99201–99215, 99401–99412) on the same day.

⚬ Are not reported in conjunction with adaptive behavior treatment (97153–97158; 0373T).

⚬ Do not include neuropsychological testing (96116, 96121), which can be reported separately.

⚬ The initial assessment (96150) may include a health-focused clinical interview, behavioral observations, psychophysiological monitoring, and completion of health-oriented questionnaires.

⚬ Code 96151 is used to report the reassessment of a patient's condition by interview and behavioral health instruments.

Examples

➤ **A 12-year-old girl undergoing treatment for acute lymphoblastic leukemia is referred to a social worker trained in health and behavior assessment or intervention procedures for assessment of pain, behavioral distress, and combativeness associated with repeated procedures and treatment.** The patient is assessed using standardized questionnaires (eg, Pediatric Pain Questionnaire, Coping Strategies Inventory). The child's parents are also interviewed.

Code 96150 would be reported with, for example, *ICD-10-CM* code C91.00, acute lymphoblastic leukemia, without remission. One unit of service would be reported for each 15 minutes of face-to-face time with the patient and/or parents. Time must be documented and does not include time spent before or after face-to-face services.

➤ **Same patient as previous example.** Results from the health and behavior assessment are used to develop a treatment plan. Thirty minutes is spent with the patient discussing the behavior and suggested coping skills.

Code 96152 with 2 units of service would be reported with the same diagnosis as used in the initial assessment.

➤ **A 10-year-old boy diagnosed with localization-related symptomatic epilepsy with simple partial seizures 2 years ago has undergone health and behavior assessment after parents noted the boy was afraid to go to school, where he fears being in trouble and failing.** Based on the assessment conducted at a previous encounter, the clinical psychologist works with the boy to develop new coping skills and improve self-management. Parents are urged to meet with the boy's teacher about adherence to an existing behavioral intervention plan and recommended revisions. A total of 55 minutes is spent face-to-face with the boy and his parents.

Code 96154 is reported with 4 units of service (3 full 15-minute periods and 1 unit for the last 10 minutes because the midpoint of 8 minutes beyond the last full period was passed). *ICD-10-CM* code G40.109 (localization-related [focal] [partial] symptomatic epilepsy and epileptic syndromes with simple partial seizures, not intractable, without status epilepticus) is reported.

Psychiatric Services

Psychiatry services include diagnostic services, psychotherapy, and other services to an individual, a family, or a group. Comprehensive services may be provided by a multidisciplinary team (eg, a psychiatrist, developmental-behavioral pediatrician, nurse practitioner, psychologist, clinical social worker, and/or clinical counselor). However, in many parts of the country, children's mental and behavioral health professionals are not available. General pediatricians often must take on management of minor mental health problems and, when possible, consult with a mental/behavioral health professional at a distant location or arrange for services via telemedicine services.

An emerging method of delivering mental health services is psychiatric collaborative care management (PCCM), in which care is directed by a primary care pediatrician or QHP and provided in collaboration with a psychiatric consultant. See the Psychiatric Collaborative Care Management Services section later in this chapter for more information.

Interactive Complexity

+90785   Interactive complexity

Psychiatric services to children may include interactive complexity. According to *CPT®*, psychiatric procedures may be reported "with interactive complexity" when at least one of the following is present:

* The need to manage maladaptive communication (related to, eg, high anxiety, high reactivity, repeated questions, or disagreement) among participants that complicates delivery of care.
* Caregiver emotions or behavior interfering with the caregiver's understanding and ability to assist in the implementation of the treatment plan.
* Evidence or disclosure of a sentinel event and mandated report to third party (eg, abuse or neglect with report to state agency) with initiation of discussion of the sentinel event and/or report with patient and other visit participants.
* Use of play equipment, other physical devices, interpreter, or translator to communicate with the patient to overcome barriers to therapeutic or diagnostic interaction between the physician or other QHP and a patient who
  * Is not fluent in the same language as the physician or other QHP, or
  * Has not developed, or has lost, either the expressive language communication skills to explain his/her symptoms and response to treatment or the receptive communication skills to understand the physician or other QHP if he/she were to use typical language for communication

Add-on code 90785 is reported when interactive complexity complicates delivery of psychiatric services, including diagnostic psychiatric evaluation (90791, 90792), psychotherapy (90832, 90834, 90837), psychotherapy when performed with an E/M service (90833, 90836, 90838), and group psychotherapy (90853).

* Interactive complexity indicates an *increased complexity of work* as opposed to an extended duration of services.
* Interactive complexity is not billed in conjunction with psychotherapy for crisis (90839, 90840).
* Interactive complexity applies only to the psychiatric portion of a service including both psychiatric and E/M components. Code 90785 is never reported alone and is not reported in conjunction with E/M services alone.
* Do not report code 90785 in conjunction with adaptive behavior treatment (97153–97158; 0373T).

Examples

➤ **A 10-year-old patient undergoes psychiatric evaluation.** The child is accompanied by divorced parents, reporting declining grades, temper outbursts, and bedtime difficulties. Parents are extremely anxious and repeatedly ask questions about the treatment process. Each parent continually challenges the other's observations of the patient.

Codes **90791** (psychiatric diagnostic evaluation) and **90785** (interactive complexity) are reported.

➤ **A 6-year-old girl is seen for psychotherapy.** The child was placed in foster care following hospitalization for head injuries sustained due to physical abuse and neglect by her mother and the mother's boyfriend. The service includes the psychologist's review of the child's medical record and telephone interviews with the child's social worker and teacher. The mother refuses a request for interview. The psychologist interviews the foster mother, who expresses concerns that the child is grieving the loss of contact with 2 half-siblings who are in their father's custody and is fearful of making emotional connections with her foster parents. The psychologist uses play to gain trust and evaluate the child. The psychologist and foster mother agree on a treatment plan and then discuss the plan with the child in terms she can understand. Following the service, the psychologist provides a report to the patient's social worker.

Codes **90791** (psychiatric diagnostic evaluation) and **90785** (interactive complexity) are reported.

Psychiatric Diagnostic Evaluation

90791 Psychiatric diagnostic evaluation
90792 Psychiatric diagnostic evaluation with medical services

Psychiatric diagnostic evaluation (**90791**) and psychiatric diagnostic evaluation with medical services (**90792**) include an integrated biopsychosocial assessment, including history, mental status, and recommendations. When medical services (medical assessments and physical examination other than mental status, when indicated) are included, code **90792** is reported.

- Psychiatric diagnostic evaluation or reevaluation (**90791, 90792**) is reported once per day. Do not report psychotherapy codes (**90832–90839**) on the same date of service as **90791** or **90792**.
- The same individual may not separately report E/M services on the same date as psychiatric diagnostic evaluation.
- Report code **90785** for interactive complexity in addition to code **90791** or **90792**, when applicable.
- Health plans may not cover mental health consultation, testing, or evaluation that is performed to assess custody, visitation, or parental rights. Verify health plan contractual obligations prior to providing services that may lack medical necessity and determine if a waiver of liability must be signed by the patient(s) prior to beginning the service. A waiver of liability is the patient's agreement to pay out of pocket for services not covered by his or her health plan.

> **||||||| Coding Pearl |||||||**
>
> When services are requested for purposes that a health plan may consider not medically necessary (eg, evaluation of parent seeking child custody or visitation, services that exceed those authorized by a payer), failure to obtain the responsible party's signature on a waiver of liability *prior to the service* may release the patient from the obligation to pay based on contractual agreement between the provider and health plan. Modifier **GA** (waiver of liability statement issued as required by payer policy, individual case) may be appended to the code reported to indicate the waiver is on file.

Examples

➤ **A 14-year-old girl is referred by her primary care pediatrician for evaluation and treatment of depression with suicidal ideation.** The psychologist obtains information on the presenting problem and situation. A statement of need and expectations is documented. Current symptoms and behaviors are documented. The patient has no history of previous psychiatric treatment. The patient denies previous substance abuse treatment and current use of alcohol or drugs. Her current medication regimen of fluoxetine 10 mg once a day is documented. She has no current medical problems and is not allergic to any medications. The patient's family and social status (current and historical), school status/functioning, and resources are obtained and documented. A diagnosis of moderate major depressive disorder, single episode, and parent-child relationship problem is documented.

Code 90791 is reported in conjunction with *ICD-10-CM* codes F32.1 (major depressive disorder, single episode, moderate) and Z63.8, other specified problems related to primary support group.

➤ **A 15-year-old girl was admitted through the emergency department (ED) following a suicide attempt.** The girl is evaluated by a psychiatrist for admission to inpatient psychiatric care. The psychiatrist performs a psychiatric diagnostic evaluation of this patient, who previously attempted suicide at age 13 and has a history of recurrent major depressive disorder. The patient also expresses fear that she may be pregnant and has been exposed to a sexually transmitted infection. Medical history includes nausea with vomiting for the last week and last menstrual period 6 weeks ago. Laboratory tests are ordered to rule out pregnancy and/or infection, and consultation with a gynecologist is ordered. Diagnoses are severe major depressive disorder without psychosis (F33.2), nausea with vomiting (R11), and pregnancy test, unconfirmed (Z72.40).

Code 90792 is reported for combined psychiatric and medical evaluations.

➤ **A 17-year-old girl wishes to be evaluated for purposes of determining her ability to accept responsibility for herself.** The girl is seeking emancipation from her mother, who is currently living with an abusive boyfriend and will not allow her to move in with her aunt while finishing high school. An attorney has advised obtaining a psychological evaluation to support the girl's claims that she is psychologically prepared to take this action. The girl's health plan considers this service not medically necessary but allows for patient payment when a waiver of liability is obtained prior to the service. She agrees to sign the waiver and pay for the service. An evaluation is completed, and a report of the evaluation is provided to the girl and her attorney.

The service is reported to the health plan with modifier GA (waiver of liability statement issued as required by payer policy, individual case) appended to code 90791.

Psychotherapy

CPT® defines psychotherapy as the treatment of mental illness and behavioral disturbances in which the physician or QHP, through definitive therapeutic communications, attempts to alleviate the emotional disturbances, reverse or change maladaptive patterns of behavior, and encourage personality growth and development. Services include ongoing assessment and adjustment of psychotherapeutic interventions and may include involvement of informants in the treatment process.

Codes differentiate psychotherapy services to individuals (with and without E/M services), an individual family or groups of families, and groups of patients. Codes for each are provided in the following discussions. In addition, separate codes (90839, 90840) are reported for psychotherapy for crisis (see the Psychotherapy for Crisis section later in this chapter).

Pertinent instructions for coding for all psychotherapy services are
☀ Psychotherapy times are for face-to-face services with a patient and/or family member. The patient must be present for all or some of the service except when reporting family psychotherapy without the patient present (90846). This allows for the participation of others in the psychotherapy session for the patient as long as the patient remains the focus of the intervention. Documentation must support that the patient was present for a significant portion of the session.

> **||||||||| Coding Pearl |||||||||**
>
> Progress notes for psychotherapy services should include
> - Start and stop times of psychotherapy
> - Service type
> - Diagnosis
> - Interval history (eg, increase/decrease in symptoms, current risk factors)
> - Names and scores of standardized rating scales used in monitoring progress
> - Therapeutic interventions (eg, type of therapy, medications)
> - Summary of goals and progress
> - An updated treatment plan
> - Date and signature of performing provider

Chapter 14: Mental and Behavioral Health Services

⁕ Psychotherapy documentation must include the time of service, preferably with start and stop times documented. Other documentation elements include diagnosis, interval history, therapeutic interventions, summary of goals and progress toward goals, and an updated treatment plan. *These elements should be documented in the progress note in the patient record rather than the protected psychotherapy notes.* Psychotherapy notes are not disclosed for purposes of receiving or supporting accurate payment.

⁕ For psychotherapy with biofeedback, see codes **90875** and **90876** (see Psychotherapy With Biofeedback section later in this chapter).

⁕ Psychotherapy differs from family psychotherapy (**90846**, **90847**), which uses family psychotherapy techniques to benefit the patient (eg, attempting to improve family communication or alter family interactions that negatively affect the patient; encouraging interactions to improve family functioning). Family psychotherapy includes sessions with the entire family as well as sessions that may not include the patient.

⁕ In reporting, choose the code closest to the actual time (**Table 14-5**). Do not report psychotherapy of less than 16 minutes' duration.

Table 14-5. Reporting Psychotherapy Services

Duration of Psychotherapy	CPT® Codes
<16 min	Do not report.
16–37 min	90832, 90833
38–52 min	90834, 90836
53–89 min	90837, 90838
≥26 min	90846, 90847

Abbreviation: CPT, Current Procedural Terminology.

⁕ Do not report psychotherapy codes in conjunction with codes for adaptive behavior assessment or treatment services (**97153–97158**, **0362T**, **0373T**).

⁕ Psychotherapy of more than 45 minutes is often considered unusual and may require health plan precertification.

Psychotherapy With Evaluation and Management

+90833   Psychotherapy, 30 minutes with patient when performed with an evaluation and management service

+90836   45 minutes with patient when performed with an evaluation and management service

+90838   60 minutes with patient when performed with an evaluation and management service

Psychiatrists and other physicians who provide a combination of psychotherapy and E/M services (eg, **99213**) on the same date may report an E/M code and an add-on code for psychotherapy (**90833**, **90836**, **90838**).

⁕ To report both E/M and psychotherapy, the 2 services must be significant and separately identifiable.

⁕ Time may not be used as the basis of E/M code selection. Evaluation and management code selection must be based on the level of key components of history, examination, and medical decision-making when reported in conjunction with psychotherapy.

⁕ Prolonged services *may not* be reported when psychotherapy with E/M (**90833**, **90836**, **90838**) is reported.

Example

➤ **An 8-year-old boy presents for psychotherapy.** The psychiatrist provides psychotherapy services with face-to-face time of 40 minutes and also provides an E/M service to reevaluate the effectiveness and patient reaction to current medications. The E/M service includes problem-focused history and examination and straightforward medical decision-making. Codes reported are **99212** and **90836**.

The time of 40 minutes is only the face-to-face time of psychotherapy services and does not include the time of the E/M service. Because the midpoint between 30 and 45 minutes was passed, code 90836 (45 minutes) is reported in lieu of 90833 (30 minutes). No modifier is required (eg, modifier 25) because the add-on codes were assigned values taking into account the overlapping practice expense of the 2 services (eg, same clinical staff and examination room).

Psychotherapy Without Evaluation and Management

90832	Psychotherapy, 30 minutes with patient and/or family member
90834	45 minutes with patient and/or family member
90837	60 minutes with patient and/or family member
+90863	Pharmacologic management, including prescription and review of medication, when performed with psychotherapy services

When psychotherapy is provided without an E/M service on the same date, codes 90832, 90834, and 90837 are reported based on the face-to-face time of service. To accommodate reporting of pharmacologic management by psychologists who have prescribing privileges but who cannot provide E/M services, add-on code 90863 is reported in addition to the appropriate code for psychotherapy without E/M. Physicians and QHPs providing pharmacologic management report the service with an E/M code.

* Prolonged services in the office or other outpatient setting (99354, 99355) or inpatient or observation setting (99356, 99357) may be reported in addition to the psychotherapy service code 90837 when 90 minutes or longer of face-to-face time with the patient and/or family member is spent performing psychotherapy services, which are not performed with an E/M service.

* Code 90863 is an add-on code and may only be reported in addition to one of the stand-alone psychotherapy codes (ie, 90832, 90834, 90837). Time spent providing medication management is not included in the time spent in psychotherapy.

Example

➤ **An 8-year-old boy presents for psychotherapy.** The licensed clinical psychologist (whose state scope of practice includes prescribing authority) provides psychotherapy services with face-to-face time of 40 minutes and also provides a pharmacologic management service to reevaluate the effectiveness and patient reaction to current medications. Codes reported are 90834 and 90863.

Only a psychologist with prescribing authority may provide pharmacologic management. Other QHPs may provide psychotherapy but must collaborate with a physician or advance practice professional who provides pharmacologic management.

Psychotherapy With Biofeedback

90875	Individual psychophysiological therapy incorporating biofeedback training by any modality (face-to-face with the patient), with psychotherapy (eg, insight oriented, behavior modifying or supportive psychotherapy); 30 minutes
90876	45 minutes

When psychotherapy incorporates biofeedback training, code 90875 or 90876 is reported based on the face-to-face time of the combined services. Do not separately report codes for psychotherapy (90832–90838) or biofeedback training (90901).

Example

➤ **A child with chronic pain is provided psychotherapy and biofeedback training to help her cope with and control her pain.** The face-to-face time of service is 45 minutes.

Code 90876 is reported for the combined services. Were biofeedback training provided on a date when no psychotherapy was provided, code 90901 would be reported. Time of service is not a factor in reporting code 90901.

Psychotherapy for Crisis

90839   Psychotherapy for crisis; first 60 minutes
+90840   each additional 30 minutes (List separately in addition to code 90839)

Psychotherapy for crisis is provided on an urgent basis to a patient requiring mobilization of resources to defuse a crisis and restore safety and implementation of psychotherapeutic interventions to minimize the potential for psychological trauma. This includes assessment and history of a crisis state, a mental status examination, and a disposition. The presenting problem is typically life-threatening or complex and requires immediate attention to a patient in high distress.

- Codes 90839 and 90840 are reported based on the total face-to-face time the physician or QHP spends with the patient and/or family providing psychotherapy for crisis on a single date of service. Time is cumulative for all psychotherapy for crisis on the same date even if time is not continuous.
  - ❖ Code 90839 is reported for the first 30 to 74 minutes of psychotherapy for crisis on a single date of service. For psychotherapy for crisis with face-to-face time of less than 30 minutes' duration, report individual psychotherapy codes (90832 or 90833).
  - ❖ Add code 90840 for each additional block of time (each 30 minutes beyond the first 74 minutes and once for up to 30 minutes of the last full 30-minute period).
- Do not report psychotherapy for crisis (90839, 90840) for service of less than 30 minutes or on the same date as other psychiatry services (90785–90899).

Example

➤ **Parents of a 16-year-old established patient with depression and history of substance abuse phone his psychologist's office requesting an immediate appointment because the patient has phoned his mother at work saying he planned to kill himself.** The patient's grandfather has arrived at the patient's home to find the patient distraught and prepared to follow through with self-harm. The psychologist is consulted and speaks to the mother to determine the nature of the crisis. The parents agree to evaluation and possible inpatient admission. The psychologist meets the family in the ED of the hospital, examines the patient, obtains agreement for inpatient treatment, and makes arrangements for admission. The total face-to-face time of the encounter is 45 minutes.

Code 90839 is reported. Although the code descriptor states "first hour," the instructions for reporting psychotherapy for crisis instruct that code 90839 is reported for the first 30 to 74 minutes of face-to-face service.

Family and Group Psychotherapy

90846   Family psychotherapy (without the patient present)
90847   Family psychotherapy (conjoint psychotherapy) (with patient present)
90849   Multiple-family group psychotherapy

While family members may act as informants during individual psychotherapy, psychotherapy using family psychotherapy techniques is reported with codes 90846 and 90847 based on whether or not the patient is present for the service. The focus of family psychotherapy is on family dynamics and/or subsystems within the family (eg, parents, siblings). Family therapy is focused on improving the patient's functioning by working with the patient in the context of the family.

- Do not report family psychotherapy for services of fewer than 26 minutes.
- Prolonged service may also be reported in conjunction with code 90847 (family psychotherapy [conjoint psychotherapy] [with patient present], 50 minutes) when 80 minutes or longer of face-to-face time with the patient and family are spent performing psychotherapy.
- Codes for individual psychotherapy (90832–90838) may be reported on the same day as family psychotherapy codes 90846 and 90847 when the services are separate and distinct. Append modifier 59 (distinct procedural service) to the group psychotherapy code when both services are reported on the same date.
- When multiple families participate in family psychotherapy at the same session, code 90849 is reported once for each family.

❋ Psychotherapy to a group of individual patients includes discussion of individual and/or group dynamics. Processes may include interpersonal interactions, support, emotional catharsis, and reminiscing.

90853   Group psychotherapy (other than of a multiple-family group)

❋ Report code 90853 with 1 unit of service for each group member. Documentation should support the individual patient's involvement in the group session, the duration of the session, and issues that were presented.

❋ No time is assigned to code 90853. This service is reported with 1 unit of service regardless of the time of service.

Other Psychiatric Services

The following services are often bundled under payer contracts (ie, considered components of other services) or non-covered. However, check plan benefits, especially for Medicaid patients, as there may be circumstances in which these services are separate benefits. Plan-specific modifiers are often required when coverage of the following services is a health plan benefit:

90882   Environmental intervention for medical management purposes on a psychiatric patient's behalf with agencies, employers, or institutions

90885   Psychiatric evaluation of hospital records, other psychiatric reports, psychometric and/or projective tests, and other accumulated data for medical diagnostic purposes

90887   Interpretation or explanation of results of psychiatric, other medical examinations and procedures, or other accumulated data to family or other responsible persons, or advising them how to assist patient

90889   Preparation of report of patient's psychiatric status, history, treatment, or progress (other than for legal or consultative purposes) for other individuals, agencies, or insurance carriers

Code 90889 should not be reported in conjunction with psychological or developmental testing, as the codes for these services include time for report writing.

Evaluation and Treatment of Substance Abuse

The initial evaluation of a child for alcohol and/or substance abuse is often in the context of an E/M service. When more than 50% of the physician/QHP time with the patient is spent in counseling and/or coordinating care, E/M codes are selected based on the total face-to-face time of the service in a non-facility setting or total unit/floor time in a facility setting (eg, ED, hospital unit).

> |||||||||| **Coding Pearl** ||||||||||
>
> Document the names and results of any standardized rating scales used during the initial evaluation. Each completed, scored, and documented standardized scale may be properly reported. Payers, however, may limit the number of scales they will pay for on a single date of service. See the discussion of Medically Unlikely Edits in Chapter 2, Modifiers and Coding Edits, for more information.

ICD-10-CM *Coding for Use, Abuse, and Dependence*

The guidelines for *ICD-10-CM* offer specific guidance for reporting diagnoses of mental and behavioral disorders due to psychoactive substance use.

❋ Code Z71.41 is reported as the first-listed code when an encounter is primarily focused on alcohol abuse counseling and surveillance. An additional code for alcohol abuse or dependence (F10.-) is additionally reported.

❋ Code Z71.51 is reported as the first-listed code when an encounter is primarily for drug abuse counseling and surveillance of drug abuser. Codes for drug abuse or dependence (F11–F16, F18, or F19) are reported in addition to code Z71.51.

❋ The codes for psychoactive substance *use* disorders (F10.9-, F11.9-, F12.9-, F13.9-, F14.9-, F15.9-, F16.9-) are to be used only when the psychoactive substance use is associated with a physical, mental, or behavioral disorder and such a relationship is documented by the provider. Note that codes for inhalant use (F18.9-) and polysubstance or indiscriminate drug use (F19.9-) are not included in this instruction.

- Subcategories of codes for mental and behavioral disorders due to psychoactive substance use indicate use, abuse, and dependence of various psychoactive substances. These categories do not include abuse of non-psychoactive substances such as antacids, laxatives, or steroids that are reported with category F55. Each subcategory offers a spectrum of use, abuse, and dependence with extended information such as with intoxication, with withdrawal, with delusions, etc.

- When documentation refers to use of, abuse of, and dependence on the same substance (eg, alcohol, opioid, cannabis), only one code should be assigned to identify the pattern of use based on the following hierarchy:
  - ❖ If both use and abuse are documented, assign only the code for abuse.
  - ❖ If both abuse and dependence are documented, assign only the code for dependence.
  - ❖ If use, abuse, and dependence are all documented, assign only the code for dependence.
  - ❖ If both use and dependence are documented, assign only the code for dependence.

- Selection of codes for substance abuse or dependence "in remission" for mental and behavioral disorders due to psychoactive substance use (categories F10–F19 with -.11, -.21) requires the provider's clinical judgment. The appropriate codes for "in remission" are assigned only on the basis of provider documentation unless otherwise instructed by the classification.
  - ❖ Mild substance use disorders in early or sustained remission are classified to the appropriate codes for substance abuse in remission, and moderate or severe substance use disorders in early or sustained remission are classified to the appropriate codes for substance dependence in remission.

Management/Treatment of Alcohol and Substance Use Disorders

Coding for management/treatment of alcohol and substance use disorders is largely payer driven. Psychotherapy codes may be applicable, or E/M codes may be selected based on time of counseling and/or coordination for ongoing counseling on alcohol and/or substance use disorders. However, many health plans and Medicaid programs require use of HCPCS codes for reporting assessments and management/treatment of alcohol and/or substance use disorders.

Examples of HCPCS codes include

H0001	Alcohol and/or drug assessment
H0005	Alcohol and/or drug services; group counseling by a clinician
H0007	Alcohol and/or drug services; crisis intervention (outpatient)
H0014	Alcohol and/or drug services; ambulatory detoxification
H0016	Alcohol and/or drug services; medical/somatic (medical intervention in ambulatory setting)
H0022	Alcohol and/or drug intervention service (planned facilitation)
H0047	Alcohol and/or other drug abuse services, not otherwise specified
T1006	Alcohol and/or substance abuse services, family/couple counseling
T1007	Alcohol and/or substance abuse services, treatment plan development and/or modification

Individual health and Medicaid plans may define the services reported with HCPCS codes differently. Prior authorization of services is often required.

General behavioral health integration (GBHI) care management services (99484) may also be provided for substance use disorders; see that section later in this chapter for a discussion.

Alcohol and/or Substance Abuse Screening/Testing

Presumptive Drug Class Screening

Presumptive drug class screening is typically used to identify possible use or nonuse of a drug or drug class. These tests are often used to verify compliance with treatment, identify undisclosed drug use, and monitoring for relapse in patients with known abuse or dependence.

Urine is often the specimen used for testing in outpatient settings. *ICD-10-CM* codes for abuse or dependence (F10–F19) or counseling (eg, Z71.51) are often sufficient to support the need for testing. However, payer policies may vary, so it is advisable to verify each plan's policy and any coding requirements.

> **|||||||| Coding Pearl ||||||||**
>
> Codes for findings of drugs and other substances not normally found in blood (R78.-) are not reported in conjunction with codes for substance use (F10–F19).

When the specimen used for alcohol/drug testing is blood, report *ICD-10-CM* code **Z02.83** (encounter for blood-alcohol and blood-drug test). When blood test findings are positive in a patient not diagnosed with substance use (**F10–F19**), report codes from category **R78.-** (findings of drugs and other substances, not normally found in blood) in addition to code **Z02.83**.

When findings of blood alcohol testing are positive, codes in category **Y90.-** are used to report the alcohol level. Codes in category **Y90** are reported secondary to codes for associated alcohol-related disorders. See **tables 14-6 and 14-7** for a listing of related codes in categories **R78** and **Y90**.

Table 14-6. *International Classification of Diseases, 10th Revision, Clinical Modification* Abnormal Finding Drug Blood Test

R78	Findings of drugs and other substances, not normally found in blood
R78.0	Finding of alcohol in blood (Use additional external cause code [Y90.-] for detail regarding alcohol level.)
R78.1	Finding of opiate drug in blood
R78.2	Finding of cocaine in blood
R78.3	Finding of hallucinogen in blood
R78.4	Finding of other drugs of addictive potential in blood
R78.5	Finding of other psychotropic drug in blood
R78.6	Finding of steroid agent in blood
R78.89	Finding of other specified substances, not normally found in blood
R78.9	Finding of unspecified substance, not normally found in blood

Table 14-7. *International Classification of Diseases, 10th Revision, Clinical Modification* Blood Alcohol Level

Y90	Evidence of alcohol involvement determined by blood alcohol level[a]
Y90.0	Blood alcohol level of <20 mg/100 mL
Y90.1	Blood alcohol level of 20–39 mg/100 mL
Y90.2	Blood alcohol level of 40–59 mg/100 mL
Y90.3	Blood alcohol level of 60–79 mg/100 mL
Y90.4	Blood alcohol level of 80–99 mg/100 mL
Y90.5	Blood alcohol level of 100–119 mg/100 mL
Y90.6	Blood alcohol level of 120–199 mg/100 mL
Y90.7	Blood alcohol level of 200–239 mg/100 mL
Y90.8	Blood alcohol level of ≥240 mg/100 mL
Y90.9	Presence of alcohol in blood, level not specified

[a] *Code first any associated alcohol-related disorders (F10).*

Presumptive drug class screening includes all drugs and drug classes performed by the respective methodology (eg, dipstick kit with direct optical observation) on a single date of service. Sample validation is included in presumptive drug screening service. Venipuncture to obtain samples for drug testing may be separately reportable with code **36415** (collection of venous blood by venipuncture).

When testing is performed with a method using direct optical observation to determine the result, code **80305** is reported. Tests that have a waived status under the Clinical Laboratory Improvement Amendments may be reported with modifier **QW** (waived test).

80305   Drug test(s), presumptive, any number of drug classes, any number of devices or procedures; capable of being read by direct optical observation only (eg, utilizing immunoassay [eg, dipsticks, cups, cards, or cartridges]), includes sample validation when performed, per date of service

When a reader is used to determine the result of testing (eg, a dipstick is inserted into a machine that determines the final reading), code **80306** is reported.

Chapter 14: Mental and Behavioral Health Services

Chapter 14: Mental and Behavioral Health Services

80306   read by instrument assisted direct optical observation (eg, utilizing immunoassay [eg, dipsticks, cups, cards, or cartridges]), includes sample validation when performed, per date of service

Testing that uses a chemistry analyzer or more effort than tests represented by codes **80305** and **80306** is reported with code **80307**.

80307   by instrument chemistry analyzers (eg, utilizing immunoassay [eg, EIA, ELISA, EMIT, FPIA, IA, KIMS, RIA]), chromatography (eg, GC, HPLC), and mass spectrometry either with or without chromatography, (eg, DART, DESI, GC-MS, GC-MS/MS, LC-MS, LC-MS/MS, LDTD, MALDI, TOF); includes sample validation when performed, per date of service

Some plans require use of HCPCS codes for reporting alcohol/drug screening or testing. Code **H0048** allows for reporting of the collection and handling of specimens other than blood for alcohol and/or drug testing. Code **H0003** is used to report the analysis of a screening test for alcohol and/or drugs.

H0003   Alcohol and/or drug screening; laboratory analysis of specimens for presence of alcohol and/or drugs

H0048   Alcohol and/or other drug testing: collection and handling only, specimens other than blood

> ||||||||| **Coding Pearl** |||||||||
>
> *International Classification of Diseases, 10th Revision, Clinical Modification* code **F40.231** (fear of injections and transfusions) may be used for patients who have "needle phobia."

Examples

➤ **A psychologist is consulted by an ED physician to evaluate and recommend treatment options for an intoxicated 17-year-old patient who presented with a scalp laceration.** Although not notably intoxicated at the encounter, the patient admits to alcohol dependence since age 14 and intoxication on arrival to the ED. His blood alcohol level on admission was 22 mg/100 mL. The psychologist recommends treatment for alcoholism through a local community health center. The diagnosis documented is alcohol dependence with intoxication.

   ICD-10-CM codes reported are **F10.229** (alcohol dependence with intoxication, unspecified) and **Y90.1** (blood alcohol level of 20–39 mg/100 mL).

➤ **A patient who is dependent on cannabis is seen in follow-up.** A urine sample is tested for the presence of drugs and is negative. The patient's diagnosis is cannabis dependence, in remission.

   Codes **Z02.83** (encounter for blood-alcohol and blood-drug test) and **F12.21** (cannabis dependence, in remission) are reported.

Definitive Drug Testing

When necessary to identify specific drugs or metabolites, a definitive drug test may be ordered. Definitive drug identification methods are able to identify individual drugs and distinguish between structural isomers but not necessarily stereoisomers. Definitive drug tests are reported with codes **80320–80373** based on drug classes (eg, alcohol[s] or non-opioid analgesics) as identified in the Definitive Drug Classes Listing in the Pathology and Laboratory section of *CPT®* references.

Behavioral Health Integration

Behavioral health integration includes PCCM (**99492–99494**) and GBHI services (**99484**). These services are differentiated by the required elements of service. Psychiatric collaborative care management services include a defined team of health care professionals providing care using a specific care method. General behavioral health integration services do not include specific types of providers or a specified method of delivery.

   If the treating physician or other QHP personally performs behavioral health care manager (BHM) activities and those activities are not used to meet the criteria for a separately reported code, his or her time may be counted toward the required BHM time to meet the elements of **99484** and **99492–99494**.

Psychiatric Collaborative Care Management Services

99492   Initial psychiatric collaborative care management, first 70 minutes in the first calendar month of behavioral health care manager activities, in consultation with a psychiatric consultant, and directed by the treating physician or other qualified health care professional, with the following required elements:

- outreach to and engagement in treatment of a patient directed by the treating physician or other qualified health care professional;
- initial assessment of the patient, including administration of validated rating scales, with the development of an individualized treatment plan;
- review by the psychiatric consultant with modifications of the plan if recommended;
- entering patient in a registry and tracking patient follow-up and progress using the registry, with appropriate documentation, and participation in weekly caseload consultation with the psychiatric consultant; and
- provision of brief interventions using evidence-based techniques such as behavioral activation, motivational interviewing, and other focused treatment strategies.

99493   Subsequent psychiatric collaborative care management, first 60 minutes in a subsequent month of behavioral health care manager activities, in consultation with a psychiatric consultant, and directed by the treating physician or other qualified health care professional, with the following required elements:

- tracking patient follow-up and progress using the registry, with appropriate documentation;
- participation in weekly caseload consultation with the psychiatric consultant;
- ongoing collaboration with and coordination of the patient's mental health care with the treating physician or other qualified health care professional and any other treating mental health providers;
- additional review of progress and recommendations for changes in treatment, as indicated, including medications, based on recommendations provided by the psychiatric consultant;
- provision of brief interventions using evidence-based techniques such as behavioral activation, motivational interviewing, and other focused treatment strategies;
- monitoring of patient outcomes using validated rating scales; and
- relapse prevention planning with patients as they achieve remission of symptoms and/or other treatment goals and are prepared for discharge from active treatment.

+99494   Initial or subsequent psychiatric collaborative care management, each additional 30 minutes in a calendar month of behavioral health care manager activities, in consultation with a psychiatric consultant, and directed by the treating physician or other qualified health care professional (List separately in addition to code for primary procedure)

(Use 99494 in conjunction with 99492, 99493)

> |||||||||| **Coding Pearl** ||||||||||
>
> Psychiatric collaborative care management includes use of validated rating scales in monitoring patient outcomes. Do not separately report use of standardized rating scales (eg, 96127).

Psychiatric collaborative care management services are reported by a supervising physician or QHP for services by a BHM working under the supervision of the reporting physician or QHP. Psychiatric collaborative care management services are provided to patients who have a new or existing psychiatric disorder that requires a behavioral health assessment; care plan implementation, revision, or monitoring; and provision of brief interventions. These services require a team effort of 3 health care professionals: a treating physician or QHP, a BHM, and a psychiatric consultant. The treating physician or QHP reports codes 99492–99494 when all requirements for reporting are met. Evaluation and management and other services may be reported separately by the same physician or QHP during the same calendar month.

Each team member's role is defined in *CPT®* as follows:

- The treating physician or QHP directs the BHM and continues to oversee the patient's care, including prescribing medications, providing treatments for medical conditions, and making referrals to specialty care when needed. The treating physician or QHP engages the services of the psychiatric consultant who does not directly bill for PCCM services (ie, the treating physician's or QHP's practice contracts with the psychiatric consultant for this component of the PCCM service).

- The treating physician or QHP acts in a supervisory role to the BHM (may be a direct employee or contractual employee but should represent a practice expense similar to other clinical staff and AHPs). If the treating physician or QHP personally performs behavioral health care management activities and those activities are not used to meet criteria for a separately reported service, his or her time may be counted toward the required time for PCCM. As the reporting or billing provider for PCCM services, the treating physician or QHP is ultimately responsible for delivery, documentation, and billing of PCCM services in compliance with *CPT* and payer policies.

- The BHM is an AHP or clinical staff member with master- or doctoral-level education *or* specialized training in behavioral health who provides behavioral health care management services under the treating physician's or QHP's supervision and in consultation with a psychiatric consultant. The BHM provides the following services, as needed:
  - ❖ Assessment of needs including the administration of validated rating scales
  - ❖ Development of a care plan
  - ❖ Provision of brief interventions face-to-face and non–face-to-face
  - ❖ Ongoing collaboration with the treating physician or QHP
  - ❖ Consultation with the psychiatric consultant at least weekly (typically non–face-to-face)
  - ❖ Maintenance of a registry

- The psychiatric consultant is a medical professional trained in psychiatry or behavioral health *and qualified to prescribe a full range of medications*. The psychiatric consultant typically does not see the patient or prescribe medications, except in rare circumstances. The psychiatric consultant advises and makes recommendations to the treating physician or QHP (typically via consultation with the BHM). The psychiatric consultant's services include recommending the following services, as needed:
  - ❖ Psychiatric and other medical differential diagnosis
  - ❖ Treatment strategies addressing appropriate therapies
  - ❖ Medication management
  - ❖ Medical management of complications associated with treatment of psychiatric disorders
  - ❖ Referral for specialty services

- The psychiatric consultant may directly provide and separately report E/M or psychiatric services, such as psychiatric evaluation (**90791**, **90792**) to a patient within a calendar month when the same patient receives PCCM services. Activities for services reported separately are not included in the services reported with codes **99492–99494**.

  Reporting requirements for PCCM services include

- Psychiatric collaborative care management services are time-based services and are subject to the *CPT* midpoint rule for reporting time. Time of service is met when the midpoint is passed. Documentation must support provision of PCCM services for
  - ❖ 36 minutes or more to report a 70-minute service (**99492**)
  - ❖ 31 minutes or more to report a 60-minute service (**99493**)
  - ❖ 16 minutes or more beyond the last full service period to report an additional 30 minutes of service (**99494**)
  - ❖ When service time does not meet the midpoint (ie, 36 minutes for **99492**, 31 minutes for **99493**), do no report PCCM.

- Psychiatric collaborative care management services are provided for an episode of care defined as beginning when the treating physician or QHP directs the patient to the BHM and ending when
  - ❖ The attainment of targeted treatment goals, which typically results in the discontinuation of care management services and continuation of usual follow-up with the treating physician or other QHP
  - ❖ Failure to attain targeted treatment goals culminating in referral to a psychiatric care provider for ongoing treatment
  - ❖ Lack of continued engagement with no PCCM services provided over a consecutive 6-month calendar period (break in episode)

Chapter 14: Mental and Behavioral Health Services

- A new episode of care starts after a break in episode of 6 calendar months or more.
- Medical necessity of PCCM services may be supported by documentation of a newly diagnosed condition, a patient's need for help engaging in treatment, or a patient who has not responded to standard care delivered in a nonpsychiatric setting or who requires further assessment and engagement prior to consideration of referral to a psychiatric care setting. (These are typical patient scenarios. Other reasons for services may support medical necessity.) Where health plans implement specific coverage criteria and/or prior authorization for PCCM services, documentation of the patient's behavioral health conditions, psychosocial needs, and other factors influencing patient care may help support the necessity of services.
- Unlike CCM services, PCCM services do not require establishment of a care plan for *all* the patient's health care needs. Psychiatric collaborative care management services are directed to behavioral health needs. Patients may or may not have comorbid conditions that affect treatment and management.
- The BHM may provide and report other services (within his/her scope of practice) in the same calendar month as PCCM. These may include psychiatric diagnosis, psychotherapy, smoking and tobacco use cessation counseling (99406, 99407), and alcohol and/or substance abuse structured screening and brief intervention services (99408, 99409).
- Provision of PCCM services may support quality initiatives such as use of an electronic clinical data system to track care and administration of a validated rating scale (eg, Patient Health Questionnaire-9) during a 4-month period for patients diagnosed with major depression or dysthymia.
- Psychiatric collaborative care management services may be reported in the same month as CCM services (99487, 99489–99491) when the requirements for each service are met without overlap.

Example

➤ **A pediatrician orders PCCM services for a 15-year-old patient diagnosed with moderate depression, single episode.** A licensed clinical psychologist acting as the BHM meets with the patient to discuss PCCM services and perform an initial assessment. Standardized assessment instruments are used to further assess the patient's health, and a treatment plan including psychotherapy is agreed on. After the meeting, the BHM enters the patient information into a registry, which will be used to track her medication compliance and progress. Later, the BHM has a regularly scheduled conference call with a consulting psychiatrist who reviews the patient's assessment and approves of the treatment plan. The supervising pediatrician is also consulted and approves the treatment plan. The BHM, whose scope of practice includes psychotherapy, provides 3 individual psychotherapy sessions within the calendar month in addition to PCCM services. The BHM will separately report the psychotherapy services in addition to PCCM. During the calendar month, the BHM documents 60 minutes of time spent in PCCM services.

PCCM 60 minutes in first calendar month of service Psychotherapy without E/M service	**ICD-10-CM** F32.1 (major depressive disorder, single episode, moderate)
	CPT® 99492 (initial month PCCM service, first 70 minutes) 90832, 90834, or 90837 (psychotherapy based on time of service; 30, 45, or 60 minutes)

Teaching Point: *CPT* instructs that time of service for PCCM services is met when the midpoint is passed. In this example, the 60 minutes spent by the BHM supports reporting of code 99492, which includes the first 70 minutes of PCCM services in the initial month of service. No time spent in provision of psychotherapy may be attributed to the time of PCCM services. If psychotherapy services were not within the scope of practice for the BHM, the patient might be referred to another provider (eg, the consulting psychiatrist), who would report the services rendered.

General Behavioral Health Integration Care Management

#99484   Care management services for behavioral health conditions, at least 20 minutes of clinical staff time, directed by a physician or other qualified health care professional, per calendar month, with the following required elements:

- ❋ Initial assessment or follow-up monitoring, including the use of applicable validated rating scales;
- ❋ Behavioral health care planning in relation to behavioral/psychiatric health problems, including revision for patients who are not progressing or whose status changes;
- ❋ Facilitating and coordinating treatment such as psychotherapy, pharmacotherapy, counseling and/or psychiatric consultation; and
- ❋ Continuity of care with a designated member of the care team

General behavioral health integration care management (99484) is reported by physician or QHP for supervision of clinical staff who provide at least 20 minutes of GBHI services within a calendar month to a patient with a behavioral health condition (includes substance abuse). A treatment plan must be documented addressing the patient's behavioral health condition(s), but a comprehensive health care plan is not required. General behavioral health integration is an outpatient service.

CPT® does not define the education or credentials of clinical staff who may provide services described by code 99484. Clinical staff providing GBHI services are not required to have qualifications that would permit them to separately report services (eg, psychotherapy), but, if qualified and they perform such services, they may report such services separately. The time of the separately reported service is not used to support reporting 99484.

Services must be provided under general physician supervision and in accordance with the licensing and scope of practice requirements of the state where services are provided. The individual supervising and reporting GBHI care management services must be able to report E/M services.

All the required elements of service listed in the code descriptor must be provided and documented.

Example

➤ **A 15-year-old presents to the primary care pediatrician with vague complaints of stomachaches, fatigue, excessive sleep, and atypically poor grades.** The primary care physician diagnoses the patient with a behavioral health disorder and recommends that the patient receive behavioral health care management as part of the treatment plan. Clinical staff provide behavioral health care planning and coordination of care with a psychologist in another practice as directed by the pediatrician. At least 20 minutes of clinical staff time is documented for contacts with the patient and psychologist throughout the calendar month to assess progress using standardized rating scales and coordinating care, including facilitating access to community resources, as needed.

If clinical staff time of fewer than 20 minutes is documented in a calendar month, code 99484 is not reported. Code 99484 does not include requirements for a BHM or collaboration with a psychiatrist.

- ❋ *Use of validated rating scales is required and is not separately reported* (ie, do not report code 96127 for rating scales administered during the period of behavioral health care management services).
- ❋ Time may be non–face-to-face or face-to-face but may more typically be non–face-to-face. Clinical staff must be available to provide face-to-face services to the patient when requested.
- ❋ The reporting individual may separately report E/M and/or psychiatric services on the same date or in the same calendar month as GBHI services when performed, but these services cannot be used to support reporting of GBHI (ie, time of separately reported services is not counted toward the time of GBHI services).
- ❋ General behavioral health integration care management for behavioral health conditions (99484) may be reported in the same month as CCM services (99487, 99489–99491) when the requirements for each service are met without overlap.

* The reporting individual may personally provide GBHI services and combine the time of service with that of clinical staff to support reporting code 99484. However, the time of services that are separately reported (eg, 15 minutes spent providing an E/M service reported with code 99213) cannot be included in the time supporting 99484.
* Behavioral health integration care management (99484) and PCCM (99492–99494) may not be reported by the same professional in the same month.
* Clinical staff time spent coordinating care with the ED may be reported using 99484, but time spent while the patient is an inpatient or is admitted to observation status may not be reported using 99484.

Chapter 14: Mental and Behavioral Health Services

Part 3:
Primarily for
Hospital Settings

Part 3: Primarily for Hospital Settings

Hospital Care of the Newborn

Contents

Perinatal Care

This chapter focuses on coding for care of the typical newborn and those with conditions not requiring intensive monitoring or critical care. See Chapter 18, Critical and Intensive Care, for intensive or critical care services provided to a neonate.

The American Academy of Pediatrics (AAP) Section on Neonatal-Perinatal Medicine, in conjunction with state chapters and councils of the AAP, has developed strategies that have been successful in addressing payment concerns for neonatal care. Contact your state chapter, its pediatric council, your section district AAP Executive Committee representative, a neonatal trainer, or the AAP Committee on Coding and Nomenclature for assistance in addressing any payment inequities for neonatal services in your state.

Definitions of the Perinatal and Neonatal Periods

For coding purposes, the *perinatal period* commences at 32 completed weeks of gestation through the 28th day following birth (World Health Organization definition). Based on this definition, the *neonatal period* begins at birth and continues through the completed 28th day after birth, ending on the 29th calendar day after birth. The day of birth is considered day 0 (zero). Therefore, the day after birth is considered day 1. This definition is important to diagnosis code selection for conditions that originate in the perinatal period. (This is also important for selection of codes for neonatal critical care and initial intensive care. See Chapter 18, Critical and Intensive Care, for more information on codes for these services.)

> 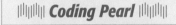 **Coding Pearl**
>
> *International Classification of Diseases, 10th Revision, Clinical Modification* codes for fetal conditions affecting management of the mother (categories **O35** and **O36**) are reported only when the fetal condition is actually responsible for modifying the management of the mother (ie, requiring diagnostic studies, additional observation, special care, or termination of pregnancy). That a fetal condition exists does not justify assigning a code to the mother's record.

Attendance at Delivery and Newborn Resuscitation

99464   Attendance at delivery (when requested by the delivering physician or other qualified health care professional) and initial stabilization of newborn

99465   Delivery/birthing room resuscitation, provision of positive pressure ventilation and/or chest compressions in the presence of acute inadequate ventilation and/or cardiac output

Code **99464** is not reported when hospital-mandated attendance is the only underlying basis for providing the service. When physician on-call services are mandated by the hospital (eg, attending specific types of deliveries, such as all repeat cesarean deliveries) and are not physician requested, report code **99026** (hospital-mandated on-call service; in hospital, each hour) or **99027** (hospital-mandated on-call service; out of hospital, each hour). See Chapter 16, Noncritical Hospital Evaluation and Management Services, for guidelines for use of codes **99026** and **99027**.

Attendance at delivery (**99464**)

- Service is only reported when requested by the delivering physician and indicated for a newborn who may require immediate intervention (ie, stabilization, resuscitation, or evaluation for potential problems).
- Medical record documentation must include the request for attendance at the delivery and substantiate the medical necessity of the services performed. If there is no documentation by the delivering physician for attendance at delivery, the verbal request and the reason for the request should be documented in the attendance note.
- Includes initial drying, stimulation, suctioning, blow-by oxygen, or continuous positive airway pressure (CPAP) or high-flow air/oxygen without positive-pressure ventilation (PPV); a cursory visual inspection of the neonate; assignment of Apgar scores; and discussion of the care of the newborn with the delivering physician and parents. A quick look into the delivery room or examination after stabilization is not sufficient to report **99464**.

Chapter 15: Hospital Care of the Newborn

- Any *medically necessary* procedures to complete the resuscitation that are provided in the delivery room may be reported separately (eg, direct laryngoscopy without intubation). Procedures performed only due to hospital protocol would not be separately reported.
- May be reported in addition to initial normal newborn (**99460**), initial sick newborn (**99221–99223**), initial intensive care of the neonate (**99477**), or critical care (**99468**; **99291**, **99292**) codes.

When qualifying resuscitative efforts are provided, code **99465** (delivery/birthing room resuscitation) is reported instead. Codes **99464** and **99465** *cannot be* reported on the same day of service.

Attendance at delivery with neonatal resuscitation (**99465**)

- Includes bag-and-mask or bag-to-endotracheal tube ventilation (PPV) and/or cardiac compressions.
- May be reported when positive-pressure breaths are administered by the T-piece resuscitator to a neonate exhibiting inadequate ventilation and/or cardiac output in lieu of a manual bag-mask resuscitator (documentation should support ventilatory or cardiac dysfunction and the necessity and provision of PPV). Do not report when T-piece resuscitator is used to provide CPAP only. See Chapter 18, Critical and Intensive Care, for further information.
- Other life support procedures that are performed as a necessary part of the resuscitation may be reported separately, such as **31500**, intubation, endotracheal, emergency procedure; **31515**, laryngoscopy, direct, for aspiration; **36510**, catheterization of umbilical vein for diagnosis or therapy, newborn; and **94610**, surfactant administration.
  - ❖ It is important to document why the newborn required a procedure and not assume the payer will infer that it was necessary for resuscitation.
  - ❖ Services that are performed prior to transfer to the neonatal intensive or critical care unit but are not a necessary part of resuscitation (eg, catheter placed for convenience) or later as part of intensive or critical care services may not be separately reported.
- May be reported in addition to any initial care service, including initial critical care (**99468**; **99291**, **99292**) or initial neonatal intensive care (**99477**). Payers may require modifier **25** (significant, separately identifiable evaluation and management [E/M] service) appended to the code for E/M services reported in addition to code **99464** or **99465**. However, National Correct Coding Initiative (NCCI) edits do not bundle these services.

> **~ More From the AAP ~**
>
> Read more about code **99465** and continuous positive airway pressure/T-piece ventilation in "Newborn Resuscitation and the T-piece" in the May 2015 *AAP Pediatric Coding Newsletter* at http://coding.aap.org (subscription required).

Examples

➤ **A physician attends a repeat cesarean delivery.** The services are provided because they are mandated by hospital policy. The delivering physician did not request the services.

Code **99026** (hospital-mandated on-call service; in hospital, each hour) is reported. This may be used for tracking purposes or in financial arrangements with the hospital.

➤ **A physician is called at the request of an obstetrician to stand by during a delivery and spends 30 minutes waiting for the delivery before she attends the delivery of a typical newborn and admits him to her service.**

Codes **99464** (attendance at delivery) and **99460** (initial hospital or birthing center care, per day, for the E/M of normal newborn infant) are reported.

Standby services requiring prolonged attendance, each 30 minutes (**99360**), are not reported in addition to attendance at delivery but may be reported with the newborn resuscitation services (**99465**) per *Current Procedural Terminology* (*CPT*) guidelines.

➤ **A physician provides brief resuscitation services, including PPV, to a neonate with mild primary apnea who recovers quickly and is later released to the newborn nursery for close monitoring over the next 4 hours.** The neonate shows no further signs of distress.

Codes **99465** and **99460** (initial newborn care) are reported. (Neonatal resuscitation is likely followed by initial neonatal intensive or critical care more often than normal newborn care.)

➤ **A neonatologist is asked to be present at delivery by the delivering physician.** The neonatologist documents a comprehensive examination of the neonate, in addition to the maternal and fetal history, and provides all the elements required for reporting of attendance at delivery. The neonate is typical and admitted to the newborn nursery under the orders of her general pediatrician.

Code **99464** is the only code reported by the neonatologist. Although a history and examination were performed, this does not equate to initial hospital care of the newborn, which is reported by the attending physician who provides a comprehensive history and examination, ordering of screening tests and prophylactic interventions, and counseling the family on topics such as newborn feeding, sleep, and safety.

Coding Conundrum: When a Physician Arrives After Delivery, What Service Can Be Reported?

There are no specific time requirements for reporting attendance at delivery. Remember, this service requires a request for attendance at delivery by the delivering physician and includes physician work to perform the initial drying, stimulation, suctioning, blow-by oxygen, or continuous positive airway pressure without positive-pressure ventilation; a cursory visual inspection of the neonate; assignment of Apgar scores; and discussion of the care of the newborn with the delivering physician and parents. When a physician arrives in the delivery room after the delivery and some or all this work has been performed, should attendance at delivery be reported? Physicians might want to consider

- When the newborn continues to require intervention or stabilization in the delivery room, code **99464** (attendance at delivery) may be reported if the physician work and medical necessity are related to the delivery, not a component of a sick, intensive, or critical admission, and the nature of the intervention is documented in the medical record.
- When the work provided in the delivery room is related more to the initial hospital care (neonate is examined and the physician sends him to the well-baby nursery), only the initial normal newborn code (**99460**) is reported.

For example, attendance at delivery was requested by the delivering physician and the physician arrives after the delivery.

→ The 1-minute Apgar score has been assigned and the neonate has been dried, stimulated, and suctioned by the nurses and is ready to be sent to the newborn nursery by the time the physician appears in the delivery room. The delivering physician acknowledges that assistance is no longer needed. The physician will report initial normal newborn care (**99460**) after completing his or her initial examination of the newborn. However, if the physician is not the attending pediatrician, no service can be reported.

→ In the previous example, the delivering physician continues to want assistance. The physician assigns the 5-minute Apgar score, performs a cursory examination, and discusses the care of the newborn with the delivering physician and parents. Code **99464** can be reported because most of the basic elements of the attendance at delivery were performed and documented in the medical record.

A stillborn neonate for whom unsuccessful resuscitation services are provided will be billed to the mother's insurer.

A stillborn neonate examined after birth at the request of the obstetrician should be reported on the mother's insurance as a consultation, with a report sent to the obstetrician.

Normal Newborn Care

99460	Initial hospital or birthing center care, per day, for evaluation and management of normal newborn infant
99461	Initial care, per day, for evaluation and management of normal newborn infant seen in other than hospital or birthing center

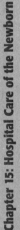

99462	Subsequent hospital care, per day, for evaluation and management of normal newborn
99463	Initial hospital or birthing center care, per day, for evaluation and management of normal newborn infant admitted and discharged on the same date
99238	Hospital discharge day management; 30 minutes or less
99239	more than 30 minutes

Codes 99460, 99462, 99463, 99238, and 99239 are used to report E/M services provided to the healthy newborn in a hospital setting (including birthing room deliveries). They are reported when the neonate is cared for in the mother's room (rooming-in), a labor and delivery room, a postpartum floor, or a traditional newborn nursery and when a normal neonate is cared for after the mother is discharged (eg, awaiting adoption). Normal newborn codes are also used to report services to neonates who are being observed for onset of jaundice, low glucose, or other conditions or problems but are presently asymptomatic. A *normal newborn* is defined as a newborn who

- Transitions to life in the usual manner
- Requires delivery room intervention but is normal after transition
- May require some testing or monitoring (eg, bilirubin, complete blood cell count [CBC], culture)
- Will not require significant intervention
- Is being observed for illness but is not sick
- Is late preterm but requires no special care
- Is in house with sick mother/twin

Guidelines for reporting include

- The neonate is considered admitted at the time of arrival to the nursery.
- Code 99463 (history and examination of the normal newborn, including discharge) should be reported when an initial history and physical examination and the discharge management are performed *on the same calendar date* for a normal newborn.
- Code 99460 (history and examination of the normal newborn, initial service) is reported only once on the first day that the physician provides a face-to-face service in the facility. This date may not necessarily correlate with the date the patient is born or the hospital admission date.
- Code 99462 (subsequent hospital care, normal newborn) is reported once per calendar date on the date(s) subsequent to the initial normal newborn care service but *not* on the discharge date.
- Any additional procedures (eg, circumcision) should be reported in addition to normal newborn care codes. Modifier 25 (significant, separately identifiable E/M service) should be appended to the E/M code when a procedure is performed on the same day of service.
- Discharge management services performed on a day subsequent to initial newborn care are reported with code 99238 (hospital discharge day management; 30 minutes or less) or 99239 (hospital discharge day management; more than 30 minutes), when discharging a normal newborn. Include time spent in final examination of the patient, discussion of the hospital stay, instructions for continuing care, and preparation of discharge records, prescriptions, and referral forms. Time must be documented when reporting 99239.

> |||||||| **Coding Pearl** ||||||||
>
> Normal newborn codes can be reported for care provided to neonates who are acting normally but recovering from fetal stress or a low Apgar score or who are being observed for a potential problem but are asymptomatic.

International Classification of Diseases, 10th Revision, Clinical Modification (ICD-10-CM) codes from category Z38 are used to report live-born neonates according to type of birth and are the first-listed codes for care by the attending or admitting physician during the entire birth admission. Category Z38 codes for single live-born infant are shown in **Table 15-1**.

See the *ICD-10-CM* manual for Z38 codes for multiple-birth neonates.

Table 15-1. *International Classification of Diseases, 10th Revision, Clinical Modification Codes for Single Live-born Neonates*
Z38.00   Single liveborn infant, delivered vaginally
Z38.01   Single liveborn infant, delivered by cesarean
Z38.1   Single liveborn infant, born outside hospital
Z38.2   Single liveborn infant, unspecified as to place of birth

Report *ICD-10-CM* code **Z76.2** (encounter for health supervision and care of other healthy infant and child) when a healthy newborn continues to receive daily visits pending discharge of the mother, adoption, or other reasons. Code **Z76.2** is useful for indicating the reason for an extended stay of a healthy newborn.

Examples

➤ **The physician is not present at a repeat cesarean delivery of a healthy term boy.** The nursery calls the office and relates that the newborn has been admitted and seems fine. The physician's standing admission orders are followed, and the physician examines the newborn the following morning. The physician reviews the record, examines the neonate, and speaks with the mother. The newborn and his mother remain in the hospital 2 additional days, when both are then discharged home. Discharge management takes 25 minutes.

Diagnosis code for all days	*ICD-10-CM* **Z38.01** (single liveborn by cesarean section)
 Day 1 of hospital stay Day 2 Day 3 Day 4	*CPT®* No charge (no face-to-face services provided) **99460** (initial normal newborn care) **99462** (subsequent normal newborn care) **99238** (hospital discharge day management; 30 minutes or less)

➤ **A baby is born vaginally in the hospital on March 3 at 4:00 pm.** The pediatrician first sees the baby on March 4 and determines, after initial hospital assessment, that the newborn is ready for discharge. A history and examination of the newborn, discussion of the hospital stay with the parents, instructions for continuing care, family counseling, and preparation of the final discharge records are performed.

ICD-10-CM	*CPT*
Z38.00 (single liveborn, delivered vaginally)	**99463** (initial normal newborn care and discharge on the same date)

➤ **A subsequent hospital visit is performed in the well-baby nursery on a 2-day-old who is being observed due to risk of jaundice; however, no interventions are noted, and baby is doing well.**
Code **99462** (subsequent normal newborn care) is reported.

➤ **A neonate fails a routine hearing examination.** During a subsequent newborn care visit, the attending physician spends 15 minutes discussing the results with the parents and refers to an audiologist for testing to confirm or rule out hearing abnormality.

ICD-10-CM	*CPT*
Z38.00 (single liveborn, delivered vaginally) **R94.120** (abnormal auditory function study)	**99462** (subsequent normal newborn care)

Chapter 15: Hospital Care of the Newborn

Teaching Point: Only code **Z38.00** would be reported when the result of an auditory screening is normal. The audiologist performing the screening would report code **Z13.5**, encounter for screening for eye and ear disorders.

Hospital Care of the Ill Neonate

Diagnosis Codes for Perinatal Conditions

There are some important guidelines for reporting conditions that originate in the perinatal period. In *ICD-10-CM*, these conditions are classified to Chapter 16 and codes **P00–P96**. Codes in this chapter are used only on the neonate's record and not that of the mother. Other important guidelines include

- Perinatal condition codes are assigned for any condition that is clinically significant.
- In addition to clinical indications for reporting codes from other chapters, perinatal conditions are considered clinically significant if the condition has implications for future health care needs. Other clinical indications that apply to all conditions are those requiring
  - ❖ Clinical evaluation
  - ❖ Therapeutic treatment
  - ❖ Diagnostic procedures
  - ❖ Extended hospital stay
  - ❖ Increased nursing care and/or monitoring
- Should a condition originate in the perinatal period and continue throughout the life of the patient, the perinatal code should continue to be used regardless of the patient's age.
- If a newborn has a condition that could be due to the birth process or community acquired and documentation does not indicate which it is, the condition is reported as due to the birth process. Community-acquired conditions are reported with codes other than those in *ICD-10-CM* Chapter 16.
- Codes in categories **P00–P04**, newborn affected by maternal factors and by complications of pregnancy, labor, and delivery, may be reported when the conditions are suspected but have not yet been ruled out. However, if a neonate is suspected of having an abnormal condition that, after examination and observation, is ruled out, assign codes for signs and symptoms or, in the absence of signs or symptoms, a code from category **Z05** (encounter for observation and evaluation of newborn for suspected diseases and conditions ruled out).

> |||||||||| **Coding Pearl** ||||||||||
>
> The ordering of codes for neonates at the birth hospital are as follows:
> 1. Birth outcome (**Z38-**, reported only by the attending/admitting physician)
> 2. Codes from the perinatal chapter (**P00–P96**)
> 3. Codes from the congenital anomalies chapter (**Q00–Q99**)
> 4. All other chapters

Examples

➤ **The pediatrician admits a 3,500-g term neonate born vaginally to a mother who developed a low-grade fever during labor.** The neonate is hypothermic. A comprehensive history, including review of the maternal, prenatal, labor, and delivery history; history of present illness; and social and family history, is performed. A comprehensive examination is performed. Complete blood cell count and blood cultures are obtained, and antibiotics are started. On day 1, medical decision-making (MDM) is of high complexity due to a new problem with additional workup and a potential illness that may pose a threat to life.

On day 2, the physician performs a problem-focused interval history and examination and reviews laboratory results. Infection is ruled out. The problem (hypothermia) has resolved, laboratory results were reviewed with no abnormal findings, and prescription drugs were managed (stop antibiotics). The overall level of MDM for the encounter on day 2 is straightforward.

ICD-10-CM	CPT®
Day 1 **Z38.00** (single liveborn, delivered vaginally) **P80.8** (other hypothermia of newborn) **Day 2** **Z38.00** (single liveborn, delivered vaginally) **Z05.1** (observation and evaluation of newborn for suspected infectious condition ruled out)	**Day 1** **99223** *MDM:* High complexity *History:* Comprehensive *Physical examination:* Comprehensive **Day 2** **99231**

Teaching Point: If test results are positive, use a diagnosis code appropriate to the findings and procedure codes for the appropriate level of subsequent hospital or intensive care. If the neonate had required intensive observation, frequent interventions, and other intensive care services, code **99477** (initial hospital care, per day, for the E/M of the neonate, 28 days of age or younger, who requires intensive observation, frequent interventions, and other intensive care services) would have been reported in lieu of **99223**.

➤ **A neonate was born to a mother who tested positive for group B β-hemolytic streptococcal infection and received 2 doses of prophylactic intravenous (IV) administration of penicillin during labor.** The newborn appeared typical in the delivery room and was admitted to the newborn nursery. A comprehensive maternal history and physical examination with review of intrapartum laboratory values were performed. The newborn is monitored for 48 hours with no indication of illness. On day 2, the patient is found to be a normal newborn.

ICD-10-CM	CPT
Day 1 **Z38.00** (single liveborn, delivered vaginally) **P00.89** (newborn affected by other maternal conditions) **Day 2** **Z38.00** (single liveborn, delivered vaginally) **Z05.1** (observation and evaluation of newborn for suspected infectious condition ruled out)	**Day 1** **99460** **Day 2** **99462**

Teaching Point: Note that on day 1, the patient was suspected of being affected by a localized maternal infection (**P00.89**), but by day 2, the condition was ruled out (**Z05.1**). Initial and subsequent normal newborn care codes are reported rather than initial and subsequent hospital care because the neonate, while at risk for infection in this case, was not treated but observed and did not develop infection.

◉ Codes in category **P05** are reported for the newborn affected by fetal growth restriction or slow intrauterine growth.
   ❖ Codes in subcategory **P05.0** are used to report the neonate is light for dates but not small. (See definitions in the *International Classification of Diseases, 10th Revision, Clinical Modification* Codes for Small and/or Light for Gestational Age box later in this chapter.)
   ❖ Codes in subcategory **P05.1** are used to report the neonate is small or small and light for dates.

> ⦙⦙⦙⦙⦙ **Coding Pearl** ⦙⦙⦙⦙⦙
>
> Codes in category **Z05** (encounter for observation and evaluation of newborn for suspected diseases and conditions ruled out) may be reported for inpatient or outpatient services when a suspected disease or condition is ruled out at the encounter.

CPT copyright 2018 American Medical Association. All rights reserved.

> ### International Classification of Diseases, 10th Revision, Clinical Modification Codes for Disorders of Newborn Related to Length of Gestation and Fetal Growth
>
> Codes in subcategory **P07.0-** (extremely low birth weight newborn) and **P07.1-** (other low birth weight newborn) are not reported in conjunction with codes in category **P05**, disorders of the newborn due to slow fetal growth and fetal malnutrition. However, subcategory **P07.2-** (extreme immaturity of newborn) and **P07.3-** (preterm newborn) may be reported in addition to category **P05**.

☀ Code **P05.2** is provided for reporting fetal (intrauterine) malnutrition affecting a newborn who is not light or small for gestational age.

> ### International Classification of Diseases, 10th Revision, Clinical Modification Codes for Small and/or Light for Gestational Age
>
> *International Classification of Diseases, 10th Revision, Clinical Modification* (ICD-10-CM) codes for small and/ or light for gestational age are aligned to the World Health Organization definitions of these conditions. In the United States, many clinicians use the term *small for gestational age* for all newborns below the 10th (or fifth) percentile for gestational age and then subcategorize as *symmetric* when weight, length, and head circumference are all below the 10th percentile and *asymmetric* when only the weight is below the 10th percentile. Asymmetric fetal growth would fall in the light for gestational age group, whereas symmetric fetal growth would fall in the small for gestational age group. *Note that head circumference percentile is not a factor in choosing the correct code.*
>
> The World Health Organization provides definitions to support diagnostic selection for these conditions.
>
> *Light for gestational age:* Usually referred to as weight below but length above the 10th percentile for gestational age.
>
> *Small for gestational age:* Usually referred to as weight and length below the 10th percentile for gestational age.
>
> *ICD-10-CM* includes codes **P05.09** (newborn light for gestational age, 2500 grams and over) and **P05.19** (newborn small for gestational age, other) to allow for identification of all infants with fetal growth and malnutrition, fetal growth retardation, and preterm birth.

☀ Codes from category **P07**, disorders of newborn related to short gestation and low birth weight, are reported based on the recorded birth weight and estimated gestational age to indicate these conditions as the cause of morbidity or additional care of the newborn.

    ❖ When both are documented, weight is sequenced before age.

    ❖ These codes may be reported for a child or an adult who was preterm or had a low birth weight as a newborn and this is affecting the patient's current health status.

    Codes in subcategory **P07.3-** (preterm newborn) should be reported for infants born at 36 weeks' gestation who stay in the newborn nursery.

Hospital Evaluation and Management Services to the Newborn

Initial Hospital Care

Codes **99221–99223** are used to report the initial hospital care of a sick neonate who does not require intensive observation and monitoring or critical care services. Refer to Chapter 16, Noncritical Hospital Evaluation and Management Services, and **Table 16-2** for the specific coding and documentation requirements for reporting initial hospital care.

Example

➤ **The pediatrician sees a newborn boy admitted to the well-baby nursery.** He was born to a mother with blood type O+ who has a history of 2 previous newborns with jaundice secondary to ABO incompatibility. Umbilical cord blood sent for blood typing and direct antibody (antiglobulin/Coombs) test shows the baby is A+ DAT+. At 8 hours of age, the neonate appears jaundiced. A bilirubin and CBC with a reticulocyte count are ordered, results are evaluated, the newborn's risks for kernicterus are discussed with the family, and phototherapy is started. The pediatrician performs a comprehensive history and physical examination. Medical decision-making is of moderate complexity for this new problem with moderate risk.

| MDM: Moderate
History: Comprehensive
Physical examination: Comprehensive | **ICD-10-CM**
Z38.00 (single liveborn, delivered vaginally)
P55.1 (hemolytic disease due to ABO isoimmunization) |
| | **CPT®**
99222 |

Teaching Point: When reporting initial hospital care, all 3 key components (history, physical examination, MDM), or average total floor/unit time if more than 50% of time spent is in counseling and/or coordination of care, must be met. The level of service is based on all hospital care services on the same date by the same physician or physicians of the same group practice and same specialty. If the minimum key components are not sufficiently met (eg, an expanded history is performed), the initial care must be reported using subsequent hospital care codes (**99231–99233**). See Chapter 16, Noncritical Hospital Evaluation and Management Services.

Subsequent Hospital Care and Discharge Management

Subsequent hospital care codes (**99231–99233**) are reported for each day of service subsequent to initial care for the newborn who continues to be sick (ie, not a typical neonate but not in critical condition and not requiring intensive observation and interventions). Code **99238** or **99239** (hospital day discharge management) is reported on the day the newborn is discharged (when on a separate day from the initial hospital care).

❋ When a neonate is not treated but only observed for the potential development of illness, normal newborn codes would be reported.

❋ If the neonate is sick but improves and requires no more care than a normal newborn, the subsequent normal newborn care code (**99462**) should be reported.

It is useful to consider the typical patient when reporting subsequent hospital care. These are

❋ **99231:** Usually, the patient is stable, recovering, or improving.

❋ **99232:** Usually, the patient is responding inadequately to therapy or has developed a minor complication.

❋ **99233:** Usually, the patient is unstable or has developed a significant complication or a significant new problem.

Refer to Chapter 16, Noncritical Hospital Evaluation and Management Services, and **Table 16-3** for detailed coding and documentation requirements for codes **99231–99233**. Chapter 16 also includes more information on discharge day management codes **99238** and **99239**.

|||||||| *Coding Pearl* ||||||||

Payers that utilize the Medicare or Medicaid National Correct Coding Initiative (NCCI) will not allow separate payment of

- Normal newborn hospital care (**99460, 99462, 99463**) *by the same physician or a physician of the same specialty and same group practice on the same date* as initial hospital care (**99221–99223**)
- Initial hospital care (**99221–99223**) *by the same physician or a physician of the same specialty and same group practice on the same date* as initial inpatient neonatal critical care (**99468**)
- Subsequent hospital care (**99231–99233**) *by the same physician or a physician of the same specialty and same group practice on the same date* as subsequent normal newborn care (**99462**)

When reporting to these payers, report only the most extensive level of care provided; the code in column 1 of the NCCI edit table is considered the more comprehensive code.

Examples

➤ **The physician performs a follow-up visit for a neonate who was on IV antibiotics until this morning and is breastfeeding well, with no further fevers.** Vital signs and general appearance and examination of the heart, lungs, abdomen, and skin are performed. Blood and urine cultures remain negative after 48 hours. Intravenous antibiotics are discontinued. Patient will be discharged the next day if no contraindications. Diagnosis is single live-born neonate by cesarean delivery with suspected infection ruled out.

MDM: Low complexity—established problem improving, review of laboratory data, prescription drug management *History:* Expanded problem focused *Physical examination:* Expanded problem focused	***ICD-10-CM*** **Z38.00** (single liveborn, delivered vaginally) **Z05.1** (observation and evaluation of newborn for suspected infectious condition ruled out)
	CPT® **99232**

Teaching Point: Two of 3 key components are required to support the level of subsequent hospital care provided. If the payer requires MDM as 1 of the 2 key components met for subsequent hospital care, this service would be reported with code **99231** because MDM was low.

➤ **The physician performs a follow-up visit for a neonate who was on IV antibiotics until this morning and is breastfeeding well, with no further fevers.** Vital signs and general appearance and examination of the heart, lungs, abdomen, and skin are performed. Blood and urine cultures remain negative after 48 hours. Intravenous antibiotics are discontinued. Patient is discharged home with instructions for home care and follow-up. Thirty-five minutes was spent on the floor reviewing the hospital course, expected follow-up, and signs and symptoms of possible sepsis or infection with the mother.

Time (35 minutes unit/floor time dedicated to the patient) is the key controlling factor.	***CPT*** **99239** (more than 30 minutes)

Teaching Point: If time spent in discharge day management is not documented, code **99238** must be reported.

Prolonged Services

+99356   Prolonged service in the inpatient or observation setting, requiring unit/floor time beyond the usual service; first hour (30–74 min)

+99357   each additional 30 minutes

99358   Prolonged evaluation and management service before and/or after direct patient care; first hour

+99359   each additional 30 minutes

☀ If direct (face-to-face) prolonged services in the inpatient setting (**99356**, **99357**) are required on the same day as a consultation (**99241–99245**, **99251–99255**), an initial hospital service (**99221–99223**), or a subsequent hospital service (**99231–99233**), they may be reported in addition to the basic E/M service (an add-on code).

☀ Direct prolonged services are not reported with normal newborn codes, intensive care codes, or neonatal/pediatric critical care codes because these services do not include an assigned typical time by *CPT.*

The specific coding guidelines for reporting face-to-face (**99354–99357**) and non–face-to-face (**99358** and **99359**) prolonged service codes are detailed in Chapter 16, Noncritical Hospital Evaluation and Management Services. Prolonged clinical staff services (**99415** and **99416**) are not reported for inpatient care.

Examples

➤ **The physician performs an expanded problem-focused history and physical examination on a term neonate born via cesarean delivery who is experiencing mild tachypnea on a subsequent day.** The physician obtains and reviews a chest radiograph and CBC and requests that an oxygen saturation (Spo_2) monitor be placed on the neonate for 5 minutes. The chest radiograph and CBC are normal and the Spo_2 is persistently greater than 95%. The physician spends 65 minutes of total time on the floor with the patient, speaking with the mother and reviewing the chart.

MDM: Low complexity *History:* Expanded problem focused *Physical examination:* Expanded problem focused	**CPT** **99232** (average time is 25 minutes) **99356** (direct prolonged services, first 30–74 minutes)

Teaching Point: In addition to code **99232**, code **99356** will be reported based on total documented time spent on the floor or unit dedicated to the one patient. Time is not the controlling factor in selection of the subsequent hospital care code because there is no documentation of time spent counseling and coordinating care.

➤ **An infant is transferred from a Level III neonatal intensive care unit, following a 30-day hospital stay, to a community Level II unit to complete her recovery before home discharge.** A large volume of records accompanies the infant. A comprehensive history and physical examination are performed on admission; MDM is moderately complex. The provider spends another 1 hour and 20 minutes reviewing the extensive transfer records while off the unit.

MDM: Moderate complexity *History:* Comprehensive *Physical examination:* Comprehensive	**CPT**® **99222** **99358** (prolonged non–face-to-face services, first hour) **99359** (each additional 30 minutes)

Teaching Point: This service included 80 minutes of prolonged services. Code **99358** represents the first 60 minutes. Code **99359** is reported for the final 15 to 30 minutes of prolonged services; in this example, the final 20 minutes. If fewer than 75 minutes of prolonged services were provided, code **99359** would not be reported because this code is reported for time that goes at least 15 minutes beyond the first hour or final 30 minutes.

Consultations

A consultation is reported when a physician or other appropriate source requests an opinion and/or advice from another physician or appropriate source. This request must be in writing or given verbally by the requestor. The consulting physician renders advice, records it, and returns a report to the requesting physician or appropriate source.

Chapter 16, Noncritical Hospital Evaluation and Management Services, details the specific reporting, documentation, and coding requirements for the selection of consultation codes or other E/M service codes when consultation codes are not recognized.

See **Table 16-4** for inpatient consultation codes.

Example

➤ **At the request of a primary care physician, a neonatologist evaluates a 35-weeks' gestation neonate with recurrent hypoglycemia.** A detailed history is obtained from the mother, and consistent with the obstetric notes, she has no history of diabetes. Family history is negative for previous neonates with hypoglycemia or other metabolic diseases. Review of labor and delivery records is unremarkable. After birth, the newborn had 3 documented preprandial blood glucose concentrations less than 40 mg/dL and responded well to oral feeding. A detailed physical examination was performed. Gestational age assessment by physical examination and growth parameters was consistent with 35 weeks' gestation. The neonatologist recommends more frequent feeding and rechecking blood glucose before feeds until 4 consecutive preprandial glucose concentrations are greater than 60 mg/dL. The neonatologist spends 10 minutes explaining the findings and reassuring the baby's parents. The neonatologist writes a detailed chart note and discusses her recommendations with the pediatrician by phone.

| MDM: Moderate complexity
History: Detailed
Physical examination: Detailed | **ICD-10-CM**
P70.4 (hypoglycemia, newborn)
P07.38 (preterm newborn, gestational age 35 completed weeks) |
| | **CPT**
99253
or, if payer does not recognize consultations,
99221 (initial hospital care) |

Coding for Transitions to Different Levels of Neonatal Care

During a hospital stay, a newborn or readmitted neonate may require different levels of care. A normal newborn may end up becoming sick, intensively ill, or critical during the same hospital stay. Neonates who were initially sick may also improve to require lower levels of care (eg, normal neonatal care).

It is important to remember

☀ Normal newborn care (**99460** or **99462**) may be reported in addition to hospital care (**99221–99223**), initial intensive care (**99477**), or initial critical care (**99468**) or time-based critical care (**99291**, **99292**) on the same day when a patient qualifies for normal newborn care earlier in the day and, at a subsequent encounter on the same day, becomes ill and requires an additional encounter at a higher service level. *CPT*® instructs to report the appropriate E/M code with modifier **25** for these services in addition to the normal newborn code.

Examples

➤ **A neonate who was initially normal becomes ill 5 hours after birth.** A pediatrician, who provided initial newborn care earlier the same day, provides a second E/M service to evaluate the neonate's condition and determines that a transfer to a neonatal intensive care unit is necessary. Following transfer, a neonatologist provides initial intensive care to the newborn.

| The pediatrician reports
99460
99223 25 | The neonatologist reports
99477 |
| | |

    Teaching Point: The second E/M service on the same date as the initial newborn care is reported with modifier **25** appended.

➤ **A neonate who was initially normal becomes ill several hours after Physician A provided normal newborn care.** Physician B of another specialty assumes management of the newborn's care and provides an initial hospital care service with a comprehensive history and examination and moderate MDM.

| Physician A reports
99460 | Physician B reports
99222 |

    Teaching Point: No modifier is required because the physicians are not of the same specialty.

❖ Once an initial-day care code for a higher service level has been reported, an initial code for a lower service level within the same hospital stay will not be reported. If a patient has required intensive care (**99477**) but no longer qualifies for intensive care and is transferred to the care of a primary care pediatrician, the receiving physician will report sick visit codes. The receiving physician will not report initial hospital care (**99221–99223**) for the first encounter; rather, the physician will report subsequent hospital care (**99231–99233**) based on the level of service provided.

Examples

➤ **A neonate (2,600 g) is transferred from neonatal intensive care by an intensivist to a pediatric hospitalist to complete her recovery before home discharge.** On the day of transfer, the intensivist provides intensive care from midnight to noon and determines the neonate no longer requires intensive care. The hospitalist provides a face-to-face visit to the neonate, documenting a detailed interval history, comprehensive examination, and moderate-complexity MDM, and 75 minutes of time on the unit reviewing the patient's record and consulting with the family.

The intensivist reports	The hospitalist reports
99480 (subsequent intensive care, per day, for the E/M of the recovering infant [present body weight of 2501-5000 grams])	**99233** (subsequent hospital care)

Teaching Point: The hospitalist may not report initial hospital care for services to the patient who has received prior initial hospital services (eg, initial neonatal intensive care).

➤ **A pediatrician attends the delivery of a hypoxic neonate and provides neonatal resuscitation, including intubation and umbilical vein catheterization.** The pediatrician arranges for transport to another facility and, while awaiting arrival of a transport team, spends 35 minutes providing critical care. A neonatologist accompanying the transport team assumes care of the neonate at the birth facility and provides critical care prior to and during transport for a total of 100 minutes. The transporting neonatologist then provides initial neonatal critical care at the receiving facility and initiates total body hypothermia.

The physician reports
99465 (delivery/birthing room resuscitation)
99291 25 (critical care, E/M of the critically ill or critically injured patient; first 30–74 minutes)
31500 (endotracheal intubation, emergency)
36510 (catheterization of umbilical vein for diagnosis or therapy, newborn)

Teaching Point: The physician reports all services provided on that date. Because initial neonatal critical care (**99468**) will be reported by the attending physician at the receiving facility, the physician does not report this service.

❖ See Chapter 18, Critical and Intensive Care, for information on reporting intensive or critical care on dates when the level of care changes or the patient is transferred.

> ### ~ *More From the AAP* ~
>
> See the American Academy of Pediatrics *Newborn Coding Decision Tool* for an easy reference for coding for inpatient care of the newborn (available for purchase online at https://shop.aap.org).

Other Newborn Hospital Care

Circumcision

54150   Circumcision, using clamp or other device with regional dorsal penile or ring block

❖ If the circumcision using a clamp or other device is performed without dorsal penile or ring block, append modifier **52** (reduced services) to **54150**.

❉ Medicare has a global period of 0 (zero) assigned to code **54150**. When performing a circumcision and a separately identifiable E/M service on the same day (eg, **99462**, subsequent normal newborn care; **99238**, discharge services <30 minutes), append modifier **25** to the E/M code. Link the appropriate *ICD-10-CM* code (eg, **Z38.00**) to the E/M service and link *ICD-10-CM* code **Z41.2** (encounter for routine and ritual male circumcision) to the circumcision code.

54160	Circumcision, surgical excision other than clamp, device, or dorsal slit; neonate (28 days of age or less)
54161	older than 28 days

Unlike code **54150**, Medicare has a global period of 10 days assigned to codes **54160** and **54161**. A physician who performs a procedure with a 10-day global period must append modifier **24** (unrelated E/M service by the same physician or other QHP during a postoperative period) to the E/M code for subsequent newborn or hospital care or discharge management (eg, **99238 24**) provided in the 10-day period following the procedure for general care of the newborn unrelated to the procedure.

When circumcisions are performed in the office

❉ If a payer does not base payment on a global surgical package, a supply code for the surgical tray can be reported with code **99070**. The description of the supply (circumcision tray) would need to be included on the claim form.

❉ Anesthetic creams (eutectic mixture of local anesthetics) are included in the circumcision code itself and should not be reported unless a third-party payer pays separately for topical anesthetic agents. In that case, they would be reported with code **99070**.

Car Safety Seat Testing

New in 2019! Codes **94780** and **94781** (car seat testing) are reported for monitoring to determine if *an infant through 12 months of age* may be safely transported in a car seat or must be transported in a car bed. These services are most commonly provided to infants who required critical care during their initial hospital stay. Car seat testing codes may be reported in addition to the subsequent hospital or discharge day management codes when performed and documented. *Note:* These codes cannot be reported in addition to critical or intensive care services. Time spent in car seat testing would not be counted as time spent in discharge day management. Car seat testing may also be provided to an infant in an outpatient setting to determine if the infant can safely move from car bed to car seat transportation. See Chapter 18, Critical and Intensive Care, for more information on car seat testing.

CHAPTER 16

Noncritical Hospital Evaluation and Management Services

Contents

Coding for Noncritical Hospital Evaluation and Management Services

Evaluation and management (E/M) codes for noncritical hospital care services require adherence to the 1995 or 1997 Centers for Medicare & Medicaid Services (CMS) *Documentation Guidelines for Evaluation and Management Services*. (See Chapter 6, Evaluation and Management Documentation Guidelines, for specific documentation requirements.) This chapter includes tables with descriptions of the required key components (ie, history, physical examination, medical decision-making [MDM], and time) for all the E/M services that are reported in the observation and inpatient hospital setting.

Here are basic guidelines for reporting noncritical observation and inpatient hospital E/M services. There are no distinctions between new and established patients.

- Codes are reported based on the cumulative services (performance of the required key components and/or time when appropriate) provided by an individual physician or physicians or other qualified health care professionals (QHPs)
  - ❖ Of the same specialty within a group
  - ❖ With the same tax identification number
  - ❖ During a calendar day
- Services may be performed and reported by any physician of any specialty (eg, hospitalist, primary care physician, specialist).
- Any procedure or other service with a *Current Procedural Terminology* (CPT®) code may be reported separately when performed by the reporting provider or group and documented.

Table 16-1 provides the key components and specific detail of required elements within each level of history and physical examination (eg, problem focused, expanded) and MDM (eg, straightforward, moderate) of an E/M code. Services may be reported using either the 1995 or 1997 documentation guidelines. The nature of the presenting problem (ie, reason for the encounter) is included as a contributory factor for levels of MDM but is not 1 of the 3 required elements.

Time-Based Code Selection

- Time in the observation and inpatient setting is defined as floor or unit time (dedicated to the one patient) and includes time spent
  - ❖ At the patient's bedside
  - ❖ Counseling family or patient (or those who may have assumed responsibility for the care of the patient [eg, foster parents, legal guardians, persons acting in loco parentis])
  - ❖ On the floor documenting care, performing the history and examination, and reviewing diagnostic tests
  - ❖ Coordinating care with care team members
- When time is used as the controlling factor in the selection of the code, the time spent and the notation that more than half the time was spent in counseling and/or coordination of care *must be documented* in the medical record. See Chapter 1, The Basics of Coding, for further discussion of code selection based on time; see also the Prolonged Evaluation and Management Services Provided in the Inpatient Setting section later in this chapter for discussion of prolonged services.

Table 16-1. Evaluation and Management Key Components[a]

History (must meet or exceed HPI, ROS, and PFSH)	Problem focused	Expanded	Detailed	Comprehensive
	HPI: 1–3 elements ROS: 0 PFSH: 0	HPI: 1–3 elements ROS: 1 PFSH: 0	HPI: 4+ elements or status of 3 chronic or inactive conditions ROS: 2–9 PFSH: 1	HPI: 4+ elements or status of 3 chronic or inactive conditions ROS: 10+ PFSH: 3
Examination	**Problem focused** 1995: 1 body area/organ system 1997: Performance and documentation of 1–5 elements identified by a bullet (●) in ≥1 areas or systems	**Expanded** 1995: Limited examination—affected body area/organ system and other related areas/systems 1997: Performance and documentation of at least 6 elements identified by a bullet (●) in ≥1 areas or systems	**Detailed** 1995: Extended examination—affected body area(s) and other symptomatic or related organ system(s) 1997: Performance and documentation of at least 2 elements identified by a bullet (●) in at least 6 areas or systems or at least 12 elements identified by a bullet (●) in at least 2 areas or systems	**Comprehensive** 1995: 8+ organ systems or complete examination of a single organ system 1997: Multisystem examination—9 systems or areas with performance of all elements identified by a bullet (●) in each area/system examined and documentation of at least 2 elements identified by a bullet (●) of each area(s) or system(s) Single organ system examination—Performance of all elements identified by a bullet (●) and documentation of every element in box with shaded border and at least 1 element in box with unshaded border
MDM (must meet 2 of 3—diagnoses/options, data, and risk)	**Straightforward** # diagnoses/options: Minimal Data: Minimal Risk: Minimal Presenting problem: Usually self-limited or minor severity	**Low complexity** # diagnoses/options: Limited Data: Limited Risk: Low Presenting problem: Usually moderate severity	**Moderate complexity** # diagnoses/options: Multiple Data: Moderate Risk: Moderate Presenting problem: Usually moderate to high severity	**High complexity** # diagnoses/options: Extensive Data: Extensive Risk: High Presenting problem: Usually moderate to high severity

Abbreviations: HPI, history of present illness; MDM, medical decision-making; PFSH, past, family, and social history; ROS, review of systems.

[a] See Chapter 6, Evaluation and Management Documentation Guidelines, for a detailed description of the guidelines and components of evaluation and management services with documentation requirements and tips.

Observation Care

- Hospital observation services are provided to patients who require monitoring for possible inpatient admission. For example, a patient with dehydration who requires hydration and is not quite sick enough to be at an inpatient level of care in the hospital would be admitted to observation.

- Hospitals do not need to designate a separate area for these patients; rather, designation of observation versus inpatient status is dependent on the physician's order and patient's diagnosis(es) and severity of illness.

- Initial observation care is reported by the admitting physician or QHP using codes 99218–99220. Subsequent-day observation care is reported with codes 99224–99226 and observation care discharge management with code 99217.

- Physicians of specialties other than the supervising physician (ie, attending physician) who provide care in the observation setting report outpatient consultation (99241–99245) or subsequent observation care codes. (See the Coding Conundrum: 2 Physicians Providing Initial Observation or Inpatient Hospital Day Services box later in this chapter for Medicare and *CPT* guidance.)

- Admission (ie, initial care) and discharge services (observation or inpatient status) provided on the same day are reported with codes 99234–99236.

- When the patient's status changes from observation to inpatient status or the reverse (eg, physician is asked by utilization review staff to change status from inpatient to observation), the physician should write an order to reflect the change and report only the code that reflects care consistent with the patient's final status on that date.

- Typical times have not been established for code 99217, so time spent in discharge management is not a factor in the selection of this code.

Coding Conundrum: 2 Physicians Providing Initial Observation or Inpatient Hospital Day Services

When Payers Follow Medicare Rules

Initial observation services: The admitting physician will report the initial observation care codes (**99218–99220**). Other physicians (ie, physicians belonging to a different group practice or of a different specialty) providing initial services to a patient in observation will report a new or established office or outpatient evaluation and management (E/M) code (**99201–99215**) based on the performance and documentation of the required key components.

Initial inpatient hospital services: Initial inpatient hospital care codes (**99221–99223**) may be reported by every physician who performs initial hospital care. The admitting physician will append modifier **AI** (principal physician of record) to codes **99221–99223**.

When Payers Do Not Follow Medicare Rules

Initial observation services: The admitting physician will report the initial observation care codes (**99218–99220**). The office or outpatient consultation codes (**99241–99245**) may be reported by other physicians if the service was requested by a physician or other appropriate source, opinion and/or advice was rendered by the consulting physician, and a written report was generated from the consulting physician to the referring physician. When the criteria for reporting a consultation are not met, the subsequent observation E/M codes (**99224–99226**) would be reported based on the level of care provided and documented.

Initial inpatient hospital services: The admitting physician will report the initial hospital care codes (**99221–99223**). Inpatient consultation codes (**99251–99255**) may be reported by other physicians if the requirements for reporting the services are met (ie, requested, opinion/advice rendered, written report to requesting source). Otherwise, subsequent hospital care E/M codes (**99231–99233**) are reported.

Chapter 16: Noncritical Hospital Evaluation and Management Services

Initial Observation Care

99218–99220　Initial observation care, per day, for the evaluation and management of a patient

See the full code descriptors in **Table 16-2**. The examples included here and throughout the chapter are coded based on the 1995 E/M documentation guidelines.

Initial observation care codes are reported

* On the first day that the admitting physician provides face-to-face services to the patient in the observation setting

* Using the code that reflects the overall care provided to the patient on that calendar date (See the Unique Considerations for Hospital Services box later in this chapter for more details about coding for initial observation care initiated elsewhere [eg, office, emergency department (ED)].)

Table 16-2. Initial Observation Care (99218–99220), Inpatient Hospital Care (99221–99223), and Observation or Inpatient Care Admission and Discharge Same Day (99234–99236)

Key Components (For a description of key components, see Table 16-1.)
3 of 3 key components must be performed to at least the degree specified for the codes in each row.

CPT® Code/Timeᵃ	Medical Decision-making	History (cc required for each level)	1995 Examinationᵇ
99218 (I) 30 min 99221 (I) 30 min 99234 (A&D) 40 min	Straightforward to low complexity PP: Usually low severity	HPI: ≥4 or 3 cc; ROS: 2–9; PFSH: 1/3	2–7 detailed
99219 (I) 50 min 99222 (I) 50 min 99235 (A&D) 50 min	Moderate complexity PP: Usually responding inadequately to therapy or minor complication	HPI: ≥4 or 3 cc; ROS: ≥10; PFSH: 3/3	≥8 body areas/ systems
99220 (I) 70 min 99223 (I) 70 min 99236 (A&D) 55 min	High complexity PP: Usually patient is unstable or develops significant complication or new problem.	HPI: ≥4 or 3 cc; ROS: ≥10; PFSH: 3/3	≥8 body areas/ systems

Abbreviations: A&D, admission and discharge on same day; cc, chronic conditions; CPT, Current Procedural Terminology; HPI, history of present illness; I, initial day; PFSH, past, family, and social history; PP, presenting problem; ROS; review of systems.

ᵃ Typical time is an average and represents a range of times that may be higher or lower depending on clinical circumstances. The presenting problem is considered to be a contributory factor and does not need to be present to the degree specified.

ᵇ Number of body areas or organ systems examined; see **Table 16-1** for details.

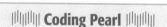

||||||||| Coding Pearl |||||||||

Under Medicare policy, when a patient is admitted to observation or inpatient care for fewer than 8 hours on the same calendar date, only the initial observation (**99218–99220**) or inpatient care (**99221–99223**) shall be reported by the physician. A separate code for discharge services (**99217** or **99234–99236**) is not reported. Medicaid or private payers may or may not limit reporting.

When "observation status" is initiated in the course of an encounter in another site of service (eg, ED, physician's office), all E/M services performed by the same physician (or physicians of the same specialty in the same group practice) are considered part of the initial observation care when performed on the same calendar date.

Important guidelines to remember include

- ☀ If the patient is admitted for observation and subsequently is formally admitted to the hospital on the same day, only the initial inpatient hospital code (**99221–99223**) is reported.
- ☀ Physicians from other groups providing services on the same date will report other appropriate outpatient E/M services based on the services provided and payer requirements. Chapter 7, Evaluation and Management Services in the Office and Outpatient Clinics, addresses the guidelines for selection of codes **99241–99245** and **99201–99215**.
- ☀ Place of service code **22** (on campus—outpatient hospital) is reported with observation service codes. (See Chapter 4, The Business of Medicine: Working With Current and Emerging Payment Systems, for more information on place of service codes.)
- ☀ Selection of the code is dependent on the performance and documentation of all 3 key components. Time may be used as the key controlling factor in the selection of the code if more than 50% of the total face-to-face encounter and/or floor/unit time is spent in counseling and/or coordination of care.
- ☀ Observation care codes are not reported for initial care of hospital-born neonates.

Use **Table 16-2** to help you in the selection of the appropriate codes in the following clinical examples:

Examples

➤ **A 3-year-old girl is admitted to observation for vomiting and diarrhea with dehydration.**
History: Parents report vomiting and diarrhea for 2 days and the patient is not keeping liquids down. She has been sluggish with decreased urine output. She has no respiratory symptoms or rashes and remainder of a complete system review is negative. She attends child care where several children have had similar symptoms. Past and family histories are noncontributory. Immunizations including rotavirus are up-to-date.

> ||||||| **Coding Pearl** |||||||
>
> Report code **A08.4**, viral intestinal infection, unspecified, as the infectious agent had not been identified at the end of this encounter.

   Physical examination: Detailed-level examination includes vital signs, general appearance, extended examination of abdomen (notations of no masses or tenderness, no enlargement of liver or spleen, and no hernia), and examination of related organ systems (ears, nose, mouth, and throat; lymphatic; cardiovascular; respiratory; and skin).

   Assessment/plan: Assessment is moderate dehydration secondary to acute viral gastroenteritis. The plan is to rehydrate with intravenous (IV) fluids and monitor electrolytes, urine output, and weight. Stool is to be tested for rotavirus. Appropriate infection precautions are taken.

MDM: Moderate complexity History: Comprehensive Physical examination: Detailed	***International Classification of Diseases, 10th Revision, Clinical Modification (ICD-10-CM)*** **A08.4** (viral intestinal infection, unspecified) **E86.0** (dehydration)
	CPT® **99218** (requires at least detailed history and examination and straightforward or low MDM)

   Teaching Point: Remember, all 3 key components must be met for the level of initial observation care reported. The level of history is comprehensive with extended history of present illness (duration: 2 days; severity: not keeping liquids down; associated signs and symptoms: sluggish; context: possible exposure at child care), complete review of systems, and complete past, family, and social history (social: attends child care; past and family: noncontributory). (*Note:* Some payers may not accept "noncontributory" as sufficient for documentation of past and family histories without further documentation. This would reduce the level of history to detailed but would not affect the level of service in this example.) The examination is detailed. Medical decision-making is moderate based on a new problem with additional workup and risk associated with an undiagnosed new problem. The detailed examination limits reporting of this service to code **99218**, even though the history and MDM meet or exceed requirements for code **99219**.

➤ **A 3-year-old girl is admitted to observation for vomiting and diarrhea with dehydration.**
History: Parents report that she has vomited about 10 times over the last 24 hours with frequent watery, non-bloody stools. She has become sluggish and has a decreased urinary output. She is unable to keep any liquids down. She had a fever to 38.3°C (101.0°F) last night and was given acetaminophen but vomited it back up. Past history includes no food intolerances and no surgeries. Family history includes a maternal aunt who is lactose intolerant. Social history includes child care attendance, no recent travel, and no tobacco use in the home.

   Physical examination: Comprehensive-level examination includes vital signs, general appearance, and examination of the mucous membranes, neck, lymph nodes, ears, eyes, heart, lungs, gastrointestinal system, and skin.

   Assessment/plan: Assessment is moderate dehydration secondary to acute viral gastroenteritis. The plan is to rehydrate with IV fluids; order complete blood cell count, stool studies, and electrolytes; and monitor urine and weight. Stool is to be tested for rotavirus. Appropriate infection precautions are taken.

MDM: Moderate complexity *History:* Comprehensive *Physical examination:* Comprehensive	***ICD-10-CM*** A08.4 E86.0 (dehydration)
	CPT 99219 (requires at least comprehensive history and examination and moderate MDM)

   Teaching Point: The examination in this example includes 8 organ systems (constitutional; eyes; ears, nose, mouth, and throat; lymphatic; cardiovascular; respiratory; gastrointestinal; and skin) to support a comprehensive examination.

➤ **An established patient presents to her physician's office on Monday.** During the evaluation of the patient, the physician decides to admit to observation care for further treatment and monitoring for acute pyelonephritis and dehydration. The physician does not see the patient in the observation setting until the next morning (Tuesday) but phones in orders and keeps in touch with the nursing staff. On Tuesday, the physician performs an initial observation care service (detailed history and examination, moderate-complexity MDM) on the patient and determines the patient is not improving enough to be discharged.

Monday's visit	***ICD-10-CM*** N10 (acute pyelonephritis) E86.0 (dehydration)
	CPT® 99212–99215 (office E/M, established patient)
Tuesday's visit	***CPT*** 99218 (initial observation care) Same diagnosis codes as Monday's visit

   Teaching Point: Initial observation care and initial inpatient care (99218–99220, 99221–99223) require a face-to-face service with the patient by the reporting physician in the facility. Entry of the history, physical examination, and orders directly into a facility electronic health record by online connection without a face-to-face visit in the facility does not support reporting. Also, an outpatient office building connected physically to the hospital does not count as seen in facility.

➤ **Same patient; however, the physician sees the patient in the office and in the hospital on the same day.** The combined E/M service in the office and hospital results in a comprehensive history and physical examination with moderately complex MDM.

Monday's services	**CPT** **99219** (initial observation care)

Subsequent Observation Care

99224–99226   Subsequent observation care, per day, for the evaluation and management of a patient

- Codes include all E/M services by a physician or physician group provided on a given day.
- Level of service reported will be dependent on the total services provided and documented.
- Codes require that 2 of the 3 key components be performed and documented. Some payers may require MDM as 1 of the 2 key components performed and documented.
- Time may be used as the key controlling factor in the selection of the code if more than 50% of the total face-to-face encounter (ie, floor/unit time) is spent in counseling and/or coordination of care.
- The history component required for subsequent observation visits is considered interval history (ie, new history obtained since the last physician assessment, including history of present illness and problem-pertinent system review). A past, family, and social history is not required.
- Because the individual documentation for each encounter should contain all information necessary to determine the level of service provided, it is important to document the chief complaint and other factors of the patient presentation that affect management at each encounter.

When reporting subsequent observation services, the status of the patient is often an indicator of the medically necessary level of service. *CPT* indicates the patient status for each level of subsequent observation care.

99224   Usually, the patient is stable, recovering, or improving.

99225   Usually, the patient is responding inadequately to therapy or has developed a minor complication problem.

Use **Table 16-3** to help you select the appropriate codes in the clinical example.

Example

➤ **7:00 am: A 3-year-old girl is seen for subsequent observation care for vomiting and diarrhea with dehydration.** She is experiencing occasional diarrhea and vomiting but is now tolerating sips of liquids. The patient has a low-grade fever without abdominal discomfort. Vital signs are stable, and examination of skin, heart, lungs, and abdomen is normal. Diagnostic test results are negative. The plan is to continue IV fluids until vomiting and diarrhea decrease and patient is eating soft foods.

MDM: Straightforward or low complexity *History:* Expanded problem focused *Physical examination:* Expanded problem focused	**ICD-10-CM** **E86.0** (dehydration) **R19.7** (diarrhea) **R11.10** (vomiting)
	CPT **99225**

Teaching Point: The patient in this example is improving. Medical decision-making is straightforward or low depending on whether tests reviewed were from one or more sections of *CPT* (laboratory, radiology, or medicine). A payer may require MDM as 1 of the 2 key components to support subsequent observation care, which would reduce the level of service to **99224**.

Table 16-3. Subsequent Observation or Inpatient Care

Key Components (For a description of key components, see Table 16-1.)
2 of 3 key components must be performed to at least the degree specified for the codes in each row.

CPT® Code/Time[a]	Medical Decision-making[b]	History[c] (cc required for each level)	1995 Examination[b]
99224 15 min 99231 15 min	Straightforward to low complexity PP: Usually stable, recovering, or improving	HPI: 1–3; ROS: 0; PFSH: 0	1 body area/system
99225 25 min 99232 25 min	Moderate complexity PP: Usually responding inadequately to therapy or minor complication	HPI: 1–3; ROS: 1; PFSH: 0	2–7 limited
99226 35 min 99233 35 min	High complexity PP: Usually patient is unstable or develops significant complication or new problem.	HPI: ≥4 or 3 cc; ROS: 2–9; PFSH: 0	2–7 detailed

Abbreviations: cc, chief complaint; CPT, Current Procedural Terminology; HPI, history of present illness; PFSH, past, family, and social history; PP, presenting problem; ROS, review of systems.

[a] Typical time is an average and represents a range of times that may be higher or lower depending on clinical circumstances. When counseling and/or coordination of care dominates the encounter, time shall be the controlling factor.

[b] The presenting problem is considered to be a contributory factor and does not need to be present to the degree specified.

[c] Past, family, and social histories are not required for interval history.

Observation Care Discharge Day Management

99217   Observation care discharge day management

Code 99217 is to be used to report all services provided to a patient on discharge from "observation status" (ie, final examination of the patient, discussion of the hospital stay, counseling, instructions for continuing care, and preparation of discharge records) if the discharge is on a day other than the initial date of observation status.

◉ Performance of the key components is not required.

◉ Observation care discharge services are not assigned a typical time.

◉ A face-to-face encounter is required on the date that code 99217 is reported. Even if some of the discharge work was performed on the day prior to discharge, code 99217 would be reported on the discharge date, if a face-to-face encounter occurred on that date.

Example

➤ **Same patient as previous example (ie, patient with dehydration).** Patient is fully alert and interactive. She experienced no vomiting overnight; diarrhea has decreased. The patient has a low-grade fever with no abdominal pain. She is tolerating fluids and had cereal this morning. Parents are now comfortable with discharge home.

Physical examination: Vital signs and examination of skin, heart, lungs, and abdomen.

Assessment/plan: Assessment is resolving gastroenteritis, most likely viral. Instructions for home care and follow-up are given.

ICD-10-CM	CPT®
K52.9 (acute gastroenteritis)	99217 (observation care discharge day management)

Observation or Inpatient Hospital Care Services (Including Admission and Discharge Services)

When a patient is admitted and discharged from observation or inpatient services on the *same date of service,* report codes 99234–99236.

* Selection of the code is based on the performance and documentation of all 3 key components and includes the combined services provided by the same physician or physician of the same specialty within a group during a calendar day.
* Time may be used as the key controlling factor in the selection of the code if more than 50% of the total face-to-face encounter (eg, floor/unit time) is spent in counseling and/or coordination of care.
* Except where payer guidance specifies otherwise, reporting of initial observation or inpatient care is based on the date of the face-to-face assessment and not the date of admission or designation of a status by a facility on physician order.

Use **Table 16-2** to review the required components used to select level of service in the following examples:

Examples

➤ **6:00 am: A 3-year-old girl is admitted to observation for vomiting and diarrhea with dehydration.** Encounter includes comprehensive history and examination and MDM of moderate complexity. Physician returns to the hospital at 7:00 pm.

  7:00 pm: Patient has occasional diarrhea without vomiting and is now tolerating sips of liquids. She has a low-grade fever without abdominal discomfort. Vital signs are stable, and examination of skin, heart, lungs, and abdomen is normal. Diagnostic test results are negative. Diagnosis is resolving viral gastroenteritis. Parents are comfortable with taking child home. Discharge instructions are given.

  Face-to-face services performed include initial care and discharge management. A code from the 99234–99236 series would be reported because observation admission and discharge services were provided on the same date. Diagnosis is resolving viral gastroenteritis.

| *MDM:* Moderate complexity
History: Comprehensive
Physical examination: Comprehensive | **ICD-10-CM**
A08.4 (viral gastroenteritis) |
| | **CPT**
99235 |

  Teaching Point: Physicians participating in quality initiatives may elect to additionally report *CPT* Category II performance measure codes to indicate specific elements of care were provided (eg, 4058F, pediatric gastroenteritis education provided to caregiver). Category II codes are not used for direct fee-for-service payment. For more on Category II codes, see Chapter 3, Coding to Demonstrate Quality and Value.

➤ **On Monday evening, a physician admits a 4-year-old patient by phone to observation care after an urgent care encounter for acute viral laryngotracheitis (croup).** On Tuesday morning, the physician performs a face-to-face service in the observation setting. The physician performs a comprehensive history and physical examination with low-complexity MDM. Later that day, the physician determines the patient has improved enough to be discharged and performs the discharge service.

Monday's service	**CPT®** There is no *CPT* code to report for this service.
Tuesday's visit *MDM:* Low complexity *History:* Comprehensive *Physical examination:* Comprehensive	**ICD-10-CM** J05.0 (croup)
	CPT 99234 (observation care, same-day admission and discharge)

Teaching Point: If reporting to a payer that has adopted Medicare policy on same-date admission and discharge services, the physician must document that the patient was in observation or inpatient status for a minimum of 8 hours and no more than 24 hours. Therefore, it is important that the physician document the length of time spent in observation or inpatient status when admission and discharge occur on the same date of service. See the Reporting to Payers Using Medicare Policy section later in this chapter for more information on Medicare requirements.

➤ **An established patient is seen in the physician's office with acute viral laryngotracheitis (croup) and admitted for observation at 6:00 pm on Tuesday.** The attending physician telephones the observation admission orders and does not see the child again until the next morning (Wednesday). On Wednesday, the physician completes a history and physical examination and discharges the child.

Tuesday's visit	**ICD-10-CM** J05.0 (croup)
	CPT 99211–99215 (office E/M, established patient)
Wednesday's visit	**CPT** 99234–99236 (observation care, same-day admission and discharge) Same diagnosis code as was reported for Tuesday's visit

➤ **A 4-year-old patient with croup is admitted from the ED at 6:00 am on Monday.** A physician from a different group than the ED physician sees the child that morning and performs the initial history and physical examination. Another physician from the attending physician's group practice returns to the hospital at 5:00 pm and, after evaluation of the child, discharges the patient home. The combined service is a comprehensive history and physical examination with moderate-level MDM.

MDM: Moderate complexity *History:* Comprehensive *Physical examination:* Comprehensive	**ICD-10-CM** J05.0 (croup)
	CPT 99235 (observation care, same-day admission and discharge)

➤ **A 14-year-old patient is seen in the ED at 8:00 am on Monday after falling while riding his skateboard to school.** Witnesses reported brief loss of consciousness and the emergency medical technician reported disorientation at the time of transport. The ED physician consults the patient's pediatrician, who orders observation care to rule out clinically significant brain injury. The pediatrician visits the patient and provides initial observation care, including a comprehensive history and physical examination with moderate-level MDM, finding the patient has a moderately severe headache and mild nausea. Later the same day, the patient experiences seizures and repeated vomiting. After reexamining the patient, the pediatrician orders admission, computerized tomography, and a neurologic consultation. The pediatrician's combined services include a comprehensive history and examination and high-complexity MDM. Assessment is closed head injury with concussion.

If payer or state mandates require reporting of all external cause of injury information, document and report the cause, intent (when applicable), place of occurrence, activity, and patient status (eg, employee, volunteer, at leisure) at the time of the event. Place of occurrence, activity, and status are reported only for the initial encounter for care of an injury.

MDM: High complexity *History:* Comprehensive *Physical examination:* Comprehensive	**ICD-10-CM** S06.0X1A (initial encounter for concussion with loss of consciousness of 30 minutes or less) R56.1 (post-traumatic seizures) V00.131A (initial encounter for fall from skateboard)
	CPT® 99223 (initial hospital care)

Teaching Point: Observation care is not separately reported when initial hospital care is provided on the same date by the same physician or physicians of the same group and specialty.

Reporting to Payers Using Medicare Policy

Medicaid and private payers may adopt a Medicare policy that limits reporting of codes 99234–99236 to services provided to a patient who was admitted to observation or inpatient status for at least 8 hours and not more than 24 hours. Under this policy, when a patient is admitted to observation or inpatient care for fewer than 8 hours on the same calendar date, only the initial observation (99218–99220) or inpatient care (99221–99223) shall be reported by the physician. A separate code for discharge services is not reported.

> ~ **More From the AAP** ~
>
> For more information on reporting observation care services, see "Observation Care Services: *CPT* or Medicare" in the August 2014 *AAP Pediatric Coding Newsletter*™ at http://coding.aap.org (subscription required).

Medicare also requires that there must be a medical observation record for the patient that contains dated and timed physician's orders for the observation services the patient is to receive, nursing notes, and progress notes prepared by the physician indicating physical presence and personal performance of services. This record must be in addition to any record prepared as a result of an ED or outpatient clinic encounter.

Inpatient Hospital Care

Initial Inpatient Hospital Care

99221–99223   Initial hospital care, per day, for the evaluation and management of a patient

- Initial inpatient hospital service codes are used to report initial face-to-face services provided to a hospital inpatient.
- Initial inpatient encounters by more than one physician must be reported based on payer guidelines. (See the Coding Conundrum: 2 Physicians Providing Initial Observation or Inpatient Hospital Day Services box earlier in this chapter.)
- Selection of the code is based on performance and documentation of the 3 key components or time, if more than 50% of the encounter is spent in counseling and/or coordination of care (see **Table 16-2**).
- If the level of history and physical examination performed and documented is expanded or problem focused, initial inpatient hospital care must be reported using subsequent hospital visit codes 99231–99233 because the required key components for code 99221 (ie, at least a detailed history and detailed examination) have not been met.
- The code is reported on the first day that a face-to-face (physician–patient) service is provided.
- The date of initial hospital care that the physician reports does not need to correlate with the facility's date of admission.

◉ Report only an initial hospital care code when a patient is admitted to inpatient status from observation status.

Use **Table 16-2** to review the required components used to select level of service in the following examples:

Examples

➤ **An 8-week-old is seen in the ED and admitted by Physician A.** Over the past 2 days, the mother reported that the infant seemed warm to the touch, fed much less than normal, and had been harder to arouse. The mother had noticed only 2 wet diapers and one stool in the past 24 hours.

Review of systems: Fever; no history of heart murmur; no apnea or cyanosis; no wheeze or respiratory distress. *Past, family, and social history:* Full-term male; no reported problems with pregnancy or delivery; delivered by repeat cesarean. No maternal complications with delivery; rupture of membranes at the time of cesarean delivery, no fever prior to cesarean delivery; no prior ED visits or hospitalizations since birth hospitalization, no sick contacts at home, and lives with parents and 2 older female siblings. Two-month well-child vaccinations were received last week. *Physical examination:* Comprehensive examination includes vital signs with rectal temperature 38.0°C (100.4°F) and general appearance with examination of head, mucous membranes, clavicles, heart, lungs, abdomen, hips, genitalia, and skin.

Assessment: Laboratory evaluation: complete blood cell count with white blood cells 12,000, no left shift on differential; urinalysis normal or negative with pH 7.0, specific gravity 1.020; fever. Concern for sepsis or serious bacterial infection; doubt pyelonephritis given normal urinalysis; less likely meningitis given normal examination and not ill appearing; doubt bronchiolitis given lack of viral symptoms.

Plan: 8-week-old with fever, dehydration, and lethargy. Admit for IV antibiotics and IV fluids, pending culture results. Continue breastfeeding ad-lib. Discussed differential diagnoses, working diagnosis, current diagnostic and treatment plans, and anticipated hospital course with parents.

MDM: Moderate complexity *History:* Detailed *Physical examination:* Comprehensive	**ICD-10-CM** **R50.9** (fever, unspecified) **E86.0** (dehydration) **R53.83** (lethargy)
	CPT® **99221**

➤ **Later that same calendar day, Physician B from the same group practice sees the infant.** She performs a more comprehensive history, examines the infant, and spends 20 minutes talking with the parents.

MDM: Moderate complexity *History:* Comprehensive *Physical examination:* Comprehensive	**ICD-10-CM** **R50.9** **E86.0** (dehydration) **R53.83** (lethargy)
	CPT **99222**

Teaching Point: The total E/M services provided on this date now meet the guidelines for a comprehensive history. Physician B may now report the service with code **99222**. Physician A would submit no bill for his work that day.

If Physician A performed a comprehensive history and physical examination with moderate-complexity MDM at the initial hospital visit and documented that he spent 25 minutes on the floor with the patient and family, the service would be reported with code **99222**. However, later that same calendar day, Physician B (same specialty and from the same practice) sees the patient. She documents that 35 of her 40 minutes on the floor were spent counseling the parents and coordinating the patient's care. The code for all the care provided on that calendar day would now be reported using code **99223** based on the documented floor/

unit time (total of 65 minutes between the 2 physicians, with 35 minutes spent in counseling/coordination of care). Physician A would submit no bill, and Physician B would submit the bill for the calendar day's service. Coding based on time is further discussed in Chapter 1, The Basics of Coding.

Subsequent Hospital Care

99231–99233   Subsequent hospital care, per day, for the evaluation and management of a patient
- Codes include all E/M services by a physician or physician group provided on a given subsequent day.
- The level of service reported will be dependent on the total services provided and documented.
- Selection of the code is based on performance and documentation of 2 of the 3 key components or time if more than 50% of the encounter is spent in counseling and/or coordination of care (see **Table 16-3**).
- The history component required for subsequent hospital visits is considered interval history (ie, new history information obtained since the last physician assessment, including chief complaint, history of present illness, and problem-pertinent system review).

Use **Table 16-3** to help you in the selection of the appropriate codes in the following examples:

> **|||||||| Coding Pearl ||||||||**
>
> Past, family, and social history is not required as part of an interval history.

Examples

➤ *Continuing from previous example.* **No reported problems overnight; breastfeeding well; continues to have low-grade fever (38.2°C [100.7°F] maximum temperature) overnight; no reported apnea or cyanosis; no respiratory distress. Drinking better, more wet diapers, more alert.**

Physical examination: Expanded-level examination, including vital signs and general appearance, heart, lungs, genitourinary, and skin.

Laboratory: No growth in blood or urine cultures at less than 24 hours.

Assessment/plan: Continued fever. Concern for sepsis; suspect viral etiology given negative workup so far for common serious bacterial infections, such as pyelonephritis and bacteremia. Continue IV antibiotics until culture results are negative for 48 hours; continue breastfeeding ad-lib. Spoke with mom and reviewed overnight events, morning laboratory results, current plan, and possible discharge home tomorrow.

MDM: Straightforward *History:* Expanded interval history *Physical examination:* Expanded	**ICD-10-CM** R50.9 (fever)
	CPT® 99232

Teaching Point: Time cannot be used as the controlling factor in selection of the code because the documentation does not indicate the total floor/unit time or time spent in counseling and/or coordination of care.

In this example, the risk is moderate with an undiagnosed problem requiring IV antibiotics. However, the diagnosis and management options are limited to an established problem that is stable. The amount and complexity of data reviewed was limited to laboratory results. With 2 of 3 elements required to support the level of MDM, it is straightforward. A payer may require MDM as 1 of 2 key components supporting subsequent hospital care. This example would be limited to code 99231 if MDM were a required component.

➤ **Same progress note as in previous vignette but with additional documentation.**

Spoke with mom for 30 minutes and reviewed overnight events, morning laboratory results, and current plan; anticipate discharge home tomorrow. Total visit time: 40 minutes.

Time would be used as the controlling factor in selection of the code because a total of 40 minutes was spent on the unit/floor with the patient and more than 50% of the time was spent in counseling. The appropriate code would be **99233**.

Hospital Discharge Day Management

99238   Hospital discharge day management; 30 minutes or less
99239   more than 30 minutes

Codes **99238** (≤30 minutes) and **99239** (>30 minutes) are reported by the attending physician providing discharge services on a day subsequent to the date that the admission service was provided.

- ⦿ A face-to-face physician-patient encounter in the hospital is required.
- ⦿ Reporting is based on the total time (time does not have to be continuous) spent performing all final discharge services, including, as appropriate, examination of the patient, discussion of the hospital stay, patient and/or family counseling, instructions for continuing care to all relevant caregivers, and preparation of referral forms, prescriptions, and records.
- ⦿ May be used to report discharge services provided to patients who die during their hospital stay.
- ⦿ Services are reported on the day the physician sees the patient and performs discharge services, even if the patient leaves the hospital on a different day.
- ⦿ Only the attending physician or physician providing services on behalf of the attending physician (eg, covering physician, physician of same group and same specialty) may report discharge management services. If another physician is providing concurrent care, his or her services would be reported using subsequent hospital visit codes (**99231–99233**).
- ⦿ Time spent in discharge services must be documented in the medical record to report code **99239**. If the total time spent performing the discharge management is not documented in the medical record, report code **99238** instead of **99239**. Only time spent on the day of discharge may be counted.
- ⦿ Time spent on the day of discharge performing separately reported services (eg, car safety seat testing) is not included in the discharge day management time.

> |||||||| **Coding Pearl** ||||||||
>
> If the total time spent in performing discharge management is not documented in the medical record, report code **99238** instead of **99239**.

> |||||||| **Coding Pearl** ||||||||
>
> Only unit or floor time spent on the date of the discharge management is reported with codes **99238** and **99239**. Do not include time spent documenting discharge on a date after the service was rendered.

Example

➤ *Continuing from previous example.* **Patient continued on IV antibiotics until this morning; breastfeeding well; no more fevers.** Vital signs and general appearance and examination of the heart, lungs, abdomen, and skin are performed. Blood and urine culture results remain negative after 48 hours. Intravenous antibiotics are discontinued. Patient is discharged home with instructions for home care and follow-up. The physician spent 35 minutes on the floor reviewing the hospital course, expected follow-up, and signs and symptoms of possible sepsis or infection with mother.

This visit would be reported with code **99239** because 35 minutes was spent in the provision of discharge management services and the time was documented in the medical record.

Unique Considerations for Hospital Services

Admission to the hospital after a visit in the office and hospital rounds by more than one physician can create unusual circumstances. Proper coding in these situations will be contingent on whether the attending physician and colleagues provide coverage, bill under the same group name and tax identification number, or bill independently using individual tax identification numbers.

Office Visit and Initial Hospital Care on Same Day of Service

The primary care physician examines the patient in the office and a colleague admits the patient to the hospital later the same day for the same problem. If using independent billing numbers, each physician would submit a separate bill (ie, the primary care physician would bill for the office visit; the colleague would bill for the observation or inpatient hospital admission). If using the same billing number, services should be combined into one initial hospital care code encompassing the combined work of the 2 encounters. If the 2 encounters are not related and have different diagnoses, there is a legitimate reason to submit a claim for 2 distinct evaluation and management (E/M) services on the same day, even by the same provider, but be prepared to justify payment. Alternatively, bundle the 2 encounters, including all appropriate *International Classification of Diseases, 10th Revision, Clinical Modification* codes. If 2 distinct E/M services are reported on the same day of service by the same provider, append modifier **25** to the second service.

Two Hospital Visits on Same Day of Service

The primary care physician admits the patient to the hospital in the morning and a colleague is called to see the patient in the evening. If using independent National Provider Identifiers, separate bills are submitted. If using the same National Provider Identifier, the services are combined.

When office or outpatient E/M and hospital admissions occur on the same calendar day, coding will depend on whether the admitting physician and/or physician of the same group and specialty provides face-to-face care in the hospital setting.

Office Visit Without Face-to-face Encounter in Hospital

The primary care physician examines an established patient in the office and determines the patient needs admission. The admission history and physical examination are performed, and a treatment plan and orders are sent to the hospital. The physician remains in communication with the hospital nurses that night as the child improves and sees the child the next morning on rounds—he is stable but not ready for discharge. The office visit on day 1 would be reported with code **99212–99215** (office/outpatient E/M service, established patient) based on the performance and documentation of the required key components. The second day's work is reported using initial hospital care or observation care codes (**99221–99223** or **99218–99220**) based on the level of work (ie, history, physical examination, and medical decision-making or time) performed on the hospital floor on that day of service. If the work performed on the second day did not meet the required key components, the service would be reported using subsequent-day codes (**99224–99226, 99231–99233**).

Office Visit and Inpatient Encounter on Same Day of Service

The physician (or physician of the same group) provides face-to-face services in the hospital later that same day. The level of initial hospital care service will then be based on the combination of the E/M services provided during that calendar day.

Coordinating billing is important. The office billing manager should have all hospital charges for each patient by the end of the next business day to coordinate billing and avoid delays in claims submissions.

Teaching Physician Encounter on Day After Admission

If a resident provides the only face-to-face encounter on the date a patient is admitted to inpatient or observation status and the attending physician provides an initial face-to-face encounter on the next day, the physician reports the encounter based on the extent of work performed. If documentation clearly supports the work of an initial encounter (**99221–99223** or **99218–99220**), this service may be reported because these services are reported for the initial encounter without regard to the date of admission. However, if the encounter involves a more limited interval assessment, subsequent encounter services (**99231–99233** or **99224–99226**) or same-day admission and discharge services (**99234–99236**) are likely more appropriate.

Discharge Versus Subsequent Hospital Services

Codes 99238 and 99239 are underused and often reported incorrectly. Subsequent hospital visit codes should not be reported on the day of discharge alone or in addition to the discharge code. Code 99239 is one of the most underreported *CPT*® codes, even though it often more accurately reflects the service performed! Physicians often spend more than 30 minutes in discharge management, especially when the patient is seen several times that day. Time spent in charting *on the day of discharge* is counted in the total unit/floor time.

Note: The 2019 relative value units (RVUs) were not available at time of publication.

CPT Code	2018 Medicare RVUs
99231	1.11
99232	2.06
99233	2.95
99238	2.07
99239	3.05

Teaching Point: The RVUs for discharge service codes reflect the additional services provided on the day of discharge.

Consultations

CPT® defines *consultations* as services provided by a physician at the request of another physician or "other appropriate source" to provide advice or opinion about the management or evaluation of a specific problem. Medicare does not recognize consultation codes but pays for the services using codes for other E/M services. Detailed information on the *CPT* and CMS Medicare guidelines for reporting consultations for office and outpatient consultations appears in Chapter 7, Evaluation and Management Services in the Office and Outpatient Clinics. Please review those guidelines carefully as general guidelines that apply for all consultations.

Consultation codes should not be reported by the physician who has agreed to accept transfer of care before an initial evaluation. Consultation codes are appropriate to report if the decision to accept transfer of care cannot be made until after the initial consultation evaluation, regardless of site of service. See Chapter 7 for the definition of *transfer of care* versus *consultation*.

Guidelines Used by Payers That Do Not Follow Medicare Consultation Guidelines

Consultations for Patients in Observation

99241–99245   Office consultation for a new or established patient (includes consultations in other outpatient settings)

- Level of care is determined by performing and documenting the required 3 key components (history, physical examination, and MDM) or time (**Table 16-4**) as described for other E/M services that are assigned a typical time. Follow-up visits that are initiated by the physician consultant are reported using codes for subsequent observation care services (99224–99226).
- If an additional request for an opinion or advice on the same or a new problem is received from the attending physician and documented in the medical record, office or outpatient consultation codes, unlike inpatient consultation codes, may be used again.
- When reporting prolonged physician care with consultations that are performed in the observation care setting, report the office or other outpatient setting prolonged services code (99354, 99355) in addition to the appropriate outpatient consultation code (99241–99245) or appropriate other outpatient service code (99201–99205, 99212–99215). See Chapter 7, Evaluation and Management Services in the Office and Outpatient Clinics, for more information.

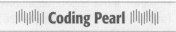

> ||||||| **Coding Pearl** |||||||
>
> Consultation codes are not reported when a transfer of care occurs before the patient is seen.

Use **Table 16-4** to help you in the selection of the appropriate codes in the following example:

Example

➤ **A 14-year-old is admitted to observation for closed head trauma and possible concussion after a fall from his skateboard with brief loss of consciousness.** The attending physician consults a pediatric neurologist for her opinion and advice. The neurologist performs a detailed history and physical examination, reviews computed tomography images, and orders additional diagnostic studies. Documentation of the written report is included in the shared medical record. Assessment is concussion with brief loss of consciousness. The neurologist reports the service with

MDM: Moderate *History:* Detailed *Physical examination:* Detailed	**ICD-10-CM** **S06.0X1A** (initial encounter for concussion with loss of consciousness of 30 minutes or less) **V00.131A** (initial encounter for fall from skateboard)
	CPT **99243** or, if payer does not recognize consultations, **New Patient** **Established Patient** **99203** (office/outpatient E/M) **99214** (office/outpatient E/M)

Table 16-4. Observation (99241–99245) and Inpatient (99251–99255) Consultation Codes

Key Components (For a description of key components, see Table 16-1.)
3 of 3 key components must be performed to at least the degree specified under the code.

CPT® Code/Timeª	Medical Decision-making	History (cc required for each level)	1995 Examinationᵇ
99241 15 min 99251 20 min	Straightforward	HPI: 1–3; ROS: 0; PFSH: 0	1 body area/system
99242 30 min 99252 40 min	Straightforward	HPI: 1–3; ROS: 1; PFSH: 0	2–7 limited
99243 40 min 99253 55 min	Low complexity	HPI: ≥4 or 3 cc; ROS: 2–9; PFSH: 1/3	2–7 detailed
99244 60 min 99254 80 min	Moderate complexity	HPI: ≥4 or 3 cc; ROS: ≥10; PFSH: 3/3	≥8 body areas/systems
99245 80 min 99255 110 min	High complexity	HPI: ≥4 or 3 cc; ROS: ≥10; PFSH: 3/3	≥8 body areas/systems

Abbreviations: cc, chronic conditions; CPT, Current Procedural Terminology; HPI, history of present illness; PFSH, past, family, and social history; ROS; review of systems.

ª *Typical time is an average and represents a range of times that may be higher or lower depending on clinical circumstances. The presenting problem is considered to be a contributory factor and does not need to be present to the degree specified.*

ᵇ *Number of body areas or organ systems examined; see* **Table 16-1** *for details.*

Inpatient Consultations

99251–99255   Inpatient consultation for a new or established patient

* Codes **99251–99255** are to be used only once by the reporting physician for an individual hospital patient for a particular admission. There are no specific guidelines for the length of stay.

* Follow-up visits provided in the hospital by the same physician must be reported using subsequent care codes (**99231–99233**). Examples of a follow-up visit might be to complete the initial consultation when test results become available or in response to a change in the patient's status.

* If a consultation is requested by the attending physician for the same patient on a completely different problem during the same hospital stay, subsequent hospital care codes (**99231–99233**) must be reported. The subsequent role of a consultant in the ongoing care of the patient must be made clear in the medical record by the attending physician. If the attending physician turns over the care of the patient to the consultant, the consultant, now the new attending physician, should use subsequent hospital care codes (**99231–99233**) to indicate the level of service provided.

* The attending physician and consultant may continue to provide care to the patient. Each would code for subsequent hospital care as long as the problems they manage are different. (The attending and consulting physicians should use different *diagnosis* codes to indicate they are managing different problems. However, sometimes, the diagnosis will be the same.)

* If a patient is readmitted for the same or different problem (a new hospital stay), an initial inpatient consultation code may be reported if it meets the definition and requirements for reporting a consultation.

* When an inpatient consultation is performed on a date a patient is admitted to the hospital, all E/M services provided by the consultant (including any outpatient encounters) related to the admission are reported with the inpatient consultation service code. If a patient is admitted after an outpatient consultation (eg, office, ED) and the patient is not seen on the unit on the date of admission, only the outpatient consultation code is reported.

Use **Table 16-4** to help you in the selection of the appropriate codes in the following examples:

Examples

➤ **A 3-month-old patient is seen by the pediatrician in the ED and is subsequently admitted for bilious vomiting, dehydration, and possible bowel obstruction.** A gastroenterologist is consulted and, following workup, diagnoses volvulus due to congenital malrotation of the intestine. He documents his written report in the medical record, speaks to the parents, and agrees to follow the patient. The gastroenterologist reports his consultation service with

MDM: High complexity *History:* Comprehensive *Physical examination:* Comprehensive	**ICD-10-CM** **K56.2** (volvulus) **Q43.3** (congenital malformations of intestinal fixation)
	CPT® **99255** or, if payer does not recognize consultations, **99223** (initial hospital visit)

Teaching Point: Follow-up visits by the gastroenterologist are reported using the appropriate-level subsequent inpatient hospital codes (**99231–99233**).

> ||||||||| **Coding Pearl** |||||||||
>
> A diagnosis of congenital volvulus would be reported with *International Classification of Diseases, 10th Revision, Clinical Modification* code **Q43.8**, other specified congenital malformation of the intestine.

➤ **A neonatologist is asked by an obstetrician to consult with a mother in preterm labor with triplets at 23 weeks' gestation.** She is being treated with steroids and magnesium sulfate. The neonatologist reviews the maternal prenatal and hospital record, interviews the mother, and meets with both parents to discuss fetal and neonatal risks and likely hospital course and complications if delivered in the next few days. The neonatologist spends a total of 65 minutes of floor/unit time devoted to this patient's consultation, which is dominated by discussing morbidity and mortality risks and resuscitation and possible treatment.

Inpatient floor/unit time (65 minutes) is the key controlling factor.	**ICD-10-CM** O60.02 (preterm labor without delivery, second trimester) O30.102 (triplet pregnancy, unspecified number of placenta and unspecified number of amniotic sacs, second trimester)
	CPT 99253 (typical time 55 minutes) or, if payer does not recognize consultations, 99223 (average 70 minutes)

Teaching Point: Pediatric hospital care may, at times, begin prior to birth with services provided to the mother during the peripartum period. Although it is atypical for pediatric claims to be submitted for services to adult patients, these services rendered to the mother are an exception. Services provided prior to delivery are reported as services to the mother (ie, to the mother's health insurance plan).

Guidelines Used by Payers That Follow Medicare Consultation Guidelines

Medicare guidelines require that consultations provided to patients in observation status will be reported with office or outpatient E/M codes 99201–99215. If the patient is new to the physician (ie, has not received any face-to-face professional services from the physician or another physician of the same specialty who belongs to the same group practice within the past 3 years), codes 99201–99205 are reported based on the performance and documentation of the required key components. If the patient does not meet the requirements of a new patient, an established patient office or outpatient E/M code is reported.

Consultations provided to inpatient hospital patients are reported using initial inpatient hospital care codes (99221–99223). The admitting physician must report the initial hospital care services with modifier AI (principal physician of record) appended to the appropriate code to distinguish the services from the consulting physician. Subsequent face-to-face services, including new consultations within the same admission, are reported with subsequent hospital care codes 99231–99233.

Check with your commercial payers to learn if they follow Medicare consultation guidelines or have otherwise adopted consultation guidelines that differ from *CPT®*.

Concurrent Care

Concurrent care is defined by *CPT* as the provision of similar services to the same patient by more than one physician on the same day. Concurrent care may be provided by physicians from different practices or physicians of the same practice but different specialties. When concurrent care is provided, the diagnosis code(s) reported by each physician should reflect the medical necessity for the provision of services by more than one physician on the same *date* of service. Although it is easier to justify concurrent care when each treating physician reports different diagnoses, if the *diagnosis* code is reported for the same condition, it does not prevent billing for the services.

> **~ More From the AAP ~**
>
> For more information on concurrent care, see "Concurrent Care: A Refresher" in the May 2014 *AAP Pediatric Coding Newsletter*™ at http://coding.aap.org (subscription required).

Example

➤ The attending physician wants the consultant to provide ongoing management of one problem (eg, heart failure) while the attending physician provides ongoing management for other active problems (eg, pneumonia, inadequate weight gain).

Both physicians would report subsequent hospital care codes and link the *CPT* codes to the appropriate *diagnosis* codes. (See the claim form example in Chapter 1 for an example of linking diagnosis to procedure codes on a claim.)

Interprofessional Telephone/Internet/Electronic Health Record Consultation

A consultation request by a patient's attending or primary physician or other QHP soliciting opinion and/or treatment advice by telephone, Internet, or electronic health record from a physician with specialty expertise (consultant) is reported by the consultant with interprofessional consultation codes 99446–99451. This consultation does not require face-to-face contact with the patient by the consultant. The patient may be in the inpatient or outpatient setting. For information on reporting interprofessional consultation or on services provided via an interactive audiovisual telemedicine system, see Chapter 20, Digital Medicine Services: Technology-Enhanced Care Delivery.

Prolonged Evaluation and Management Services Provided in the Inpatient Setting

According to *CPT,* the prolonged services inpatient add-on codes 99356 and 99357 may be reported in addition to observation codes (99218–99220, 99224–99226, 99234–99236) because, although observation care services are performed in an "outpatient" setting, the intraservice times for the codes are defined as unit or floor time rather than face-to-face time as required in the office or outpatient setting. Prolonged service codes (**tables 16-5 and 16-6**) are reported when a physician provides services that are 30 minutes or more beyond the usual service duration described in an E/M code or other codes with a published maximum time. The codes for prolonged service are subdivided into the following categories: service with direct (ie, face-to-face) patient contact and service without direct patient contact.

Refer to Chapter 7, Evaluation and Management Services in the Office and Outpatient Clinics, for details of the specific requirements for reporting physician prolonged services in the office or outpatient setting.

- Direct prolonged services (99356 and 99357) may only be reported in conjunction with the following codes: 99221–99223 (initial hospital care), 99218–99220 (initial observation care), 99234–99236 (admission/discharge same day), 99224–99226 (subsequent observation care), 99231–99233 (subsequent hospital care), 99251–99255 (inpatient consultations), 99304–99310 (nursing facility services), 90837 (psychotherapy without E/M, 60 minutes), and 90847 (family psychotherapy [conjoint psychotherapy] [with patient present], 50 minutes).

- Direct prolonged services (99356 and 99357) may not be reported in conjunction with observation or inpatient discharge management (99217, 99238, or 99239), critical care (99291, 99292; 99466, 99467; 99468–99476), or intensive care (99477–99480) because none of these E/M services has an assigned typical time.

- Direct patient contact time in the inpatient facility is defined as floor or unit time dedicated to the patient. (*Note:* Medicare policy is that time spent reviewing charts or discussion of a patient with house medical staff and not with direct face-to-face contact with the patient, or waiting for test results, changes in the patient's condition, end of a therapy, or use of facilities, cannot be billed as direct prolonged services. It is important to be aware of Medicaid and private payers that adopt Medicare policy.)

- When an E/M service is reported using time as the key or controlling factor, prolonged services can be reported only when the prolonged service exceeds 30 minutes beyond the highest level of E/M service (eg, 99220, 99223).

Table 16-5. Prolonged Services in Inpatient or Observation Settings

Code	Description of Prolonged Services
+99356	Prolonged service in the inpatient or observation setting, requiring unit/floor time beyond the usual service; first hour (30–74 min) (List separately in addition to the code for inpatient evaluation and management service.) (Use code 99356 in conjunction with codes 90837, 99218–99220, 99221–99223, 99224–99226, 99231–99233, 99234–99236, 99251–99255, 99304–99310.)
+99357	each additional 30 minutes (List separately in addition to the code for prolonged physician service.) (Use code 99357 in conjunction with code 99356.)
99358	Prolonged evaluation and management service before and/or after direct patient care; first hour
+99359	each additional 30 minutes (Use code 99359 in conjunction with code 99358.)

- The medical record must reflect the total time of the service and medical need for the service.
- Non-direct prolonged physician services (99358 and 99359) may be reported on a different date than the related primary service. The related primary service may be an E/M service (with or without an assigned typical time), a procedure, or other service.
- Non-direct prolonged E/M services must relate to a face-to-face service that has occurred or will occur and must be relative to ongoing care.

Table 16-6. Coding Direct Prolonged Services for Inpatient and Observation Care

Total Duration of Prolonged Services, min	Code(s)
<30	Not reported separately
30–74	99356 × 1
75–104	99356 × 1 and 99357 × 1
≥105 (≥1 h 45 min)	99356 × 1 and 99357 × 2 (or more for each additional 30 min)

Examples

➤ The pediatrician spends 40 minutes reviewing extensive medical records that are received the day after a patient is admitted.

Code 99358 would be reported. Prolonged service of less than 30 minutes' total duration would not be separately reported.

➤ A 10-year-old patient is admitted to the care of a neurologist following a first-time seizure that occurred shortly after waking in the morning. The neurologist completes a comprehensive history and physical examination. Results of an electroencephalogram are reviewed. The diagnosis is juvenile myoclonic epilepsy. Later that same day, the neurologist visits the patient and spends 60 minutes discussing the patient's test results and the anticipated plan of care with the parents and documents the total unit/floor time of 120 minutes in the medical record.

The neurologist reports her services with codes 99223 and 99356.

Teaching Point: The neurologist reports initial inpatient hospital code 99223 based on the key components of comprehensive history and examination and high-complexity MDM. The typical time assigned to code 99223 is 70 minutes. This leaves an additional 50 minutes of unit/floor time that may be appropriately reported with prolonged services code 99356.

Hospital-Mandated On-Call Services

99026   Hospital mandated on-call service; in-hospital, each hour
99027   out of hospital, each hour

❖ Codes 99026 and 99027 describe services provided by a physician who is on call per hospital mandate as a condition of medical staff privileges.

❖ Used to report on-call time spent by the physician when he or she is not providing other services.

❖ Time spent performing separately reportable services should not be included in time reported as mandated on-call services.

❖ Most payers do not cover these services because they consider this a contract issue between the hospital and physician. However, these codes may be used for tracking purposes.

Critical Care and Continuing Intensive Care Services

Specific guidelines for reporting hourly and inpatient neonatal and pediatric critical care are provided in Chapter 18, Critical and Intensive Care.

Medical Team Conferences

99366   Medical team conference with interdisciplinary team of health care professionals, face-to-face with patient and/or family, 30 minutes or more, participation by nonphysician qualified health care professional

99367   Medical team conference with interdisciplinary team of health care professionals, patient and/or family not present, 30 minutes or more; participation by physician

99368   Medical team conference with interdisciplinary team of health care professionals, patient and/or family not present, 30 minutes or more; participation by nonphysician qualified health care professional

   Codes 99366–99368 are used to report participation by physicians or nonphysician providers (NPPs) in conferences to coordinate or manage care and services for established patients with chronic or multiple health conditions (eg, cerebral palsy) or with congenital anomalies (eg, craniofacial abnormalities). Code 99367 is the only code that may be reported by a physician, and it can only be reported when the patient and/or family is not present at the team conference. When the physician or QHP who may report E/M services (eg, advanced practice nurse) participates in a medical team conference with the patient and/or family present, the appropriate-level E/M code (eg, 99231–99233) will be reported based on the place of service and total face-to-face time spent in counseling and/or coordination of care.

   See Chapter 12, Managing Chronic and Complex Conditions, for a complete summary of the reporting requirements.

Advance Care Planning

99497   Advance care planning, including the explanation and discussion of advance directives such as standard forms (with completion of such forms, when performed), by the physician or other qualified health care professional; first 30 minutes, face-to-face with the patient, family member(s) and/or surrogate

+99498   each additional 30 minutes (List separately in addition to code for primary procedure)

   Codes 99497 and 99498 include

❖ Face-to-face service by a physician or QHP to a patient, family member, or surrogate spent in counseling and discussion of advance directives

❖ Completion of forms, when applicable (eg, Health Care Proxy, Durable Power of Attorney for Health Care, Living Will, and Medical Orders for Life-Sustaining Treatment)

Face-to-face time spent by the physician or QHP is required and the total time must be documented.

Active management of problems is not included in advance care planning. Other E/M services provided on the same date as advance care planning may be separately reported, with the exceptions of hourly critical care services (99291 and 99292), inpatient neonatal and pediatric critical care (99468 and 99469; 99471–99476), and initial and continuing intensive care services (99477–99480). Do not report codes 99497 and 99498 in conjunction with codes 99291 and 99292, 99468 and 99469, 99471–99476, or 99477–99480.

Example

> **An adolescent with metastatic cancer wishes to discuss and be involved in planning her care.** Her oncologist spends 50 minutes face-to-face with the patient and her parent assessing their understanding of the diagnosis and prognosis, the continued hope that treatment is successful, and the patient's wishes to be included in decisions about her care. A plan of care is developed and documented and an appointment with the supportive care team at the hospital is scheduled to provide additional counseling and support services to the patient and family.
>
> The oncologist may report codes 99497 and 99498 for the 50 minutes of face-to-face time spent providing the advance care planning. Because the *CPT®* prefatory language and code descriptors for advance care planning do not include other instruction on the time required for reporting, these services may be reported based on general *CPT* instruction to report when the midpoint is passed (eg, 1 unit of 99498 may be reported for 46–75 minutes). Exceptions may apply for payers with policy requiring that the time be met or exceeded.

Continuing Care After Hospitalization

A key goal of many quality improvement programs is avoidance of readmittance and/or ED visits following hospitalization. In recent years, *CPT* and payers have recognized a need for codes to capture services related to care coordination and management of chronic and episodic conditions that may lead to emergency and inpatient care. For physicians continuing patient care after hospital discharge, services such as transitional care management and chronic care management offer opportunities to provide and be compensated for care aimed at reducing the risk of decline, exacerbation, and/or functional decline.

See Chapter 12, Managing Chronic and Complex Conditions, for more information on transitional and chronic care management services.

Teaching Points: Progression of Care

Selecting the appropriate level of service from the appropriate family of codes will be dependent on the child's condition, type of service (observation vs inpatient), and intensity of the service provided and documented on a particular day of service. The following scenarios indicate the category of codes that should be reported based on the progression of care provided (**Figure 16-1**). Remember that the level of service reported is based on all the face-to-face care provided during the calendar day.

See the progression of care when reporting daily hospital care and neonatal and pediatric critical care or neonatal intensive care in Chapter 18, Critical and Intensive Care.

Figure 16-1. Coding Progression—Same-Date Evaluation and Management Services by the Admitting Physician

Report only the applicable service that is farthest to the right.
(Applies to encounters for the same or related problem by the *same individual or physicians and/or qualified health care professionals of the same group practice and specialty*)

| Office or Other Outpatient E/M
99201–99215
Outpatient Consultation
99241–99245
Emergency Department
99281–99285 | Initial Observation Care
99218–99220
Subsequent Observation Care
99224–99226 | Initial Hospital Care
99221–99223
Same-Date Admission and Discharge
99234–99236 |

Examples

➤ **The patient receives E/M services in the office and is sent to the hospital on the same day.**

If the patient is examined in the office or outpatient setting, admitted to the hospital for observation or as an inpatient, and not seen in the hospital on the same day, report the appropriate office or outpatient code (**99201–99215**) or consultation code (**99241–99245**) as applicable.

If the patient is examined in the office or outpatient setting, admitted to the hospital for observation or as an inpatient, and seen in the hospital on the same day, report the appropriate initial observation or inpatient hospital code (**99218–99220** or **99221–99223**) based on all the E/M services provided on that calendar day.

If the patient is admitted by Physician A and discharged on the same day by Physician B (from the same practice and of the same specialty), a code for same-day admission and discharge observation or inpatient services (**99234–99236**) is reported based on the combined services.

➤ **The patient receives an initial face-to-face E/M service in the observation setting.**

If the patient is admitted to observation and not discharged or admitted to inpatient status on the same date, the appropriate initial observation code (**99218–99220**) is reported by the attending physician.

If the patient is admitted and discharged on the same day, a code for admission and discharge observation or inpatient services (**99234–99236**) is reported.

If the patient is admitted for observation and subsequently formally admitted to the hospital on the same day, only the initial inpatient hospital code (**99221–99223**) is reported.

If the patient was admitted to observation care status and is seen the following day and not discharged, codes **99224–99226** are reported for the subsequent-day encounter.

If the patient is placed in observation status and then admitted as an inpatient the next day, initial observation (**99218–99220**) and initial hospital care (**99221–99223**) codes are reported with the appropriate dates of service. If the level of service performed during the initial hospital care does not meet the requirements for the initial hospital care (all 3 key components or time requirements), report the appropriate subsequent hospital care code (**99231–99233**).

If the patient is discharged from observation status on a day subsequent to the admission, observation care discharge management (**99217**) is reported.

➤ The patient receives face-to-face E/M services in the inpatient hospital setting.

If the patient is evaluated in the hospital and not discharged on the same date, the appropriate initial hospital care code (99221–99223) is reported for the first face-to-face E/M service.

If the patient is admitted and discharged on the same day, a code for admission and discharge observation or inpatient services (99234–99236) is reported.

If the patient is followed on subsequent days, codes 99231–99233 are reported for each subsequent day of service.

If the patient is discharged on a day subsequent to the initial service, discharge code 99238 or 99239 is reported.

> ⦀⦀ **Coding Pearl** ⦀⦀
>
> If the patient's condition deteriorates and he or she requires *critical care services,* coding will be dependent on the age of the child. If the child is 6 years or older, hourly critical care services will be reported (**99291** and **99292**) in addition to codes **99231–99233**. See Chapter 18, Critical and Intensive Care, for guidelines used to report critical are.
>
> For infants weighing 5,000 g or less, if the patient's condition declines and he or she requires *intensive care services,* see Chapter 18 for specific details about coding intensive care services.

Transfer of Service

Transfer of Service in the Observation or Inpatient Status		
Example	**Physician A reports**	**Physician B reports**
The patient is examined by Physician A in the office or outpatient setting and sent to the hospital to be admitted by Physician B from a different group or specialty (eg, hospitalist or other physician from a group with a different tax identification number than physician A).	All E/M and other services that he or she provided in the office (eg, 99201–99215)	The appropriate initial hospital observation or inpatient service code (99218–99220, 99221–99223) or if discharged on the same date (99234–99236)
Physician A admits the patient during a face-to-face visit and then transfers care (not a consultation) to a physician of a different specialty.	Physician A reports 99218–99220 or 99221–99223 and, if care is provided on subsequent days prior to transfer, subsequent observation (99224–99226) or subsequent inpatient (99231–99233) care.	Subsequent observation (99224–99226) or subsequent inpatient (99231–99233) care until the day of discharge (observation [99217] or hospital [99238–99239])
Physician A admits the patient (face-to-face visit) and requests an opinion or advice from Physician B, who may be from the same or different group or specialty, and the requirements for a consultation are performed.	Physician A reports initial hospital care (99221–99223) and if care is provided on subsequent days prior to discharge (99231–99233) and 99238 or 99239 on the date of discharge.	In observation (99241–99245 or 99201–99215) or inpatient (99251–99255 or 99221–99223) and if subsequent care is provided, 99231–99233. If care is transferred, 99238 or 99239 is reported for discharge day management services.
Physician A admits the patient by phone and then transfers care (not a consultation) to a physician of a different group in the hospital.	There is nothing to report for an admission by phone unless the time spent could be reported by a non–face-to-face code such as non-direct prolonged services (99358, 99359) if >30 min is spent.	The appropriate initial hospital observation or inpatient service code (99218–99220, 99221–99223) or if discharged on the same date (99234–99236)

If both physicians are from the same group, additional justification may be required to support payment for services by both physicians. See Chapter 18, Critical and Intensive Care, for guidelines for reporting concurrent critical care or transfer of care of the critically ill infant or child.

Split/Shared Billing

A split/shared E/M service is one in which a physician and a QHP, such as a nurse practitioner or physician assistant, from the *same group practice* each personally perform a medically necessary and substantive portion of one or more face-to-face E/M encounters on the same date.

The following requirements apply to all split/shared services:

- A portion of the key components of the service must be provided face-to-face by the physician to report under the physician's National Provider Identifier.
- Split/shared services were defined and implemented for services to Medicare beneficiaries. Private payers may adopt the same or a similar policy.
- The physician and QHP must document and sign their portion of the service.
- A physician cannot merely sign off on the documentation of the NPP's work.
- If the E/M service is reported based on counseling and/or coordination of care, only the physician's time is used to select the level of service if billing under that physician.
    - ❖ The physician must document his or her total time, the portion of time (ie, >50%) spent in counseling and/or coordination of care, and a summary of the issues discussed or coordination of care provided.
- Shared services are not permitted if the QHP is a hospital employee.
- Services may be reported by the QHP or physician (if QHP may bill).
- Shared services are allowed when sick hospital care services are reported (combined physician and NPP time) and with discharge services.
- Critical care is never a split/shared service because critical care services reflect the work of only one individual.

Split/shared billing differs from incident-to billing, which is only allowed in the outpatient setting. See Chapter 13, Allied Health and Clinical Staff Services, for more information on incident-to rules.

Example

➤ **A pediatrician and NPP from the same group practice see a patient on the same date.** The NPP provides and documents initial hospital care, including a comprehensive history, detailed examination, and MDM of moderate complexity. Later that day, the pediatrician is called to see the patient, who is exhibiting new symptoms, and to review new laboratory test results. Taking into account both services, which have been individually documented and signed, the examination and history are comprehensive and MDM is of high complexity.

   Teaching Point: Because both providers are from the same group practice and have signed off on their individually provided services, the services may be shared and billed under the physician as code **99223**.

CHAPTER 17

Emergency Department Services

Contents

Reporting the Diagnosis Code for Emergency Department (ED) Visits

While several symptoms may be listed as the "chief complaint" as part of the emergency department (ED) triage process, the physician must designate only one sign, symptom, disease, or injury as the chief complaint. The hospital depends on the physician's designation of the chief complaint because only one diagnosis code may be reported for this category on the hospital claim form. This diagnosis is used to help support the urgency of the ED visit under prudent layperson guidelines. This may be different from conditions that are "present on admission" that must now be tracked by hospitals.

Reporting External Cause of Injury

States may require EDs to report codes describing the circumstances of an injury. These codes are referred to as *external cause* codes in *International Classification of Diseases, 10th Revision, Clinical Modification (ICD-10-CM)*. These codes capture the cause, intent, place of occurrence, activity of the patient at the time of the event, and patient status (eg, employee, military, volunteer, student). External cause codes provide information that is valuable for research on the cause and occurrence of injuries and evaluation of injury prevention strategies (eg, reduced reporting of injuries due to automobile crashes following mandates to use seat belts and car seats). While the physician may not be required to add the specific external cause code with the discharge diagnosis, there should be sufficient documentation in the record so that a coder can extract the proper diagnosis code.

Key points for reporting external cause codes include

- External cause codes may be reported in conjunction with any health condition that is related to an external cause (eg, adverse effect of medical treatment).
- External cause codes are never the principal or first-listed diagnosis code.
- In *ICD-10-CM,* only external cause codes for the cause and intent of an injury or illness are reported for the duration of treatment, with the seventh character of the code indicating whether an encounter is for initial care, subsequent care, or care for sequela (late effect) of the injury or illness.
- External cause codes indicating place of occurrence, activity, and patient status are reported only at the initial encounter for treatment.
- If the intent (eg, accident, self-harm, assault) of the cause of an injury or other condition is unknown or unspecified, code the intent as *accidental.*
- No external cause code should be assigned when the cause and intent of an illness or injury are included in another reported code (eg, T58.11XA, initial encounter for toxic effect of carbon monoxide from utility gas, accidental).
- No external cause code should be assigned when an injury is ruled out after examination and observation (eg, Z04.1, encounter for examination and observation following transport accident).

Reporting Suspected or Confirmed Abuse

T76.02X-	Child neglect or abandonment, suspected
T76.12X-	Child sexual abuse, suspected
T76.32X-	Child psychological abuse, suspected
T74.02X-	Child neglect or abandonment, confirmed
T74.12X-	Child physical abuse, confirmed
T74.22X-	Child sexual abuse, confirmed
T74.32X-	Child psychological abuse, confirmed
T74.4XX-	Shaken infant syndrome
Z04.42	Encounter for examination and observation following alleged child rape (ruled out)
Z04.72	Encounter for examination and observation following alleged child physical abuse (ruled out)

The appropriate seventh character is to be added to each code from categories **T74** and **T76**.

A	Initial encounter
D	Subsequent encounter
S	Sequela

Suspected (**T76.-**) or confirmed abuse (**T74.-**) is reported as the first-listed diagnosis when this is the reason for the encounter. Codes for associated mental health or injury are reported secondary to the code for suspected or confirmed abuse.

- Codes are selected based on documentation. The record should clearly state whether abuse is suspected, ruled out, or confirmed.
- If a suspected case of child abuse, neglect, or mistreatment is ruled out during an encounter, code **Z04.72** (encounter for examination and observation following alleged child physical abuse, ruled out) should be used, not a code from **T76**.
- When reporting confirmed abuse, report also codes for assault (**X92–Y04, Y08–Y09**) and perpetrator (**Y07.-**).

> |||||||| **Coding Pearl** ||||||||
>
> Seventh character **A** is often reported for management of injuries other than fracture in the emergency department. It may be helpful to remember that seventh character **A** (initial encounter) is reported for active treatment and not for care during the healing phase of an injury.

ED Evaluation and Management Codes

- Evaluation and management (E/M) codes **99281–99285** are only reported when care is provided in an ED. An ED is defined as an organized hospital-based facility for the provision of unscheduled episodic services to patients who present for immediate medical attention. The facility must be available 24 hours a day, 7 days a week.
  - ❖ Some states allow for nonhospital-based "freestanding" EDs. Payers may or may not allow the use of ED codes in these circumstances. Government payers (eg, Medicaid, Tricare) will not pay freestanding EDs that are not off-site hospital based.
- Services performed in an urgent care center, a nonhospital facility, or a facility that is not open for 24 hours a day should be reported with the appropriate *Current Procedural Terminology* (*CPT*®) office or outpatient visit codes (**99201–99215**) and with the appropriate place of service code (eg, **20** for urgent care facility). These facilities are not considered a "freestanding" ED.
- Selection of the appropriate E/M code is primarily driven by the risk involved in the presenting problem, evaluation measures, and/or treatment options.
- Performance and documentation of all 3 key components (history, physical examination, and medical decision-making [MDM]) are used to select the level of an ED E/M code.

> |||||||| **Coding Pearl** ||||||||
>
> Services provided in an urgent care center or nonhospital-based facility are not reported with codes **99281–99285**.

Emergency Department Caveat: Code 99285

The emergency department evaluation and management code **99285** allows an exception to the "3 key components" rule (Level 5 caveat) for patients whose clinical condition, mental status, or lack of available history may not permit obtaining a comprehensive history and/or physical examination. Therefore, code **99285** may be reported for patients presenting with a high-severity condition that requires a high level of medical decision-making when circumstances prevent the physician from obtaining a comprehensive history and/or completing a comprehensive physical examination. When such urgency exists, the physician must document the condition or reason why a comprehensive history and/or physical examination could not be obtained.

- Because of the unpredictability and inconsistency in the intensity of these services, there are no time values assigned to this family of codes. Therefore, time spent in counseling and/or coordination of care *cannot* be used as a key or controlling factor in the selection of the code, nor can prolonged services be reported with ED codes.

- There is no differentiation between new or established patients for ED encounters. All problems for encounters in the ED are considered new to the attending physician for purposes of determining MDM.
- The ED codes are not reported if the treating ED physician admits the patient to his or her service for observation or inpatient status on the same date of service as the ED encounter. Only the appropriate initial observation (99218–99220), initial hospital care (99221–99223), or initial observation or inpatient hospital admission and discharge, same day (99234–99236), codes are reported instead of ED codes. All the E/M work performed in the ED should be combined with any additional work performed for admission (and, when appropriate, discharge) when selecting the correct code and level of care.

Table 17-1 summarizes the key components required for each ED E/M code based on the 1995 and 1997 Centers for Medicare & Medicaid Services *Documentation Guidelines for Evaluation and Management Services.* Also refer to Chapter 6, Evaluation and Management Documentation Guidelines, for more details on E/M coding guidelines. Medical necessity is an overarching criterion for selecting the level of E/M service. Physicians should always consider whether the nature of the presenting problem supports the medical necessity of services rendered when selecting the level of E/M service.

Table 17-1. Emergency Department Services

Key Components

3 of 3 key components must be performed to at least the degree specified for each code. All patients in the emergency department are considered new patients.

Code	MDM	History	Physical Examination
99281	**Straightforward** # diagnoses/options: Minimal Data: Minimal Risk: Minimal	**Problem focused** HPI: 1–3 elements ROS: 0 PFSH: 0	**Problem focused** **1995:** One body area/organ system **1997:** Performance and documentation of 1–5 elements identified by a bullet (●) in ≥1 areas or systems
99282	**Low complexity** # diagnoses/options: Limited Data: Limited Risk: Low	**Expanded problem focused** HPI: 1–3 elements ROS: 1 PFSH: 0	**Expanded problem focused** **1995:** Limited examination—affected body area/organ system and 1–6 other related areas/systems **1997:** Performance and documentation of at least 6 elements identified by a bullet (●) in ≥1 areas or systems
99283	**Moderate complexity** # diagnoses/options: Multiple Data: Moderate Risk: Moderate	**Expanded problem focused** HPI: 1–3 elements ROS: 1 PFSH: 0	**Expanded problem focused** **1995:** Limited examination—affected body area/organ system and 1–6 other related areas/systems **1997:** Performance and documentation of at least 6 elements identified by a bullet (●) in ≥1 areas or systems
99284	**Moderate complexity** # diagnoses/options: Multiple Data: Moderate Risk: Moderate	**Detailed** HPI: 4+ elements or status of 3 chronic or inactive conditions ROS: 2–9 PFSH: 1	**Detailed** **1995:** Extended examination—affected body area(s) and 1–6 other symptomatic or related organ system(s) **1997:** Performance and documentation of at least 2 elements identified by a bullet (●) in at least 6 areas or systems or at least 12 elements identified by a bullet (●) in at least 2 areas or systems

Table 17-1. Emergency Department Services (*continued*)

Key Components

3 of 3 key components must be performed to at least the degree specified for each code. All patients in the emergency department are considered new patients.

Code	MDM	History	Physical Examination
99285	**High complexity** # diagnoses/options: Extensive Data: Extensive Risk: High	**Comprehensive** HPI: 4+ elements or status of 3 chronic or inactive conditions ROS: 10+ PFSH: 2 Or clinical condition or mental status did not permit performance of history (must document reason that comprehensive history could not be performed).	**Comprehensive** **1995:** 8+ organ systems or complete examination of a single organ system **1997:** <u>Multisystem examination</u>—At least 9 organ systems or body areas with performance of all elements identified by a bullet (●) in each area/system examined Documentation is expected for at least 2 elements identified by a bullet (●) of each area(s) or system(s). <u>Single organ system examination</u>—Performance of all elements identified by a bullet (●) and documentation of every element in each box with a shaded border and at least one element in a box with an unshaded border Or clinical condition or mental status did not permit performance of examination.

Abbreviations: HPI, history of present illness; MDM, medical decision-making; PFSH, past, family, and social history; ROS, review of systems.

Examples

➤ **A 18-month-old girl presents with pulling at left ear, fever, and irritability.** Parents noticed that the child had a fever (temporal artery 39.5°C [103.1°F]) the prior evening and administered ibuprofen. Fever returned during the night, and the child has had 2 additional doses of ibuprofen, with the last dose provided 2 hours ago. The patient did not sleep well and has been alternately fussy and rather lethargic today. She has had some nasal congestion over the past week and shows little appetite today. The pediatrician diagnosed bilateral otitis media 1 month ago that was treated with amoxicillin. The patient has had no prior hospitalizations and has no known drug allergies and no tobacco exposure. She attends child care. Her sibling has a history of ear infections requiring tube placement. Based on this information the physician determines that fever is the chief principal complaint for the encounter.

Review of systems (ROS): Positive for fever, pulling at left ear, seasonal allergies, decreased appetite, and irritability. A review of the eyes is negative for purulent discharge; the parents deny cough, vomiting, diarrhea, and signs of abdominal pain.

Examination: The patient weighs 12.2 kg (26.9 lb), is 86 cm (33.9") tall, and has a temperature of 38.2°C (100.8°F). She is alert and fussy but appears to be in no acute distress; she appears well developed and well nourished. The patient's eyelids and conjunctiva are normal; pupils are equal, round, and reactive to light and accommodation. Her ears are typical externally; otoscopic examination reveals the right tympanic membrane is slightly erythematous, and the left tympanic membrane is erythematous, bulging with decreased mobility and suppurative fluid noted. On examination of the nose, it is noted that the membranes are swollen and erythematous and there is opaque white mucous. The patient's throat is clear, her thyroid is normal, and neck is supple with no lymphadenopathy and no meningeal signs. Respiratory rate is typical, clear to auscultation; the patient's heart has typical rate and rhythm and no murmurs. She has typical cervical, axillary, supraclavicular, suboccipital, and periauricular nodes and no rashes.

The diagnosis is left acute suppurative otitis media. The physician discusses the following plan with the parents: amoxicillin/clavulanate, 600 mg/5 mL twice daily for 10 days, with follow-up with primary care in 14 days. A patient education handout is provided to the parents.

ICD-10-CM	CPT®
H66.005 (acute suppurative otitis media without spontaneous rupture of ear drum, recurrent, left ear) R50.9 (fever)	99283 or 99284 (See Teaching Point for rationale.) *History:* Detailed *Examination:* Comprehensive *MDM:* Moderate complexity

Teaching Point: This example includes a chief complaint of pulling at ear, fever, and irritability. The history of present illness (HPI) includes location of left ear; timing of last evening; associated signs and symptoms of fever, not sleeping well, and little appetite; and a modifying factor of ibuprofen for fever. With 4 elements, the level of HPI is extended. The ROS is extended. A complete ROS may be documented for an encounter (eg, all others reviewed and negative), but pertinent positives and negatives related to the chief (principal) complaint should determine the level of the ROS. Past (otitis media 1 month ago), family (sibling: otitis media), and social (child care; no tobacco exposure) history are documented, although only 2 of 3 must be documented for a complete history for ED visits. The level of history is detailed. Examination of 8 organ systems (constitutional [vitals, general appearance]; eyes; ears, nose, mouth, and throat; neck [supple, no meningeal signs]; cardiovascular; respiratory; lymphatic [neck]; and skin) is comprehensive. The finding of otitis media (suppurative fluid) is documented and supports the discharge diagnosis. Medical decision-making is moderately complex with a new problem to the examiner with no additional workup and moderate risk. With all 3 key components required to support the level of ED service, this encounter could be reported with code 99284. However, a payer may consider the presenting problem of otitis media to be self-limiting and insufficient to support the medical necessity of the level of service supported by the 3 key components. The physician must use clinical judgment in deciding the medically necessary level of service based on the complete patient presentation (eg, age, medical history, general appearance of the patient) and may choose to report 99283.

➤ **A 7-year-old patient presents to the ED with acute exacerbation of asthma.** Parents report that the patient began wheezing and complained of chest tightness about 1 hour ago. Treatment with rescue medication did not provide significant relief. The patient was hospitalized for severe exacerbation of asthma 1 year ago but, until now, has not required further emergency or hospital care. The patient has no known drug allergies. Father smokes but never in the home or near the child. Mother has seasonal allergies.

Examination: Patient appears ill and anxious. He is currently receiving oxygen by face mask. His respiratory rate is 28 breaths per minute, pulse is 110 beats per minute, and oxygen saturation is 93%. The patient weighs 22.5 kg (49.6 lb) and is 124 cm (48.8") tall. Pupils are equal, round, and reactive to light and accommodation. There is mild swelling of the nasal mucosa, tympanic membranes are clear, and oropharynx is dry but otherwise normal. The patient's neck is supple, with no lymphadenopathy. He is wheezing throughout expiration and speaks in partial sentences, with visible subcostal retractions. Patient has mild tachycardia and no rubs or murmur. His abdomen is soft and nontender. He has no rashes.

After 2 intermittent inhalation treatments over the course of an hour, the patient's symptoms are relieved. The patient is discharged to home with instruction to continue albuterol every 4 hours, and his pediatrician is notified of the ED encounter and need for follow-up the next day.

Discharge diagnosis is asthma with acute exacerbation.

ICD-10-CM	CPT®
J45.901 (unspecified asthma with [acute] exacerbation)	99281 *History:* Problem focused *Examination:* Comprehensive *MDM:* Moderate complexity

Teaching Point: The documentation in this example illustrates how failure to document even one *pertinent* portion of the history can significantly affect code selection. This example includes a chief complaint of acute exacerbation of asthma. The HPI includes 4 elements: location (chest tightness), signs and symptoms (wheezing), time (1 hour ago), and modifying factors (rescue medication did not provide relief). The HPI is extended. *No ROS is documented.* Past (hospitalized 1 year ago; no known drug allergies), social (father smokes), and family (mother has allergies) history is documented. The past, family, and social history (PFSH) is complete. With extended HPI, no ROS, and complete PFSH, the overall history is problem focused. The examination is comprehensive, with 8 organ systems, based on the 1995 guidelines. Medical decision-making is moderately complex with a new problem, no additional workup, tests in the medicine section of *CPT* performed, and risk associated with an exacerbation of a chronic illness. The overall level of service is 99281, which includes at least a problem-focused history, problem-focused examination, and MDM of straightforward complexity. If the history had included review of 2 to 9 systems, code 99284 would have been supported by a detailed history, comprehensive examination, and moderate-complexity MDM. While only medically necessary history should be counted when determining a level of E/M service, it is likely that an expanded ROS would be obtained for this presentation. Failure to document the ROS has a significant effect on the level of service reportable for the encounter.

➤ **A 2-year-old girl presents via ambulance following an automobile crash along with her mother, the driver, who sustained bruising and minor cuts.** The mother requests that the child be examined for any possible injuries. An expanded problem-focused history is obtained. Examination of the head, neck, chest, abdomen, musculoskeletal system, and skin reveals no signs of injury. The child is released to the family.

ICD-10-CM	CPT®
Z04.1 (examination and observation following transport accident without abnormal findings)	99283 *History:* Expanded problem focused *Examination:* Expanded problem focused *MDM:* Moderate complexity

Teaching Point: *ICD-10-CM* code Z04.1 is reported to indicate the reason for the encounter with a child who presents with no apparent complaints. If the child displayed any signs of injury, these would be reported in lieu of code Z04.1. Remember, do not report an external cause code.

Comanagement of ED Patients

Only one physician should report an ED E/M service for a patient who receives care in the ED. In general, this will be the emergency physician or pediatric emergency medicine specialist who is staffing the ED. At times, other physicians (eg, generalists, specialists) may have to provide care for a patient in the ED. When this occurs, the code(s) used by each physician will depend on several factors.

- Is the physician managing the patient in the ED, or was the physician called in by the ED physician?
- Did the physician personally perform any procedures in the ED or only direct the ED staff?
- Was the patient sent home, transferred to another facility, or kept at the hospital for observation or admission?
- Was the patient stable or critically ill or injured?

Follow these guidelines to determine which codes will be reported.

Examples

➤ **You are the primary physician managing the patient in the ED (ie, the ED physician or a physician meeting his or her patient in the ED).**
Codes 99281–99285 (ED E/M service) will be reported.

➤ **You are the primary physician managing the patient in the ED (ie, the ED physician or a physician meeting his or her patient in the ED) and you call in another physician to see the patient.**

The type of service reported will depend on whether the other physician is providing consultative services, a specific intervention (eg, diagnostic or therapeutic procedure), or primary management of the patient. The ED physician will typically report the ED E/M code and the other physician will report services as follows:

❖ *Consultation:* An outpatient consultation (**99241–99245**) may be reported when the ED physician requests the opinion of and/or advice from the other physician (and the request is documented in the medical record), the consulting physician provides an opinion and/or advice (including the initiation of diagnostic and/or therapeutic services), and a written report is documented (may be part of the ED medical record). If a payer follows Medicare guidelines and does not cover consultations, services should be reported using the office or outpatient E/M codes (**99201–99215**). See Chapter 7, Evaluation and Management Services in the Office and Outpatient Clinics, for detailed requirements for reporting consultations. No matter which code set you report, place of service code **23** (ED) would be used. (See later in this list for reporting consultation with admission to observation or inpatient status.)

❖ *Procedure:* The second physician may report the diagnostic and/or therapeutic procedure requested by the ED physician that is provided to the patient in the ED (eg, fracture reduction by an orthopedic surgeon; wound repair by a plastic surgeon; echocardiogram performed by a cardiologist; imaging interpretation by a radiologist; lumbar puncture performed by a pediatrician, hospitalist, or neonatologist).

❖ *Assume management:* If the second physician is called in to take over management of the patient's care (not a consultation) and the patient is sent home, an office or outpatient code (**99201–99215**) would be reported with place of service code **23** (ED). This would also be the case when an insurance carrier does not recognize consultation codes and the patient is sent home.

❖ *Observation or inpatient admission:* If the other physician admits the child to the hospital for observation or inpatient services after stabilization and/or provision of care in the ED, he or she would report *only* the appropriate initial observation, hospital inpatient, or pediatric critical care or intensive care code (**99218–99220, 99221–99223, 99468, 99471, 99475, 99477**) as appropriate based on all the E/M services provided in the ED and as part of the initial service. That could also apply if

— The admitting physician is a member of the same physician group as the ED physician, but the admitting physician is providing different services and is not considered the exact same specialty.

— The other physician transferred the child to another facility where the child would be under his or her care (or a member of his or her group and same specialty).

❖ *Critical care:* If the patient is critically ill or injured, the physicians managing the patient's care may report their services using time-based critical care codes **99291** and **99292** (see Table 18-2).

➤ **You are the primary physician managing the patient in the ED (ie, the ED physician or a physician meeting his or her patient in the ED) and you treat a patient and request an opinion and/or advice from another physician who provides consultative services. A third physician admits the child to the hospital.**

Each physician will report the appropriate service (ie, ED physician reports code **99281–99285**, consulting physician reports code **99241–99245** [or **99201–99215** if the payer follows Medicare rules], and admitting physician reports an appropriate initial code [eg, **99218–99220, 99221–99223**]) so long as the physicians are not in the same group practice and of the exact same specialty.

Use **Table 17-1** to help you in the selection of the appropriate level of ED E/M service in the following examples:

➤ **The ED physician is treating a 6-year-old who was struck by a car while riding a bicycle on a neighborhood street.** The patient is brought in by emergency medical services (EMS) from the scene with concern for closed head trauma (no known loss of consciousness [LOC] is reported), a friction burn on her right shoulder, multiple abrasions on her forearm and elbow, and large contusions on her left hip and thigh. The child is not accompanied by a parent. While, initially, there was a concern that the child might be in imminent risk of a life-threatening condition, following further assessment, imaging studies, and consultation with a trauma surgeon, the ED physician determines there is no risk of deterioration and the child is clinically stable. No history, other than that obtained from EMS, is available prior to the *trauma service* evaluation. There was high-complexity MDM. No separately billable procedures were performed. The child is admitted for observation by a hospitalist for a concussion.

Physician	ICD-10-CM	CPT®
ED physician	S06.0X0A (concussion without loss of consciousness, initial encounter) T22.151A (friction burn, first degree, right shoulder, initial encounter) S50.811A (abrasion, right forearm, initial encounter) S50.311A (abrasion, right elbow, initial encounter) S70.02XA, S70.12XA (contusions, left hip and thigh, initial encounter) V13.4XXA (pedal cycle driver injured in collision with car in traffic accident, initial encounter) Y92.414 (local residential or business street as the place of occurrence of the external cause)	99285 (ED visit code)
Trauma surgeon	S06.0X0A (concussion with no LOC, initial encounter) T22.151A, S50.811A, S50.311A, S70.02XA, S70.12XA, V13.4XXA, Y92.414	99241–99245 (office or other outpatient consultation [likely 99244 or 99245])
Hospitalist	S06.0X0A (concussion with no LOC, initial encounter) T22.151A, S50.811A, S50.311A, S70.02XA, S70.12XA, V13.4XXA, Y92.414	99218–99220 (initial observation care)

Teaching Point: The Level 5 caveat regarding unobtainable history would apply because this patient's condition was initially felt to be unstable and no other history, other than that from EMS, was available.

➤ **The ED physician evaluates a 10-month-old for fever, vomiting, and lethargy.** A comprehensive history and physical examination are performed and there is high-complexity MDM. Because of a concern for meningitis, the on-call pediatrician is consulted and is asked to perform a lumbar puncture and to determine the child's disposition. The pediatrician does the procedure, confirms the course of treatment by the ED physician, and admits the infant as an inpatient to his or her service.

ICD-10-CM	CPT®
Both physicians report R50.9 (fever) R11.10 (vomiting) R53.83 (lethargy)	The ED physician reports 99285 (ED visit code) The pediatrician reports 99221–99223 25 (initial inpatient hospital care) 62270 (lumbar puncture)

Teaching Point: A code for meningitis is not reported by the physician because this condition has not been confirmed.

Directing Emergency Medical Technicians

99288   Physician or other qualified health care professional direction of emergency medical systems (EMS) emergency care, advanced life support

- Report code 99288 (physician direction of EMS) when
  - ❖ The physician directing the services is in the hospital and in 2-way communication with EMS personnel who are in the prehospital setting providing advanced life support that requires direct or online medical control.
  - ❖ The documentation includes the times of all contacts, any orders provided, and/or directions provided to the EMS team.
- Code 99288 may be reported on the same day as ED E/M or hourly critical care services. Modifier 25 would be appended to code 99288 to alert payers that this was a significant and separately identifiable service from ED E/M (99281–99285) or the critical care (99291, 99292) service provided.
- The supervising physician cannot report the actual procedures and interventions performed by the EMS team because he or she is not physically present during the transport.
- Code 99288 is designated as a bundled procedure (included in the work value of other services) by Medicare. There are no relative values assigned under the Medicare Resource-Based Relative Value Scale. Check with your major payers and negotiate for coverage of this service.
- See codes 99485 and 99486 in Chapter 18, Critical and Intensive Care, for information on supervision of inter-facility transport of a critically ill or injured patient, 24 months or younger, via direct 2-way communication with a transport team.
- When a qualified health care professional (QHP) (eg, nurse practitioner) provides critical care services during transport, and those services will be reported under the QHP's National Provider Identifier or by the employing hospital, the ED physician does not report 99288.

Critical Care in the ED

99291   Critical care, E/M of the critically ill or critically injured patient; first 30 to 74 minutes
+99292   each additional 30 minutes (Use in conjunction with 99291.)

A critical illness or injury is defined in *CPT®* as one that acutely impairs one or more vital organs such that there is a high probability of imminent or life-threatening deterioration of the patient's condition. Guidelines for reporting critical care codes 99291 (critical care, E/M of the critically ill or injured patient; first 30–74 minutes) and 99292 (each additional 30 minutes) are described in detail in Chapter 18, Critical and Intensive Care.

- Time-based critical care codes (99291, 99292) should be used to report the provision of critical care when performed in the ED. The patient's condition must meet the specific *CPT* definition of a critically ill or injured patient. The global codes for pediatric or neonatal critical care should not be reported by a physician providing critical care in the ED unless that physician (eg, an intensivist) will continue to provide critical care services in the inpatient setting.
- Critical care may be reported on the same day as an ED E/M code when provided by the same physician when 2 independent services are provided. Modifier 25 should be appended to the ED E/M code when this occurs. Here are examples of critical care and ED E/M services that may be separately reportable when provided on the same date. (*Note:* Payers that use Medicare or Medicaid National Correct Coding Initiative [NCCI] edits will not allow separate payment for codes 99281–99285 and 99291 and 99292 on the same date of service by the same physician or physicians of the same specialty and same group practice.)
  - ❖ A child injured in an accident arrives at the ED. The ED physician evaluates the child's injuries and orders a surgical consultation. While the surgeon is in route to the facility, the patient's condition deteriorates and the ED physician provides 40 minutes of critical care before the patient is transferred to the surgeon's care.
  - ❖ A child arrives to the ED in critical condition. The ED physician provides 45 minutes of critical care services. After the child's condition improves, the ED physician obtains a comprehensive history, completes a detailed examination, and arranges admission to the intensive care unit by a hospitalist.

- Time spent providing critical care does not need to be continuous and includes time at the bedside as well as time in the ED reviewing data specific to the patient, discussing the patient with other physicians, and discussing the patient's management or condition with the patient's family. Time of any learner (eg, student, resident) involved in the patient's care may not be reported by the attending physician. Only the time specifically spent by the attending physician may be reported.

- Time reported for critical care must be devoted to the critically ill or injured patient. Therefore, the "critical care clock" stops when attention is turned to the care of another patient or the physician is not readily available in the ED.

- Those procedures not bundled with codes 99291 and 99292 and when personally performed by the reporting provider may be reported separately (eg, starting an intravenous line on a child younger than 3 years, placing an intraosseous or central venous line, endotracheal intubation, cardiopulmonary resuscitation [CPR], cardioversion). Time spent performing these separately reported services must be subtracted from the critical care time calculated and reported. See **Table 18-1** for a list of services and procedures that are included in hourly critical care codes.

Examples

➤ **The ED physician performs a comprehensive history and physical examination on a 13-month-old patient with severe stridor and respiratory distress believed to be secondary to croup.** Medical decision-making is highly complex. The patient's condition does not improve with nebulized epinephrine and then worsens, evidenced by progressive lethargy. The patient goes into respiratory failure and 75 minutes of critical care is provided. Ten minutes of the critical care time is spent performing endotracheal intubation.

ICD-10-CM	CPT
J96.00 (acute respiratory failure) J05.0 (croup)	99285 25 (ED visit code) 99291 25 (critical care, first 30–74 minutes) 99292 (critical care, each additional 30 minutes) 31500 (endotracheal intubation, emergency)

Teaching Point: Endotracheal intubation is not bundled with critical care; therefore, time spent in the provision of the service (10 minutes for this patient) is not considered in the total critical care time, so only the base code, 99291, can be used. Modifier 25 is appended to codes 99285 and 99291 to indicate they were significant and separately identifiable services.

➤ **The ED physician saw a 10-year-old for moderate asthma exacerbation in the morning.** The child responded well to an aerosolized bronchodilator treatment and was discharged home. The child returns to the ED a few hours later with a more severe exacerbation and is seen by the same physician. The child now has respiratory failure with hypoxia. The child receives oxygen, a continuous bronchodilator nebulizer treatment, and, subsequently, a parenteral bronchodilation drug. The child improves enough to be admitted to a monitored medical ward bed with diagnosis of respiratory failure due to status asthmaticus. The ED physician spends a total of 60 minutes in patient-directed critical care.

ICD-10-CM	CPT®
J96.01 (acute respiratory failure with hypoxia) J45.42 (moderate persistent asthma with status asthmaticus)	99284 25 99291

Teaching Point: The patient received oxygen, continuous inhalation treatment, and parenteral bronchodilator in the ED. However, these services include no professional component. The facility will report the services because the cost of supplies and clinical staff time are an expense to the facility.

➤ **A 13-month-old with apparent sepsis and hypotension is brought to the ED.** The child requires placement of an intraosseous needle to achieve vascular access and, subsequently, receives parenteral fluids, antibiotics, and vasopressors. The child suffers cardiopulmonary arrest, prompting the ED physician to intubate the child. Cardiopulmonary resuscitation is performed for 20 minutes. The child is in the ED for a total of 45 minutes before transfer to the intensive care unit.

ICD-10-CM	CPT
I46.9 (cardiac arrest) If the physician included sepsis in the diagnosis, this would be reported.	99285 25 92950 (CPR) 36680 (placement of intraosseous needle) 31500 (endotracheal intubation, emergency)

    Teaching Point: Critical care time does not accrue during the performance of non-bundled, separately billable procedures. Because CPR is a separately billable, non-bundled procedure, the ED physician did not spend a minimum of 30 minutes providing critical care. Because the E/M service is reported rather than critical care, coding is based on documented key components of history, examination, and MDM. However, the caveat for code 99285 allows reporting based on the extent of history and examination possible within the constraints imposed by the urgency of the patient's clinical condition and mental status.

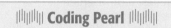

> **Coding Pearl**
>
> If septic shock was specified as the cause of cardiac arrest, codes **A41.9**, sepsis, unspecified organism; **R65.21**, severe sepsis with septic shock; and **I46.8**, cardiac arrest due to other underlying condition, would be reported.

Reporting Procedures in the ED

Many procedures performed in the ED have an associated global period assigned by payers. The global period affects reporting of pre- and post-procedural care. (See Chapter 19, Common Surgical Procedures and Sedation in Facility Settings, for the definition of the *CPT* surgical package and Medicare global period.)

    To report an E/M service in addition to a procedure, there must be documentation of performance of a significant and separately identifiable E/M service beyond the pre- and post-procedural work typical for the procedure. Post-procedural prescriptions for pain control or prophylactic antibiotics may be included in the procedure performed.

    Table 17-2 contains a list of procedures (with assigned Medicare global periods) commonly performed in the ED.

    Any separately identifiable procedure that is personally performed by the physician may be reported, with the exception of

- Procedures that are bundled in time-based critical care codes (See Table 18-1 for a list of services and procedures that are included in hourly critical care codes.)
- Services performed by hospital personnel because they are billed by the hospital facility (If a nurse or allied health care professional assists in part of a procedure, the ED physician may bill for the professional services if he or she provides the primary or key component of the procedure.)
- Hydration, infusion, and/or injection procedures (96360–96379) because the physician work associated with the procedures involves only confirmation of the treatment plan and not direct supervision of staff
- Procedures involving use of hospital-owned equipment (eg, pulse oximetry), unless the procedure includes a technical and professional component (If performed and documented, the professional component may be reported with modifier 26 [professional component] appended to the procedure code.)

Table 17-2. Common Emergency Department Procedures		
Procedure	**CPT® Code**	**Global Period (d)ª**
Arterial puncture	36600	NA
Bladder aspiration	51100	0
Burn care, >10% TBSA	16030	0
Burn care, 5%–10% TBSA	16025	0
Burn care, <5% TBSA	16020	0
Cardiopulmonary resuscitation	92950	0
Cardioversion	92960	0
Chest tube insertion	32551	0
Dislocation, shoulder, reduction	23650	90
Endotracheal intubation (open procedure), emergency	31500	0
Foreign body removal, conjunctiva	65205	0
Foreign body removal, ear	69200	0
Foreign body removal, nose	30300	10
Foreign body removal with incision, subcutaneous, simple	10120	10
Fracture, clavicle	23500	90
Fracture, finger distal, each	26750	90
Fracture, finger shaft, each	26720	90
Gastric intubation and aspiration(s), therapeutic, including lavage (if performed)	43753	0
Incision and drainage, abscess, simple	10060	10
Incision and drainage, finger, complicated (eg, felon)	26011	10
Incision and drainage, perianal abscess	46050	10
Intraosseous needle placement	36680	0
Laceration repair, simple ≤2.5 cm, face/ears/lips	12011	0
Repair, simple ≤2.5 cm, scalp/trunk/extremities	12001	0
Repair, simple 2.6–5.0 cm, face/ears/lips	12013	0
Repair, simple 2.6–7.5 cm, scalp/trunk/extremities	12002	0
Laceration repair, intermediate ≤2.5 cm, face/ears/lips	12051	10
Repair, intermediate ≤2.5 cm, hands/feet/neck	12041	10
Repair, intermediate ≤2.5 cm, scalp/trunk/arms/legs	12031	10
Repair, intermediate 2.6–5.0 cm, face/ears/lips	12052	10
Repair, intermediate 2.6–7.5 cm, hands/feet/neck	12042	10
Repair, intermediate 2.6–7.5 cm, scalp/trunk/extremities	12032	10
Lumbar puncture	62270	0
Nursemaid elbow reduction	24640	10
Pleural drainage, percutaneous, with insertion of indwelling catheter; without imaging guidance	32556	0

Table 17-2. Common Emergency Department Procedures (*continued*)

Procedure	CPT® Code	Global Period (d)ᵃ
Pleural drainage, percutaneous, with insertion of indwelling catheter; with imaging guidance	32557	0
Puncture aspiration of abscess, hematoma, bulla, or cyst	10160	10
Repair, nail bed	11760	10
Splint, finger	29130	0
Splint, short arm	29125	0
Splint, short leg	29515	0
Strap, ankle	29540	0
Strap, knee	29530	0
Strap, shoulder	29240	0
Subungual hematoma evacuation	11740	0
Thoracentesis, needle or catheter, without imaging	32554	0
Thoracentesis, needle or catheter, with imaging	32555	0
Venipuncture, >3 y requiring physician skill	36410	NA
Venipuncture, requiring physician skill, femoral/jugular <3 y	36400	NA

Abbreviations: CPT, Current Procedural Terminology; NA, not applicable; TBSA, total body surface area.

ᵃ *Procedures noted with global period NA have an X or M status in the Medicare Physician Fee Schedule.*

Point-of-Care Ultrasound

Point-of-care ultrasound services performed by the ED physician (**Table 17-3**) are separately reportable in addition to the ED E/M service when *all 3 of the following conditions apply:*

- Thorough evaluation of organ(s) or anatomical region is performed.
- There is permanent image documentation (with measurements, when clinically indicated).
- A written report equivalent to that typically produced by a radiologist is documented.

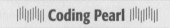

|||||||||| Coding Pearl |||||||||||

Use of handheld or portable ultrasound that does not include all 3 of the listed elements is not separately reported.

Without all these elements, the examination is not separately reported and would be considered part of any E/M service provided. (*Exception:* Permanent image documentation is not required for ophthalmic ultrasound for biometric measurement.) Use of handheld or portable ultrasound that does not include all 3 of the previously listed elements is not separately reported.

Bedside ultrasound services in the ED are reported by the physician with the professional service only modifier (**26**). (See the Modifiers Used With ED Codes section later in this chapter for more information.) The technical component (eg, equipment cost, facility overhead costs) is typically reported by the facility. (Payers may limit physicians to reporting of the professional component only for all facility-based services even if the physician performs the ultrasound and/or owns the equipment used for the service. The technical component includes all associated overhead costs. Check individual payer policies for reporting.)

One use of point-of-care ultrasound in the ED is the focused assessment with sonography for trauma (FAST) examination. This may consist of 2 distinct components: limited transthoracic echocardiogram and limited abdominal ultrasound. When 2 distinct procedures are performed, 2 codes are reported.

76705   Ultrasound, abdominal, real-time with image documentation; limited

93308   Echocardiography, transthoracic, real-time with image documentation (2D), includes M-mode recording, when performed, follow-up or limited study

Table 17-3. Common Point-of-Care Procedures

76536	Ultrasound, soft tissues of head and neck (eg, thyroid, parathyroid, parotid), real time with image documentation
76604	Ultrasound, chest (includes mediastinum when performed), real time with image documentation
76700	Ultrasound, abdominal, real time with image documentation; complete
76705	Ultrasound, abdominal, real time with image documentation; limited (eg, single organ, quadrant, follow-up)
76770	Ultrasound, retroperitoneal (eg, renal, aorta, nodes), real time with image documentation; complete
76775	Ultrasound, retroperitoneal (eg, renal, aorta, nodes), real time with image documentation; limited
76857	Ultrasound, pelvic (nonobstetric), real time with image documentation; limited or follow-up (eg, for follicles, presence of urine in bladder)
76870	Ultrasound, scrotum and contents[a]
76881	Ultrasound, complete joint (eg, joint space and peri-articular soft tissue structures), real-time with image documentation[b]
76882	Ultrasound, limited, joint or other nonvascular extremity structure(s) (eg, joint space, peri-articular tendon[s], muscle[s], nerve[s], other soft tissue structure[s], or soft tissue mass[es]), real-time with image documentation[b]
76885	Ultrasound, infant hips, real time with imaging documentation; dynamic (requiring physician or other qualified health care professional manipulation)
76886	Ultrasound, infant hips, real time with imaging documentation; limited, static (not requiring physician or other qualified health care professional manipulation)
76937	Ultrasound guidance for vascular access requiring ultrasound evaluation of potential access sites, documentation of selected vessel patency, concurrent real-time ultrasound visualization of vascular needle entry, with permanent recording and reporting (List separately in addition to code for primary procedure.)
93976	Duplex scan of arterial inflow and venous outflow of abdominal, pelvic, scrotal contents and/or retroperitoneal organs; limited study[a]

[a] Evaluation of vascular structures using both color and spectral Doppler is separately reportable. However, color Doppler alone, when performed for anatomical structure identification in conjunction with a real-time ultrasound examination, is not reported separately.

[b] Code 76881 requires ultrasound examination of all the following joint elements: joint space (eg, effusion), periarticular soft-tissue structures that surround the joint (eg, muscles, tendons, other soft tissue structures), and any identifiable abnormality. When fewer than all the required elements for a "complete" examination (76881) are performed, report the "limited" code (76882).

When a limited ultrasound examination of the chest is included (eg, for pneumothorax), report code 76604 (ultrasound, chest [includes mediastinum when performed], real-time with image documentation). Limited studies are defined in *CPT®* as those that include examination of less than the required elements for a "complete" examination (eg, limited number of organs, limited portion of region evaluated). See your *CPT* reference for required components of complete examinations.

Ultrasound guidance for vascular access may be reported with code 76937. This service must include ultrasound evaluation of potential access sites, documentation of selected vessel patency, concurrent real-time ultrasound visualization of vascular needle entry, and permanent recording and reporting. This code is reported separately in addition to a code for primary vascular access procedure (eg, 36555). Do not report 76937 if ultrasound guidance is not used for vascular needle placement (ie, vessel identification only), as this is not a separately reportable service. (If the same physician will provide neonatal or pediatric critical care on the same date, the vascular access procedure will not be

> **~ More From the AAP ~**
>
> Read more about reporting ultrasound services in the November 2015 *AAP Pediatric Coding Newsletter*™ at http://coding.aap.org (subscription required).

separately reported. However, ultrasound guidance is not bundled to neonatal and pediatric critical care and may be separately paid.)

When ultrasound guidance is used for needle placement for procedures such as aspiration of an abscess, code **76942** is reported. Do not report code **76942** in conjunction with a service for which the code descriptor of the service includes ultrasound guidance (eg, joint aspiration). Code **76937** (ultrasound guidance for vascular access) is not reported in conjunction with code **76942**.

Example

> **A child is seen in the ED for injuries sustained in a traffic accident.** The physician performs a trauma assessment, including a FAST examination. This examination may consist of 2 distinct components: limited transthoracic echocardiogram and limited abdominal ultrasound. When 2 distinct procedures are performed, 2 codes are reported.
>
> The physician reports **76705 26** (ultrasound, abdominal, real-time with image documentation; limited) and **93308 26** (echocardiography, transthoracic, real-time with image documentation [2D], includes M-mode recording, when performed, follow-up or limited study). Modifier **26** signifies the physician is reporting the professional component of each service. The facility will report the same codes with modifier **TC** to indicate reporting of the technical component of each service. When applicable and all requirements for reporting are met, an ultrasound performed with physician-owned equipment is reported without a modifier (ie, modifier **26** is not applicable).

Modifiers Used With ED Codes

Physicians need to understand when it is appropriate to report modifiers in addition to E/M or procedural service codes. Modifiers **25** (significant, separately identifiable E/M service) and **57** (decision for surgery) may be appended to ED E/M codes to indicate E/M beyond the preservice work of a procedure. Procedures performed in the ED may require reporting of modifiers such as **26** (professional component) or **59** (distinct procedural service) or, when accepted by the payer in lieu of modifier **59**, modifier **XE** (separate encounter), **XP** (separate practitioner), **XS** (separate structure), or **XU** (unusual nonoverlapping service). **Table 17-4** lists modifiers commonly used in the ED. (See Chapter 2, Modifiers and Coding Edits, for more detail on the use of modifiers.)

Examples

> **A child is seen in the ED for left shoulder pain that occurred following a fall while playing soccer at a community sports field.** The child is examined for additional injuries (expanded problem-focused history, detailed examination). Radiograph interpreted by a radiologist reveals a mid-shaft clavicle fracture. The physician places the patient in a sling and refers the patient to another physician for follow-up care.

ICD-10-CM	CPT®
S42.022A (displaced fracture of left clavicle, initial encounter) **W18.30XA** (unspecified fall on same level, initial encounter) **Y93.66** (activity, soccer) **Y92.322** (soccer field as place of occurrence)	**99283 25** **23500 54** (closed treatment of clavicular fracture, without manipulation)

Teaching Point: The use of modifier **54** (surgical care only) alerts payers that another physician will report postsurgical care. Alternatively, the ED physician may report the ED E/M code based on the level of service performed and documented and allow another physician to report the global fracture care. Medical decision-making for the ED visit is moderate based on a new problem without additional workup (the diagnosis is known at the end of the encounter, though treatment will follow) and moderate risk related to the decision for closed treatment of a fracture without manipulation.

‖‖‖‖‖ **Coding Pearl** ‖‖‖‖‖

A fracture not specified as displaced or non-displaced should be reported as displaced.

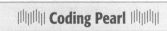

Modifier	When to Use
Table 17-4. Common Modifiers Used in the Emergency Department	
24	An unrelated E/M service is provided during the global period of a previously performed procedure by the same physician or group.
25	A significant, separately identifiable E/M service is performed by the same physician on the same day of the procedure or other service.
26	Reporting professional component only of a service for which payment includes equipment (or technical services) cost (eg, radiograph)
32	A service is mandated by third-party payer, regulation, or governmental entity.
51	Multiple procedures are performed on the same day other than E/M, physical medicine and rehabilitation services, or provision of supplies (eg, vaccines).
54	Only the surgical care component of a procedure was provided. Another physician will provide postoperative care.
57	Decision for surgery was made. Some payers may require this modifier be appended to the E/M code only with procedures with 90-day global periods.
59	Distinct procedural service (non-E/M) was performed on the same day as another procedural service and was at a different encounter or a different surgery or procedure, or performed on a different body site or organ system.
63	Procedures (**20000–69999**) performed on an infant weighing <4 kg if the code descriptor does not include a descriptor of "young infant or neonate"
76	The same physician repeats a procedure or service on the same date of service.
77	Another physician repeats a procedure or service already performed by another physician on the same day of service.
79	An unrelated procedure is performed during the global period of a previously provided procedure by the same physician or group.
XE	The service was provided at a separate encounter on the same date.
XP	The non-E/M service or procedure was performed by a separate practitioner of the same group on the same date.
XS	The procedure or service was performed on a separate structure.
XU	Unusual nonoverlapping service

Abbreviation: E/M, evaluation and management.

➤ **The ED physician evaluates a 6-year-old with a small (<2.5 cm) simple laceration on her right cheek that occurred when she fell, striking her face on the edge of a table at home.** The wound is clean, there is no concern for other associated injury, and her immunization status is up-to-date. The parents are concerned about scarring and request a plastic surgeon to do the repair. The on-call surgeon is consulted and responds to the ED. The surgeon evaluates and repairs the wound with sutures in the ED. The ED physician documents a detailed history and physical examination with diagnoses of laceration, right cheek, and closed head injury without LOC. Instructions are provided to parents about home monitoring following a head injury.

Although the ED physician documented a detailed history and physical examination, the MDM would only rise to moderate complexity (new problem with no additional workup, potential for associated head injury). The surgeon does not report a consultation because the surgical service was at the request of the family and not the ED physician.

> |||||||| **Coding Pearl** ||||||||
>
> Place of occurrence (**Y92.009**), activity, and external cause status codes are reported only at the initial encounter for treatment, so no seventh code character is required.

ICD-10-CM	CPT®
S01.411A (laceration without foreign body, right cheek, initial encounter) **S09.90XA** (unspecified injury of head) **W01.190A** (fall on same level from slipping, tripping, and stumbling with subsequent striking against furniture, initial encounter) **Y92.009** (occurred at home) **Y99.8** (other external cause status)	ED physician reports **99283 25** Surgeon reports **12011** (laceration repair)

Teaching Point: No modifiers are required for these services because the ED physician provided only the ED E/M service and not the procedure. The scenario does not indicate the surgeon provided any E/M service beyond the typical preservice work of the laceration repair.

➤ **The ED physician is caring for a 9-year-old who has a 4-cm–long, deep laceration of the right calf and a separate 1-cm–long laceration of the right ankle from broken glass in his backyard.** The physician performs a detailed history and physical examination. A radiograph of the extremity shows no retained radiopaque foreign bodies. The child's immunizations are current, with the last tetanus booster less than 5 years ago. The physician irrigates, carefully explores both wounds, and performs a 2-layer repair on the calf. The ankle laceration requires only single-layer closure. The child is discharged with appropriate follow-up plans.

ICD-10-CM	CPT
S81.811A (laceration without foreign body, right lower leg, initial encounter) **S91.011A** (laceration without foreign body, right ankle, initial encounter) **W25.XXXA** (contact with sharp glass, initial encounter) **Y92.007** (garden or yard of noninstitutional residence)	**99283 25** **12032** (intermediate repair of the extremities, 2.6–7.5 cm) **12001 59** or **XS** (simple repair of the extremity, ≤2.5 cm)

Teaching Point: Modifier **25** is used to indicate the ED E/M service was significant and separately identifiable from the preservice work of the laceration repairs. A modifier is required to indicate the simple repair was performed on a separate site from the intermediate or layered closure. Verify payer policy on reporting of modifier **59** (distinct procedural service) versus **XS** (separate structure). (See Chapter 2, Modifiers and Coding Edits, for more information on these modifiers.)

When multiple lacerations require the same type of repair (simple, intermediate, or complex) and are of body areas described by a single code (eg, intermediate repair of scalp, arms, and/or legs), sum the lengths of the repairs and report a single code for the repairs. See Chapter 10, Surgery, Infusion, and Sedation in the Outpatient Setting, for more examples of coding for laceration repairs.

> ⦚⦚⦚⦚ **Coding Pearl** ⦚⦚⦚⦚
>
> *International Classification of Diseases, 10th Revision, Clinical Modification* codes for poisoning include intent. If intent is unknown, assign a code for accidental intent. No external cause code is required for poisonings, toxic effects, adverse effects, and underdosing codes.

Sedation

Moderate Sedation

Moderate sedation (**99151–99157**) (**Table 17-5**) is a drug-induced depression of consciousness during which patients may respond purposefully to verbal commands, alone or accompanied by light tactile stimulation. Moderate sedation may be necessary for the performance of certain procedures in the ED.

Chapter 17: Emergency Department Services

- ⦿ Codes are selected based on intraservice time. Intraservice time
  - ❖ Begins with the administration of the sedating agent(s)
  - ❖ Ends when the procedure is completed, the patient is stable for recovery status, and the physician or other QHP providing the sedation ends personal continuous face-to-face time with the patient
  - ❖ Includes ordering and/or administering the initial and subsequent doses of sedating agents
  - ❖ Requires continuous face-to-face attendance of the physician or other QHP
  - ❖ Requires monitoring patient response to the sedating agents, including
    - — Periodic assessment of the patient
    - — Further administration of agent(s) as needed to maintain sedation
    - — Monitoring of oxygen saturation, heart rate, and blood pressure
- ⦿ Moderate sedation services of less than 10 minutes' intraservice time are not separately reported.

Coding and documentation requirements for reporting this service are detailed in Chapter 19, Common Surgical Procedures and Sedation in Facility Settings.

Table 17-5. Moderate Sedation

Moderate Sedation	First 10–22 min Intraservice Time	Each Additional 15 min Intraservice Time
Moderate sedation services provided by the same physician or other qualified health care professional performing the diagnostic or therapeutic service that the sedation supports, requiring the presence of an independent trained observer to assist in the monitoring of the patient's level of consciousness and physiological status; initial 15 minutes of intra-service time, patient younger than 5 years of age	99151	+99153
5 years or older	99152	+99153
Moderate sedation services (other than those services described by codes 00100–01999) provided by a physician other than the health care professional performing the diagnostic or therapeutic service that the sedation supports; younger than 5 years	99155	+99157
5 years or older	99156	+99157

Example

> A 10-year-old presents to the ED with left forearm pain after falling from her bicycle. She fell onto a concrete patio at her house but did not hit her head. The injury occurred 1 hour ago and was iced by the mother, but pain and swelling continued
>
> *Review of systems:* Pain is limited to lower left arm and wrist; patient has no headache and no nausea or vomiting. She has had no past surgeries or hospitalizations; she has no known allergies; and her immunizations are up-to-date. The patient is active in gymnastics and dance. Family history is reviewed and is noncontributory. Detailed examination includes constitutional, head, eyes, neck, musculoskeletal, cardiovascular, and respiratory elements. Imaging shows a Salter-Harris type II physeal fracture of the left distal radius (interpreted by the radiologist). An orthopedic surgeon is consulted and requests that the ED physician provide moderate sedation for closed reduction in the ED. The ED physician documents 25 minutes of moderate sedation, beginning with administration of the sedating agent and ending when the patient is sufficiently recovered that the physician's continuous face-to-face monitoring is no longer necessary. The ED physician reports

ICD-10-CM	CPT
S59.222A (Salter-Harris type II physeal fracture, lower left radius) **V18.000A** (pedal cycle rider injured noncollision transport accident, nontraffic accident) **Y92.018** (other place of single-family house)	**99283 25** **99156** (moderate sedation by other than physician performing procedure, first 15 minutes) **99157** (moderate sedation, each additional 15 minutes)

Teaching Point: The orthopedic surgeon will separately report the fracture reduction procedure (eg, **25605**, closed treatment with manipulation) and, if applicable, any medically necessary E/M service beyond the preservice work of the procedure (modifier **57** may be required to indicate that the physician determined the need for the procedure at this encounter).

Deep Sedation

Deep sedation or analgesia is a drug-induced depression of consciousness during which patients cannot be easily aroused but respond purposefully after repeated verbal or painful stimulation (eg, purposefully pushing away the noxious stimuli). The ability to independently maintain ventilatory function may be impaired. Patients may require assistance in maintaining a patent airway, and spontaneous ventilation may be inadequate. Cardiovascular function is usually maintained. A state of deep sedation may be accompanied by partial or complete loss of protective airway reflexes.

Although ED physicians may provide deep sedation, payment for these services is limited.

Deep sedation provided by a physician also performing the services for which the sedation is being provided is reported by appending modifier **47** (anesthesia by surgeon) to the procedure code for the service for which sedation is required. Many health plans do not pay separately for anesthesia by the physician or surgeon performing the procedure.

National Correct Coding Initiative edits do not allow payment of an ED visit (**99281–99285**) and deep sedation when provided by the same ED physician or 2 ED physicians of the same group practice. No modifier will override the NCCI edits. Payers that have adopted Medicare or Medicaid NCCI edits will deny the ED visit when reported on the same date as deep sedation.

Please see Chapter 19, Common Surgical Procedures and Sedation in Facility Settings, for more information on deep sedation.

Special Service Codes

99053   Service(s) provided between 10:00 pm and 8:00 am at 24-hour facility, in addition to basic service

99056   Service(s) typically provided in office, provided out of office at request of patient, in addition to basic service

99060   Service(s) provided on an emergency basis, out of office, which disrupts other scheduled office services, in addition to basic service

Special service codes may be used to report services that are an adjunct to the basic service provided. *CPT®* guidelines do not restrict the reporting of adjunct special service codes in the ED. However, third-party payers will have specific policies for coverage and payment. Communicate with individual payers to understand their definition or interpretation of the service and coverage and payment policies.

These codes are intended to describe services that are provided outside the normal time frame and location.

Code **99053** would be reported when services are provided between the designated time limits in an ED.

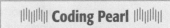

> |||||||| **Coding Pearl** ||||||||
>
> It would not be appropriate for an emergency department (ED) physician to report code **99056** or **99060** for services provided in the ED.

Chapter 17: Emergency Department Services

CPT does not restrict reporting of any procedure or service to any specific specialty. However, it would be inappropriate for an ED physician to report code **99056** or **99060** for services provided in the ED.

If appropriate, a non-ED physician could report *CPT* code **99056** or **99060** when he or she provides services in the ED in addition to an outpatient office or clinic visit, ED visit, or consultation E/M code.

Continuum Models for Asthma, Head Injury, and Laceration

Three common conditions seen in the ED follow in a teaching tool called the Continuum Model. Each condition—asthma, head injury, and laceration—is described across the continuum of codes **99281–99285** plus critical care. Although the actual assignment of a code for an individual patient may vary from the examples, members of the American Academy of Pediatrics Committee on Coding and Nomenclature have generally agreed that these examples provide an accurate representation of how one condition typically flows across the family of codes.

It is important to remember that all 3 key components (history, examination, MDM) must be met to support the code selected. Past, family, and social history elements are required only for codes **99284** (1 of 3) and **99285** (2 of 3).

Continuum Model for Asthma			
CPT® Code Vignette	**History**	**Physical Examination (systems)**	**Medical Decision-making (1. diagnoses; 2. data; 3. risk)**
99281 Stable asthma, noncustodial parent concerned about continuous use of control medication	**Problem focused** CC: asthma medication concern HPI: duration of medication use, no side effects ROS: constitutional, respiratory	**Problem focused** Constitutional (vitals, general appearance) and respiratory systems (effort and auscultation)	**Straightforward** 1. Established problem, stable 2. Asthma control test reviewed 3. Anticipatory guidance with routine follow-up
99282 Stable asthma, out of medication	**Expanded problem focused** CC: out of asthma medication HPI: stable but out of medication, no use of rescue inhaler ROS: normal ENMT, infrequent nighttime cough, all others reviewed and normal PFSH: current medications reviewed, no hospitalizations	**Expanded problem focused** Constitutional (height, weight, temperature), respiratory system (effort and auscultation), eyes, and ENMT (nasal and oral mucosa)	**Low complexity** 1. Established problem, stable 2. Review and evaluation of asthma control test 3. Alteration in medication regimen and/or refills
99283 Known asthma with URI symptoms	**Expanded problem focused** CC: asthma with stuffy nose and sinus pressure HPI: stuffy nose for 2 days, sinus pressure today, dry cough this afternoon relieved by inhalation treatment ROS: no fever; denies postnasal drip, shortness of breath, and wheezing; no body aches PFSH: current medications and allergies updated, asthma diagnosed in 2016, to ED twice last year for asthma symptoms	**Expanded problem focused** Constitutional (temperature, weight, height, pulse oxygen), eyes, ENMT, respiratory (effort and auscultation), and other pertinent organ systems	**Moderate complexity** 1. Self-limited problem and one established problem with mild exacerbation or new problem with no additional workup 2. Asthma control test, pulse oxygen 3. ≥1 chronic illnesses with mild exacerbation, progression *or* side effects of treatment and/or prescription drug management

Continuum Model for Asthma (*continued*)

CPT Code Vignette	History	Physical Examination (systems)	Medical Decision-making (1. diagnoses; 2. data; 3. risk)
99284 Known asthma with moderate exacerbation	**Detailed** CC: shortness of breath, wheezing HPI: timing of symptom onset, context (exposure to flowers), modifying factors (used rescue inhaler and inhalation treatment at home), severity (worse than prior episodes) ROS: feels tired and scared, no fever, denies dizziness or fainting, no ear or throat pain, chest feels tight, no GI or GU complaints PFSH: medications and allergies updated	**Detailed** Constitutional (temperature, blood pressure, pulse oxygen, general appearance), ENMT, neck, respiratory, cardiovascular, and skin	**Moderate complexity** 1. New problem to examiner with or without additional workup planned 2. Pulmonary function testing, chest radiograph 3. Continuous or back-to-back inhalation treatments until improved
99285 Known asthma with moderate to severe exacerbation	**Comprehensive** CC: unable to catch breath HPI: duration and severity of symptoms, medications used, other signs and symptoms ROS: constitutional, eyes, ENMT, respiratory, cardiovascular, and at least 5 more (all others reviewed and negative) PFSH: medications and allergies updated, no tobacco use or exposure	**Comprehensive** Constitutional, eyes, ENMT, respiratory, cardiovascular, GI, neurologic, skin	**High complexity** 1. New problem, additional workup planned (transfer to hospitalist for observation care) 2. Blood gases, pulmonary function testing, chest radiograph 3. Severe exacerbation of chronic condition
99291, 99292 **Critical Care** Known asthma unstable with marked distress and (impending) respiratory failure			**High complexity** 1. Severe exacerbation with high probability of imminent or life-threatening deterioration requires >30 min of directed patient care. 2. Assess, manipulate, and support vital system function(s) to treat respiratory failure and/or to prevent further life-threatening deterioration of the patient's condition. (Usually requires use of additional therapies such as ketamine, magnesium sulfate, parenteral adrenergic agents, and/or heliox; ET intubation; or BiPAP.)

Abbreviations: *BiPAP, bi-level positive airway pressure; CC, chief complaint; CPT, Current Procedural Terminology; ENMT, ear, nose, mouth, throat; ET, endotracheal; GI, gastrointestinal; GU, genitourinary; HPI, history of present illness; PFSH, past, family, and social history; ROS, review of systems; URI, upper respiratory infection.*

Chapter 17: Emergency Department Services

Continuum Model for Head Injury

CPT® Code Vignette	History	Physical Examination (systems)	Medical Decision-making (1. diagnoses; 2. data; 3. risk)
99281 Repaired scalp laceration, well healed, presents for suture removal	**Problem focused** CC: suture removal HPI: wound repair 10 days ago, no complaints	**Problem focused** Limited skin	**Straightforward** 1. Established problem, improved 2. No tests ordered/ reviewed 3. Suture removal
99282 Minor head trauma without local bruising, swelling, or laceration, no neurologic changes	**Expanded problem focused** CC: bumped head HPI: context (injury mechanism), timing	**Expanded problem focused** Examination of skin and neurologic system	**Low complexity** 1. New problem, no additional workup 2. No tests ordered/ reviewed 3. Acute uncomplicated injury
99283 Minor head trauma with local bruising, swelling, or laceration, no neurologic changes; GCS 15	**Expanded problem focused** CC: hit in head HPI: injury mechanism, timing, associated signs and symptoms ROS: neurologic, musculoskeletal	**Expanded problem focused** Eyes, ENMT, skin, and neurologic system	**Moderate complexity** 1. New problem, no additional workup 2. No tests ordered/ reviewed 3. Acute complicated injury
99284 Head trauma with signs of concussion	**Detailed** CC: head injury with LOC HPI: mechanism of injury, associated signs and symptoms (pain, loss of recall), duration of LOC (<5 min), severity (no focal neurologic changes; GCS ≥13) PFSH: medications, allergies, past illnesses/ injuries	**Detailed** Eyes, ENMT, neck, respiratory, cardiovascular, skin, neurologic, and other pertinent systems	**Moderate complexity** 1. New problem, no additional workup planned. 2. Radiology and laboratory tests may be obtained. Neurology or neurosurgical consultation may be obtained. 3. Acute complicated injury.
99285 Head trauma with signs of concussion including LOC (<5 min), brief seizure, and/or persistent emesis; closed skull fracture and/or focal neurologic changes may be present; GCS 9–12	**Comprehensive** CC: head trauma with LOC HPI: mechanism of injury, associated signs and symptoms (pain, emesis), duration of LOC (<5 min), severity (GCS 9–12) ROS: ≥10 systems PFSH: medications, allergies, past illnesses/ injuries, family or social history (eg, bleeding disorders, use of drugs or alcohol)	**Comprehensive** Constitutional, eyes, ENMT, respiratory, cardiovascular, gastrointestinal, neurologic, skin	**High complexity** 1. New problem, no additional workup planned. 2. History obtained from someone other than patient. Radiology and laboratory tests may be obtained/reviewed. Neurology or neurosurgical consultation may be obtained. 3. Acute injuries that may pose a threat to life or bodily function.

Continuum Model for Head Injury (*continued*)

CPT® Code Vignette	History	Physical Examination (systems)	Medical Decision-making (1. diagnoses; 2. data; 3. risk)
99291, 99292 **Critical Care** Head trauma with persistent LOC and/or seizures; open or closed skull fracture and/or focal neurologic changes may be present; GCS ≤8			**High complexity** 1. Critically ill, unstable patient; requires >30 min of directed patient care. 2. Physician assesses, manipulates, and supports vital system function(s) to treat single or multiple vital organ system failure and/or to prevent further life-threatening deterioration of the patient's condition.

Abbreviations: CC, chief complaint; CPT, Current Procedural Terminology; ENMT, ear, nose, mouth, throat; GCS, Glasgow Coma Scale; HPI, history of present illness; LOC, loss of consciousness; PFSH, past, family, and social history; ROS, review of systems.

Continuum Model for Laceration

These codes reflect E/M services only and not any procedure the same physician may provide. The physician needs to be aware that the pre-procedural and intra-procedural global periods may include some of the medical decision-making indicated with each code, thus reducing the level of E/M service provided, and that any E/M service reported with a procedure must meet the requirement for a significant, separately identifiable service.

CPT® Code Vignette	History	Physical Examination (systems)	Medical Decision-making (1. diagnoses; 2. data; 3. risk)
99281 Repaired scalp laceration, well healed, presents for suture removal	**Problem focused** CC: suture removal HPI: wound repair 10 days ago, no complaints	**Problem focused** Limited skin	**Straightforward** 1. Established problem, stable 2. No tests ordered/reviewed 3. Minimal risk—suture removal
99282 Uncomplicated laceration of single body area or organ system	**Expanded problem focused** CC: laceration HPI: location, context (mechanism of injury), timing ROS: skin or musculoskeletal	**Expanded problem focused** Skin and/or musculoskeletal, neurologic systems	**Low complexity** 1. New problem, laceration 2. No tests ordered/reviewed 3. Acute uncomplicated injury

Chapter 17: Emergency Department Services

Continuum Model for Laceration (*continued*)

These codes reflect E/M services only and not any procedure the same physician may provide. The physician needs to be aware that the pre-procedural and intra-procedural global periods may include some of the medical decision-making indicated with each code, thus reducing the level of E/M service provided, and that any E/M service reported with a procedure must meet the requirement for a significant, separately identifiable service.

CPT® Code Vignette	History	Physical Examination (systems)	Medical Decision-making (1. diagnoses; 2. data; 3. risk)
99283 Uncomplicated laceration of single body area or organ system with minor associated injury (eg, minor head injury) *or* Uncomplicated lacerations of >1 body area or organ system *or* Minimally complicated laceration (eg, small foreign body, delay in seeking care) of single body area or organ system	**Expanded problem focused** CC: laceration(s) HPI: location, context (mechanism of injury), timing ROS: skin or musculoskeletal	**Expanded problem focused** Constitutional, skin and/or musculoskeletal, neurologic systems	**Moderate complexity** 1. New problem(s). 2. Radiograph of affected area may be ordered/ viewed. 3. Acute complicated injury.
99284 Uncomplicated laceration of single body area or organ system with other associated injury (eg, mild concussion) *or* Minimally complicated lacerations (eg, small foreign body) of >1 body area or organ system *or* Complicated laceration (eg, infection, GSW, deep knife wound) of single body area or organ system without immediate threat to life or limb	**Detailed** CC: injuries HPI: location, context (mechanism of injury), timing, associated signs and symptoms ROS: constitutional, skin, musculoskeletal, neurologic PFSH: medications and allergies	**Detailed** Eyes, neck, respiratory, cardiovascular, skin, musculoskeletal, neurologic	**Moderate complexity** 1. New problem. 2. Radiograph of affected area may be ordered/ viewed. 3. Acute complicated injury.
99285 Uncomplicated laceration of ≥1 body area or organ system with significant associated injury (eg, multiple trauma) *or* Complicated laceration (eg, GSW, deep knife wound) of >1 body area or organ system without immediate threat to life or limb	**Comprehensive** CC: injuries HPI: location, context (mechanism of injury), timing, associated signs and symptoms ROS: ≥10 systems PFSH: medications, allergies, and pertinent family history of tobacco, alcohol, or substance use	**Comprehensive** Constitutional, eyes, ENMT, respiratory, cardiovascular, musculoskeletal, neurologic, skin	**High complexity** 1. New problem 2. Tests ordered/reviewed (radiology and/or laboratory) 3. Acute injury that may pose a threat to life or bodily function or emergency major surgery

Continuum Model for Laceration (*continued*)

These codes reflect E/M services only and not any procedure the same physician may provide. The physician needs to be aware that the pre-procedural and intra-procedural global periods may include some of the medical decision-making indicated with each code, thus reducing the level of E/M service provided, and that any E/M service reported with a procedure must meet the requirement for a significant, separately identifiable service.

CPT® Code Vignette	History	Physical Examination (systems)	Medical Decision-making (1. diagnoses; 2. data; 3. risk)
99291, 99292 **Critical Care** Uncomplicated or complicated laceration of ≥1 body area or organ system with significant associated injury (eg, multiple trauma) with immediate threat to life or limb			**High complexity** 1. Critically ill, unstable patient; requires >30 minutes of directed patient care. 2. Physician assesses, manipulates, and supports vital system function(s) to treat single or multiple vital organ system failure and/or to prevent further life-threatening deterioration of the patient's condition.

Abbreviations: CC, chief complaint, CPT, Current Procedural Terminology; E/M, evaluation and management; ENMT, ear, nose, mouth, throat; GSW, gunshot wound; HPI, history of present illness; PFSH, past, family, and social history; ROS, review of systems.

CHAPTER 18

Critical and Intensive Care

Contents

This chapter focuses on the correct coding for critical and intensive care, including attendance at delivery, neonatal resuscitation, hourly critical care, critical care of the neonate and child younger than 6 years, and intensive care of the recovering or low birth weight neonate and infant. Services commonly reported before and after intensive or critical care services, such as care during emergency transport, consultations, and medical team care conferences, are included.

Evaluation and management (E/M) of the child who no longer requires intensive or critical care is discussed in Chapter 16, Noncritical Hospital Evaluation and Management Services.

Attendance at Delivery and Newborn Resuscitation

Attendance at Delivery

99464   Attendance at delivery (when requested by the delivering physician or other qualified health care professional) and initial stabilization of newborn

Attendance at delivery (99464) is only reported when the physical presence of the provider is requested by the delivering physician and indicated for a newborn who may require immediate intervention (ie, stabilization, resuscitation, or evaluation for potential problems). See coding examples in Chapter 15, Hospital Care of the Newborn.

Code 99464 is not reported when hospital-mandated attendance is the only underlying basis for providing the service. When physician on-call services are not requested by the delivering physician but, rather, are mandated by the hospital (eg, attending specific types of deliveries without physician request, such as all repeat cesarean deliveries), report code 99026 (hospital-mandated on-call service; in hospital, each hour) or 99027 (hospital-mandated on-call service; out of hospital, each hour). See Chapter 16, Noncritical Hospital Evaluation and Management Services, for guidelines on the use of codes 99026 and 99027.

Attendance at delivery (99464)
- Service is only reported when requested by the delivering physician.
- Medical record documentation must include the request for attendance at the delivery and substantiate the medical necessity of the services performed. If there is no documentation by the delivering physician for attendance at delivery, the verbal request and the reason for the request should be documented in the attendance note.
- Includes initial drying, stimulation, suctioning, blow-by oxygen, or continuous positive airway pressure (CPAP) without positive-pressure ventilation (PPV); a cursory visual inspection of the neonate; assignment of Apgar scores; and discussion of the care of the newborn with the delivering physician and parents. A quick look in the delivery room or examination after stabilization is not sufficient to support reporting of 99464.
- Any medically necessary procedures to complete the resuscitation that are provided in the delivery room may be reported separately (eg, direct laryngoscopy without intubation).
- May be reported in addition to the initial normal newborn (99460), initial sick newborn (99221–99223), initial intensive care of the neonate (99477), or critical care (99468; 99291, 99292) codes.

When qualifying resuscitative efforts are provided, code 99465 (delivery/birthing room resuscitation) is reported instead. Codes 99464 and 99465 cannot be reported on the same day of service.

Neonatal Resuscitation

99465   Delivery/birthing room resuscitation, provision of positive pressure ventilation and/or chest compressions in the presence of acute inadequate ventilation and/or cardiac output

Attendance at delivery with neonatal resuscitation (99465)
- Includes bag-and-mask or bag-to-endotracheal tube ventilation (PPV) and/or cardiac compressions.
- Is reported when positive-pressure breaths are administered by the T-piece resuscitator in lieu of a manual bag-mask resuscitator (see Coding Conundrum: T-Piece Positive-Pressure Ventilation box later in this chapter).

- Does not include other life support procedures that are performed as a necessary part of the resuscitation and may be reported separately (eg, 31500, intubation, endotracheal, emergency procedure; 31515, laryngoscopy, direct, for aspiration; 36510, catheterization of umbilical vein for diagnosis or therapy, newborn; 94610, surfactant administration).

- May be reported in addition to any initial care service, including initial critical care (99468), hourly critical care (99291, 99292), initial neonatal intensive care (99477), or normal newborn care (99460) if the resuscitation results in a stable term neonate.

- Medically necessary procedures (eg, intubation, umbilical line placement) essential to successful resuscitation (and not performed as a convenience before admission to the neonatal intensive care unit [NICU]) that are performed in the delivery room prior to admission may also be reported in addition to code 99468 or 99477. Medical record documentation must clearly support that the services are provided as part of the pre-admission or pre-global service.

Example

▶ **A neonatologist attends the cesarean delivery of a 27-weeks' gestation neonate at the request of an obstetrician, who suspects an abruption.** The neonate has no spontaneous activity. The resuscitation includes PPV, intubation, and placement of an umbilical vein catheter. The newborn is stabilized and admitted to the NICU, where the neonatologist administers surfactant and performs an umbilical artery catheterization.

The intubation and umbilical vein catheterization are separately reported procedures provided as part of the resuscitation and not as a convenience to the physician prior to admission.	**Current Procedural Terminology (CPT®)** 99465 (delivery/birthing room resuscitation) 31500 (endotracheal intubation, emergency) 36510 (catheterization of umbilical vein for diagnosis or therapy, newborn) 99468 25 (initial neonatal critical care)

Modifier 25 is appended to code 99468 to signify a significant, separately identifiable E/M service provided in addition to codes 31500 and 36510 because these services are bundled by National Correct Coding Initiative (NCCI) edits. (For more on edits, see Chapter 2, Modifiers and Coding Edits.) Codes 99465 and 99468 are not bundled by NCCI edits, but individual payers may require modifier 25 to designate separately identifiable critical care services on the same date. The surfactant administration and umbilical artery catheterization are not separately reported when performed in conjunction with neonatal critical care.

Coding Conundrum: T-Piece Positive-Pressure Ventilation

A frequently asked question is whether code **99465** can be reported if the T-piece resuscitator is used to provide continuous positive airway pressure (CPAP) only. Clearly, from the definitions given previously, the answer is no. If CPAP is provided to the neonate and she responds with an adequate respiratory effort, code **99464** should be reported. On the other hand, if the neonate is apneic or, in the judgment of the provider, exhibiting inadequate respiratory effort, positive-pressure breaths administered by the T-piece resuscitator in lieu of a manual bag-mask resuscitator would justify reporting code **99465**. It is important for the documentation to explicitly state that the neonate demonstrated respiratory and/or cardiac instability requiring intervention, including apnea or inadequate respiratory effort to support gas exchange; that the provider instituted positive-pressure ventilation (PPV); and the neonate's response to the PPV.

Definition of Perinatal Period

The World Health Organization defines the *perinatal period* as the time from the 22nd week of completed gestation through the 28th day following birth (28 completed days after birth). Based on this definition, the perinatal period continues through the 28th day after birth, ending on the 29th calendar day after birth. The day of birth is considered day 0 (zero); therefore, the day after birth is considered day 1.

In addition to assigning *International Classification of Diseases, 10th Revision, Clinical Modification* codes for perinatal diagnoses, this definition affects reporting of the initial- and subsequent-day neonatal and pediatric critical care codes 99468–99472 and code 99477 for the initial hospital care of the neonate, 28 days or younger, who requires intensive observation, frequent interventions, and other intensive care services.

Critical Care Services

Critical Illness or Injury

- A *critical illness or injury* is defined by *CPT*® as one that acutely impairs one or more vital organs such that there is a high probability of imminent or life-threatening deterioration of the patient's condition.
- Critical care involves high-complexity medical decision-making (MDM) to assess, manipulate, and support vital organ system function(s); treat single or multiple organ system failure; and/or prevent further life-threatening deterioration of the patient's condition.
- Immaturity alone, or any of the specific procedures, equipment, or therapies associated with care of the immature neonate, does not define critical care.
- Coding critical care is not determined by the location in which the care is delivered but by the nature of the care being delivered and the condition of the patient requiring care.
- Services qualify as critical care *only if both* the injury or illness *and* the treatment being delivered meet the following criteria:
  - ❖ The illness or injury acutely impairs one or more vital organs as defined previously.
  - ❖ The treatment delivered involves high-complexity MDM to prevent life-threatening deterioration of the patient's condition.
- Critical care is not limited to an inpatient setting or a critical care area, and a physician of any specialty can provide these services. Services must be provided directly by the physician or other qualified health care professional (QHP).

Coding Conundrum: Applying the Critical Care Definition

The physician must use his or her experience and judgment in assigning the *Current Procedural Terminology*® definition of critical care. In summary, these are patients presently at clear risk of death or serious morbidity, requiring close observation and frequent interventions and assessments, and where the high-complexity medical decision-making (MDM) is apparent in the medical record documentation. No single criterion places or excludes a patient from this category, and the patient is not required to demonstrate all the characteristics listed in this chapter. The most convincing way to demonstrate the appropriate application of a critical care code is to clearly document in the medical record the child's condition, noting the risks to the patient, frequency of needed assessments and interventions, degree of and type of organ failure(s) the patient is presently experiencing, and complexity of the MDM. While immaturity commonly leads to many levels of organ dysfunction that will increase the risk of a critical illness in a newborn, neither immaturity alone nor any of the specific procedures or therapies associated with care of the immature neonate or infant qualifies alone for reporting critical care.

Chapter 18: Critical and Intensive Care

Hourly Critical Care

99291 Critical care, E/M of the critically ill or critically injured patient; first 30 to 74 minutes

+99292 each additional 30 minutes (Use in conjunction with **99291**.)

Guidelines for reporting codes **99291** and **99292**

- ☀ Reported when critical care is provided for 30 minutes or more.
  - ❖ In the outpatient setting (eg, emergency department [ED], office, clinic) *regardless of age*
  - ❖ To an inpatient 6 years or older (Daily critical care of a child younger than 6 years is discussed later in this chapter.)
  - ❖ Concurrently by a second physician from a different specialty to a critically ill or injured child aged 5 years or younger
  - ❖ To an inpatient aged 5 years or younger when the patient is being transferred to another facility where the receiving physician of the same specialty but different medical group will be reporting the daily inpatient critical care service codes (**99468** and **99469**; **99471** and **99472**; **99475** and **99476**)
  - ❖ By the physician physically transporting a critically ill child older than 2 years (Refer to codes **99466** and **99467** for face-to-face transport care of the critically ill or injured patient 24 months or younger.)
- ☀ These are bundled codes (many procedures typically performed are included in the work valuation of the code and cannot be reported separately) (**Table 18-1**). (See also Procedures *Not* Bundled With Critical/Intensive Care Services section later in this chapter for commonly provided services not bundled with hourly and/or neonatal and pediatric critical care services.)

Table 18-1. Critical Care Bundled Services

CPT® Code and Procedure	Hourly Critical Care 99291, 99292	Pediatric Transport 99466, 99467	Neonatal/Pediatric Critical and Intensive Care 99468–99476, 99477–99480
Interpretation and Monitoring			
71045 X-ray, chest; single view	x	x	x
71046 X-ray, chest; 2 views	x	x	x
93561 Cardiac output measurement	x		x
93562 subsequent measurement of cardiac output	x	x	x
94760 Pulse oximetry; single determination	x	x	x
94761 multiple determinations (eg, during exercise)			
94762 by continuous overnight monitoring			
Vascular Access Procedures			
36000 Introduction of needle or intracatheter, vein	x	x	x
36140 Catheterization extremity artery		x	
36400 Venipuncture, <3 years, requiring physician or QHP skill; femoral or jugular vein		x	x
36405 scalp vein			
36406 other vein			
36410 Venipuncture, ≥3 years, requiring physician or QHP skill	x		x
36415 Collection of venous blood by venipuncture	x	x	x

Table 18-1. Critical Care Bundled Services (*continued*)			
CPT® Code and Procedure	Hourly Critical Care 99291, 99292	Pediatric Transport 99466, 99467	Neonatal/Pediatric Critical and Intensive Care 99468–99476, 99477–99480
Vascular Access Procedures (*continued*)			
36420 Venipuncture, cutdown; younger than age 1 year			x
36430 Transfusion, blood or blood components			x
36440 Push transfusion, blood, 2 years or younger			x
36510 Catheterization of umbilical vein, newborn			x
36555 Insertion of non-tunneled CICC; <5 years of age			x
36591 Collection blood from venous access device	x	x	x
36600 Arterial puncture, withdrawal of blood for diagnosis	x	x	x
36620 Arterial catheterization, percutaneous			
36660 Catheterization, umbilical artery, newborn			x
Other Procedures			
31500 Endotracheal intubation, emergency			x
43752 Nasogastric/orogastric intubation, fluoroscopic guidance	x	x	x
43753 Gastric intubation including lavage if performed	x	x	x
51100 Aspiration of bladder; by needle			x
51701 Insertion of non-indwelling bladder catheter			x
51702 Temporary indwelling bladder catheter; simple			x
62270 Spinal puncture, lumbar, diagnostic			x
92953 Temporary transcutaneous pacing	x	x	x
94002 Ventilation initiation; inpatient/observation, initial day 94003 each subsequent day	x	x	x
94004 Ventilation initiation; nursing facility, per day	x		x
94375 Respiratory flow volume loop			x
94610 Intrapulmonary surfactant administration			x
94660 CPAP initiation and management	x	x	x
94662 CNP, initiation and management	x	x	x
94780 Car seat/bed testing, infants through 12 months; 60 minutes 94781 each additional full 30 minutes			x

Abbreviations: CICC, centrally inserted central venous catheter; CNP, continuous negative pressure ventilation; CPAP, continuous positive airway pressure; CPT, Current Procedural Terminology; QHP, qualified health care professional.

Chapter 18: Critical and Intensive Care

⁑ Procedures not included as bundled may be reported separately (eg, lumbar puncture, endotracheal intuba-tion, thoracentesis). The reported time of critical care *cannot* include any time spent performing procedures or services that are reported separately.

⁑ Reporting is time based. **Table 18-2** lists times and billing units. The total floor or unit time devoted to the patient in the provision of critical care is used in code selection. Critical care time includes physician–patient face-to-face time or time spent on the patient's *unit or floor* directly related to the patient's care (eg, hands-on care at the bedside, reviewing test results, discussing care with other medical staff or family, docu-menting services in the medical record).

⁑ Time spent in the provision of critical care does not need to be continuous. The cumulative time of critical care provided on a single date of service is used to calculate the units of service provided. However, when a *continuous period* of critical care occurs before and after midnight, report the total time on the date that the period of care was initiated. Do not report a second initial hour of critical care for the period beginning at midnight.

⁑ The physician must be immediately available to the patient during time reported as critical care. No time spent in activities that take place out of the unit, off the patient's floor, or consulting with other caregivers from home are included in critical care time.

⁑ Code **99291** is reported once on a given date of service when 30 to 74 minutes of critical care is performed. If less than 30 minutes of critical care is provided, an appropriate E/M service (eg, **99201–99215** for office services, **99221–99233** for inpatient hospital care) is reported.

⁑ Code **99292** is reported with 1 unit for each additional period up to 30 minutes beyond the previous period. See **Table 18-2** for reporting the correct codes based on the total duration of critical care. *Time spent provid-ing critical care services must be documented in the medical record.*

Table 18-2. Reporting Hourly Critical Care Services	
Duration of Face-to-face Critical Care	*CPT*® **Codes**
<30 min	Do not report as critical care; included in the reported E/M service.
30–74 min	99291
75–104 min	99291 × 1 unit plus 99292 × 1 unit
105–134 min	99291 × 1 unit plus 99292 × 2 units

Abbreviations: CPT, Current Procedural Terminology; *E/M, evaluation and management.*

⁑ Critical care is not permitted to be reported as a split/shared service (ie, the times of a physician and QHP cannot be combined and reported as a single service). The time required to report code **99291** must be met by a single physician. If multiple providers from the same group practice and same specialty care for a patient after a single physician has provided the initial 30 minutes of critical care, combine the total time and report with code **99292** as appropriate. Do not report **99291** more than once per day. All services must be reported under the name and National Provider Identifier of a single physician.

⁑ Time-based critical care services (**99291**, **99292**) may be reported by an individual of a *different specialty* from either the same or different group on the same day that neonatal or pediatric critical care services are reported by another individual (**99468–99476**).

⁑ A teaching physician may report time-based critical care services only when he or she was present for the entire period for which the claim is submitted and that time is supported in documentation of the service.

⁑ When inpatient and outpatient critical care services are provided to a neonate, an infant, or a child younger than 6 years on the same date by the same physician (or physician of the same group and specialty), only the *inpatient* critical care codes are reported (**99468–99476**).

⁑ Other significant, separately identifiable E/M services (eg, **99212–99215**, **99281–99285**) can be reported in addition to time-based critical care services as appropriate. Do not count time spent in separately reported E/M services in critical care time.

Examples

➤ **A 3-week-old exposed to a sick sibling at home acquires respiratory syncytial virus and is seen in the ED for respiratory distress.** The ED physician provides an hour of critical care before the neonate is admitted to the NICU by the neonatologist.

Code **99291** with 1 unit of service (30–74 minutes) is reported by the ED physician. The neonatologist will report the appropriate level of daily hospital, intensive, or critical care.

➤ **A 4-month-old is admitted with fever, lethargy, and poor feeding. Laboratory work, cultures, and intravenous (IV) fluids are begun.** Later that afternoon, the infant decompensates, developing desaturation, apnea, and falling blood pressures. The pediatrician returns to the bedside; 3 hours are spent at the hospital stabilizing the infant, directing nursing staff, discussing management options with the tertiary care facility, speaking with the parents, and monitoring the infant while awaiting the transport team to take the infant to a hospital where the pediatrician does not practice.

Care is reported with an initial hospital care code (**99221–99223**) along with **99291** and **99292** with 4 units of service for the 180 minutes of critical care services. It would be appropriate to report the critical care time in addition to the initial hospital care code by the transferring pediatrician, for 165 to 194 minutes of care on the same date of service.

Procedures Not *Bundled With Critical/Intensive Care Services*

When reporting hourly critical or neonatal and pediatric critical and intensive care services, many services commonly provided with these codes are not bundled into the intensive or critical care services. However, claim edits may require appending a modifier to indicate the services were distinct. Examples of procedures that are not bundled with critical care services include (not all-inclusive)

- Thoracentesis (**32554** without imaging guidance, **32555** with imaging guidance) (via needle or pigtail catheter)
- Percutaneous pleural drainage with insertion of indwelling catheter (**32556** without imaging guidance, **32557** with imaging guidance)
- Complete (double volume) exchange transfusion (**36450**, newborn; **36455**, other than newborn)
- Partial exchange transfusion (**36456**)
- Abdominal paracentesis (**49082**, **49083** with imaging guidance)
- Bone marrow aspiration (**38220**)
- Circumcision (**54150**)
- Cardioversion (**92960**)
- Cardiopulmonary resuscitation (**92950**)
- Extracorporeal membrane oxygenation (**33946–33949**)
- Peripherally inserted central catheter (PICC) (NCCI edits do bundle the PICC codes [**36568, 36569**] with all neonatal and pediatric critical care codes. However, a modifier can override when appropriate. See Chapter 2, Modifiers and Coding Edits, for more information on NCCI edits.)
- Insertion of non-tunneled centrally inserted central venous catheter, older than 5 years (**36556**)
- Replacement (rewire) of non-tunneled centrally inserted central venous catheter (**36580**)
- Therapeutic apheresis (**36511–36514**)
- Insertion of cannula for hemodialysis, other purpose (separate procedure); vein to vein (**36800**)
- Placement of needle for intraosseous infusion (**36680**)
- Initiation of selective head or total body hypothermia in the critically ill neonate (**99184**) (Report only once at initiation of service.)

> 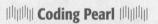 **Coding Pearl** ||||||||
>
> Do not report code **32551** for percutaneous pleural drainage, as this code represents an open procedure. See Chapter 19, Common Surgical Procedures and Sedation in Facility Settings, for more information on reporting thoracentesis, pleural drainage, and thoracostomy procedures.

Chapter 18: Critical and Intensive Care

Payer edits may vary, and certain services are bundled unless performed for diagnostic purposes rather than monitoring. The following instructions from the Medicaid NCCI manual demonstrate reporting of diagnostic services:

Lumbar puncture (62270) and suprapubic bladder aspiration (51100) are separately reportable with hourly critical care (99291, 99292) but are *not separately reportable* with the pediatric and neonatal critical care service codes (99468–99472, 99475, 99476) and the intensive care services codes (99477–99480).

Diagnostic rhythm electrocardiogram (ECG) codes 93040–93042 are reported only when there is a sudden change in a patient status associated with a change in cardiac rhythm that requires a diagnostic rhythm ECG and return to the critical care unit. When separately reporting a diagnostic ECG, do not include the time for this service in the time spent providing critical care. Modifier 59 is appended to the ECG code when indicated by patient status and performed on the same date as critical care services.

Transesophageal echocardiography (TEE) monitoring (93318) *without probe placement* is not separately reportable by a physician performing critical care E/M services. However, if a physician places a transesophageal probe to be used for TEE monitoring on the same date of service that the physician performs critical care E/M services, code 93318 may be reported with modifier 59. The time necessary for probe placement shall not be included in the critical care time reported with *CPT*® codes 99291 and 99292, as is true for all separately reportable procedures performed on a patient receiving critical care E/M services. Diagnostic TEE services may be separately reportable by a physician performing critical care E/M services. (*American Academy of Pediatrics [AAP] Tip:* Payers may require modifier 25 to be appended to the codes for critical care services rather than appending modifier 59 to the procedure code. Modifier 59 is intended to distinguish 2 distinct non-E/M services.)

Many practice management and billing systems include claim scrubbers that provide an alert that claim edits apply and a modifier may be appropriate based on clinical circumstances. Payers may also offer online tools for determining when code pair edits apply.

Example

➤ **During an encounter with an adolescent who dove into a lake, hit his head, and was unconscious when pulled from the water, a physician spends 10 minutes performing cardiopulmonary resuscitation (CPR) and then another 45 minutes providing critical care before the patient is transferred to another facility.** Critical care service (99291) time is documented and distinctly identifiable in the patient record from the time spent performing the separately reportable CPR (92950), for which start and stop times were documented.

Neonatal and Pediatric Daily Critical Care Codes

Codes are
- Reported for critical care of children younger than 6 years in the inpatient setting.
- Global—encompass all E/M services by a single provider (or provider of the exact same specialty in the same group) on one calendar date. Other physicians and QHPs providing critical care must report hour critical care code 99291 or 99292. (See exceptions under the Guidelines for Reporting Neonatal or Pediatric Inpatient Critical Care section later in this chapter.)
- Bundled—have commonly performed procedures included in the E/M codes.
- Not time based. Prolonged services *may not* be reported in conjunction with neonatal or pediatric critical care services.
- Not based on typical E/M rules and the performance and documentation of key components (history, physical examination, MDM, and/or time).
- Reported based on postnatal age (see the Definition of Perinatal Period section earlier in this chapter) and initial or subsequent care (**Table 18-3**).

Guidelines for Reporting Neonatal or Pediatric Inpatient Critical Care

* The physician primarily responsible for the patient on the date of service should report the neonatal or pediatric critical care codes. (A neonatal nurse practitioner [NNP] may be primarily responsible and report pediatric critical care if independent billing is allowed by state regulations, services are within scope of practice, and the NNP has hospital privilege credentials for the service.) When the physician and NNP provide critical care services to a patient only one may report the code.

* This includes most E/M services and bundled procedures provided on a calendar day. If critical care is provided in the outpatient and inpatient setting by the same physician or physician of the same specialty and group, only the inpatient code is reported.

* Codes may be reported in addition to normal newborn care (99460 or 99462) when the patient receives normal newborn care and then, at a subsequent separate encounter the same day, requires critical care. A neonatologist may also provide a consultation (99251–99255) at the request of the attending physician early in the day and later provide critical or intensive care services. However, the neonatologist would report only critical or intensive care services if a transfer of care occurs at the initial encounter.

* Codes are reported only once per day, per patient.

* When the same physician or physicians of the same specialty and group practice provide pediatric critical care during transport of a child 24 months or younger (99466, 99467; 99485, 99486) and critical care after admission to the receiving facility, both services are reported and modifier 25 is appended to the transport code.

* Initial critical care codes (99468, 99471, 99475) are only reported once per calendar day and once per hospital stay for a given patient. If the patient has to be readmitted to critical care during the same hospital stay, report a subsequent critical care code (99469, 99472, 99476).

Table 18-3. Neonatal and Pediatric Global Critical Care			
Inpatient Neonatal Critical Care	28 Days or Younger	29 Days Through 24 Months of Age	2 Through 5 Years of Age
Initial inpatient neonatal critical care	99468	99471	99475
Subsequent inpatient neonatal critical care	99469	99472	99476

* Subsequent critical care may be reported on multiple days even if there is no change in the patient's condition as long as the patient continues to meet the critical care definition and documentation supports this level of service.

* Procedures bundled in these codes must not be reported separately. The services and procedures that are included with neonatal critical care codes are identified in **Table 18-1**.

* Care may be provided on any unit in a hospital facility.

* Care must be provided by the reporting physician but also includes the services provided by the health care team functioning under the direct supervision of the physician or an advanced nurse practitioner who is employed by the physician or physician group and when allowed under state licensure requirements. See the Critical and Intensive Care Supervision Requirements section later in this chapter and Appendix V, Global Per Diem Critical Care Codes: Direct Supervision and Reporting Guidelines.

* Medical record documentation must support the need for and meet the definition of critical care (eg, complex MDM, high probability of imminent or life-threatening deterioration, organ system failure).

Subsequent-day neonatal and pediatric intensive care codes (99478–99480) are reported when critical care is no longer required, the neonate requires more intensive care than typically provided under routine subsequent hospital care (99231–99233), and the neonate weighs 5,000 g or less on the day the code is reported. Once the neonate weighs at least 5,001 g and critical care services are no longer required, report subsequent-day inpatient hospital visit codes (99231–99233).

Chapter 18: Critical and Intensive Care

Coding Conundrum: Selecting the Appropriate Code

Many diagnoses or conditions, such as respiratory distress, infection, seizures, mild to moderate hypoxic-ischemic encephalopathy, and metabolic disorders, can be reported with codes **99468**, **99477**, or **99221–99223**. The patient's clinical status, required level of monitoring and observation, and present body weight will determine which of these code sets is chosen. Selection of the service must be justified by medical record documentation.

Critical and Intensive Care Supervision Requirements

The American Medical Association/Specialty Society Relative Value Scale Update Committee (RUC) makes valuation recommendations based on surveys in which physicians who perform services are presented with a vignette describing the typical patient and the face-to-face physician work associated with that service. The neonatal and pediatric critical and intensive care code vignettes describe hands-on care by the attending physician (intraservice work) as well as the preservice and post-service work associated with this service. Neither the vignette nor the intent of the codes was to imply that 24-hour in-house attendance was a requirement of this code set. However, the codes' values were established assuming the physician is physically present and participating directly in the patient's care for a significant portion of the reported service. Documentation in the patient's chart should reflect this active participation, including documentation of hands-on care, such as a personal physical examination. Supervision of all the care from a distance without face-to-face care is not reported as critical or intensive care. (Refer to Appendix V, Global Per Diem Critical Care Codes: Direct Supervision and Reporting Guidelines.)

The vignettes also include the phrase "repeated examinations over a 24-hour period," which was included to indicate that these neonates or infants do not receive "continuous" care but rather are typically evaluated during numerous intervals over a 24-hour period, depending on the clinical needs of the patient. In some cases, the neonate's or infant's level of illness requires in-house attending presence for extended periods, while in other situations, only daytime presence is required. While the critical care team is present with the neonate or infant for the full 24 hours, overnight in-house care by the reporting physician is determined by the complexity of the total population of neonates cared for in a nursery or the changes in a specific neonate's or infant's condition that cannot be adequately assessed or managed over the telephone.

Under the heading Inpatient Neonatal and Pediatric Critical Care Service, *CPT®* states that codes 99468, 99469, and 99471–99476 are used to report services provided by a physician "directing the inpatient care" of a critically ill neonate, infant, or child through 5 years of age. The medical record documentation must support the physician's presence and supervision of the team as well as the critical nature of the child's disease. As noted previously, the directing physician is not required to be present or in the facility for the total 24 hours of daily care. Rather, because neonatal and pediatric critical and intensive care may require numerous encounters to reevaluate and manage the patient each day, neonatal and pediatric critical and intensive care codes encompass all the sick care provided within a calendar day.

Neonatal Critical Care

99468   Initial inpatient neonatal critical care, per day, for the evaluation and management of a critically ill neonate, 28 days of age or younger

99469   Subsequent inpatient neonatal critical care, per day, for the evaluation and management of a critically ill neonate, 28 days of age or younger

Selection of the appropriate code will depend on the newborn's or infant's condition and the intensity of the service provided and documented on a particular day of service.

In some situations, the neonate will be normal at birth and, many hours later, show signs of an illness. *CPT®* guidelines specify that only one initial hospital service may be reported for the same patient on the same day of service by the same physician or physician of the same specialty within the same group. However, if 2 distinct, medically necessary services are provided, both services may be reported. Each service should be reported with the appropriate diagnosis code to support the service (eg, diagnosis codes for well newborn and the defined illness). In other situations, a newborn's illness or condition progresses during the hospital stay, requiring a higher intensity of service by the same physician or another physician from a different group or specialty. When all the neonate's care on the same date of service is related to the same condition or disease but the level of illness and required care progresses through the day, only a single code representing the highest level of service performed and documented is reported if all the care was provided by a single physician or physicians of the same specialty and group practice. However, when the intensity of care progresses over the day and services are provided by physicians from different groups or specialties or the patient is transferred to another facility, each physician reports a different level of service.

Examples

> **A term 3,500-g neonate is born cyanotic following a vaginal delivery.** He has minimal respiratory distress and appears otherwise vigorous. He is brought to the NICU, where a chest radiograph shows dramatic cardiomegaly and a marked increase in pulmonary markings. An umbilical artery catheter and umbilical vein catheter are inserted to determine blood gases. An ECG is performed, and a pediatric cardiologist is consulted to obtain an emergency echocardiogram.

It is important to remember that respiratory support (ie, mechanical ventilation) is not required to report critical care services. In this case, serious cyanosis and clear evidence of cardiac decompensation qualify as critical care. Code 99468 would be reported for initial date of neonatal critical care services. The umbilical vessel catheterizations are bundled with 99468. Depending on the findings on the echocardiogram and a need for cardiac intensive care, the cardiologist may report hourly critical care for any additional time beyond the echocardiogram. If critical care is not provided, the cardiologist would report consultative services (99251–99255) or subsequent hospital care (if requirements for reporting a consultation are not met). (See Chapter 16, Noncritical Hospital Evaluation and Management Services, for more information on reporting consultations and reporting to payers who do not recognize consultation codes.) If the neonate were transferred to a cardiac center by the neonatologist, the neonatologist would report time-based critical care codes (99291, 99292) for the care provided prior to the transfer.

> **A 3-day-old recovering from respiratory distress syndrome with a present body weight of 1,600 g is still unstable but is weaned off the ventilator to CPAP.** He is continued on total parenteral nutrition by central vein and IV antibiotics.

Code 99469 is reported because the medical record continues to document the neonate's instability and the continued need for critical care services.

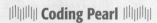

Coding Pearl

Report first a code from category **Z38** (liveborn infants according to place of birth and type of delivery) when care is provided by the attending physician during the birth admission. Codes for abnormal conditions are reported secondary to the code for live birth. When a neonate is transferred to another facility after birth, the admission to the receiving facility is not a birth admission and **Z38** codes are not reported.

Coding Conundrum: Apnea in Neonates

Apnea in neonates may be an expected component of preterm birth and may be effectively managed by manual stimulation, pharmacological stimulation, high-flow nasal oxygen, or continuous positive airway pressure. At other times, this symptom will be associated with a serious underlying problem(s) and is a reflection of the instability of a critically ill neonate and will require one or more of the same interventions. The physician must employ his or her best clinical judgment and clearly document the factors that make the patient's present condition critical (or require intensive care). The same requirements for organ failure, risk of imminent deterioration, and complex medical decision-making apply. With apnea and many other conditions, it is the total picture of the neonate with the diagnosis, clinical presentation, and immediate threat to life, amount of hands-on and supervisory care provided by the physician, and the level of intervention needed to manage that neonate's conditions on a given day that drive the correct code selection. In all cases, when critical care codes are reported, the documentation must support the physician's judgment that the patient is critically ill and services provided are commensurate with the condition on that day of service on which critical care codes are reported.

Chapter 18: Critical and Intensive Care

Pediatric Critical Care

99471   Initial inpatient pediatric critical care, per day, for the evaluation and management of a critically ill infant or young child, 29 days through 24 months of age

99472   Subsequent inpatient pediatric critical care, per day, for the evaluation and management of a critically ill infant or young child, 29 days through 24 months of age

99475   Initial inpatient pediatric critical care, per day, for the evaluation and management of a critically ill infant or young child, 2 through 5 years of age

99476   Subsequent inpatient pediatric critical care, per day, for the evaluation and management of a critically ill infant or young child, 2 through 5 years of age

Codes 99471–99476 are used to report direction of the inpatient care of a critically ill infant or young child outside of the neonatal period. Services are provided to patients who are at least 29 days of age (postnatal age with day of birth being 0 [zero]) until the child reaches 6 years of age. Initial pediatric critical care for children of these ages is reported with code 99471 (29 days through 24 months of age—up to, but not including, the second birthday) or 99475 (2 through 5 years of age—up to, but not including, the sixth birthday). Initial pediatric critical care codes (99471, 99475) are only reported once, per calendar day, per hospital stay for a given patient. If the patient has been sent to another inpatient unit for continued care and then requires readmission to critical care during the same hospital stay, report a subsequent critical care code (99472, 99476) on the readmission date and each subsequent date the child remains critical. Subsequent days of care for the infant or child who remains critical are reported with code 99472 or 99476. These subsequent-day codes may be reported only by a single individual and only once per day, per patient, in a given setting.

Examples

➤ **A 22-month-old with developmental delays and a seizure disorder is initially treated by the ED physician for status epilepticus (1 hour of critical care).** Although seizures were initially controlled, the pharmacologic management led to irregular respiratory activity, lethargy, and hypotension. The patient was admitted to the pediatric intensive care unit at 11:00 pm that evening by the critical care attending physician, who intubated her, placed her on a ventilator, began fluid expansion, used dobutamine to control her blood pressure, and made arrangements for a bedside electroencephalogram (EEG).

The ED physician would report 1 hour of critical care (99291). The pediatrician or intensivist would report his or her services with the initial inpatient pediatric critical care code (99471) for that calendar day, even though only 1 hour of care was provided. One hour later, after midnight, a new date of service would begin. The intubation is bundled with 99471 and cannot be separately billed.

➤ **A primary care pediatrician admits a 4-year-old to observation for symptoms of lower respiratory infection.** Later the same day, the patient becomes hemodynamically unstable and the pediatrician provides 35 minutes of critical care services before transferring the patient's care to a pediatric intensivist. The pediatric intensivist assumes management of the critically ill patient at 10:00 pm.

The pediatrician reports initial observation care (99218–99220) based the level of service provided and appends modifier 25 to indicate that this service is significant and separately identifiable from critical care services reported with code 99291. The intensivist reports code 99475 (initial inpatient pediatric critical care, per day, for the E/M of a critically ill infant or young child, 2 through 5 years of age).

Patients Critically Ill After Surgery

Postoperative care of a surgical patient is included in the surgeon's global surgical package. For some neonatal surgical care (eg, codes 39503 [repair of diaphragmatic hernia], 43314 [esophagoplasty, thoracic approach; with repair of tracheoesophageal fistula], or 49605 [repair of large omphalocele or gastroschisis; with or without prosthesis]), some critical care days are included in the work values assigned to these surgical procedures.

However

* If a second physician provides care for the routine postoperative patient, the surgeon must append modifier **54** (surgical care only) to the surgical code. (A formal transfer of care should be documented.)

* If the surgeon provides and reports the complete surgical care package, a request for consultation from another specialist may be made.

* If the patient's course is not typical and an unexpected complication occurs that requires the concurrent care of another specialist, both may report their service. For example, if the surgeon first requests a consultation, an initial consultation code (or other appropriate E/M code based on the payer's payment policy for consultations) would be reported by the consultant. If the surgeon requests concurrent care for a specific medical problem, time-based critical care (**99291, 99292**) or subsequent hospital care (**99231–99233**) codes would be reported dependent on the child's condition and care provided. The diagnosis code representing the condition or symptom being treated should be reported with the concurrent *CPT*® code. The rationale for the need for concurrent care must be documented in the surgeon's notes.

Remote Critical Care Services

G0508   Telehealth consultation, critical care, physicians typically spend 60 minutes communicating with the patient via telehealth (initial)

G0509   Telehealth consultation, critical care, physicians typically spend 50 minutes communicating with the patient via telehealth (subsequent)

Remote critical care is the direct delivery by a physician(s) of medical care for a critically ill or critically injured patient from an off-site location (ie, when a critically ill or injured patient requires additional critical care resources that are not available on-site). Previously, Category III codes **0188T** and **0189T** were reported for remote real-time critical care services. *Codes* **0188T** *and* **0189T** *are deleted in 2019.* To report neonatal and pediatric critical care via telemedicine in 2019 *CPT* instructs to report code **99499** (unlisted evaluation and management service). Other payers may allow reporting with codes **G0508** or **G0509** with place of service **02**. It is recommended that practices verify health plan policies regarding provision of critical care services via telemedicine before initiating these services.

See Chapter 20, Digital Medicine Services: Technology-Enhanced Care Delivery, for more information on reporting telemedicine services, including remote critical care.

Neonatal and Pediatric Intensive Care

99477   Initial hospital care, per day, for the evaluation and management of the neonate, 28 days of age or younger, who requires intensive observation, frequent interventions, and other intensive care services

99478   Subsequent intensive care, per day, for the evaluation and management of the recovering very low birth weight infant (present body weight less than 1500 grams)

99479   Subsequent intensive care, per day, for the evaluation and management of the recovering low birth weight infant (present body weight of 1500-2500 grams)

99480   Subsequent intensive care, per day, for the evaluation and management of the recovering infant (present body weight of 2501-5000 grams)

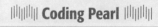

Coding Pearl

Continuing intensive care services provided to an infant weighing more than 5,000 g (approximately 11.02 lb) are reported with subsequent hospital care codes (**99231– 99233**). Documentation of these services must support 2 of 3 key components or the total unit or floor time and time spent counseling and/or coordinating care.

Neonatal and pediatric intensive care codes (**99477–99480**) may be used to report care for neonates or infants who are not critically ill but have a need for intensive monitoring, observation, and frequent assessments by the health care team and supervision by the physician. This includes

* Neonates who require intensive but not critical care services from birth

Chapter 18: Critical and Intensive Care

- Neonates who are no longer critically ill but require intensive physician and health care team observation and interventions
- Recovering low birth weight infants who require a higher level of care than that defined by other hospital care services

These neonates often have a continued need for oxygen, parenteral or gavage enteral nutrition, treatment for apnea of prematurity, and thermoregulation from an Isolette or radiant warmer, and may be recovering from cardiac or surgical care. The intensive services described by these codes include intensive cardiac and respiratory monitoring, continuous and/or frequent vital sign monitoring, heat maintenance, enteral and/or parenteral nutritional adjustments, and laboratory and oxygen saturation monitoring when provided.

- Code 99477 is used to report the more intensive services that an ill but not critically ill neonate (28 days or younger) requires on the day of admission to inpatient care.
- Services are typically (but not required to be) provided in a NICU or special care unit and require a higher intensity of care than would be reported with codes 99221–99223 (initial hospital care of sick patient).
- Patients are under constant observation by the health care team under direct physician supervision.
- These are global codes and include all the E/M services (and bundled procedures) provided to the neonate on that date of service, excluding normal newborn care (99460–99462), when performed. Attendance at delivery (99464) or newborn resuscitation (99465) may be reported in addition to code 99477, when performed. Append modifier 25 to code 99477 when reporting on the same date as 99460–99462, 99464, or 99465. Note: Payers that have adopted the Medicare NCCI edits will not allow payment of codes 99460–99462 and 99477 for services by the same physician or physicians of the same specialty and group practice on the same date. Only code 99477 is reported under these circumstances. See more about NCCI edits in Chapter 2, Modifiers and Coding Edits.
- These are bundled services and include the same procedures that are bundled with neonatal and pediatric critical care services (99468–99476). See Table 18-1 for a list of all the services and procedures that are included.
- Code 99477 should also be used to report readmission to a facility (after initial discharge) of an ill neonate (aged 28 days or younger) if the neonate requires intensive (not critical) care services.
- If the infant is older than 28 days at admission but weighs less than 5,000 g, codes 99221–99223 should be used for intensive care on the date of hospital admission (typically 99223, assuming documentation of comprehensive history and physical examination and high-level MDM) and 99478–99480 for subsequent days, as long as the infant continues to require intensive care.
- Table 18-4 illustrates codes for subsequent-day neonatal and pediatric intensive care services (99478–99480) by present body weight.

Table 18-4. Neonatal and Pediatric Subsequent-Day Intensive Care				
Description	Present Weight <1,500 g	Present Weight 1,500–2,500 g	Present Weight 2,501–5,000 g	Present Weight ≥5,001 g
Subsequent intensive care	99478	99479	99480	99231–99233

- Codes 99478–99480 are reported once per calendar day of subsequent intensive (but not critical) care for the E/M of the recovering infant weighing 5,000 g or less. Selection of the code will be dependent on the *present* body weight of the infant, not the infant's age, on the date of service. Therefore, code selection may change from one day to the next depending on the infant's present body weight and condition.
- Once the baby's weight exceeds 5,000 g, subsequent hospital care codes (99231–99233) are reported until the date of discharge (99238, 99239).

Examples

➤ **A 1,500-g neonate has mild respiratory distress.** She is on 30% oxygen by nasal cannula, a cardiorespiratory monitor, and continuous pulse oximetry. Laboratory tests and radiographs are ordered, and IV fluids and antibiotics are started. Frequent monitoring and observation are required and ordered.

    Code 99477 (initial hospital care for the ill neonate, 28 days of age or less, who requires intensive observation and monitoring) would be reported by the admitting physician.

➤ **A 1,150-g neonate, now 5 days old, is receiving 30% oxygen and continues on IV fluids, small trophic feeds, and caffeine for apnea.**

    Code 99478 would be reported.

➤ **A 15-day-old, 1,600-g neonate remains in an Isolette for thermoregulation and is on methylxanthines for intermittent apnea and bradycardia, for which the neonate requires continuous cardiorespiratory and pulse oximetry monitoring.** The physician adjusts the neonate's continuous gavage feeds based on tolerance and weight.

    Code 99479 would be reported. In these examples, the neonate is not critically ill but continues to require intensive monitoring and constant observation by the health care team under direct physician supervision.

➤ **A baby requires intensive care and weighs 2,500 g on Monday.** The following day, she continues to require intensive care and her weight is 2,504 g.

    Code 99479 would be reported for the care provided on Monday. Code 99480 would be reported for the continuing intensive care provided the following day.

Coding for Transitions to Different Levels of Neonatal Care

During a hospital stay, a newborn or readmitted neonate may require different levels of care. A normal newborn may end up becoming sick, intensively ill, or critical during the same hospital stay. Neonates who were initially sick may also improve to require lower levels of care (eg, normal neonatal care).

    An initial-day critical or intensive care code (eg, 99468, 99477) is reported only once per hospital stay. If the patient recovers and is later stepped up again to that higher level of care, only the subsequent-level codes (99469, 99478–99480) are reported.

    Figure 18-1 provides an illustration of coding for a newborn who transitions from critical care to intensive care and hospital care before discharge. Note that all services take place during the same admission and the physicians are of 2 different specialties (eg, general pediatrics and neonatology). Each physician individually reports the services provided, and each may only report one initial hospital or intensive or critical care service. See also the AAP *Newborn Coding Decision Tool* (available for purchase at https://shop.aap.org) for numerous scenarios of coding for newborn care throughout admissions and transfers of care.

Example

➤ **A neonate (2,600 g) becomes critically ill on a date after being transferred from neonatal critical care by a neonatologist to a hospitalist pediatrician (same facility) to complete her recovery before home discharge.** Care is again transferred to the same neonatologist or neonatologist of the same group practice for critical care services.

The neonatologist reports
99469 (subsequent inpatient neonatal critical care, per day, for the E/M of a critically ill neonate, 28 days of age or younger)

The hospitalist reports
99233 (subsequent hospital care)
or, if 30 minutes or more of critical care services were rendered
99291, **99292** (hourly critical care services)

Teaching Point: The neonatologist may not report initial neonatal critical care for services to the patient who has received prior initial hospital services (eg, initial neonatal intensive care). If the patient initially met the requirements for subsequent intensive care rather than subsequent hospital care, code **99480** would be reported in lieu of code **99233**.

~ **More From the AAP** ~

See the American Academy of Pediatrics *Newborn Coding Decision Tool* for an easy reference to coding for inpatient care of the newborn (available for purchase online through https://shop.aap.org).

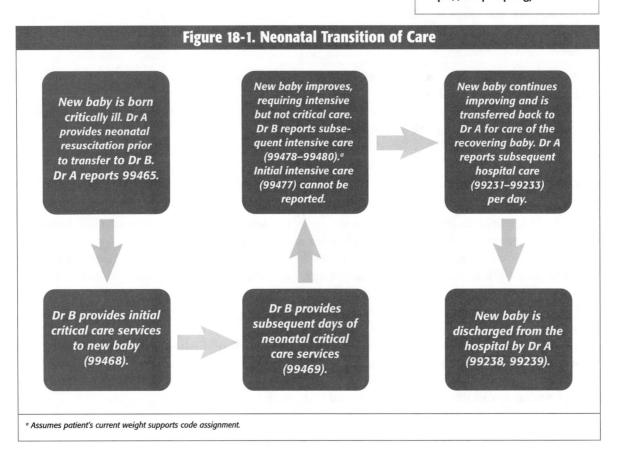

Figure 18-1. Neonatal Transition of Care

New baby is born critically ill. Dr A provides neonatal resuscitation prior to transfer to Dr B. Dr A reports 99465.

New baby improves, requiring intensive but not critical care. Dr B reports subsequent intensive care (99478–99480).ᵃ Initial intensive care (99477) cannot be reported.

New baby continues improving and is transferred back to Dr A for care of the recovering baby. Dr A reports subsequent hospital care (99231–99233) per day.

Dr B provides initial critical care services to new baby (99468).

Dr B provides subsequent days of neonatal critical care services (99469).

New baby is discharged from the hospital by Dr A (99238, 99239).

ᵃ *Assumes patient's current weight supports code assignment.*

Emergency Medical Services Supervision and Patient Transport

Direction of Emergency Medical Services

99288   Physician or other qualified health care professional direction of emergency medical systems (EMS) emergency care, advanced life support

Guidelines for reporting code 99288 (direction of emergency medical systems emergency care, advanced life support) by physician or QHP include

⁕ May be reported by any physician of any specialty or QHP when advanced life support services are provided via 2-way voice communications (eg, cardiac and/or pulmonary resuscitation; administration of IV fluids, antibiotics, or surfactant).

⁕ This code reflects all the services provided by the directing physician and is not based on any time require-ments. Code 99288 may be reported when less than 16 minutes is spent in physician non–face-to-face supervision of inter-facility transport of a critically ill or injured pediatric patient (ie, requirements for reporting 99485 are not met).

⁕ The directing physician should maintain documentation of the times of all contacts, orders, and/or directions for treatment or management of the patient.

⁕ Services or procedures performed by emergency medical services (EMS) personnel are not reported by the physician because he or she was not physically present.

⁕ When an advance practice professional provides and reports face-to-face services during transport, the physi-cian would not report 99288.

⁕ The appropriate diagnoses are linked to the service.

⁕ If, after directing EMS personnel, the physician performs the initial critical care, code 99468 (initial inpa-tient neonatal critical care) would also be reported with modifier 25 appended to indicate that 2 separate and distinct E/M services were provided by the same physician on the same day of service.

There is no assigned Medicare relative value unit (RVU) to this service, so it is "carrier priced" and payments will vary by payer.

Medicare considers code 99288 a bundled service and does not pay separately for the service. Check with your state Medicaid program and other payers to determine their coverage policy.

See the Non–face-to-face Pediatric Critical Care Patient Transport section later in this chapter for discussion of physician non–face-to-face supervision of inter-facility transport of a critically ill or injured pediatric patient 24 months or younger (99485, 99486).

Pediatric Critical Care Patient Transport

Face-to-face Critical Care Patient Transport

99466   Critical care face-to-face services, during an interfacility transport of critically ill or critically injured pediatric patient, 24 months of age or younger; first 30–74 minutes of hands-on care during transport

99467   each additional 30 minutes (List separately in addition to code 99466)

Codes 99466 and 99467 are used to report the physical attendance and direct face-to-face care provided by a physician or QHP during the inter-facility transport of a critically ill or injured patient aged 24 months or younger.

⁕ The patient's condition must meet the *CPT*® definition for critical care.

⁕ Face-to-face time begins when the physician or practitioner assumes primary responsibility for the patient at the referring hospital or facility and ends when the receiving hospital or facility accepts responsibility for the patient's care. Only the time the physician spends in direct face-to-face contact with the patient during transport should be reported.

⁕ Less than 30 minutes of face-to-face time cannot be reported.

⁕ Code 99466 is used to report the first 30 to 74 minutes of physician face-to-face time with the critically ill or injured patient during the transport.

⁕ Code 99467 is used to report each additional 30 minutes of physician face-to-face time of critical care pro-vided on the same day of service.

⁕ Codes include the bundled services listed in **Table 18-1**. Codes 99466 and 99467 may be reported sepa-rately from any other procedures or services that are not bundled and performed on the date of transfer. The time involved in performing any procedures that are not bundled and reported separately should not be included in the face-to-face transport time.

☀ Procedures or services that are performed by other members of the transport team with the physical presence, participation, and supervision of the accompanying physician may be reported by the physician. Documentation must support the physician's participation.

☀ Medical record documentation must include the total face-to-face time spent with the patient, the critical nature of the patient's condition, and any performed procedures that are not bundled.

☀ The pediatric critical care transport codes are preadmission codes and may be reported in addition to neonatal (99468) or pediatric (99471) initial-day critical care codes. For payers that have adopted NCCI edits, modifier 25 is required to indicate the significant and separately identifiable E/M services. Append modifier 25 to code 99466 when reporting in conjunction with daily critical care codes.

☀ Face-to-face critical care services provided during an inter-facility transport to a child older than 24 months are reported with hourly critical care codes (99291 and 99292).

☀ If an NNP employed by the neonatal group is on the transport team, the NNP may report codes 99466 and 99467 if independent billing by an NNP is allowed by the state and the activities are covered in the scope of practice. The neonatologist from that same group would not report codes 99485 and 99486 (physician direction of pediatric critical care transport) or 99288 (physician direction of EMS emergency care). The facility (hospital) could also report these services if the NNPs are employed by the hospital. In this case, the neonatologist would report codes 99485 and 99486.

☀ CPT® does not include specific codes for face-to-face transport of a patient when criteria for critical care are not met. When face-to-face care during transport of a patient is medically necessary but not critical care, report code 99499 (unlisted E/M service).

Example

➤ **A 3,000-g, 38-weeks' gestation neonate born at a community hospital with meconium aspiration syndrome requires ventilator care and transport to a Level III unit where extracorporeal membrane oxygenation (ECMO) is also available.** The receiving neonatologist accompanies the transport nurse and therapist. Ground transport takes 40 minutes one way. On arrival, the neonatologist spends 60 minutes face-to-face evaluating and stabilizing the newborn. The newborn is intubated, surfactant is administered, umbilical venous and arterial catheters are inserted, and parents are counseled. The neonatologist spends 5 minutes intubating and administering the surfactant and 20 minutes placing the umbilical venous and arterial catheters. The newborn is then transferred to the neonatal transport van and back to the receiving nursery. Total time from bedside back to the receiving nursery is 60 minutes. Frequent assessments and alterations in drugs, fluids, and ventilator settings are performed on the transport back. The neonatologist spent a total of 120 minutes of face-to-face critical care time with the neonate; 25 minutes is subtracted for the performance of non-bundled procedures. The neonatologist continues care of the newborn in the NICU.

> **99466 25**
> **99467 25** × 1 unit
> **31500** (endotracheal intubation, emergency)
> **94610** (surfactant administration)
> **36510** (catheterization of umbilical vein)
> **36660** (catheterization of umbilical artery)
> **99468 25** (initial neonatal critical care)

Modifier 25 is appended to each of the services to designate a significant and separately identifiable E/M service provided by the same physician on the same date of service. Endotracheal intubation is bundled with daily neonatal critical care but is separately reported when provided during transport of the critically ill or injured neonate.

Non–face-to-face Pediatric Critical Care Patient Transport

#99485   Supervision by a control physician of interfacility transport care of the critically ill or critically injured pediatric patient, 24 months of age or younger, includes two-way communication with transport team before transport, at the referring facility and during the transport, including data interpretation and report; first 30 minutes

#99486   each additional 30 minutes (List separately in addition to code 99485)

Code 99485 is used to report the first 30 minutes of a control physician's non–face-to-face supervision of inter-facility critical care transport of a patient 24 months or younger, which includes all 2-way communication between the control physician and the specialized transport team prior to transport, at the referring facility, and during transport to the receiving facility. Each additional 30-minute period of communication is reported with add-on code 99486. These codes do not include communication between the control physician and referring facility before or following patient transport.

- The patient's condition must meet the *CPT*® definition of critical care.
- Only report for patients 24 months or younger who are critically ill or injured.
- The control physician does not report any services provided by the specialized transport team.
- The control physician only reports cumulative time spent communicating with the specialty transport team members during an inter-facility transport. Communication between the control physician and the referring facility before or following patient transport is not counted.
- Reportable time begins with the initial discussions with the transport team, including discussions of best mode of transport and strategies for therapy on arrival. Time ends when the patient's care is handed over to the receiving facility team.
- Code 99485 is used to report the first 16 to 45 minutes of direction on a given date and should only be used once even if time spent by the physician is discontinuous.
- Code 99486 is used in conjunction with 99485 for each additional 30 minutes.
- Do not report 99485 or 99486 for services of 15 minutes or less or any time when a provider from the same group is also reporting 99466 or 99467.
- Time spent with the individual patient's transport team and reviewing data submissions should be recorded. Time spent discussing the patient with the referring physician or facility is not counted.
- Services represented by codes 99485 and 99486 are preadmission services and may be reported by the same or different individual of the same specialty and same group when neonatal or pediatric critical care services (99468–99476) are reported for the same patient on the same day.

Example

➤ **A community pediatrician asks to refer a newborn with cyanosis, tachycardia, and possible congenital cardiac disease.** The neonatologist dispatches the transport team, consisting of a hospital-employed transport nurse and a respiratory therapist. On the trip to the referring hospital, the neonatologist converses by telephone for 10 minutes with the team, explaining the newborn's condition and formulating an initial treatment plan. After arrival, the nurse evaluates the neonate and telephones the neonatologist to discuss the findings. The decision is made to provide prostaglandin to maintain ductal patency and avoid oxygen therapy. Because of the critical nature of the newborn, the neonatologist elects to remain on the telephone until therapy is completed (15 minutes). The team then leaves the referring hospital. On the return trip, telephone contact lasting 10 minutes is again made to update the physician on the neonate's condition, vital signs, and overall physical status. The team then completes the transport without further incident.

The neonatologist spent a total of 35 minutes in direct 2-way telephone communication with the team in 3 discrete episodes. The neonatologist carefully documents in the medical record the time spent and what decisions were made in each contact. Code 99485 is used to report this service.

Total Body Systemic and Selective Head Hypothermia

99184   Initiation of selective head or total body hypothermia in the critically ill neonate, includes appropriate patient selection by review of clinical, imaging and laboratory data, confirmation of esophageal temperature probe location, evaluation of amplitude EEG, supervision of controlled hypothermia, and assessment of patient tolerance of cooling
(Do not report 99184 more than once per hospital stay)

Examples

➤ **A term neonate born with evidence of hypoxic-ischemic encephalopathy is admitted to the NICU and receives critical care services.** Laboratory, EEG, blood gas, and imaging studies confirm the neonate meets objective criteria for *total body cooling.* Continuous total body cooling is undertaken.

Code 99184 is reported for total body systemic hypothermia in addition to 99468, initial day of neonatal critical care.

➤ **A term neonate born with evidence of hypoxic-ischemic encephalopathy is admitted to the NICU and receives critical care services.** Laboratory, EEG, blood gas, and imaging studies confirm the neonate meets objective criteria for *selective head cooling.* Continuous selective head cooling is undertaken.

Code 99184 is reported for selective head hypothermia in addition to 99468, initial day of neonatal critical care.

When total body systemic or selective head hypothermia is used in treatment of a critically ill neonate, code 99184 represents the work of initiating the service.

Documentation for use of total body systemic hypothermia and selective head hypothermia should include the neonatal criteria that support initiating this service.

◉ During either cooling approach, monitoring includes
  ❖ Radiographic confirmation of core temperature probe
  ❖ Continuous core temperature assessment and adjustment
  ❖ Repeated assessment of skin integrity
  ❖ Recurrent objective evaluation of evolving neurologic changes (eg, Sarnat score), which may also include assessment of continuous amplitude EEG monitoring
◉ In addition, cooling-related laboratory evaluations are required to monitor for cooling-specific complications, including metabolic and coagulation alterations.

Extracorporeal Membrane Oxygenation (ECMO) or Extracorporeal Life Support (ECLS) Services

Prolonged ECMO and extracorporeal life support (ECLS) services provide cardiac and/or respiratory support, allowing the heart and/or lungs to rest and recover when sick or injured. These services commonly involve multiple physicians and supporting health care personnel to manage each patient. Extracorporeal membrane oxygenation and ECLS codes differentiate components of initiation and daily management of ECMO and ECLS from daily management of a patient's overall medical condition.

These services include cannula insertion (33951–33956), ECMO or ECLS initiation (33946 or 33947), daily ECMO or ECLS management (33948 or 33949), repositioning of the ECMO or ECLS cannula(e) (33957–33964), and cannula removal (33965–33986). Each physician providing part of the ECMO/ECLS services may report the services they provide except when prohibited by *CPT®* instruction (eg, cannula repositioning is not reported by the same or another physician on the same date as initiation of ECMO/ECLS).

Example

➤ **Venoarterial ECMO is initiated for a patient with cardiac and respiratory failure.** Physician A inserts the cannulae. Physician B manages the initial transition to ECMO, including working with physician A, ECMO specialists, and others to initiate an ongoing assessment of anticoagulation, venous return, cannula positioning, and optimal flow. Physician B is also providing daily management of the patient's overall care. When ECMO is discontinued, physician A returns and removes the cannulae.

Physician A will report codes for insertion and removal of the ECMO cannulae (eg, 33952 and 33966). Physician B will report initiation of venoarterial ECMO (33947), the appropriate hospital and/or critical care codes for overall management of the patient for each day provided (eg, 99291, 99292, or 99231–99233), and daily management of ECMO (33949) for each day provided.

ECMO/ECLS Initiation and Daily Management

33946	Extracorporeal membrane oxygenation (ECMO)/extracorporeal life support (ECLS) provided by physician; initiation, venovenous
33947	initiation, venoarterial
33948	daily management, each day, venovenous
33949	daily management, each day, venoarterial

Initiation of the ECMO or ECLS circuit and setting parameters (33946, 33947) involves determining the necessary ECMO or ECLS device components, blood flow, gas exchange, and other necessary parameters to manage the circuit.

Daily care for a patient on ECMO or ECLS includes managing the ECMO or ECLS circuit and related patient issues. These services may be performed by one physician while another physician manages the overall patient medical condition and underlying disorders. Regardless of the patient's condition, the basic management of ECMO and ECLS is similar.

- Do not report modifier 63 (procedure performed on infants less than 4 kg) when reporting codes 33946–33949.
- The physician reporting daily ECMO or ECLS oversees the interaction of the circuit with the patient, management of blood flow, oxygenation, carbon dioxide clearance by the membrane lung, systemic response, anticoagulation and treatment of bleeding, cannula positioning, alarms and safety, and weaning the patient from the ECMO or ECLS circuit when heart and/or lung function has sufficiently recovered.
- Daily management of the patient may be separately reported using the relevant hospital observation services, hospital inpatient services, or critical care E/M codes (99218–99220, 99221–99223, 99231–99233, 99234–99236, 99291, 99292, 99468–99480).
- Daily management (33948 or 33949) or cannula repositioning (33957–33959, 33962–33964) may not be reported on the same date as initiation (33946 or 33947) by the same or different physician.

ECMO/ECLS Cannula Insertion, Repositioning, and Removal

Table 18-5. Insertion of ECMO or ECLS Cannula(e)			
ECMO/ECLS Provided by Physician	**Birth Through 5 Years of Age**	**6 Years and Older**	**Do Not Report With**
Insertion of peripheral (arterial and/or venous) cannula(e), percutaneous (includes fluoroscopic guidance when performed)	33951	33952	33957–33964
Insertion of peripheral (arterial and/or venous) cannula(e), open	33953	33954	33957–33964, 34812, 34820, 34834
Insertion of central cannula(e) by sternotomy or thoracotomy	33955	33956	33957–33964, 32100, 39010

Abbreviations: ECLS, extracorporeal life support; ECMO, extracorporeal membrane oxygenation.

Chapter 18: Critical and Intensive Care

Table 18-6. Repositioning ECMO or ECLS Cannula(e)[a]

ECMO/ECLS Provided by Physician	Birth Through 5 Years of Age	6 Years and Older	Do Not Report With
Reposition peripheral (arterial and/or venous) cannula(e), percutaneous (includes fluoroscopic guidance when performed)	33957	33958	33946, 33947, 34812, 34820, 34834
Reposition peripheral (arterial and/or venous) cannula(e), open (includes fluoroscopic guidance when performed)	33959	33962	33946, 33947, 34812, 34820, 34834
Reposition of central cannula(e) by sternotomy or thoracotomy (includes fluoroscopic guidance when performed)	33963	33964	33946, 33947, 32100, 39010

Abbreviations: ECLS, extracorporeal life support; ECMO, extracorporeal membrane oxygenation.

[a] Repositioning of cannula(e) at the same session, as insertion is not separately reported.

Table 18-7. Removal of ECMO or ECLS Cannula(e)[a]

ECMO/ECLS Provided by Physician	Birth Through 5 Years of Age	6 Years and Older	Do Not Report With
Removal of peripheral (arterial and/or venous) cannula(e), percutaneous	33965	33966	N/A
Removal of peripheral (arterial and/or venous) cannula(e), open	33969	33984	34812, 34820, 34834, 35201, 35206, 35211, 35216, 35226
Removal of central cannula(e) by sternotomy or thoracotomy	33985	33986	35201, 35206, 35211, 35216, 35226

Abbreviations: ECLS, extracorporeal life support; ECMO, extracorporeal membrane oxygenation; N/A, not applicable.

[a] Report only the insertion when cannula(e) is replaced in the same vessel.

Codes for insertion, repositioning, and removal of ECMO and ECLS are reported based on the patient's age, with separate codes for procedures on newborns through 5 years of age and on patients 6 years and older. Codes for these services are shown in **tables 18-5, 18-6,** and **18-7.** While typically only performed by surgeons, other pediatric providers may perform as well.

- Do not separately report repositioning of the ECMO or ECLS cannula(e) (33957–33964) at the same session as insertion (33951–33956).
- Fluoroscopic guidance used for cannula(e) repositioning (33957–33964) is included in the procedure when performed and should not be separately reported.
- Report replacement of ECMO or ECLS cannula(e) in the same vessel using the insertion code (33951–33956) only.
- If a cannula(e) is removed from one vessel and a new cannula(e) is placed in a different vessel, report the appropriate cannula(e) removal (33965–33986) and insertion (33951–33956) codes.
- Extensive repair or replacement of an artery may be additionally reported (eg, 35226, 35286, 35371, 35665).
- Direct anastomosis of a prosthetic graft to the artery sidewall to facilitate arterial perfusion for ECMO or ECLS is separately reported with code 33987 in addition to codes 33953–33956.

+33987   Arterial exposure with creation of graft conduit (eg, chimney graft) to facilitate arterial perfusion for ECMO/ECLS (List separately in addition to code for primary procedure)

> ||||||||| **Coding Pearl** |||||||||
>
> Each physician providing a part of extracorporeal membrane oxygenation/extracorporeal life support services may report the part they provided except as prohibited by *Current Procedural Terminology®* instruction.

Do not report 33987 in conjunction with 34833 (open iliac artery exposure with creation of conduit for delivery of aortic or iliac endovascular prosthesis, by abdominal or retroperitoneal incision, unilateral).

Car Seat/Bed Testing

▲94780   Car seat/bed testing for airway integrity, for infants through 12 months of age, with continual clinical staff observation and continuous recording of pulse oximetry, heart rate and respiratory rate, with interpretation and report; 60 minutes

+▲94781   each additional full 30 minutes (List separately in addition to 94780.)

Neonates who required critical care during their initial hospital stay are most often those patients who require monitoring to determine if they may be safely transported in a car seat or must be transported in a car bed. While these codes are bundled under neonatal and pediatric critical and intensive care codes, these services most often take place when a neonate is about to go home and, therefore, can be reported if hospital care services (99231–99233) or hospital discharge services (99238, 99239) are being reported instead.

To report codes 94780 and 94781, the following conditions must be met:

- The patient must be an infant (12 months or younger). Assessment after the patient is 29 days or older may be necessary.
- Continual clinical staff observation with continuous recording of pulse oximetry, heart rate, and respiratory rate is required.
- Inpatient or office-based services are reported.
- Vital signs and observations must be reviewed and interpreted and a written report generated by the physician.
- Codes are reported based on the total observation time spent and documented.
- These codes may be reported with discharge day management (99238, 99239), normal newborn care services (99460, 99462, 99463), or subsequent hospital care codes (99231–99233).
- Codes 94780 and 94781 may not be reported with neonatal or pediatric critical or intensive care services (99468–99472, 99477–99480).
- If less than 60 minutes is spent in the procedure, code 94780 may not be reported.
- Each additional full 30 minutes (ie, not less than 90 minutes) is reported with code 94781.
- Do not include the time of car seat/bed testing in time attributed to discharge day management services (99238, 99239).

Examples

➤ A neonate born at 26 weeks' gestation requires a car seat test on the date of discharge from the hospital.

Code 94780 is reported with hospital discharge management code 99238 or 99239.

➤ A neonate born at 26 weeks' gestation requires a car seat test prior to discharge from the hospital. The newborn has received 60 minutes of testing reported with 94780 and now receives an additional 30 minutes.

Codes 94780 and 94781 are reported with a subsequent hospital care code (99231–99233) or a discharge day management code (99238 or 99239).

Sedation

Refer to Chapter 19, Common Surgical Procedures and Sedation in Facility Settings, for specific guidelines for reporting sedation services, including moderate (conscious) sedation (99151–99157) and deep sedation.

Resources

Coding Education

American Academy of Pediatrics Section on Neonatal-Perinatal Medicine coding trainers are available to provide coding education through local educational seminars and continuing education events. At least one coding trainer is appointed in each district. Each trainer is equipped with educational materials that can be used as an important resource for your state or hospital. Contact section manager Jim Couto (jcouto@aap.org) for additional information about these valuable services.

The AAP Section on Neonatal-Perinatal Medicine, in conjunction with state chapters and councils of the AAP, has developed strategies that have been successful in addressing payment concerns for neonatal care. Contact your state chapter, its pediatric council, your section district AAP Executive Committee representative, a neonatal trainer, or the AAP Committee on Coding and Nomenclature for assistance in addressing any payment inequities for neonatal services in your state.

Most of the codes used to report services for the intensive and critically ill neonate are reported based on the severity of the condition of the neonate and the intensity of the services that are required and performed. It is important to remember that specific therapies or diagnoses do not always equate to a specific level of care and, therefore, documentation of the critical status of the newborn is required.

Resource-Based Relative Value Scale

The 2018 RVUs for the services described in this chapter are included in the Resource-Based Relative Value Scale (RBRVS) brochure found at www.aap.org/cfp, or go to www.cms.gov to find the current year RVUs and Medicare conversion factor. At time of publication, the 2019 RVUs were not available; they are typically published in November for the upcoming year. The RBRVS brochure is updated accordingly.

Physician Work

The times for E/M services most commonly provided to newborns (typical time for neonatal services) based on RUC survey results for 2011 are provided in **Table 18-8**. Although not exact or applicable for every patient, they are the average times (in minutes) spent by neonatologists for the typical or average patient. This is an excellent and quick internal audit mechanism to judge the adequacy of your coding or nursery coverage.

Table 18-8. RUC Survey Times for Subsequent Hospital Care and Critical Care				
Code	**Preservice (min)**	**Intraservice (min)**	**Post-service (min)**	**Total RUC Time (min)**
99231	5	10	5	20
99232	10	20	10	40
99233	10	30	15	55
99291	15	40	15	70
99292	–	30	–	30
99468	45	180	49	274
99469	–	128	–	128
99471	30	180	30	240
99472	20	90	30	140
99475	30	105	30	165
99476	20	65	20	105
99477	30	77.5	40	147.5
99478	10	30	20	60
99479	10	30	15	55
99480	15	30	15	60

Abbreviation: RUC, American Medical Association/Specialty Society Relative Value Scale Update Committee.

Common Surgical Procedures and Sedation in Facility Settings

Contents

Chapter 19: Common Surgical Procedures and Sedation in Facility Settings

Surgical Package Rules

Current Procedural Terminology (CPT®) surgical codes (10004–69990) are packaged or global codes.

* Surgical codes include certain anesthesia services and the associated preoperative and postoperative care.
* The *CPT* definition of a surgical package differs from the Centers for Medicare & Medicaid Services (CMS) definition of a global surgical period, as seen in **Table 19-1**.
* Most state Medicaid programs follow the CMS definition.
* Each commercial insurance company will have its own policy for billing and payment of global surgical care, and most will designate a specific number of follow-up days for surgical procedures.
* The CMS-designated global periods for each *CPT* procedure code can be found on the Medicare Resource-Based Relative Value Scale Physician Fee Schedule at https://www.cms.gov/medicare/medicare-fee-for-service-payment/physicianfeesched.

When determining the postoperative period, the day after surgery is day 1 of a 10- or 90-day period.

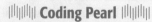 **Coding Pearl** ||||||||

Most state Medicaid programs follow the Centers for Medicare & Medicaid Services surgical package guidelines.

Table 19-1. Comparison of the *Current Procedural Terminology*® and Centers for Medicare & Medicaid Services Surgical Packages

CPT Definition of Surgical Package	CMS Medicare Global Surgery
Anesthesia Includes local infiltration, regional block, or topical anesthesia	Same
Preoperative Care <ul><li>Includes E/M service(s) subsequent to the decision for surgery (eg, assessing the site and condition, explanation of procedure, obtaining informed consent) on the day before and/or on the date of the procedure (including history and physical).</li><li>When the initial decision to perform surgery is made on the day prior to or on the day of surgery, the appropriate-level E/M visit may be reported separately with modifier 57 (decision for surgery) appended. This modifier shows the payer that the E/M service was necessary to make the decision for surgery (ie, not the routine preoperative evaluation).</li><li>When an E/M service performed on the day of the procedure is unrelated to the decision to perform surgery and is significant and distinct from the usual preoperative care associated with the procedure, it may be reported with modifier 25 (significant, separately identifiable E/M service by the same physician on the same day of the procedure or other service) appended.</li><li>Medical record documentation must support that the service was significant, separately identifiable, and medically necessary or was performed prior to the decision to perform the procedure.</li><li>Different diagnoses are not required when reporting an E/M visit and procedure.</li></ul>	Same with following exceptions: <ul><li>For "minor" procedures (ie, procedures assigned a 0- or 10-day global period or endoscopies), the E/M visit on the date of the procedure is considered a routine part of the procedure regardless of whether it is prior or subsequent to the decision for surgery. In these cases, modifier 57 is not recognized.</li><li>An E/M code may be reported on the same day as a minor surgical procedure only when a significant, separately identifiable E/M service is performed with modifier 25 appended to the E/M code.</li><li>When the initial decision to perform a major surgical procedure (ie, procedures assigned a 90-day global period) is made on the day prior to or on the day of a procedure, the E/M service may be reported appended with modifier 57. Medical record documentation should support that the decision for surgery was made during the encounter and that additional time was spent in performing counseling of the risks, benefits, and outcomes.</li></ul>

Table 19-1. Comparison of the *Current Procedural Terminology*® and Centers for Medicare & Medicaid Services Surgical Packages (*continued*)

CPT Definition of Surgical Package	CMS Medicare Global Surgery
Postoperative Care ◦ Includes all associated typical postoperative care (eg, dictation of progress notes; counseling with the patient, family, and/or other physicians; writing orders; evaluating the patient in the postanesthesia recovery area). ◦ Care for therapeutic surgical procedures includes only the care that is usually part of the surgical service. ◦ Care for diagnostic procedures (eg, endoscopies, arthroscopies, injection procedures for radiography) includes only the care that is related to the recovery from the diagnostic procedure. ◦ Care resulting from complications of surgery. ◦ Any complications, exacerbations, recurrence, treatment of unrelated diseases or injuries, or the presence of other diseases or injuries that require additional services may be reported separately.	Same ◦ Includes all additional medical or surgical services required of the surgeon during the postoperative period of the surgery because of complications that do not require additional trips to the operating room. ◦ Does not include treatment for the underlying condition or an added course of treatment that is not part of normal recovery from surgery. (See modifiers 24, 58, and 79.)
Postoperative Days Does not include any specific number of postoperative days.	◦ Designates specific postoperative periods for certain procedure codes (0 days, 10 days, 90 days). Other codes are designated YYY, which means the postoperative period is set by the carrier. There are no associated postoperative days included in the payment for codes assigned with status codes XXX (the global concept does not apply) or ZZZ (assigned to an add-on code for a service that is always related to another service to which the global period is assigned). ◦ In addition to the *CPT* code, physicians use modifier 78 for return to the operating room for a related procedure during a postoperative period. This includes return to the operating room for treatment of complications of the first procedure. ◦ For return to the operating room for staged or more extensive procedures and therapeutic procedures following a diagnostic procedure, append modifier 58. ◦ Report procedures during the postoperative period that are unrelated and not due to complications of the original procedure with modifier 79 and unrelated E/M services with modifier 24 (documentation is typically required prior to payment).

Abbreviations: CMS, Centers for Medicare & Medicaid Services; CPT, Current Procedural Terminology; *E/M, evaluation and management.*

Reporting Postoperative Care

- Report *CPT*® code **99024** (postoperative follow-up visit) for follow-up care provided during the global surgery period. Reporting of inpatient or observation follow-up visits is typically not required.
  - ❖ Reporting code **99024** allows a practice to track the number of visits performed by individuals during the postoperative period of specific procedures; calculate office overhead expenses (eg, supplies, staff, physician time) associated with the procedure; and potentially use the data to negotiate higher payment rates.
  - ❖ Payers track the postoperative care provided. If a physician is not providing or reporting the postoperative care typically performed for a procedure, payers may reduce payment for the surgical service because payment includes postoperative care as part of the procedure.
- When the physician who performed the procedure provides an unrelated evaluation and management (E/M) service during the postoperative period, modifier **24** (unrelated E/M service by the same physician during a postoperative period) should be appended to the E/M service code.
- When physicians from different practices perform part of a surgical package, the procedure should be reported with modifier **54** (surgical care only), **56** (preoperative management only), or **55** (postoperative management only). These situations require communication among the surgeon, the physician providing preoperative or postoperative care, and their respective billing personnel to ensure accurate reporting and payment. (See Chapter 2, Modifiers and Coding Edits, for a more detailed description of modifiers. For critical care following surgery, see the Patients Critically Ill After Surgery section in Chapter 18, Critical and Intensive Care.)
- When a physician other than the surgeon provides unrelated services to a patient during the postoperative period, the services are reported without a modifier. Despite the use of different National Provider Identifiers and diagnosis codes, some payers with assigned follow-up surgical periods will deny the service. The claim should be appealed for payment with a letter advising the payer that the service was unrelated to any surgery.

> ||||||||| **Coding Pearl** |||||||||
>
> Payers may reduce payment of a surgical procedure if the physician does not report code **99024**.

Multiple Procedures on the Same Date

Often, multiple, separately reportable services are provided in one session or on one date of service. However, it is important to recognize which surgical services are considered a component of another procedure and which are separately reported.

- It is not appropriate to report multiple Healthcare Common Procedure Coding System (HCPCS)/*CPT* codes when a single, comprehensive HCPCS/*CPT* code describes the procedures performed. For example, code **42820** describes tonsillectomy and adenoidectomy in a patient younger than 12 years. It would not be appropriate to separately report **42825** (tonsillectomy) and **42830** (adenoidectomy).
- Surgical access (eg, laparotomy) is integral to more comprehensive procedures (eg, appendectomy) and not separately reported.
- When the surgical approach fails, report only the code for the approach that resulted in the completed procedure. For example, if laparoscopy fails and an open approach is used to complete the procedure, report only the open procedure.
- It is advisable to adopt a process for checking the National Correct Coding Initiative (NCCI) edits prior to submitting multiple procedure codes for services on the same date, as the NCCI edits are used by many payers. For Medicaid, the NCCI manual is also informative regarding correct reporting and use of modifiers to override NCCI edits. See Chapter 2, Modifiers and Coding Edits, for more information on the NCCI.

One designation in *CPT*® helps identify procedures that are commonly performed as an integral component of another procedure. The parenthetical comment "(separate procedure)" follows the code descriptor for these services. Services designated as a separate procedure should not be reported in addition to the code for the total procedure or service of which they are considered an integral component. A procedure or service that is designated as a separate procedure may be carried out independently or considered to be unrelated or distinct from

Chapter 19: Common Surgical Procedures and Sedation in Facility Settings other procedures/services provided at that time and, in such cases, may be the only code reported or may be reported in addition to other procedures/services by appending modifier 59 (distinct procedural service).

When more than one procedure/service is performed on the same date, same session, or during a postoperative period, several *CPT* modifiers may apply. Modifier 59 is often appended to surgical procedure codes to override payer edits that otherwise would not allow payment for services that may be components of other services. It is important to carefully consider whether other modifiers are more appropriate (eg, 50, bilateral service; an anatomic modifier such as E4, lower right eyelid) to indicate a distinct service. See also modifiers XE (separate encounter), XP (separate provider), XS (separate structure), and XU (unusual nonoverlapping service) discussed in Chapter 2, Modifiers and Coding Edits.

Increased or Decreased Procedural Services

Increased Procedural Service

Modifier 22 (increased procedural service) may be appended to the code for a surgical procedure when the work required to provide the service was *significantly greater* than typically required for that procedure. To substantiate modifier 22, documentation must support that the procedure was more difficult due to one or more of the following conditions:

- Increased intensity or time
- Technical difficulty
- The severity of the patient's condition
- Significantly increased physical and mental effort

Example

➤ **An adolescent undergoes shoulder arthroscopy with capsulorrhaphy repair of a Bankart lesion and a Hill-Sachs lesion.** The surgeon reports

29806 22   Arthroscopy, shoulder, surgical; capsulorrhaphy

Teaching Point: Because the work of the procedure was significantly increased by repair of 2 lesions rather than the typical posterior capsulorrhaphy, modifier 22 is appropriately appended.

Procedures Performed on Infants Less Than 4 kg

Modifier 63 is used to identify procedures performed on neonates and infants with present body weight of up to 4 kg. This modifier signals significantly increased complexity and physician or other qualified health care professional (QHP) work commonly associated with these patients.

- Modifier 63 may only be appended to procedures/services listed in the 20100–69990 code series. This does not apply to E/M, anesthesia, radiology, pathology/laboratory, or services listed in the Medicine section of *CPT*®.
- Append modifier 63 to codes for procedures performed on these infants only when there is no instruction prohibiting reporting. Services that cannot be reported with modifier 63 are those that have been valued based on the intensity of the service in patients weighing less than 4 kg. See "Summary of *CPT* Codes Exempt from Modifier 63" in your *CPT* reference for a list of codes exempt from modifier 63.
- Payer acceptance of modifier 63 may be limited to specific procedures. Verify policies of individual health plans for reporting this modifier.

Examples

➤ **An infant weighing 3 kg undergoes transventricular valvotomy of the pulmonary valve.** The physician reports

33470   Valvotomy, pulmonary valve, closed heart; transventricular

Teaching Point: The parenthetical instruction below code 33470 ("Do not report modifier 63 in conjunction with 33470") prohibits reporting modifier 63, including when this procedure is performed on an infant weighing less than 4 kg.

➤ **A 13-day-old weighing 2.4 kg requires central venous access.** A catheter is inserted via the subclavian vein and terminates in the right atrium. The physician reports

36555 63 Insertion of non-tunneled centrally inserted central venous catheter; younger than 5 years of age

Teaching Point: The patient weighed less than 4 kg, and the procedure is not listed as modifier 63 exempt. Therefore, modifier 63 is appropriately appended to indicate the increased intensity and/or work of performing the procedure on the neonate.

Reporting Terminated or Partial Procedures

When a procedure is started but cannot be completed due to extenuating circumstances, physicians should consider the individual situation, including the reason for termination of the procedure and the amount of work that was performed, when determining how to report the service rendered.

When a procedure was performed but not entirely successful (eg, portion of foreign body removed), it may be appropriate to report the procedure code that represents the work performed without modification. Only report reduced services (modifier 52) or discontinued procedure (modifier 53) when the service was significantly reduced from the typical service. (See Chapter 2, Modifiers and Coding Edits, for more information on modifiers.)

If the work performed prior to discontinuation was insignificant, it may be appropriate to not report the procedure. When not reporting the procedure, consider whether the level of a related E/M service was increased due to the complexity of medical decision-making (MDM) associated with the attempted procedure, any complicating factors, and the revised management or treatment plan.

> ⦙⦙⦙⦙⦙⦙ **Coding Pearl** ⦙⦙⦙⦙⦙⦙
>
> For more information on reporting discontinued or incomplete procedures, see "Reporting Terminated Procedural Services" in the November 2014 *AAP Pediatric Coding Newsletter* at http://coding.aap.org (subscription required).

Reporting by Assistant Surgeon

An assistant surgeon is a physician or QHP who provides active assistance in the performance of a procedure when clinically indicated (eg, technically complex procedure).

⦾ See the Assistant Surgeon in a Teaching Facility section later in this chapter for guidance on reporting assistant surgeon services by a physician in a teaching facility.

⦾ Global rules do not apply to assistant surgeon's services. Payment is based on a percentage of the fee schedule amount allowed for the procedure performed (eg, Medicare allows 16%).

⦾ Modifiers are appended to the code(s) for the procedure on the assistant's claim.

Modifiers for Reporting Assistant Surgeon Services	
80	Assistant surgeon (use for MD or DO)
81	Minimum assistant surgeon
82	Assistant surgeon (when qualified resident surgeon not available)
AS	Physician assistant, nurse practitioner, or clinical nurse specialist services for assistant at surgery

Chapter 19: Common Surgical Procedures and Sedation in Facility Settings

❖ Reductions for multiple procedures on the same date may apply.

❖ See individual payer policies for assistant at surgery, as many limit payment to only specific procedures and/or may require documentation substantiating the need for assistance.

❖ See Chapter 2, Modifiers and Coding Edits, for discussion of other surgical modifiers (eg, **62**, 2 surgeons; **66**, surgical team).

Physicians at Teaching Hospitals Guidelines for Billing Procedures

The CMS established and maintains guidelines for documentation and billing by teaching physicians. Physicians at Teaching Hospitals guidelines for billing procedures are less complex than those for billing E/M services. Guidelines specify that

❖ When a procedure is performed by a resident, teaching physician attendance and participation are required and must be documented.

❖ The level of participation required by the teaching physician depends on the type of procedure being performed.

❖ A resident, nurse, or teaching physician may document the teaching physician's attendance.

The rules for supervising physicians in teaching settings can be obtained on the CMS Web site at http://cms.hhs.gov/manuals/downloads/clm104c12.pdf, section 100.

Modifier **GC** (services have been performed by a resident under the direction of a teaching physician) must be appended to procedure codes for services performed by a resident under the direction of a teaching physician.

Minor Procedures

❖ The CMS defines a minor procedure as one taking *5 minutes or less* to complete with relatively little decision-making once the need for the procedure is determined.

❖ Minor procedures are usually assigned a 0- to 10-day global period.

❖ Teaching physicians may bill for a minor procedure when they personally perform the service or when a resident performs the service and they are present for the entire procedure.

❖ The resident may document the procedure but must attest to the teaching physician's presence.

Interpretation of Diagnostic Radiology and Other Diagnostic Tests

❖ The teaching physician may bill for interpretation of the diagnostic service if he or she interprets tests or reviews findings with the resident.

❖ Documentation must support a personal interpretation or a review of the resident's notes with indication of agreement with the resident's interpretation.

❖ Changes to the resident's interpretation must be documented.

Endoscopy

❖ The teaching physician must be present for the entire viewing starting at the time of insertion and ending at the time of removal of the endoscope.

❖ Viewing the procedure through a monitor located in another room does not meet the requirements for billing.

❖ The presence of the teaching physician must be documented in the medical record. The teaching physician's presence must be stated.

Surgery Other Than Minor Procedures

* The teaching physician must assume the responsibility of preoperative, operative, and postoperative care of the patient. He or she must be present during all critical and key portions (as determined by the teaching physician) of the procedure. For example, if opening or closing is not considered to be key or critical, the teaching physician does not need to be present.
* The teaching physician must be immediately available to furnish services during the entire procedure.
* If circumstances prevent the physician from being immediately available, arrangements must be made with another qualified surgeon to be immediately available to assist with the procedure.
* The physician's presence for single surgical procedures may be demonstrated in notes made by the teaching physician, resident, or nurse.
* When the teaching physician is present for the entire procedure, only the written attestation of his or her presence is required.
* If the teaching physician is present during only the key or critical portions of the surgery, documentation must indicate his or her presence at those portions of the procedure (the resident may still document the operative report).
* When billing for 2 overlapping (concurrent) surgeries, the teaching physician must be present for the key or critical portions of both procedures and must personally document his or her presence. The surgeon cannot be involved in a second case until all key or critical portions in the first case have been completed.
* Arrangements may be made with another qualified surgeon to be present at one of the surgeries. The name of the other surgeon who was immediately available during overlapping surgeries must be documented.

Complex or High-risk Surgeries and Procedures

* A complex procedure or surgery is usually assigned a 90-day global period or, in the case of diagnostic procedures (eg, transesophageal echocardiography), requires the direct or personal supervision of a physician.
* A teaching physician must be present with a resident for the entire procedure when billing for a service identified by the CMS or local policy as complex and requiring personal supervision by a physician.
* Documentation must support that the teaching physician was present.

Postoperative Care

* The teaching physician determines which postoperative visits are considered key or critical and require his or her presence.
* If the teaching physician is not providing postoperative care included in the global surgery package, he or she will report the procedure(s) with modifiers 54 (surgical care only) and 56 (preoperative management only).
* Postoperative care is reported by another physician with the same surgical procedure code with modifier 55 (postoperative management only).
* The surgeon and physician providing postoperative care must keep a copy of a written transfer agreement in the patient's medical record.

Assistant Surgeon in a Teaching Facility

Medicare will not pay for the services of assistants at surgery furnished in a teaching hospital that has a training program related to the medical specialty required for the surgical procedure and has a qualified resident available to perform the service. This policy may be applied by Medicaid and other payers.

* When the Medicare Physician Fee Schedule allows payment for an assistant surgeon and a physician assists a teaching physician because no qualified resident was available, modifier 82 (assistant surgeon [when qualified resident surgeon not available]) is appended to the code for the procedure performed on the assistant surgeon's claim.

Physicians at Teaching Hospitals Guidelines: Examples of Appropriate Documentation

Minor procedures	*"Dr Teaching Physician was present during the entire procedure."* –Nurse *"Dr Teaching Physician observed me performing this procedure."* –Dr Resident
Interpretation of diagnostic radiology and other diagnostic tests	*"I personally reviewed the MRI with Dr Resident and agree with his findings."* –Dr Teaching Physician *"I personally reviewed the CAT scan with Dr Resident. Findings are indicative of (insert)."* –Dr Teaching Physician
Endoscopy	*"I was present during the entire viewing of this endoscopy."* –Dr Teaching Physician
Surgery other than minor procedures	*"Dr Teaching Physician was present during entire surgery."* –Dr Resident *"I was present and observed Dr Resident perform the key portion of this procedure."* –Dr Teaching Physician
Complex or high-risk surgeries and procedures	*"I was physically present during this entire procedure with the exception of the [opening and/or closing], as that overlapped with the key portion of another case."* –Dr Teaching Physician *"Dr Y was immediately available during the overlapping portions of this case, which included [cite specifics]."* –Dr Teaching Physician

- The unavailability of a qualified resident surgeon is a prerequisite for use of modifier 82. Documentation must specify that no qualified resident was available or that there was no residency program related to the medical specialty required for the surgical procedure.
- This modifier is only used in teaching hospitals and only if there is no approved training program related to the medical specialty required for the surgical procedure or no qualified resident was available.

Burn Care

CPT® code 16000 (initial treatment, first-degree burn, where no more than local treatment is required) is reported when initial treatment is performed for the symptomatic relief of a first-degree burn that is characterized by erythema and tenderness.

16020   Dressings and/or debridement of partial-thickness burns, initial or subsequent; small or less than 5% total body (eg, finger)

16025   medium or 5%–10% total body surface area (eg, whole face or whole extremity)

16030   large or greater than 10% total body surface area (eg, more than 1 extremity)

16035   Escharotomy; initial incision

+16036   each additional incision

Codes 16020–16030

- Are used to report treatment of burns with dressings and/or debridement of small to large partial-thickness burns (second degree), whether initial or subsequent.
- Are reported based on the percentage of total body surface area (TBSA) affected.
- The percentage of TBSA involved must be calculated and documented when reporting care of second- or third-degree burns. Pediatric physicians often use the Lund-Browder classification method for estimating the TBSA based on patient age. (The Lund-Browder diagram and classification method table are in *CPT 2019 Professional Edition*.)

- An E/M visit (critical care, emergency department [ED] services, inpatient or outpatient E/M) may be provided for evaluation of the patient's injuries and management of complications such as dehydration, shock, infection, multiple organ dysfunction syndrome, electrolyte imbalance, cardiac arrhythmias, and respiratory distress. Report the E/M code appropriate to the setting and care provided with modifier **25** appended to indicate the significant, separately identifiable E/M service is medically indicated, performed, and documented in addition to the burn care.
- Other services (eg, pulmonary testing/therapy, physical/occupational therapy) and procedures (eg, mechanical ventilation, central line placement and hyperalimentation, grafting, hyperbaric oxygenation, dialysis, tracheotomy, pacemaker insertion) should be additionally reported beyond that of local treatment of the burned surface reported by codes **16000–16036**.
- Dressing application (whether initial or subsequent) and any associated debridement or curettement is inherent in codes **16020–16030**.
- It is advisable to use *International Classification of Diseases, 10th Revision, Clinical Modification* (ICD-10-CM) category **T31**, burns classified according to extent of body surface involved, as an additional code for reporting purposes when there is mention of a third-degree burn involving 20% or more of the body surface.

    Codes **16035** and **16036**
- Are reported per incision of eschar (dead tissue cast off from the surface of the skin in full-thickness burns)
- Are not reported based on anatomic site (ie, incisions of areas of eschar on multiple body areas are totaled and reported with 1 unit of code **16035** for the first incision only and 1 unit of code **16036** for each additional incision regardless of body area)

Surgical Preparation and Skin Grafting

15002	Surgical preparation or creation of recipient site by excision of open wounds, burn eschar, or scar (including subcutaneous tissues), or incisional release of scar contracture, trunk, arms, legs; first 100 sq cm or 1% of body area of infants and children
+15003	each additional 100 sq cm, or part thereof, or each additional 1% of body area of infants and children
15004	Surgical preparation or creation of recipient site by excision of open wounds, burn eschar, or scar (including subcutaneous tissues), or incisional release of scar contracture, face, scalp, eyelids, mouth, neck, ears, orbits, genitalia, hands, feet and/or multiple digits; first 100 sq cm or 1% of body area of infants and children
+15005	each additional 100 sq cm, or part thereof, or each additional 1% of body area of infants and children

- Surgical preparation codes **15002–15005** for skin replacement surgery describe removal of nonviable tissue to treat a burn, traumatic wound, or necrotizing infection. Report codes **15002–15005** for preparation of a clean and viable wound surface for placement of an autograft, flap, or skin substitute graft or for negative pressure wound therapy (NPWT). An incisional release of scar contracture may also be used to create a clean wound bed.
    - ❖ Code selection for surgical preparation codes is based on the location and size of the defect. The Application of Skin Replacement Codes by Size of the Recipient Area box demonstrates the age groups to which a code descriptor stating "100 sq cm or 1% of body area of infants and children" is applied when determining the involvement of body size. Measurements apply to the recipient area.

Application of Skin Replacement Codes by Size of the Recipient Area	
Adults and Children 10 Years and Older	**Infants and Children Younger Than 10 Years**
100 cm²	Percentages of body surface area

   - ❖ Codes **15002–15005** are always preparation for healing by primary intention. Do not report codes **15002–15005** for chronic wounds left to heal by secondary intention.
   - ❖ Report the appropriate codes when closure is achieved by adjacent tissue transfer (codes **14000–14061**) or a complex repair (codes **13100–13153**) rather than skin grafts or substitutes.

Example

➤ **An 8-year old patient undergoes surgical preparation for skin grafting of face, front of right arm, and right hand.** The body areas are measured as face, 4% of body area; right arm, 4%; and right hand, 1%.

ICD-10-CM	CPT®
Appropriate codes for burns by depth and body area	15004 (first 1% of body areas of face and hand) 15005 x 4 (each additional 1%) 15002 59 (first 1% body area of arm) 15003 x 3 (each additional 1%)

Teaching Point: Because the face and hand are both included in the descriptor for codes 15004 and 15005, the percentages of body areas are combined. Because the preparation of an area on the arm is described by codes 15002 and 15003, the body area of the arm is not added to that of the face and hand. Modifier 59 indicates that the procedure reported with code 15002 was performed on distinct body areas not described by code 15004.

❋ Codes 16020–16030 include the application of materials (eg, dressings) not described in codes 15100–15278 (skin grafts and substitutes). See code descriptors in **tables 19-2 through 19-5**.

❖ When burn wounds are treated and subsequently require skin grafting at the same session, report the burn code along with the appropriate skin graft code.

❖ A skin graft procedure may be performed as a staged procedure (delayed) with the preparation of the recipient site being performed on one date and the graft procedure being performed on another date. In these cases, modifier 58 (staged procedure) is appended to the grafting procedure code performed during the global period.

❖ The appropriate code for harvesting cultured skin autograft is 15040 (harvest of skin for tissue cultured skin autograft, 100 sq cm or less).

❖ Debridement is considered a separate procedure only when gross contamination requires prolonged cleansing, when appreciable amounts of devitalized or contaminated tissue are removed, or when debridement is carried out separately without immediate primary closure.

❖ The Application of Skin Replacement Codes by Size of the Recipient Area box earlier in this chapter demonstrates the age groups to which a code descriptor stating "100 sq cm or 1% of body area of infants and children" is applied when determining the involvement of body size. Measurements apply to the recipient area.

❖ Procedures involving the wrist and/or ankle are reported with codes that include "arm" or "leg" in the descriptor.

❖ The physician should select the skin substitute graft application code based on the actual size of the wound, and not the amount of the skin graft substitute used. The size of the wound should be measured after wound preparation has been performed.

❖ Skin substitute graft products are reported using HCPCS codes by the party supplying the products.

Table 19-2. Codes for Skin Autografts

Body Area[a]	Split-Thickness Autograft	Epidermal Autograft	Dermal Autograft
Trunk, arms, legs	15100 Split-thickness autograft, trunk, arms, legs; first 100 sq cm or less, or 1% of body area of infants and children (except 15050) +15101 each additional 100 sq cm, or each additional 1% of body area of infants and children, or part thereof	15110 Epidermal autograft, trunk, arms, legs; first 100 sq cm or less, or 1% of body area of infants and children +15111 each additional 100 sq cm, or each additional 1% of body area of infants and children, or part thereof	15130 Dermal autograft, trunk, arms, legs; first 100 sq cm or less, or 1% of body area of infants and children +15131 each additional 100 sq cm, or each additional 1% of body area of infants and children, or part thereof
Face, scalp, eyelids, mouth, neck, ears, orbits, genitalia, hands, feet, and/or multiple digits	15120 Split-thickness autograft, face, scalp, eyelids, mouth, neck, ears, orbits, genitalia, hands, feet, and/or multiple digits; first 100 sq cm or less, or 1% of body area of infants and children (except 15050) +15121 each additional 100 sq cm, or each additional 1% of body area of infants and children, or part thereof	15115 Epidermal autograft, face, scalp, eyelids, mouth, neck, ears, orbits, genitalia, hands, feet, and/or multiple digits; first 100 sq cm or less, or 1% of body area of infants and children +15116 each additional 100 sq cm, or each additional 1% of body area of infants and children, or part thereof	15135 Dermal autograft, face, scalp, eyelids, mouth, neck, ears, orbits, genitalia, hands, feet, and/or multiple digits; first 100 sq cm or less, or 1% of body area of infants and children +15136 each additional 100 sq cm, or each additional 1% of body area of infants and children, or part thereof

[a] Sum the surface area of all wounds within the same grouping of body areas in the code descriptors. Do not sum wounds from different groupings (eg, face and arms).

Table 19-3. Codes for Tissue-Cultured Autografts

Body Area	Code
Trunk, arms, legs	15150 Tissue cultured skin autograft, trunk, arms, legs; first 25 sq cm or less +15151 additional 1 sq cm to 75 sq cm +15152 each additional 100 sq cm, or each additional 1% of body area of infants and children, or part thereof
Face, scalp, eyelids, mouth, neck, ears, orbits, genitalia, hands, feet, and/or multiple digits	15155 Tissue cultured skin autograft, face, scalp, eyelids, mouth, neck, ears, orbits, genitalia, hands, feet, and/or multiple digits; first 25 sq cm or less +15156 additional 1 sq cm to 75 sq cm +15157 each additional 100 sq cm, or each additional 1% of body area of infants and children, or part thereof

Table 19-4. Code for Full-Thickness Free Grafts

Body Area	Codes
Trunk	15200 Full thickness graft, free, including direct closure of donor site, trunk; 20 sq cm or less +15201 each additional 20 sq cm, or part thereof
Scalp, arms, and/or legs	15220 Full thickness graft, free, including direct closure of donor site, scalp, arms, and/or legs; 20 sq cm or less +15221 each additional 20 sq cm, or part thereof
Forehead, cheeks, chin, mouth, neck, axillae, genitalia, hands, and/or feet	15240 Full thickness graft, free, including direct closure of donor site, forehead, cheeks, chin, mouth, neck, axillae, genitalia, hands, and/or feet; 20 sq cm or less +15241 each additional 20 sq cm, or part thereof
Nose, ears, eyelids, and/or lips	15260 Full thickness graft, free, including direct closure of donor site, nose, ears, eyelids, and/or lips; 20 sq cm or less +15261 each additional 20 sq cm, or part thereof

Table 19-5. Codes for Skin Substitute Grafts

Body Area	Surface Area Up to 100 sq cm	Surface Area ≥100 sq cm or 1% of Body Area of Infants and Children
Trunk, arms, legs	15271 Application of skin substitute graft to trunk, arms, legs, total wound surface area up to 100 sq cm; *first 25 sq cm or less wound surface area* +15272 *each additional* 25 sq cm wound surface area, or part thereof	15273 Application of skin substitute graft to trunk, arms, legs, total wound surface area greater than or equal to 100 sq cm; *first 100 sq cm wound surface area, or 1% of body area of infants and children* +15274 *each additional* 100 sq cm wound surface area, or part thereof, or each additional 1% of body area of infants and children, or part thereof
Face, scalp, eyelids, mouth, neck, ears, orbits, genitalia, hands, feet, and/or multiple digits	15275 Application of skin substitute graft to face, scalp, eyelids, mouth, neck, ears, orbits, genitalia, hands, feet, and/or multiple digits, total wound surface area up to 100 sq cm; *first 25 sq cm or less wound surface area* +15276 *each additional* 25 sq cm wound surface area, or part thereof	15277 Application of skin substitute graft to face, scalp, eyelids, mouth, neck, ears, orbits, genitalia, hands, feet, and/or multiple digits, total wound surface area greater than or equal to 100 sq cm; *first 100 sq cm wound surface area, or 1% of body area of infants and children* +15278 *each additional* 100 sq cm wound surface area, or part thereof, or each additional 1% of body area of infants and children, or part thereof

Musculoskeletal Procedures

Fracture and Dislocation Care Codes

Codes for fracture/dislocation care
- Are listed by anatomic location.
- Are provided (in most cases) for closed or open treatment, with or without manipulation, and with or without internal fixation.
- Most include a 90-day period of follow-up care under the Medicare global package. Evaluation and management with decision for the procedure on the day before or day of the procedure is separately reportable with modifier 57 (decision for surgery) appended to the E/M code.

- Include the initial casting, splinting, or strapping.
- Do not include radiographs.
- Routine follow-up visits during the global period are reported with no charge with code 99024 (post-op follow-up visit related to the original procedure).
- Re-reduction of a fracture and/or dislocation performed by the physician or QHP who performed the initial reduction may be identified by the addition of modifier 76 to the usual procedure number to indicate repeat procedure or service by the same physician or other QHP.

Examples

➤ **A child is evaluated in the ED for an injury to the left elbow following a fall due to overturning her bicycle on the sidewalk of her apartment complex.** An orthopedic surgeon is consulted to determine if the injury requires percutaneous fixation. The orthopedic surgeon evaluates the child and diagnoses a displaced supracondylar humerus fracture. A decision is made to proceed with closed reduction and pinning. The procedure takes place on the same date. The child is admitted to the hospital for postoperative monitoring and discharged to home the next day. The orthopedic surgeon provided a consultation, procedure, and discharge day E/M services.

ICD-10-CM	CPT®
S42.412A (displaced simple supracondylar fracture without intercondylar fracture of left humerus, initial encounter for closed fracture) V18.0XXA (pedal cycle driver injured in noncollision transport accident in nontraffic accident, initial encounter) Y92.480 (sidewalk as the place of occurrence of the external cause)	99251–99255 57 (inpatient consultation) or, if the payer does not pay consultation codes, 99221–99223 57 (initial hospital care)
Same as previous	24538 (percutaneous skeletal fixation of supracondylar or transcondylar humeral fracture, with or without intercondylar extension)

Teaching Point: Because code 24538 is assigned a 90-day global period in the Medicare Physician Fee Schedule, many payers may require modifier 57 (decision for surgery) appended to the E/M code reported for the same date of service. Individual payers may have different policies. The postoperative care in the hospital is not separately reported. Follow-up visits in the office may be reported with code 99024 (postoperative follow-up visit).

Removal of Musculoskeletal Hardware

20670   Removal of implant; superficial (eg, buried wire, pin or rod) (separate procedure)
20680   deep (eg, buried wire, pin, screw, metal band, nail, rod or plate)

Codes 20670 and 20680 may be reported for removal of orthopedic hardware. Removal of a halo or tongs is included in the placement procedure. However, removal of a halo or tongs by another physician is separately reported with code 20665. (*Note:* Physicians of the same specialty and same group practice are typically considered as the same physician for billing purposes.) If it is necessary to remove an implant within the global period (eg, due to breakage), report the appropriate removal code with modifier 78 (unplanned return to the operating/procedure room by the same physician or other QHP following initial procedure for a related procedure during the postoperative period.)

Respiratory

Intubation and Airway Management

31500   Intubation, endotracheal, emergency

⊕ Moderate sedation (99151–99157) may be reported in addition to the intubation if used to sedate the patient prior to and during the intubation procedure (eg, in rapid sequence intubation) and reporting criteria are met. See the Sedation section later in this chapter for more on moderate sedation.

31502   Tracheostomy tube change prior to establishment of fistula tract

⊕ Report code 31502 when an indwelling tracheostomy tube is replaced. Routine changing of a tracheostomy tube after a fistula tract has been established is included in a related E/M service.

31505–31520   Indirect laryngoscopy

⊕ Report code 31505 for indirect diagnostic laryngoscopy. If, while performing this procedure, a foreign body is removed, report code 31511 (laryngoscopy with removal of foreign body).

⊕ Direct laryngoscopy with or without tracheoscopy: Code 31515 is reported when it is performed for aspiration.

⊕ When diagnostic direct laryngoscopy, with or without tracheoscopy, is performed on a newborn, report code 31520. Do not report modifier 63 (procedure performed on infant less than 4 kg) in conjunction with code 31520.

31525   Laryngoscopy, direct, with or without tracheoscopy; diagnostic except newborn

Thoracostomy, Thoracentesis, and Pleural Drainage

32551   Tube thoracostomy, includes connection to drainage system (eg, water seal), when performed, open (separate procedure)

32554   Thoracentesis, needle or catheter, aspiration of the pleural space; without imaging guidance

32555   with imaging guidance

32556   Pleural drainage, percutaneous, with insertion of indwelling catheter; without imaging guidance

32557   with imaging guidance

⊕ Thoracostomy (32551) represents an open procedure involving incision into a rib interspace with dissection extending through the chest wall muscles and pleura. Thoracentesis and percutaneous pleural drainage may be more commonly performed in pediatrics with the exception of neonatal and pediatric critical care.

⊕ Percutaneous image guidance cannot be reported in conjunction with code 32551, which represents an open procedure. Diagnostic ultrasound performed prior to thoracostomy to localize a collection in the pleural space is separately reportable only when the complete ultrasound study of the chest (76441) is performed with permanent recording of images.

⊕ Thoracentesis codes 32554 and 32555 represent a procedure in which the surgical technique is puncture of the pleural space to remove fluid or air. Although a catheter (eg, pigtail catheter) may be used, it is not left in place at the end of the procedure.

⊕ Percutaneous pleural drainage codes 32556 and 32557 represent procedures in which an indwelling catheter is inserted into the pleural space and remains at the end of the procedure. The catheter is secured in place and connected to a suction drainage system.

⊕ Removal of chest tubes and non-tunneled indwelling pleural catheters is included in a related E/M service and not a separately reportable procedure.

⊕ For insertion of a tunneled pleural catheter with cuff, see code 32550. For removal of a tunneled pleural catheter with cuff, see 32552.

Cardiovascular Procedures

Cardiac Catheterization

Cardiac catheterization includes introduction, positioning, and repositioning, when necessary, of catheter(s) within the vascular system; recording of intracardiac and/or intravascular pressure(s); and final evaluation and report of procedure. Diagnostic heart catheterization in a patient without congenital anomaly is reported with the following codes:

93451 Right heart catheterization including measurement(s) of oxygen saturation and cardiac output, when performed

93452 Left heart catheterization including intraprocedural injection(s) for left ventriculography, imaging supervision and interpretation, when performed

93453 Combined right and left heart catheterization including intraprocedural injection(s) for left ventriculography, imaging supervision and interpretation, when performed

⚙ Several procedures include heart catheterization when performed. Verify that multiple procedures are separately reportable per the prefatory and parenthetical instruction for these codes in your *CPT®* coding reference.

Catheterization for Congenital Anomalies

93530 Right heart catheterization, for congenital cardiac anomalies

93531 Combined right heart catheterization and retrograde left heart catheterization, for congenital cardiac anomalies

93532 Combined right heart catheterization and transseptal left heart catheterization through intact septum with or without retrograde left heart catheterization, for congenital cardiac anomalies

93533 Combined right heart catheterization and transseptal left heart catheterization through existing septal opening, with or without retrograde left heart catheterization, for congenital cardiac anomalies

It is important to note that codes **93530–93533** are reported *only when cardiac catheterization is performed for evaluation of congenital cardiac anomalies.* However, there is no age limit mentioned in the narrative description of codes **93530–93533**. As long as there is a congenital cardiac anomaly, it is appropriate to report these codes. These codes take into account

⚙ The added technical difficulty presented when structures may be in abnormal positions and locations.

⚙ Additional preservice time in reviewing noninvasive data, previous cardiac catheterizations, and previous surgeries.

⚙ Procedures may be more time consuming due to small vessels, multiple measurements that must be made, instability of patients, frequency of multiple sites of arterial-venous admixture, and performance of other required interventions.

Procedures such as percutaneous transcatheter closure of patent ductus arteriosus (**93582**) include right and left heart catheterization for congenital cardiac anomalies. Be sure to read the *CPT®* instructions for procedures performed in conjunction with congenital cardiac catheterization to determine if the catheterization is separately reportable.

Aortic Valve Replacement

#●33440 Replacement, aortic valve; by translocation of autologous pulmonary valve and transventricular aortic annulus enlargement of the left ventricular outflow tract with valved conduit replacement of pulmonary valve (Ross-Konno procedure)

▲33411 with aortic annulus enlargement, noncoronary sinus

▲33412 with transventricular aortic annulus enlargement (Konno procedure)

▲33413 by translocation of autologous pulmonary valve with allograft replacement of pulmonary valve (Ross procedure)

New in 2019 is code **33440**, which allows for reporting aortic valve replacement by translocation of the autologous pulmonary valve and transventricular aortic annulus enlargement of the left ventricular outflow tract with valved conduit replacement of pulmonary valve (combined Ross-Konno procedure).

☀ For replacement of aortic valve with transventricular aortic annulus enlargement (Konno procedure) in conjunction with translocation of autologous pulmonary valve with allograft replacement of pulmonary valve (Ross procedure), use code **33440**.

☀ Do not report aortic valve replacement with aortic annulus enlargement, noncoronary sinus (**33412**) in conjunction with aortic valve replacement by translocation of autologous pulmonary valve with allograft replacement of pulmonary valve (**33413**).

☀ See the parenthetical instruction following code **33440** in your *CPT®* coding reference for other procedures not separately reported in conjunction with code **33440**.

Example

➤ A 4-year-old established patient undergoes autologous pulmonary valve replacement of the aortic valve and a Konno aortoventriculoplasty to correct a mixed aortic valvular stenosis with regurgitation and multilevel ventricular outflow obstruction.

ICD-10-CM	CPT®
Q23.0 (congenital stenosis of aortic valve)	#●33440 (replacement, aortic valve; by translocation of autologous pulmonary valve and transventricular aortic annulus enlargement of the left ventricular outflow tract with valved conduit replacement of pulmonary valve [Ross-Konno procedure])

A single code, **33440**, is reported for the combined Ross-Konno procedure. It would be inappropriate to separately report the procedures.

Valvuloplasty

33390   Valvuloplasty, aortic valve, open, with cardiopulmonary bypass; simple (ie, valvotomy, debridement, debulking, and/or simple commissural resuspension)

33391   complex (eg, leaflet extension, leaflet resection, leaflet reconstruction, or annuloplasty)
        (Do not report **33391** in conjunction with **33390**)

Codes for open valvuloplasty of the aortic valve

☀ Are more descriptive of currently performed valvuloplasty procedures
  ❖ Code **33390** is specifically for reporting valvotomy, debridement, debulking, and/or simple commissural resuspension.
  ❖ Code **33391** represents more complex procedures not limited to the examples in the code descriptor.

☀ May be reported in conjunction with the code for transmyocardial revascularization (**33141**), operative tissue ablation and reconstruction of atria (**33255–33259**), and reoperation, valve procedure, more than 1 month after original operation (**33530**), when appropriate

Codes for aortic valve replacement (**33405, 33406, 33410**) were revised to reflect that these are open procedures.

Transcatheter Pulmonary Valve Implantation

33477   Transcatheter pulmonary valve implantation, percutaneous approach, including pre-stenting of the valve delivery site, when performed

The key instructions for reporting code **33477** are

☀ Should only be reported once per session

- Includes, when performed,
  - Percutaneous access
  - Placing the access sheath
  - Advancing the repair device delivery system into position
  - Repositioning the device as needed and deploying the device(s)
  - Angiography, radiologic supervision, and interpretation performed to guide transcatheter pulmonary valve implantation (TPVI)
  - All cardiac catheterization(s), intraprocedural contrast injection(s), fluoroscopic radiologic supervision and interpretation, and imaging guidance performed to complete the pulmonary valve procedure
  - Percutaneous balloon angioplasty of the conduit or treatment zone, valvuloplasty of the pulmonary valve conduit, and stent deployment within the pulmonary conduit or an existing bioprosthetic pulmonary valve
  - Contrast injections, angiography, road mapping, and/or fluoroscopic guidance for TPVI
  - Pulmonary conduit angiography for guidance of TPVI
  - Right heart catheterization for hemodynamic measurements before, during, and after TPVI for guidance of TPVI
- Does not include (Report separately, when performed.)
  - Codes 92997 and 92998 when pulmonary artery angioplasty is performed at a site separate from the prosthetic valve delivery site
  - Codes 37236 and 37237 when pulmonary artery stenting is performed at a site separate from the prosthetic valve delivery site
  - Same-session/same-day diagnostic cardiac catheterization services (See your *CPT*® reference for further instruction and append catheterization code with modifier 59.)
  - Diagnostic coronary angiography performed at a separate session from an interventional procedure
  - Percutaneous coronary interventional procedures
  - Percutaneous pulmonary artery branch interventions
  - Percutaneous ventricular assist device procedure codes (33990–33993), extracorporeal membrane oxygenation/extracorporeal life support procedure codes (33946–33989), or balloon pump insertion codes (33967, 33970, 33973)
  - Percutaneous peripheral bypass (33367), open peripheral bypass (33368), or central bypass (33369)

Percutaneous Transcatheter Closure of Patent Ductus Arteriosus

93582   Percutaneous transcatheter closure of patent ductus arteriosus
- Includes, when performed
  - Introduction of catheter, right heart or main pulmonary artery (36013)
  - Selective catheter placement, left or right pulmonary artery (36014)
  - Introduction of catheter, aorta (36200)
  - Aortography, thoracic, without serialography, radiological supervision and interpretation (75600)
  - Aortography, thoracic, by serialography, radiological supervision and interpretation (75605)
  - Heart catheterization or catheter placement for coronary angiography (93451–94361)
  - Heart catheterization for congenital cardiac anomalies (93530–93533)
  - Injection procedure during cardiac catheterization including imaging supervision, interpretation, and report; for supravalvular aortography (93567)
- Separately report
  - Left heart catheterization by transseptal puncture through intact septum or by transapical puncture (93462)
  - Add-on codes for injection procedures during cardiac catheterization, including imaging supervision, interpretation, and report, for
    — Selective coronary angiography during congenital heart catheterization (93563)

— Selective opacification of aortocoronary venous or arterial bypass graft(s) (ie, aortocoronary saphenous vein, free radial artery, or free mammary artery graft) to one or more coronary arteries and in situ arterial conduits (eg, internal mammary), whether native or used for bypass to one or more coronary arteries during congenital heart catheterization, when performed (93564)
— Selective left ventricular or left atrial angiography (93565)
— Selective right ventricular or right atrial angiography (93566)
— Pulmonary angiography (93568)

Vascular Access

Central Venous Access

There is no distinction between venous access achieved percutaneously or via cutdown. Report the code appropriate to the type of insertion (centrally inserted or peripherally inserted), type of catheter (eg, non-tunneled vs tunneled), device (eg, with or without port), and age of child (**tables 19-6 and 19-7**).

- In non-facility settings, code 96522 may be reported for refilling and maintenance of an implantable pump or reservoir for systemic (intra-venous [IV], intra-arterial) drug delivery.
- Irrigation of an implanted venous access device for drug delivery (96523) is only reported in non-facility settings and when no other service is reported by the same individual on the same date.
- Codes for refilling and maintenance and/or irrigation are not reported by physicians in facility settings.

> **‖‖‖‖‖‖ Coding Pearl ‖‖‖‖‖‖**
>
> If an existing central venous access device is removed and a new one *placed via a separate venous access site,* appropriate codes for both procedures (removal of old, if code exists, and insertion of new device) should be reported. See replacement codes for removal with replacement *via the same venous access site.*

Insertion or Replacement of Centrally Inserted Central Venous Access Device

- To qualify as a centrally inserted central venous access device, the entry site must be the jugular, subclavian, or femoral vein, or the inferior vena cava, and the tip of the catheter must terminate in the subclavian, bra-chiocephalic (innominate), or iliac veins; the superior or inferior vena cava; or the right atrium.
- Moderate sedation services are separately reportable with codes 99151–99157. For more information on reporting moderate sedation, see the Sedation section later in this chapter.
- Report imaging guidance for gaining access to venous entry site or manipulating the catheter into final central position (in addition to codes 36555–36558) with either
  - ❖ 76937 (ultrasound guidance for vascular access requiring ultrasound evaluation of potential access sites, documentation of selected vessel patency, concurrent real-time ultrasound visualization of vascular needle entry, with permanent recording and reporting)
  - ❖ 77001 (fluoroscopic guidance for central venous access device placement, replacement [catheter only or complete], or removal [includes fluoroscopic guidance for vascular access and catheter manipulation, any necessary contrast injections through access site or catheter with related venography radiologic supervision and interpretation, and radiographic documentation of final catheter position])
- Ultrasound guidance for peripherally inserted central venous catheter (PICC) placement should include documentation of evaluation of the potential puncture sites, patency of the entry vein, and real-time ultrasound visualization of needle entry into the vein.
- *Do not separately report ultrasound for vessel identification only.*

> **‖‖‖‖‖ Coding Pearl ‖‖‖‖‖**
>
> Midline catheters terminate in the peripheral venous system. Midline catheter insertion is not reported as a peripherally inserted central venous catheter insertion. See codes **36400–36410** for midline catheter insertion.

Insertion of Peripherally Inserted Central Venous Access Device

- To qualify as a PICC, the entry site must be the basilic, cephalic, or saphenous vein and the tip of the catheter must terminate in the subclavian, brachiocephalic (innominate), or iliac veins; the superior or inferior vena cava; or the right atrium.
- Report PICC insertion *with a subcutaneous port* with codes 36570 and 36571. Ultrasound (76937) or fluoroscopic guidance (77001) may be separately reported when performed and documented.
  - ❖ Ultrasound guidance for PICC placement should include documentation of evaluation of the potential puncture sites, patency of the entry vein, and real-time ultrasound visualization of needle entry into the vein.
- Codes 36568 and 36569 are reported for PICC insertion without a subcutaneous port *and without imaging guidance* based on the patient's age. If imaging guidance is used in PICC insertion, see codes 36572, 36573, and 36584. Do not report imaging guidance (76937, 77001) in conjunction with codes 36568 and 36569.
- Peripherally inserted central venous catheters placed using magnetic guidance or any other guidance modality that does not include imaging or image documentation are reported with codes 36568 and 36569.
- Insertion of PICC without subcutaneous port or pump *with imaging guidance* is reported with codes 36572 and 36573. Report code 36584 for replacement of PICC without subcutaneous port or pump *with imaging guidance.*
- Codes 36572, 36573, and 36584 include imaging guidance for placement or repositioning.
- Chest radiographs (71045–71048) should not be reported for the purpose of documenting the final catheter position by the same physician on the same day of service as the PICC insertion (36572, 36573, or 36584). If PICC insertion is performed without confirmation of the catheter tip location, append modifier 52 (reduced service) to the code for catheter insertion (36572, 36573, or 36584).
- Documentation of services includes
  - ❖ Images from all modalities used (eg, ultrasound, fluoroscopy) stored to the patient record
  - ❖ Associated supervision and interpretation
  - ❖ Venography performed through the same venous puncture
  - ❖ The final central position of the catheter with imaging

Table 19-6. Insertion and Replacement of Central Venous Catheter		
Insertion	**Child <5 y**	**Child ≥5 y**
Insertion non-tunneled centrally inserted central venous catheter	36555	36556
Insertion tunneled centrally inserted central venous catheter, without subcutaneous port or pump	36557	36558
Insertion tunneled centrally inserted central venous access device, with subcutaneous port	36560	36561
Insertion	**Any Age**	
Insertion tunneled centrally inserted central venous access device with subcutaneous pump	36563	
Insertion of tunneled centrally inserted central venous access device, requiring 2 catheters via 2 separate venous access sites; without subcutaneous port or pump (eg, Tesio-type catheter)	36565	
Insertion of tunneled centrally inserted central venous access device, requiring 2 catheters via 2 separate venous access sites; with subcutaneous port(s)	36566	
Replacement		
Replacement, *catheter only,* of central venous access device, with subcutaneous port or pump, central or peripheral insertion site	36578	

Table 19-6. Insertion and Replacement of Central Venous Catheter (*continued*)

Insertion (*continued*)

Replacement, *complete,* of a non-tunneled centrally inserted central venous catheter, without subcutaneous port or pump, through same venous access	36580
Replacement, *complete,* of a tunneled centrally inserted central venous catheter, without subcutaneous port or pump, through same venous access	36581
Replacement, *complete,* of a tunneled centrally inserted central venous access device, with subcutaneous port, through same venous access	36582
Replacement, *complete,* of a tunneled centrally inserted central venous access device, with subcutaneous pump, through same venous access	36583

Table 19-7. Insertion or Replacement of Peripherally Inserted Central Venous Catheter

Insertion Procedure	Child <5 y	Child ≥5 y
Insertion of peripherally inserted central venous catheter (PICC), without subcutaneous port or pump, *without imaging guidance*	▲36568	▲36569
Insertion of peripherally inserted central venous access device, with subcutaneous port	36570	36571
Insertion of peripherally inserted central venous catheter (PICC), without subcutaneous port or pump, including all imaging guidance, image documentation, and all associated radiological supervision and interpretation required to perform the insertion	#●36572	#●36573
Replacement Procedure	**Any Age**	
Replacement, catheter only, of central venous access device, with subcutaneous port or pump, central or peripheral insertion site	36578	
Replacement, complete, of a peripherally inserted central venous catheter (PICC), without subcutaneous port or pump, through same venous access, including all imaging guidance, image documentation, and all associated radiological supervision and interpretation required to perform the replacement	▲36584	
Replacement, complete, of a peripherally inserted central venous access device, with subcutaneous port, through same venous access	36585	

Repair of Central Venous Catheters

36575   Repair of tunneled or non-tunneled central venous access catheter, without subcutaneous port or pump, central or peripheral insertion site

36576   Repair of central venous access device, with subcutaneous port or pump, central or peripheral insertion site

36593   Declotting by thrombolytic agent of implanted vascular access device or catheter

36595   Mechanical removal of pericatheter obstructive material (eg, fibrin sheath) from central venous device via separate venous access

36596   Mechanical removal of intraluminal (intracatheter) obstructive material from central venous device through device lumen

75901   Mechanical removal of pericatheter obstructive material (eg, fibrin sheath) from central venous device via separate venous access, radiologic supervision and interpretation

36598   Contrast injection(s) for radiologic evaluation of existing central venous access device, including fluoroscopy, image documentation and report

Repair of a central venous catheter includes fixing the device without replacement of the catheter or port/pump.

⊛ For the repair of a multi-catheter device, with or without subcutaneous ports/pumps, use the appropriate code describing the service with 2 units of service.

⊛ Repair of any central venous access catheter *without a port or pump* is reported with code 36575.

⊛ Repair of any central venous catheter *with a port or pump* is reported with code 36576.

⊛ Code 36593 is reported for declotting of an implanted vascular device or catheter *by thrombolysis*. Code 36593 *is not reported* for declotting of a pleural catheter. Use unlisted procedure code 32999 for declotting of a pleural catheter.

⊛ Code 36595 and 36596 are reported for the procedure of *mechanical removal* of pericatheter or intraluminal obstructive material. Radiologic supervision and interpretation is separately reported with code 75901.

   ❖ Do not report code 36595 or 36596 in conjunction with code 36593 or 36598.

⊛ When the patency of a central line is evaluated under fluoroscopy, code 36598 is reported for the contrast injection, image documentation, and report. Fluoroscopy (76000) is not separately reported. See codes 75820–75827 for complete venography studies.

Removal of Central Venous Catheters

36589   Removal of tunneled central venous catheter, without subcutaneous port or pump

36590   Removal of tunneled central venous access device, with subcutaneous port or pump, central or peripheral insertion

Removal codes are reported for removal of the entire device. See replacement codes for partial replacement (catheter only) or complete exchange *in the same venous access site* of central venous access devices.

⊛ For removal of both catheters (placed from separate venous access sites) of a multi-catheter device, with or without subcutaneous ports/pumps, use the appropriate code describing the service with 2 units of service.

⊛ When removal of an existing central venous access device is performed in conjunction with placement of new device *via a separate venous access site,* report both procedures.

Arterial Access

36600   Arterial puncture, withdrawal of blood for diagnosis

36620   Arterial catheterization or cannulation for sampling, monitoring or transfusion (separate procedure); percutaneous

36625   cutdown

⊛ An arterial puncture for diagnosis is reported with code 36600.

⊛ Code 36620 is reported when a percutaneous peripheral arterial catheterization is performed.

⊛ Code 36625 is reported when a cutdown is performed.

     Removal of central venous access device

⊛ Report repairs, partial catheter replacements, complete replacements, or removal of catheters with or without subcutaneous ports or pumps with codes 36578–36590. Code 36589 is reported for removal of tunneled central venous catheter, without subcutaneous port or pump, and code 36590 for the removal of tunneled central venous catheter, with subcutaneous port or pump, central or peripheral.

⊛ If a central venous access device is removed and replaced with a new one *through a separate venous access site,* the removal and insertion of the new device should be reported.

Transfusions

36430   Transfusion, blood or blood components

36440   Push transfusion; blood, 2 years or younger

36450   Exchange transfusion, blood, newborn

36455   other than newborn

36456   Partial exchange transfusion, blood, plasma, or crystalloid necessitating the skill of a physician or other qualified health care professional; newborn

- Indirect transfusion of blood or blood products (36430) should be used only if the physician personally infuses the substance, and not if the blood is administered by nursing personnel and allowed to enter the vessel via gravity or meter flow. Push transfusion (36440) is used only for patients younger than 2 years. This code should be used only if the physician personally performs the transfusion.

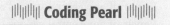

|||||||| Coding Pearl ||||||||

The placement of catheters to support exchange transfusions may be reported separately with the appropriate vascular access codes.

- Complete exchange transfusions (double volume) performed during the neonatal period are reported using code 36450; exchange transfusions for all other age groups are reported using code 36455. The assumption is that the exchange for the neonate is performed via the umbilical vein, while an exchange for an older child or adult is performed via a peripheral vessel.
- The actual placement of catheters to support the exchange transfusion may be reported separately with the appropriate vascular access codes.
- Partial exchange transfusions (eg, for hyperviscosity syndrome in the neonate) should be reported using code 36456.
- Do not report codes 36430, 36440, or 36450 with 36456.
- Do not append modifier 63 (procedure performed on infants less than 4 kg) when reporting code 36456.

Hydration, Intravenous Infusions

Services included as inherent to an infusion or injection are the use of local anesthesia, starting the IV line, access to indwelling IV lines or a subcutaneous catheter or port, flushing lines at the conclusion of an infusion or between infusions, standard tubing, syringes and supplies, and preparation of chemotherapy agents.

These codes are intended for reporting by the physician or other QHP in an office setting. *They are not reported by a physician or other QHP when performed in a facility setting* because the physician work associated with these procedures involves only affirmation of the treatment plan and direct supervision of the staff performing the services. If a significant, separately identifiable E/M service is performed, the appropriate code may be reported with modifier 25 appended. The diagnosis may be the same for the E/M service and codes 96360–96379.

Table 19-8 lists related primary and additional hydration, injection, and IV codes.

Therapeutic, Prophylactic, and Diagnostic Injections

96372	Therapeutic, prophylactic, or diagnostic injection (specify substance or drug); subcutaneous or intramuscular
96373	intra-arterial
96374	intravenous push, single or initial substance/drug
+96375	each additional sequential intravenous push of a new substance/drug (List separately in addition to 96365, 96374, 96409, or 96413)
+96376	each additional sequential intravenous push of the same substance/drug provided in a facility (List separately in addition to 96365, 96374, 96409, or 96413)

Codes 96374 and 96375 are only used when the health care professional administering the substance or drug is in constant attendance during the administration *and* must observe the patient. The IV push must be less than 15 minutes. Short infusions of less than 15 minutes are reported as a push (eg, 96374).

Codes 96372–96374

- Report code 96372 for the administration of a diagnostic, prophylactic, or therapeutic (eg, antibiotic) subcutaneous or intramuscular injection. Do not report for the administration of a purified protein derivative test.

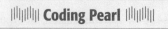

|||||||| Coding Pearl ||||||||

Short infusions of less than 15 minutes should be reported with code **96374**.

Table 19-8. Primary and Additional Hydration, Injection, and Intravenous Codes

Primary Code	Additional Codes
96360 Intravenous infusion, hydration; initial, 31 minutes to 1 hour	96361 Intravenous infusion, hydration; each additional hour
96365 Intravenous infusion, for therapy, prophylaxis, or diagnosis (specify substance or drug); initial, up to 1 hour	96366–96368, 96375 (each additional sequential intravenous push of a new substance/drug), 96376 [a] (each additional sequential intravenous push of the same substance/drug provided in a facility)
96367 Intravenous infusion, for therapy, prophylaxis, or diagnosis (specify substance or drug); additional sequential infusion of a new drug/substance, up to 1 hour	96366 Intravenous infusion, for therapy, prophylaxis, or diagnosis (specify substance or drug); each additional hour
96365, 96366, 96413, 96415, 96416	96368 Intravenous infusion, for therapy, prophylaxis, or diagnosis (specify substance or drug); concurrent infusion
96369 Subcutaneous infusion for therapy or prophylaxis (specify substance or drug); initial, up to 1 hour, including pump set-up and establishment of subcutaneous infusion site(s)	96370 Subcutaneous infusion for therapy or prophylaxis (specify substance or drug); each additional hour 96371 Subcutaneous infusion for therapy or prophylaxis (specify substance or drug); additional pump set-up with establishment of new subcutaneous infusion site(s)
96374 Therapeutic, prophylactic, or diagnostic injection (specify substance or drug); intravenous push, single or initial substance/drug	96367, 96375, 96376 [a]
96409 Chemotherapy administration; intravenous, push technique, single or initial substance/drug	96367, 96375, 96376 [a]
96413 Chemotherapy administration, intravenous infusion technique; up to 1 hour, single or initial substance/drug	96367, 96368, 96375, 96376 [a]
96415 Chemotherapy administration, intravenous infusion technique; each additional hour	96368
96416 Chemotherapy administration, intravenous infusion technique; initiation of prolonged chemotherapy infusion (more than 8 hours), requiring use of a portable or implantable pump	96368

[a] Code is only to be reported in the facility setting.

❖ Report code 96373 for an initial intra-arterial injection and 96374 for an initial injection administered by IV push. Sequential IV push of a new substance or drug is reported with add-on code 96375. Code 96375 may be reported in addition to codes for IV infusion (96365), initial IV push (96374), or chemotherapy administration (96409, 96413). Additional sequential IV push of the same substance or drug (96376) is reported only by a facility.

Each drug administered is reported separately with the appropriate infusion code.

Example

> A 3-year-old established patient is seen with a complaint of vomiting and fever for the past 24 hours. She has refused all food and liquids and last voided 12 hours prior to the visit. A detailed history and physical examination with moderate-level MDM are performed. Her diagnosis is bilateral acute suppurative otitis media and dehydration. Intravenous fluids are initiated with physiologic (normal) saline solution, and IV ceftriaxone (750 mg) is infused over 30 minutes for her otitis media. After 1 hour and 45 minutes of IV hydration, she urinates, begins tolerating liquids, and is released to home.

ICD-10-CM	CPT®
E86.0 (dehydration) H66.003 (acute suppurative otitis media without spontaneous rupture of ear drum, bilateral)	99214 25 (established patient office E/M) 96365 (IV infusion, for therapy) 96361 (IV infusion, hydration, each additional hour) J0696 (ceftriaxone sodium, per 250 mg) × 3 units J7030 (infusion, normal saline solution, 1,000 cc)

Link the appropriate diagnosis code to each procedure (eg, code H66.003 is linked to code J0696). The medication and infusion solution may need to be reported with the National Drug Code if required by the payer. The fluid used to administer ceftriaxone is not reported because it is considered incidental hydration.

Hydration

Codes 96360 (IV infusion, hydration; initial, 31 minutes to 1 hour) and 96361 (each additional hour)

- Are intended to report IV hydration infusion using prepackaged fluid and/or electrolyte solutions (eg, physiologic saline solution, D5½ physiologic saline solution with potassium).
- Typically require direct physician supervision for purposes of consent, safety oversight, or supervision of staff with little special handling for preparation or disposal of materials.
- Do not typically require advanced training of staff because there usually is little risk involved with little patient monitoring required.
- Are reported based on the actual time over which the infusion is administered and do not include the time spent starting the IV and monitoring the patient after infusion. Medical record documentation must support the service reported.
- Code 96360 may be reported for hydration infusion lasting more than 31 minutes and up to 1 hour. Code 96361 is reported for each additional hour of hydration infusion and for a final interval of greater than 30 minutes beyond the last hour reported.
- Are not reported when IV infusions are 30 minutes or less.
- Are not used to report infusion of drugs or other substances; nor are they reported when it is incidental to non-chemotherapeutic/diagnostic or chemotherapeutic services.
- Code 96361 is reported if an IV hydration infusion is provided secondary or subsequent to a therapeutic, prophylactic, or diagnostic infusion and administered through the same IV access.

Therapeutic, Prophylactic, and Diagnostic Infusions

96365	Intravenous infusion, for therapy, prophylaxis, or diagnosis (specify substance or drug); initial, up to 1 hour
+96366	each additional hour (List separately in addition to 96365 or 96367.)
+96367	additional sequential infusion of a new drug/substance, up to 1 hour (List separately in addition to 96365, 96374, 96409, 96413.)
+96368	concurrent infusion (List separately in addition to 96365, 96366, 96413, 96415, or 96416.)

Coding Conundrum: Multiple and Concurrent Infusions or Injections

When administering multiple infusions, injections, or combinations, only one "initial" service code should be reported for a given date, unless protocol requires that 2 separate intravenous (IV) sites must be used. Do not report a second initial service on the same date due to an IV line requiring a restart, an IV rate not being able to be reached without 2 lines, or accessing a port of a multi-lumen catheter. If an injection or infusion is of a subsequent or concurrent nature, even if it is the first such service within that group of services, a subsequent or concurrent code from the appropriate section should be reported. For example, the first IV push given subsequent to an initial 1-hour infusion is reported using a subsequent IV push code.

When services are performed in the physician's office, report as follows:

Initial Infusion

Physician reporting: Report the code that best describes the *key* or *primary* reason for the service regardless of the order in which the infusions or injections occur. Only one initial service code (eg, **96365**) should be reported unless the protocol or patient condition requires using 2 separate IV sites. The difference in time and effort in providing this second IV site access is also reported using the *initial* service code with modifier **59**, distinct procedural service, appended (eg, **96365**, **96365 59**).

Facility reporting: An initial infusion is based on the hierarchy. Only one initial service code (eg, **96365**) should be reported unless the protocol or patient condition requires using 2 separate IV sites. The difference in time and effort in providing this second IV site access is also reported using the *initial* service code with modifier **59**, distinct procedural service, appended (eg, **96365**, **96365 59**).

Sequential Infusion

This is an infusion or IV push of a new substance or drug following a primary or initial service. For example, if an IV push was performed through the same IV access subsequent to an IV infusion for therapy, the appropriate codes to report would be **96365** and **96375**. If an IV push was performed through a different IV access route, the services would be reported using codes **96365** and **96374**. Sequential infusions are reported only one time for the same infusate. However, if additional hours were required for the infusion, the appropriate "each additional hour" add-on code would be reported. Different infusates can be reported using the same code as the original sequential code. Hydration may not be reported concurrently with any other service. All sequential services require that there be a new substance or drug, except that facilities may report a sequential IV push of the same drug using **96376**.

Concurrent Infusion

This is an infusion of a new substance or drug infused at the same time as another drug or substance. This is not time based and is only reported once per day regardless of whether a new drug or substance is administered concurrently. Hydration may not be reported concurrently with any other service. A separate subsequent concurrent administration of another new drug or substance (the third substance or drug) is not reported.

If IV hydration (**96360**, **96361**) is given from 11:00 pm to 2:00 am, code **96360** would be reported once with **96361** with 2 units of service. However, if instead of a continuous infusion, a medication was given by IV push at 10:00 pm and 2:00 am, both administrations would be reported as initial (**96374**) because the services are not continuous. For continuous services that last beyond midnight, use the date in which the service began and report the total units of time provided continuously. Although in conflict with *CPT*® guidelines, some payers may require that the primary infusion code be reported for each day of service.

Codes **96365–96368**

* Are for infusions for the purpose of administering drugs or substances.
* Typically require direct physician supervision and special attention to prepare, calculate dose, and dispose of materials.
* If fluid infusions are used to administer the drug(s), they are considered incidental hydration and are not reported.
* Each drug administered is reported separately with the appropriate infusion code.

Other Injection and Infusion Services

96523   Irrigation of implanted venous access device for drug delivery systems

Code 96523 is used to report irrigation required for implanted venous access devices for drug delivery systems when services are provided on a separate day from the injection or infusion service. Do not report 96523 in conjunction with other services.

Ear, Nose, and Throat Procedures

30901   Central nasal hemorrhage, anterior, simple (cautery or packing)

If performing cautery or packing on both sides, report 30901 with modifier 50.

69420   Myringotomy

92511   Nasopharyngoscopy with endoscope (separate procedure)

Code 92511 is designated as a "separate procedure" and should not be reported in addition to the code for the total procedure or service of which it is considered an integral component. However, if carried out independently or considered to be unrelated or distinct from other procedures or services provided at that time, it may be reported by itself or in addition to other procedures or services by appending modifier 59 to the specific separate procedure code.

Laryngoplasty

#31551   Laryngoplasty; for laryngeal stenosis, with graft, without indwelling stent placement, younger than 12 years of age

#31552   age 12 years or older

#31553   Laryngoplasty; for laryngeal stenosis, with graft, with indwelling stent placement, younger than 12 years of age

#31554   age 12 years or older

31580   Laryngoplasty; for laryngeal web, with indwelling keel or stent insertion

31584   Laryngoplasty; with open reduction and fixation of (eg, plating) fracture, includes tracheostomy, if performed

- Do not report graft separately if harvested through the laryngoplasty incision (eg, thyroid cartilage graft).
- Report only one of the following codes for a single operative session: 31551–31554 and 31580.
- Codes for treatment of laryngeal stenosis by laryngoplasty with graft are selected based on whether or not the procedure includes indwelling stent placement and by the age of the patient (<12 years or ≥12 years).
- Open treatment of a hyoid fracture is reported with code 31584 (repair procedure on the larynx).
- To report tracheostomy, see code 31600, 31601, 31603, 31605, or 31610.
- Report laryngoplasty, not otherwise specified or for removal of a keel or stent, with code 31599.

Digestive System Procedures

Gastric Intubation and Aspiration

43752   Naso- or orogastric tube placement, requiring physician's skill and fluoroscopic guidance (includes fluoroscopy, image documentation and report)

43753   Gastric intubation and aspiration(s), therapeutic (eg, for ingested poisons), including lavage if performed

Do not report code 43752 or 43753 in conjunction with critical care codes (99291, 99292), neonatal critical care codes (99468, 99469), pediatric critical care codes (99471–99476), or pediatric intensive care service codes (99477–99480).

Note that code **43752** is reported when a physician's skill is required for placement of a nasogastric or orogastric tube using fluoroscopic guidance. This service is not separately reported when a physician's skill is not required or placement is performed without fluoroscopic guidance. Replacement of a nasogastric tube requiring physician's skill and fluoroscopic guidance may also be reported with code **43752**.

Examples

➤ **A 10-year-old is brought to the ED after having ingested drugs.** Gastric intubation and lavage are performed.

Code **43753** would be reported in addition to the appropriate E/M service (eg, ED services **99281–99285**) but is not separately reported when performed in conjunction with critical care (eg, **99291**, **99292**; **99468–99476**) or by a physician during pediatric patient transport (**99466**, **99467**).

➤ **A patient requires placement of a nasogastric tube.** Attempts by nursing staff are unsuccessful, so placement by the physician is required. The physician places the tube using fluoroscopic guidance.

Code **43752** would be reported in addition to the appropriate E/M service but is not reported when the service is performed by the physician out of convenience rather than necessity for a physician's skill. Use of fluoroscopic guidance is required and must be documented (ie, image documentation and report).

Gastrostomy Tube Replacement

● **43762**   Replacement of gastrostomy tube, percutaneous, includes removal, when performed, without imaging or endoscopic guidance; not requiring revision of gastrostomy tract

● **43763**   requiring revision of gastrostomy tract

⚙ Code **43760** is deleted in 2019. To report gastrostomy tube change without imaging or endoscopic guidance, see codes **43762** and **43763**.

⚙ See code **49450** for replacement of gastrostomy tube with fluoroscopic guidance.

⚙ See code **43246** for placement with endoscopic guidance

⚙ A significant, separately identifiable E/M service on the same date may be reported with modifier **25** appended to the E/M code (eg, **99213 25**). An E/M service should not be reported when the encounter is solely for replacement of the gastrostomy tube.

⚙ Codes **43762** and **43763** include the gastrostomy tube kit.

Enterostomy/Cecostomy With Colonic Lavage

44300   Placement, enterostomy or cecostomy, tube open (eg, for feeding or decompression) (separate procedure)

(Do not report **44300** in conjunction with **44701** for cannulation of the colon for intraoperative colonic lavage)

(For percutaneous placement of duodenostomy, jejunostomy, gastro-jejunostomy or cecostomy [or other colonic] tube including fluoroscopic imaging guidance, see **49441–49442**)

+**44701**   Intraoperative colonic lavage (List separately in addition to code for primary procedure)

(Use **44701** in conjunction with **44140**, **44145**, **44150**, or **44604** as appropriate)

(Do not report **44701** in conjunction with **44950–44960**)

⚙ Report code **44300** for enterostomy or cecostomy tube placement except when tube placement is for intraoperative colonic lavage. Codes **44300** and **44701** may be separately reported except in instances when the tube placement is for intraoperative colonic lavage.

Appendectomy

44950	Appendectomy;
+44955	when done for indicated purpose at time of other major procedure
44960	for ruptured appendix with abscess or generalized peritonitis
44970	Laparoscopy, surgical, appendectomy
44979	Unlisted laparoscopy procedure, appendix

Appendectomy is one of the most common procedures in pediatrics. As a sole procedure, appendectomy coding is fairly straightforward, with 3 code choices: **44950**, open appendectomy without ruptured appendix; **99460**, open appendectomy for ruptured appendix with abscess or generalized peritonitis; and **99470**, laparoscopic appendectomy.

CPT® instructs that incidental appendectomy (ie, not due to disease or symptom) during intra-abdominal surgery does not usually warrant reporting a code for the appendectomy procedure. If it is necessary to report an appendectomy performed during another intra-abdominal procedure, append modifier **52** (reduced service).

❖ The Medicaid NCCI manual instructs that incidental removal of a normal appendix during another abdominal surgery is not separately reportable. This instruction is likely followed by other payers.

Appendectomy performed for an indicated purpose (ie, problem with the appendix) in conjunction with another procedure is separately reported. A separate diagnosis code (distinct from the diagnoses for which other intra-abdominal procedures were performed) should be linked to the appendectomy procedure code to indicate the medical necessity of the procedure. When reporting appendectomy for an indicated purpose

❖ Report add-on code **44955** in addition the code for the primary procedure when open appendectomy is performed in conjunction with another procedure.

❖ Code **44979** must be reported for a laparoscopic appendectomy when done for an indicated purpose at the time of another major procedure.

Genitourinary System Procedures

Anogenital Examination

99170	Anogenital examination, magnified, in childhood for suspected trauma including image recording when performed

Moderate sedation may be separately reported when performed by the same physician performing the anogenital examination. Moderate sedation service of less than 10 minutes of intraservice time is not separately reported.

Example

➤ **A 6-year-old girl is brought to the ED by her mother after the mother noted blood in the child's underpants and was concerned about sexual molestation.** The physician performs a comprehensive history and physical examination. Because of the findings on general examination, the physician elects to further examine the child's genitalia with magnification to document findings that may be consistent with abuse or trauma.

ICD-10-CM	*CPT*®
Report confirmed abuse with **T74.22XA** (child sexual abuse, confirmed, initial encounter); an appropriate injury code (eg, **S39.848A**, other specified injuries of external genitals, initial encounter); a code from categories **X92–Y06** or **Y08** for assault; and a code from category **Y07** to identify the perpetrator of assault. If abuse is suspected but not confirmed, report **T76.22XA** (child sexual abuse, suspected, initial encounter) and a code for injury. If there are no findings, report **Z04.42** (encounter for examination and observation following alleged child rape or sexual abuse).	**99285** (comprehensive ED examination) **99170** (anogenital examination) If the same physician performs moderate (conscious) sedation, also report code **99152**. See more on moderate sedation in the Sedation section later in this chapter.

Lysis/Excision of Labial or Penile Adhesions

54450	Foreskin manipulation including lysis of preputial adhesions and stretching
54162	Lysis or excision of penile post-circumcision adhesions
56441	Lysis of labial adhesions

If lysis of labial or penile adhesions is performed by the application of manual pressure without the use of an instrument to cut the adhesions, it would be considered part of the E/M visit and not reported separately.

Code **54450** does not require general anesthesia. It has a relative value unit (RVU) of 2.00 when performed in a non-facility setting (eg, office). Medicare has assigned it a 0-day global surgery period. This procedure is performed on the uncircumcised foreskin and the head of the penis. Adhesions are broken by stretching the foreskin back over the head of the penis onto the shaft or by inserting a clamp between the foreskin and the head of the penis and spreading the jaws of the clamp.

Code **54162** is only reported when lysis is performed under general anesthesia or regional block, with an instrument, and under sterile conditions. This code has an RVU of 7.31 when performed in a non-facility setting (eg, office) and a Medicare 10-day global surgery period, which payers may or may not use. If post-circumcision adhesions are manually broken during the postoperative period by the physician or physician of the same group and specialty who performed the procedure, it would be considered part of the global surgical package. Report the service with *ICD-10-CM* code **N47.0**, adherent prepuce in a newborn, or **N47.5**, adhesions of prepuce and glans penis (patients older than 28 days). For repair of incomplete circumcision with removal of excessive residual foreskin, see code **54163**.

Code **56441** is performed by using a blunt instrument or scissors under general or local anesthesia. The total RVUs for this procedure in a non-facility setting are 4.09. This procedure also includes a Medicare 10-day global surgery period, which may or may not be used by payers. *ICD-10-CM* code **Q52.5** (fusion of labia) would be reported with *CPT* code **56441**. When provided without anesthesia, modifier **52** may be appended to indicate reduced services. Payer guidance may vary with regard to use of modifier **52**.

> ||||||| **Coding Pearl** |||||||
>
> A code for repair (eg, **13131**, repair, complex, forehead, cheeks, chin, mouth, neck, axillae, genitalia, hands and/or feet; 1.1 cm to 2.5 cm) is not reported in addition to code **54162** for the repair performed in conjunction with lysis or excision of penile post-circumcision adhesions.

Repair of Penis

Correction of Chordee and Hypospadias

54300	Plastic operation of penis for straightening of chordee (eg, hypospadias), with or without mobilization of urethra
54304	Plastic operation on penis for correction of chordee or for first stage hypospadias repair with or without transplantation of prepuce and/or skin flaps

Code **54300** is appropriately reported for straightening of the chordee to correct congenital concealed penis (**Q55.64**). This procedure may also be performed to correct an entrapped penis after newborn circumcision (eg, release of concealed penis with coverage of deficient penile ventral skin using penile skin-raised Byars flaps and re-circumcision).

Codes **54304–54336** describe procedures performed to correct hypospadias in either single-stage or multiple-stage procedures. Do not separately report codes **54300**, **54304**, or **54360** (plastic operation on penis to correct angulation) when reporting single-stage repair of hypospadias. Correction of penile chordee or penile curvature is included in all single-stage repairs of hypospadias. For more detailed information on reporting procedures to repair hypospadias, see the American Urological Association policy and advocacy brief, "Pediatric Hypospadias Repair: A New Consensus Document on Coding," at https://www.auanet.org/Documents/practices-resources/coding-tips/Pediatric-Hypospadias-Repair.pdf.

Negative Pressure Wound Therapy

97605   Negative pressure wound therapy (eg, vacuum assisted drainage collection), utilizing durable medical equipment (DME), including topical application(s), wound assessment, and instruction(s) for ongoing care, per session; total wound(s) surface area less than or equal to 50 square centimeters

97606   total wound(s) surface area greater than 50 square centimeters

97607   Negative pressure wound therapy, (eg, vacuum assisted drainage collection), utilizing disposable, non-durable medical equipment including provision of exudate management collection system, topical application(s), wound assessment, and instructions for ongoing care, per session; total wound(s) surface area less than or equal to 50 square centimeters

97608   total wound(s) surface area greater than 50 square centimeters

It has become common in recent years for physicians to include use of NPWT or vacuum-assisted closure in the management of traumatic and surgical wounds. Codes **97605** and **97606** represent NPWT provided via a system that includes a *non-disposable* suction pump and drainage collection device. Codes **97607** and **97608** are used for NPWT that utilizes a *disposable* suction pump and collection system. Codes **97607** and **97608** are not reported in conjunction with codes **97605** and **97606**. Payer policies may limit coverage to care of specific types of wounds that require NPWT to improve granulation tissue formation and to certain types of NPWT equipment. Be sure to verify the coverage policy of the patient's health plan prior to provision of services.

Negative pressure wound therapy

- Requires direct (one-on-one) physician or QHP contact with the patient.
- May be initiated in a hospital or surgical center setting and continued in the home setting after discharge.
- Includes application of dressings.
- Is separately reported when performed in conjunction with surgical debridement (**11042–11047**).
- Documentation should include current wound assessment, including quantitative measurements of wound characteristics (eg, site, surface area and depth), any previous treatment regimens, debridement (when performed), prescribed length of treatment, dressing types and frequency of changes, and other concerns that affect healing. Encounters for ongoing NPWT may include documentation of progress of healing and changes in the wound, including measurement, amount of exudate, and presence of granulation or necrotic tissue.
- Supplies, including dressings, are reportable with HCPCS codes (eg, **A6550**, wound care set, for NPWT electrical pump, includes all supplies and accessories). Supplies for a disposable system are reported with code **A9272**, which also includes all dressings and accessories.

Sedation

Moderate Sedation

Moderate sedation codes **99151–99153** and **99155–99157** are used for reporting moderate sedation when intraservice time is 10 minutes or more. **Table 19-9** contains sedation codes and descriptors.

Moderate sedation is a drug-induced depression of consciousness during which patients respond purposefully to verbal commands, either alone or accompanied by light tactile stimulation. No interventions are required to maintain cardiovascular functions or a patent airway, and spontaneous ventilation is adequate. Moderate sedation codes are not used to report administration of medications for pain control, minimal sedation (anxiolysis), deep sedation, or monitored anesthesia care (**00100–01999**).

Moderate sedation in the outpatient setting is typically performed by the same physician or QHP who is performing the diagnostic or therapeutic service and requires the presence of an independent trained observer. An *independent trained observer* is an individual qualified to monitor the patient during the procedure but who has no other duties (eg, assisting at surgery)

> ||||||| **Coding Pearl** |||||||
>
> Codes **99153–99157** are reported for each additional 15 minutes of intraservice time. The midpoint between the end of the previous 15-minute period must be passed to report an additional unit of intraservice time (ie, intraservice time must continue for at least 8 minutes beyond the last full 15 minutes of intraservice time).

during the procedure. In the facility setting, a physician or QHP other than the person performing the diagnostic or therapeutic service may provide moderate sedation services.

Table 19-9. Moderate Sedation		
Moderate Sedation	**First 10–22 min of Intraservice Time**	**Each Additional 15 min of Intraservice Time**
Moderate sedation services provided by the same physician or other qualified health care professional performing the diagnostic or therapeutic service that the sedation supports, requiring the presence of an independent trained observer to assist in the monitoring of the patient's level of consciousness and physiological status; initial 15 minutes of intraservice time, patient younger than 5 years of age	99151	+99153
5 years or older	99152	+99153
Moderate sedation services (other than those services described by codes 00100–01999) provided by a physician other than the health care professional performing the diagnostic or therapeutic service that the sedation supports; younger than 5 years	99155	+99157
5 years or older	99156	+99157

Codes 99151–99153 are reported when

⚬ The administration of moderate sedation is provided by the physician who is simultaneously performing a procedure (eg, fracture reduction, vessel cutdown, central line placement, wound repair).

⚬ An independent trained observer is present to assist the physician in the monitoring of the patient during the procedure or diagnostic service.

Codes 99155–99157 are reported when

⚬ A second physician or QHP other than the health care professional performing the diagnostic or therapeutic services provides moderate sedation.

⚬ Codes 99153 and 99157 are reported for each additional 15 minutes of intraservice time. The midpoint between the end of the previous 15-minute period must be passed to report an additional unit of intraservice time (ie, intraservice time must continue for at least 8 minutes beyond the last full 15 minutes of intraservice time).

Note: Documentation must include the description of the procedure, name and dosage(s) of the sedation agent(s), route of administration of the sedation agent(s), and who administered the agent (physician or independent observer); the ongoing assessment of the child's level of consciousness and physiological status (eg, heart rate, oxygen saturation levels) during and after the procedure; and the presence, name, and title of the independent observer and total time from administration of the sedation agent(s) (start time) until the physician's face-to-face service is no longer required (end time).

⚬ Codes are selected based on intraservice time. Intraservice time
  ❖ Begins with the administration of the sedating agent(s)
  ❖ Ends when the procedure is completed, the patient is stable for recovery status, and the physician or other QHP providing the sedation ends personal continuous face-to-face time with the patient
  ❖ Includes ordering and/or administering the initial and subsequent doses of sedating agents
  ❖ Requires continuous face-to-face attendance of the physician or other QHP
  ❖ Requires monitoring patient response to the sedating agents, including
    — Periodic assessment of the patient
    — Further administration of agent(s) as needed to maintain sedation
    — Monitoring of oxygen saturation, heart rate, and blood pressure
⚬ Moderate sedation service of less than 10 minutes' intraservice time is not separately reported.

- Preservice work of moderate sedation services is not separately reported and not included in intraservice time. Preservice work includes
  - Assessment of the patient's past medical and surgical history with particular emphasis on cardiovascular, pulmonary, airway, or neurologic conditions
  - Review of the patient's previous experiences with anesthesia and/or sedation
  - Family history of sedation complications
  - Summary of the patient's present medication list
  - Drug allergy and intolerance history
  - Focused physical examination of the patient, with emphasis on
    - Mouth, jaw, oropharynx, neck, and airway for Mallampati score assessment
    - Chest and lungs
    - Heart and circulation
    - Vital signs, including heart rate, respiratory rate, blood pressure, and oxygenation, with end-tidal carbon dioxide when indicated
  - Review of any pre-sedation diagnostic tests
  - Completion of a pre-sedation assessment form (with American Society of Anesthesiologists [ASA] physical status classification)
  - Patient informed consent
  - Immediate pre-sedation assessment prior to first sedating doses
  - Initiation of IV access and fluids to maintain patency
- Do not separately report or include the time of post-service work in the intraservice time. Post-service work of moderate sedation includes
  - Assessment of the patient's vital signs, level of consciousness, neurologic, cardiovascular, and pulmonary stability in the post-sedation recovery period
  - Assessment of patient's readiness for discharge following the procedure
  - Preparation of documentation for sedation service
  - Communication with family or caregiver about sedation service
- Oxygen saturation (94760–94762) cannot be reported separately.
- Codes 99151–99157 are distinguished by service provider, patient age, and time spent (see **Table 19-9**).

> **~ More From the AAP ~**
>
> For more information on coding for moderate sedation services, see "Starting Over With Moderate Sedation" in the December 2016 *AAP Pediatric Coding Newsletter* at http://coding.aap.org (subscription required).

Example

> A **5-year old** hospitalized child needs insertion of a tunneled central venous catheter (36558). A second physician will provide the moderate sedation while the first physician performs the procedure. The sedating physician administers the agent(s) and assesses the patient continuously until a safe level of moderate sedation is achieved. He or she monitors the child closely and administers additional doses of sedating and/or analgesic agent(s) as needed. The service, from the time of administration of the agent until determination that the child is stable and face-to-face physician time is no longer required, takes a total of 35 minutes. The physician providing the moderate sedation will report

ICD-10-CM	CPT
Appropriate diagnosis code	99156 (moderate [conscious] sedation services by second physician or QHP, patient 5 years or older, first 15 minutes) +99157 (moderate [conscious] sedation, each additional 15 minutes of intraservice time)

Deep Sedation

Deep sedation/analgesia is a drug-induced depression of consciousness during which patients cannot be easily aroused but respond purposefully after repeated verbal or painful stimulation (eg, purposefully pushing away the noxious stimuli). The ability to independently maintain ventilatory function may be impaired. Patients may require assistance in maintaining a patent airway, and spontaneous ventilation may be inadequate. Cardiovascular function is usually maintained. A state of deep sedation may be accompanied by partial or complete loss of protective airway reflexes.

Anesthesia services include
* Preoperative evaluation of the patient
* Administration of anesthetic, other medications, blood, and fluids
* Monitoring of physiologic parameters
* Other supportive services
* Postoperative E/M related to the surgery (ongoing critical care services by an anesthesiologist may be separately reportable)

> ‖‖‖ **Coding Pearl** ‖‖‖
>
> If surgery is canceled, subsequent to the preoperative evaluation, payment may be allowed to the anesthesiologist for an evaluation and management (E/M) service and the appropriate E/M code (eg, consultation) may be reported. See Chapter 16, Noncritical Hospital Evaluation and Management Services, for information on reporting these services.

Pediatricians who provide deep sedation services for procedures performed outside the operating suite should follow the same anesthesia policies and coding instructions as other providers of anesthesia services. *CPT®* codes for reporting anesthesia services, including deep sedation, monitored anesthesia care, or general anesthesia, are **00100–01999**. These codes are not as specific as codes for other services and generally identify a body area or type of procedure.

00102   Anesthesia for procedures involving plastic repair of cleft lip

01820   Anesthesia for all closed procedures on radius, ulna, wrist, or hand bones

Add-on codes may be reported to identify special circumstances that increase the complexity of providing anesthesia care, including

99100   Patient under 1 year or older than 70 years (not reported in conjunction with codes **00326, 00561, 00834**, or **00836**)

99116   Anesthesia complicated by total body hypothermia

99135   Anesthesia complicated by controlled hypotension

99140   Emergency conditions

> ~ **More From the AAP** ~
>
> For more information on coding for deep sedation services, see articles in the April and May 2014 *AAP Pediatric Coding Newsletter™* at http://coding.aap.org (subscription required).

Emergency is defined by *CPT* as a situation in which delay in treatment of the patient would lead to a significant increase in the threat to life or body part.

Modifiers are reported in addition to anesthesia codes to indicate the physical status of the patient. The ASA classification of the patient's physical status is represented by the following HCPCS modifiers:

P1   Normal healthy patient

P2   Patient with mild systemic disease

P3   Patient with severe systemic disease

P4   Patient with severe systemic disease that is a constant threat to life

P5   Moribund patient who is not expected to survive without the operation

P6   Declared brain-dead patient whose organs are being removed for donor purposes

Other modifiers that may be required by payers for anesthesia services by pediatric physicians are those identifying the type of anesthesia or anesthesia provider.

AA   Anesthesia services performed personally by anesthesiologist
* Payers may require this modifier for services personally rendered by physicians other than anesthesiologists. This signifies that services were not rendered by a nonphysician provider, such as a certified registered nurse anesthetist.

G8   Monitored anesthesia care for deep complex, complicated, or markedly invasive surgical procedure

G9   Monitored anesthesia care for patient who has history of severe cardiopulmonary condition

QS   Monitored anesthesia care service

      ⚙ Medicare considers deep sedation equivalent to monitored anesthesia care. Private payers may vary.

GC   This service has been performed in part by a resident under the direction of a teaching physician

  Base units for anesthesia services are published in the ASA *Relative Value Guide* and by the CMS for each anesthesia procedure code. Payers typically do not require reporting of base units on the claim for services.

⚙ Many private payers will allow additional base units for physical status modifiers **P3** (1 unit), **P4** (2 units), and **P5** (3 units).

⚙ Anesthesia time is reported in minutes unless a payer directs to report units (1 unit per 15 minutes). Start and stop times must be documented, including multiple start and stop times when anesthesia services are discontinuous.

Postoperative Pain Management

Generally, the surgeon is responsible for postoperative pain management. However, a surgeon may request assistance with postoperative pain management (eg, epidural or peripheral nerve block).

⚙ Payers may require a written request by the surgeon for postoperative pain management by the anesthesia provider.

⚙ When a catheter is placed as the mode of anesthesia (eg, epidural catheter) and retained for use in postoperative pain management, this is not separately reported.

⚙ When separately reporting postoperative pain management, append modifier **59** (distinct procedural service) to indicate the separate service and document this service distinctly (and preferably separately) from the anesthesia record.

⚙ When an epidural catheter is used for postoperative pain management, code **01996** (daily management of epidural) may be reported on days subsequent to the day of surgery. Daily management of other postoperative pain management devices may be reported with subsequent hospital care codes (**99231–99233**).

Example

➤ **An orthopedic surgeon requests preanesthetic insertion of a catheter to provide a continuous infusion of the femoral nerve for postoperative pain relief for a patient undergoing an arthroscopy of the knee with lateral meniscectomy.** The anesthesiologist uses ultrasound guidance to insert a catheter for continuous infusion prior to inducing general anesthesia for the surgical procedure.

ICD-10-CM	CPT®
Appropriate diagnosis code	**01400** (anesthesia for open or surgical arthroscopic procedures on knee joint; not otherwise specified) **64448 59** (injection, anesthetic agent; femoral nerve, continuous infusion by catheter [including catheter placement])

  Teaching Point: Because the anesthetist provided a distinct service separate from the anesthesia for the procedure, the catheter insertion is separately reported with modifier **59**. Had the procedure been performed under an epidural block and the epidural catheter left in place for postoperative pain management, no additional code would be reported.

Part 4:
Digital Medicine Services

Part 4: Digital Medicine Services

Digital Medicine Services:
Technology-Enhanced Care Delivery

Contents

This chapter provides information on coding for services that reflect and support the use of technology in enhancing care delivery. This includes face-to-face care facilitated by digital technology and services that involve collection and interpretation of physiological data. Each of the services involving digital technology has distinct service elements and periods of service.

Telemedicine

Telemedicine is the use of technology to bring a specialist in a distant location to a patient's bedside or to a setting right in the patient's own community without the need for either party to physically travel. *Telemedicine* is one term used to describe the provision of face-to-face services through the use of technology. Telemedicine may also be referred to as *telehealth;* definitions for each vary by state and payer, but telehealth is more commonly used to reference any health service provided via telecommunications. Telemedicine may be more appropriate to describe services of physicians and other qualified health care professionals (QHPs) and is the terminology used by *Current Procedural Terminology (CPT®)*. Without any consideration of state law or payer policies, telemedicine services might be loosely defined as audiovisual technology–enabled, patient-specific services provided by a physician or practitioner in a distant geographic location to a patient who requires medical expertise not otherwise available at his or her location.

Interest in telemedicine services has grown significantly in recent years. In December 2016, the Expanding Capacity for Health Outcomes (ECHO) Act was signed into law. The ECHO Act requires the secretary of Health and Human Services, in collaboration with the Health Resources and Services Administration, to study and publish a report, within 2 years of enactment, on technology-enabled learning and capacity building models and their effect on

- Addressing mental and substance use disorders, chronic diseases and conditions, prenatal and maternal health, pediatric care, pain management, and palliative care
- Addressing health care workforce issues, such as specialty care shortages and primary care workforce recruitment, retention, and support for lifelong learning
- The implementation of public health programs, including those related to disease prevention, infectious disease outbreaks, and public health surveillance
- The delivery of health care services in rural areas, frontier areas, health professional shortage areas, and medically underserved areas and to medically underserved populations and Native Americans
- Addressing other issues the secretary determines appropriate

Findings from this study will likely serve as a catalyst for additional support of telemedicine in federally funded health programs.

In addition to increased federal interest in telemedicine services, most states have enacted or have pending legislation aimed at parity in payment of telemedicine services. The American Telemedicine Association offers state legislation and regulatory trackers online at https://www.americantelemed.org/policy-page/state-policy-resource-center.

Payer Coverage

Currently, payers may restrict utilization of telemedicine services to certain settings and to patients located in rural areas that Medicare designates as a Health Professional Shortage Area. However, demonstration projects, such as those for accountable care organizations, are expanding the provision of care via telemedicine and may provide evidence to support expansion to all patients in the future. See the Medicare Telehealth Guidelines box later in this chapter for information on Medicare coverage policies, which may be adopted by other payers.

There is wide variation in how private payers and state Medicaid plans define and cover telemedicine services, making it important to identify the applicable definition and payment policies prior to delivery of services. Many states limit coverage to that delivered via interactive systems using multimedia communications equipment that includes, at minimum, audio and video equipment permitting 2-way, real-time communication between the patient and the distant site practitioner. Asynchronous or store-and-forward technology may be allowed in some areas or for certain services.

Medicare Telehealth Guidelines

Payers may adopt Medicare telehealth policies for telemedicine services. Medicare defines the term *telehealth service* as professional consultations, office visits, and office psychiatry services and any additional service specified by the secretary of Health and Human Services. These services are paid under the following conditions:

- The service is provided using an interactive 2-way telecommunications system (with real-time audio and video). An exception allows asynchronous communications in Alaska and Hawaii when participating in a demonstration project.
- The patient is at an eligible originating site (eg, office, hospital in a health professional shortage area) at the time of service.
- The physician/qualified health care professional is not in the same location as the patient. The site where the physician provides the service is referred to as a distant location.
- Subsequent hospital visits (**99231–99233**) via telehealth are limited to 1 visit every 3 days.
- An originating site fee is paid (approximately $25.76) to the office or facility where the patient is located when reported with code **Q3014**. An eligibility analyzer for checking whether an originating site is eligible for originating site payment is on the Health Resources and Services Administration Web site (https://datawarehouse.hrsa.gov/tools/analyzers/geo/Telehealth.aspx).

From a coding perspective, telemedicine services are face-to-face services reported using the same evaluation and management (E/M) codes that would be appropriate for in-person encounters.

- Usually, these are consultation services (eg, inpatient consultations [**99251–99255**]). Typically, key components or time spent in counseling and/or coordination of care may be used to select the level of E/M service provided.
- As with many services, there are combinations of *CPT* and Healthcare Common Procedure Coding System (HCPCS) codes and modifiers that may apply.
- An understanding of coverage, payment policies, and coding requirements is essential to establishing a successful telemedicine service. Coverage and reporting requirements will vary across payers, requiring verification of benefits prior to provision of services.
- The Medicare program limits payment for telemedicine services to a specific set of services.

A list of services designated as telemedicine services by *CPT®* and/or Medicare and the codes for reporting each are included in **Table 20-1**. Telemedicine services covered by Medicare are published each year as part of the update to the Medicare Physician Fee Schedule. Medicaid and/or private health plans may adopt Medicare coverage policies and/or list of covered services. **Note:** 2019 information was not available at time of publication; visit www.aap.org/cfp (access code AAPCFP24) for any updates to this list.

Table 20-1. 2018 Telemedicine Services

CY 2018 Telehealth Services (Please see coding reference for code descriptors.)	HCPCS/*CPT* Code	*CPT* Allows[a]	Medicare Allows
Advanced care planning	**99497** and **99498**		✓
Annual alcohol misuse screening, 15 min	G0442		✓
Annual behavioral therapy for cardiovascular disease, 15 min	G0446		✓
Annual depression screening, 15 min	G0444		✓
Annual wellness visit, first visit	G0438		✓
Annual wellness visit, subsequent visit	G0439		✓
Behavioral counseling for alcohol misuse, 15 min	G0443		✓
Behavioral counseling for obesity, 15 min	G0447		✓
Comprehensive assessment and care planning for chronic care management	G0506		✓

Table 20-1. 2018 Telemedicine Services (*continued*)			
CY 2018 Telehealth Services (Please see coding reference for code descriptors.)	**HCPCS/*CPT* Code**	**CPT Allows**[a]	**Medicare Allows**
Diabetes self-management training services	G0108 and G0109		✓
Electrocardiographic rhythm derived event recording	93268, 93270–93272	✓	
ESRD-related services[b]	90951, 90952, 90954, 90955, 90957, 90958, 90960, and 90961	✓	✓
ESRD-related services for home dialysis[b]	90963–90970		✓
External mobile cardiovascular telemetry with electrocardiographic recording, concurrent computerized real-time data analysis	93228 and 93229	✓	
Genetic counseling	96040	✓	
Health and behavior assessment and intervention	96150–96154	✓	✓
Health risk assessment	96160 and 96161		✓
High-intensity behavioral counseling to prevent sexually transmitted infection; 30 min	G0445		✓
Hospital subsequent care services (Payer may limit to 1 telehealth visit every 3 days.)	99231–99233	✓	✓
Inpatient consultation	99251–99255	✓	
Kidney disease education services	G0420 and G0421		✓
Medical nutrition therapy	G0270		✓
	97802–97804	✓	
Neurobehavioral status exam	96116	✓	✓
Nursing facility subsequent care services (Payer may limit to 1 telehealth visit every 30 days.)	99307–99310	✓	✓
Office consultation	99241–99245	✓	
Office or other outpatient visits	99201–99215	✓	✓
Pharmacologic management performed with psychotherapy services	90863	✓	
Pharmacologic management, telehealth, inpatient	G0459		✓
Prolonged service in the inpatient or observation setting	99356 and 99357		✓
Prolonged service in the office or other outpatient setting	99354 and 99355	✓	✓
Psychiatric diagnostic interview examination	90791 and 90792	✓	✓
Psychiatric services with interactive complexity	+90785		✓
Psychoanalysis	90845	✓	✓
Psychotherapy, family	90846 and 90847	✓	✓
Psychotherapy, individual	90832–90834 and 90836–90838	✓	✓
Psychotherapy for crisis	90839 and 90840		
Remote imaging for detection of retinal disease	92227	✓	
Remote imaging for monitoring and management of active retinal disease	92228	✓	

CY 2018 Telehealth Services (Please see coding reference for code descriptors.)	HCPCS/*CPT* Code	*CPT* Allows[a]	Medicare Allows
Remote interrogation implantable loop recorder	93298 and 93299	✓	
Self-management education and training	98960–98962	✓	
Smoking cessation services	G0436 and G0437		✓
	99406 and 99407	✓	
Structured assessment and intervention services for alcohol and/or substance (other than tobacco) abuse	G0396 and G0397		✓
	99408 and 99409	✓	
Telehealth consultation, critical care, initial, physicians typically spend 60 minutes	G0508		✓
Telehealth consultation, critical care, subsequent, physicians typically spend 50 minutes	G0509		✓
Telehealth consultations, emergency department or initial inpatient	G0425–G0427		✓
Telehealth consultations, follow-up inpatient hospital or SNF	G0406–G0408		✓
Transitional care management services	99495 and 99496	✓	✓

Abbreviations: CMS, Centers for Medicare & Medicaid Services; CPT, Current Procedural Terminology; CY, calendar year; ESRD, end-stage renal disease; HCPCS, Healthcare Common Procedure Coding System; SNF, skilled nursing facility.

[a] Append modifier 95 (telemedicine service rendered via a real-time interactive audio and video telecommunications system).

[b] For ESRD-related services, a physician, nurse practitioner, physician assistant, or clinical nurse specialist must furnish at least one "hands-on" visit (not telehealth) each month to examine the vascular access site.

Medicaid Payment

For purposes of Medicaid, telemedicine permits 2-way, real-time interactive communication between the patient and the practitioner at the distant site. This electronic communication means the use of interactive telecommunications equipment that includes, at a minimum, audio and video equipment.

States are encouraged by the Centers for Medicare & Medicaid Services to create innovative payment methodologies for services that incorporate telemedicine technology. For example, states may pay the physician or other licensed practitioner at the distant site and pay a facility fee to the originating site. States can also pay any additional costs, such as technical support, transmission charges, and equipment. These add-on costs can be incorporated into the fee-for-service rates or separately paid as an administrative cost by the state. If they are separately billed and paid, the costs must be linked to a covered Medicaid service.

States may also choose to pay for telehealth services that do not meet the definition of telemedicine services (eg, telephones, facsimile machines, e-mail systems, and remote patient monitoring devices, which are used to collect and transmit patient data for monitoring and interpretation).

States may select from a variety of HCPCS codes (eg, T1014 [telehealth transmission, per minute]; Q3014 [telehealth originating site facility fee]) and *CPT*® codes and modifiers (eg, GT, U1–UD) to identify, track, and pay for telemedicine services. HCPCS codes for reporting telemedicine services are discussed later in this chapter.

Place and Site of Service

Place of service (POS) code 02 is used to report the location where health services and health-related services are provided or received through a telecommunications system. *Telecommunications system* is not defined but should be considered to reflect use of technology as defined by the payer (eg, real-time audiovisual communications technology). It may be necessary to work with your electronic system vendors to determine the best method for ensuring that telemedicine service claims contain this POS code. In most practice management systems, the POS may be manually entered for each charge entered.

Field 32 of the 1500 paper claim form and its electronic equivalent is used to report the site of service (eg, hospital name, address, National Provider Identifier). This is typically the physical location of the physician or other provider of service at the time of service when payment is influenced by geographic location. See an individual payer's telemedicine policy to determine if there are reporting requirements for the specific site of service (eg, physical location from which services were rendered or received).

Documentation of Services

Documentation of telemedicine services should be similar to that of services provided in traditional patient care settings. For E/M services, this means that documentation supports reporting of services based on the required key components (ie, history, examination, and/or medical decision-making [MDM]) or typical time of service (when >50% of the face-to-face time of the encounter is spent in counseling and/or coordination of care). See Chapter 6, Evaluation and Management Documentation Guidelines, for more information on documentation of E/M services and instructions for reporting E/M services based on time spent in counseling and/or coordination of care.

Reporting Telemedicine With *Current Procedural Terminology*®

CPT modifier 95 is appended to the appropriate procedure code to identify telemedicine services when rendered via real-time interactive audio and video telecommunications. This modifier is not applied if the communication is not real-time interactive audio and video. Telephone care is not telemedicine.

95   Telemedicine service rendered via a real-time interactive audio and video telecommunications system: Synchronous telemedicine service is defined as a real-time interaction between a physician or other qualified health care professional and a patient who is located at a distant site from the physician or other qualified health care professional. The totality of the communication of information exchanged between the provider or other qualified health care professional and the patient during the course of the synchronous telemedicine service must be of an amount and nature that would be sufficient to meet the key components and/or requirements of the same service when rendered via a face-to-face interaction. Modifier 95 may only be appended to the services listed in Appendix P. Appendix P is the list of *CPT* codes for services that are typically performed face-to-face but may be rendered via a real-time (synchronous) interactive audio and video telecommunications system.

In addition to modifier 95, *CPT* includes Appendix P, listing all codes to which the 95 modifier is applicable, and adds a star symbol (★) to the listing of each code included in Appendix P in the main body of the manual. Appendix P codes that may be of particular interest to pediatricians include

- New and established patient office or other outpatient E/M services (99201–99205, 99212–99215)
- Subsequent hospital care (99231–99233)
- Inpatient (99251–99255) and outpatient (99241–99245) consultations
- Subsequent nursing facility care (99307–99310)
- Prolonged services in the office or outpatient setting (99354, 99355)
- Individual behavior change interventions (99406–99409)
- Transitional care management services (99495, 99496)

Appendix P also includes codes for services such as psychotherapy, health and behavior assessment and intervention, medical nutrition therapy, and education and training for patient self-management, allowing for telemedicine services provided by certain qualified nonphysician health care professionals in addition to subspecialty physicians.

Reporting Telemedicine With Healthcare Common Procedure Coding System

HCPCS uses the term *telehealth* in code descriptors. Under a Medicare demonstration project, physicians providing asynchronous telemedicine services in Alaska and Hawaii may report those services with modifier GQ appended to the appropriate code for the services rendered.

GQ   Via asynchronous telecommunications system (Medicare applies this modifier only to services provided as part of a telemedicine demonstration project in Alaska and Hawaii.)

Previously, modifier GT was required with all codes for telemedicine services submitted to Medicare and some other payers. Place of service code 02 now signifies a service provided via real-time (synchronous) telecommunications, and modifier GT is no longer required on claims for professional services submitted to Medicare. Other payers will likely also discontinue use of modifier GT. (*Note:* Critical access hospitals billing under Method II still report modifier GT because no POS code is reported on Method II claims.)

Under some plans, additional codes may be reported for overhead expenses of providing telemedicine services.

Q3014   Telehealth originating site facility fee

T1014   Telehealth transmission, per minute, professional services bill separately

For Medicare purposes, an *originating site* is the location of an eligible Medicare beneficiary at the time the service furnished via telemedicine occurs.

While *CPT* codes are accepted by most plans covering telemedicine services, payers may require HCPCS codes that are used in the Medicare program for consultations and other services with specific coverage policies (eg, inpatient telehealth pharmacologic management with no more than minimal psychotherapy). HCPCS codes are used for telemedicine consultations with Medicare beneficiaries because *CPT* consultation codes are not payable under the Medicare Physician Fee Schedule. Only specific services are eligible for Medicare payment when provided via telemedicine. The following codes do not apply in all potential settings where telemedicine might be provided (eg, Medicare does not cover telemedicine services to patients in observation settings). Exceptions apply for telemedicine services rendered as part of certain demonstration projects (eg, under telehealth waiver for patients associated with a Next Generation accountable care organization).

G0406   Follow-up inpatient consultation, limited, physicians typically spend 15 minutes communicating with the patient via telehealth

G0407   intermediate, physicians typically spend 25 minutes communicating with the patient via telehealth

G0408   complex, physicians typically spend 35 minutes communicating with the patient via telehealth

G0425   Telehealth consultation, emergency department or initial inpatient, typically 30 minutes communicating with the patient via telehealth

G0426   typically 50 minutes communicating with the patient via telehealth

G0427   typically 70 minutes or more communicating with the patient via telehealth

G0459   Inpatient telehealth pharmacologic management, including prescription, use, and review of medication with no more than minimal medical psychotherapy

G0508   Telehealth consultation, critical care, physicians typically spend 60 minutes communicating with the patient via telehealth (initial)

G0509   Telehealth consultation, critical care, physicians typically spend 50 minutes communicating with the patient via telehealth (subsequent)

When a payer uses Medicare program policies for telemedicine services, it is important to learn which services are and are not covered when delivered via telemedicine. A current listing of services covered under the Medicare program is available in Chapter 12 of the *Medicare Claims Processing Manual* (https://www.cms.gov/Regulations-and-Guidance/Guidance/Manuals/downloads/clm104c12.pdf).

Examples

➤ **A consultation is requested of a rheumatologist at a teaching facility for an inpatient in a rural hospital, 75 miles away.** Through real-time interactive technology, the physician performs a consultation, including a comprehensive history, comprehensive examination (assisted by clinical staff of the facility), and MDM of moderate complexity. The total time of the interactive communication is 30 minutes. A written report to the requesting physician is transmitted via secure electronic health information exchange.

MDM: Moderate *History:* Comprehensive *Physical examination:* Comprehensive	**CPT**® **99254 95** (inpatient consultation) or, if payer requires HCPCS codes, **G0425** (telehealth consultation, emergency department or initial inpatient, typically 30 minutes communicating with the patient via telehealth)

Teaching Point: If payer policy allows payment for overhead expenses related to telemedicine services, also report **T1014**, telehealth transmission, per minute, professional services bill separately. Because this is billed per minute, 30 units are reported. The rural hospital, as the originating facility, may also report **Q3014**, telehealth originating site facility fee.

➤ **A child with a closed head injury is held in outpatient observation at a rural health facility until evaluated via interactive audiovisual technology by a neurosurgeon who is located 500 miles away.** The child, whose current injury is the result of a car crash, has history of a concussion sustained while playing football 1 year earlier. The neurosurgeon spends 35 minutes prior to initiation of the interactive telecommunications discussing the case with the attending physician and reviewing prior medical records pertaining to the previous concussion as well as the digital images of current and past computed tomography scans. Based on the neurosurgeon's findings after review of medical records, imaging, and consultation with the patient, the patient will remain in observation at the rural facility overnight and be discharged to home if no complications occur during observation. The neurosurgeon's total time of interactive communication is 30 minutes. A follow-up visit with the neurosurgeon via telemedicine is scheduled in 7 days.

Initial outpatient consultation	**CPT** **99242 95** (office consultation for a new or established patient, typical time of 30 minutes) (HCPCS codes for telemedicine services do not include services to patients in observation. Verification of benefits and reporting requirements for telemedicine services should be conducted prior to delivery of telemedicine services.) **99358** (prolonged E/M service before and/or after direct patient care; first hour)
Follow-up visit	Report the appropriate office or other outpatient visit code (**99212–99215**) appended with modifier **95**.

Teaching Point: Because the physician spent more than 30 minutes in prolonged service related to the telemedicine service, code **99358** is reportable. Payers may or may not provide separate payment for indirect prolonged service. Modified **95** is not appended to **99358**, as this portion of the service was not face-to-face via interactive technology.

If the patient had been transferred and admitted to the neurosurgeon's care at the distant facility on the same date, all the neurosurgeon's E/M services provided on that date would be included in the initial hospital care.

➤ **An endocrinologist provides a follow-up visit for a patient who has uncontrolled diabetes mellitus type 1 and resides 3 hours away from the nearest pediatric endocrinology practice.** The patient is in her primary care physician's clinic, where clinical staff are present to assist with physical examination and other patient care that may be required during the telemedicine service. The endocrinologist spends 10 minutes prior to the visit reviewing the patient's medical records and 25 minutes face-to-face with the patient and caregivers via real-time audiovisual connection, obtaining more information and discussing options for better managing the patient's diabetes. Following the face-to-face encounter with the patient, the endocrinologist documents the service, indicating that 20 minutes of the 25-minute service were spent in counseling the patient and caregivers. A copy of the visit note is sent via secure electronic transmittal to the primary care physician. The patient's health plan accepts *CPT®* codes for telemedicine services. In addition, the health plan allows the primary care physician's clinic to report the practice expense of serving as the originating site for the encounter.

The endocrinologist reports	**99214 95** (office or other outpatient visit for the E/M of an established patient, which requires at least 2 of these 3 key components: <ul><li>a detailed history;</li><li>a detailed examination;</li><li>MDM of moderate complexity)</li></ul> (Counseling and/or coordination of care with other physicians, other QHPs, or agencies are provided consistent with the nature of the problem[s] and the patient's and/or family's needs. Usually, the presenting problem[s] are of moderate to high severity. Typically, 25 minutes are spent face-to-face with the patient and/or family.)
The ordering physician reports	**Q3014** (telehealth originating site facility fee)

Teaching Point: Because the endocrinologist's visit was predominately spent counseling and/or coordinating care, the visit is reported based on time. The time spent before and after the real-time telemedicine service with the patient is included in the preservice and post-service work of the encounter, just as it would be for an encounter in which the patient presented in the endocrinologist's office. Payment policies will vary regarding originating site fees. Practices choosing to offer telemedicine originating site services should verify the policies of plans commonly billed by the practice before initiating services.

Critical Care via Telemedicine

Codes **0188T** and **0189T** were *CPT®* Category III codes (emerging technology) previously reported for critical care via telemedicine. These codes are deleted in 2019. HCPCS codes **G0508** and **G0509** may alternatively be included as covered critical care services when provided via telemedicine.

Example

➤ **A pediatric intensivist is contacted via live audiovisual telecommunications to provide remote critical care to an infant who is entering respiratory failure due to bronchiolitis.** The intensivist views radiographs and other data from monitoring devices in addition to performing visual and audio examination of the infant. The attending physician at the hospital where the infant is an inpatient performs necessary procedures as advised by the intensivist (eg, intubation). The infant remains at the same hospital under the care of the pediatrician. A total of 65 minutes of remote critical care service is provided.

The neonatologist reports	**G0508** (telehealth consultation, critical care, physicians typically spend 60 minutes communicating with the patient via telehealth [initial])
The attending physician reports	*CPT* codes for services personally performed (eg, initial hospital care, intubation)

Teaching Point: Code **G0508** is reported only once per date of service per patient.

Remote Physiologic Monitoring

New in 2019 are codes **99453** and **99454**, which are used to report remote physiologic monitoring services during a 30-day period. Code **99091** is also revised to include collection and interpretation of physiologic data over the course of a 30-day period. Code **99090** (analysis of clinical data stored in computers) has been deleted. Also, a new code, **99457**, is added for reporting remote physiologic monitoring and treatment management services.

Remote Monitoring Setup and Supply

#●99453   Remote monitoring of physiologic parameter(s) (eg, weight, blood pressure, pulse oximetry, respiratory flow rate), initial; set-up and patient education on use of equipment

#●99454   device(s) supply with daily recording(s) or programmed alert(s) transmission, each 30 days

To report codes **99453** and **99454**, the device used must be a medical device as defined by the US Food and Drug Administration (FDA) (eg, blood glucose monitor) and the service must be ordered by a physician or QHP. Codes are used to report remote physiologic monitoring services (**99453**, **99454**) during only the initial 30-day period. Do not report when monitoring is less than 16 days.

- Do not report codes **99453** and **99454** in conjunction with codes for more specific physiologic parameters (eg, pulse oximetry [**94760**]).
- Do not report **99453** and **99454** when these services are included in other *CPT*® codes for the duration of time of the physiologic monitoring service (eg, **95250** for continuous glucose requires a minimum of 72 hours of monitoring).
- Initial setup and patient education on use of equipment (**99453**) is reported for each episode of care. For reporting remote monitoring of physiologic parameters, an episode of care is defined as beginning when the remote monitoring physiologic service is initiated and ends with attainment of targeted treatment goals.
- Do not report **99453** more than once per episode of care.

Code **99454** may be used to report the initial supply of the device for daily recording or programmed alert transmissions. This also is reported only once per episode of care.

See discussion of coding for continuous glucose monitoring and home apnea monitoring services later in this chapter for information on reporting these services.

> |||||||| **Coding Pearl** ||||||||
>
> Codes **99453** and **99454** are only reported once per episode of care. This is indicated by the word "initial," which precedes the semicolon in the code descriptor and, therefore, applies to both codes.

Examples

➤ **A child with newly diagnosed diabetes is enrolled in a remote physiologic patient monitoring program.** The patient is provided with setup and education for use of a Bluetooth-enabled glucose meter and the program's monitoring application. Daily recordings and/or programmed alerts are recorded for a 30-day period, during which the patient and caregivers are provided additional education on equipment use as needed. Codes **99453** and **99454** are reported.

Teaching Point: Monitoring via a Bluetooth-enabled glucose meter is not reported as ambulatory continuous glucose monitoring of interstitial tissue fluid via a subcutaneous sensor for a minimum of 72 hours (**95249–95251**). The Bluetooth-enabled glucose meter does not measure glucose via a subcutaneous sensor but, rather, transmits results of each single glucose reading obtained from blood specimens.

➤ **A child with poorly controlled asthma is enrolled in a remote monitoring program.** A Bluetooth-enabled handheld spirometer and tablet with monitoring software is provided to the patient by a durable medical equipment provider. The patient's physician and/or clinical staff provide education to the patient and caregivers on device use, including daily input of lung function (forced expiratory volume in first second of expiration; forced vital capacity or forced expiratory volume in 6 seconds (FEV_6), asthma symptoms, and medications. The physician reports code **99453**.

Teaching Point: Because the physician practice furnishes only the initial setup and patient education, only code 99453 is reported for the initial 16 to 30 days of monitoring. Code 99454 would be reported by the provider of the equipment and monitoring service for the initial 16 to 30 days of service. See code 99457 for reporting 20 or more minutes of remote physiologic monitoring treatment management services during a calendar month.

Remote Physiologic Monitoring Treatment Management Services

#●99457   Remote physiologic monitoring treatment management services, 20 minutes or more of clinical staff/physician/other qualified health care professional time in a calendar month requiring interactive communication with the patient/caregiver during the month

Code 99457 requires 20 or more minutes of time spent using the results of physiologic monitoring to manage a patient under a specific treatment plan. The associated monitoring device(s) must be defined as a medical device by the FDA. These services may be rendered by physicians, QHPs, and/or clinical staff working under supervision of a physician or QHP.

Documentation of remote physiologic monitoring must include

- An order by a physician or QHP
- Live interactive communication with the patient/caregiver
- Time of service of 20 or more minutes in a calendar month

Reporting instructions

- Report code 99457 once with 1 unit of service regardless of the number of physiologic monitoring modalities performed in a given calendar month.
- Do not count any time on a day when the physician or QHP reports an E/M service (office or other outpatient services 99201–99205, 99211–99215; domiciliary, rest home services 99324–99328, 99334–99337; home services 99341–99345, 99347–99350).
- Do not count any time related to other reported services (eg, 93290, interrogation of implantable cardiovascular physiologic monitor system).
- Do not report 99457 in conjunction with collection and interpretation of physiologic data (99091).
- Code 99457 may be reported during the same service period as chronic care management (99487–99490), transitional care management (99495, 99496), and behavioral health integration services (99492–99494, 99484). However, the time for each service must be distinct and not overlapping and must be separately documented.

Example

➤ **A pediatrician orders remote treatment management for type 1 diabetes in a pediatric patient.** The patient is provided a computer tablet and glucometer with a Bluetooth connection (classified as a medical device by the FDA) that transmits patient data and glucose results to the physician's practice. The patient's glucose is monitored 6 times a day with results reviewed by clinical staff in the physician practice. Interventions are provided by clinical staff and/or physicians as needed throughout a calendar month. (For example, the patient is in school when hyperglycemia is indicated by a blood glucose result. Clinical staff advise the patient and teachers on the appropriate actions as per the physician's protocol and monitor the patient until glucose readings are normalized.) Over the course of a calendar month, physician and clinical staff activities related to remote analysis and treatment management are documented in addition to the time of each service. More than 20 minutes is documented for the current calendar month.

Code 99457 is reported.

Collection and Interpretation of Digitally Stored Data

#▲99091   Collection and interpretation of physiologic data (eg, ECG, blood pressure, glucose monitoring) digitally stored and/or transmitted by the patient and/or caregiver to the physician or other qualified health care professional, qualified by education, training, licensure/regulation (when applicable) requiring a minimum of 30 minutes of time, each 30 days

Code 99091 is revised in 2019 to represent a 30-day episode of care. Collection and interpretation of physiologic data includes the physician's or QHP's time involved with data access, review, and interpretation; modification of care plan as necessary (including communication to patient and/or caregiver); and associated documentation.

◉ If the services described by code 99091 are provided on the same day the patient presents for an E/M service, these services should be considered part of the E/M service and not separately reported.

◉ Do not report 99091 in the same calendar month as, or within 30 days of reporting, care plan oversight services (99374–99380, 99399, and 99340) or remote physiologic monitoring services (99457).

◉ Do not report 99091 if other, more specific *CPT®* codes exist (eg, 93227, 93272 for cardiographic services; 95250 for continuous glucose monitoring). Do not report 99091 for transfer and interpretation of data from hospital or clinical laboratory computers.

Pediatric Home Apnea Monitoring

94772   Circadian respiratory pattern recording (pediatric pneumogram), 12-24 hour continuous recording, infant

94774   Pediatric home apnea monitoring event recording including respiratory rate, pattern and heart rate per 30-day period of time; includes monitor attachment, download of data, review, interpretation, and preparation of a report by a physician or other qualified health care professional

94775   monitor attachment only (includes hook-up, initiation of recording and disconnection)

94776   monitoring, download of information, receipt of transmission(s) and analyses by computer only

94777   review, interpretation and preparation of report only by a physician or other qualified health care professional

◉ Report code 94772 when circadian respiratory pattern recording (pediatric pneumogram), 12- to 24-hour continuous recording, is performed on an infant.

◉ Codes 94774–94777 are reported once per 30-day period.

◉ Codes 94774 and 94777 are reported by the physician.

❖ Code 94774 is reported by the physician when he or she orders home monitoring, chooses the monitor limits, and arranges for a home health care provider to teach the parents. It includes reviewing and interpreting data and preparation of the report.

❖ Code 94777 is reported when the physician receives the downloaded information on disc or hard copy or electronically, reviews the patterns and periods of abnormal respiratory or heart rate, and summarizes, in a written report, the findings and recommendations for continuation or discontinuation of monitoring. This information is provided to the primary care physician and/or the family.

◉ Codes 94775 and 94776 are reported by the home health agency because there is no physician work involved.

❖ Code 94775 is reported by the home health agency and includes connecting the child to the monitoring equipment, teaching the family how to connect and disconnect the leads, checking the proper function of the equipment, responding to alarms, and resetting the monitor.

❖ Code 94776 is reported when the monitor is downloaded by the home health care agency and analyzed by a computer and converted to a hard copy or CD-ROM and provided to the interpreting physician. This could also be sent electronically.

❖ Codes 94774–94777 are not reported in conjunction with codes 93224–93272 (electrocardiographic monitoring). The apnea recording device cannot be reported separately. When oxygen saturation monitoring is used in addition to heart rate and respiratory monitoring, it is not reported separately.

Example

➤ **An infant born at 23 weeks' gestation, now 2 months old, has chronic lung disease and requires pro-longed low-flow oxygen.** She continues to have occasional episodes of self-stimulated apnea lasting less than 15 seconds. Her physicians and parents are concerned about the possibility of unwitnessed prolonged apnea requiring intervention but agree to have her go home with heart rate and respiratory monitoring during unattended periods and sleep. The physician orders the monitor, contacts the home health agency for its provision, and instructs the home health agency to teach the parents about cardiopulmonary resuscitation, proper attachment of the monitor leads, and resetting of the monitor. The home health agency provides the physician with the downloaded recordings. The first month's data are interpreted by the physician and a written report generated. The physician counsels the parents about the need to continue monitoring.

Teaching Point: Report code **94774** and the appropriate *ICD-10-CM* code (eg, **G47.35** for congenital central alveolar hypoventilation/hypoxemia).

In subsequent months, the physician receives the downloaded recordings, interprets them, and generates reports with recommendations for continued or discontinuation of monitoring. These services are reported with code **94777**.

Ambulatory Continuous Glucose Monitoring

95250   Ambulatory continuous glucose monitoring of interstitial tissue fluid via a subcutaneous sensor for a minimum of 72 hours; physician or other qualified health care professional (office) provided equipment, sensor placement, hook-up, calibration of monitor, patient training, removal of sensor, and printout of record

#●95249   patient-provided equipment, sensor placement, hook-up, calibration of monitor, patient training, and printout of recording

95251   Ambulatory continuous glucose monitoring of interstitial tissue fluid via a subcutaneous sensor for a minimum of 72 hours; analysis, interpretation and report

⊛ When ambulatory glucose monitoring using monitoring equipment is initiated and data are captured for a minimum of 72 hours, report code **95249** or **95250** based on the supplier of the equipment (patient or physician office).

⊛ Physicians report code **95249** only if the patient brings the data receiver in to the physician's or other QHP's office with the entire initial data collection procedure conducted in the office.

⊛ Report code **95249** only once for the entire duration that a patient has a receiver, even if the patient receives a new sensor and/or transmitter. If a patient receives a new or different model of receiver, code **95249** may be reported again when the entire initial data collection procedure is conducted in the office.

⊛ Analysis, interpretation, and report (**95251**) may be performed without a face-to-face encounter on the same date of service. This service is reported only once per month.

Nonvisual Digital Evaluation and Management Services

Online Medical Services

99444   Online E/M service by a physician or other qualified health care professional who may report evaluation and management services provided to an established patient or guardian not originating from a related E/M service provided within the previous 7 days, using the Internet or similar electronic communications network

98969   Online assessment and management service provided by a qualified nonphysician health care professional to an established patient or guardian not originating from a related assessment and management service provided within the previous 7 days, using the Internet or similar electronic communications network

An online electronic medical evaluation (99444) is a non–face-to-face E/M service by a physician or other QHP who may report E/M services to a patient using Internet resources in response to a patient's online inquiry. This is in contrast to telemedicine services, which represent interactive audio and video telecommunications systems that permit real-time communication between the physician, at the distant site, and the patient, at the originating site. Code 98969 is used by a qualified allied health provider whose scope of practice does not include E/M services to report an online assessment and management service. The reporting guidelines for code 98969 are the same as those required for online services provided by the physician or QHP (99444).

> ### ~ More From the AAP ~
>
> Online transmission of personal health information requires appropriate technical safeguards, such as encryption, authentication, and integrity controls. Learn more at https://www.aap.org/en-us/professional-resources/practice-support/practice-management/HIPAA/Pages/HIPAA-and-HITECH.aspx.

The Centers for Medicare & Medicaid Services has not assigned relative value units to online medical evaluation codes and considers them noncovered services. As a result, most third-party payers do not pay for them.

Before providing online medical services, understand local and state laws, ensure that communications will be Health Insurance Portability and Accountability Act compliant, establish written guidelines and procedures, educate payers and negotiate for payment, and educate patients.

Please see Chapter 12, Managing Chronic and Complex Conditions, for more information on chronic care management services that include online services when provided during the same period.

Remote Interprofessional Consultations

▲99446   Interprofessional telephone/Internet/electronic health record assessment and management service provided by a consultative physician including a verbal and written report to the patient's treating/requesting physician/qualified health care professional; 5–10 minutes of medical consultative discussion and review

▲99447   11–20 minutes of medical consultative discussion and review

▲99448   21–30 minutes of medical consultative discussion and review

▲99449   31 minutes or more of medical consultative discussion and review

#●99451   Interprofessional telephone/Internet/electronic health record assessment and management service provided by a consultative physician including a written report to the patient's treating/requesting physician or other qualified health care professional, 5 or more minutes of medical consultative time

#●99452   Interprofessional telephone/Internet/electronic health record referral service(s) provided by a treating/requesting physician or qualified health care professional, 30 minutes

A consultation request by a patient's attending or primary physician or other QHP soliciting opinion and/or treatment advice by telephone, Internet, or electronic health record (EHR) from a physician with specialty expertise (consultant) is reported by the consultant with interprofessional consultation codes 99446–99451. This consultation does not require face-to-face contact with the patient by the consultant. The patient may be in the inpatient or outpatient setting.

New in 2019 is a code for reporting the attending or primary care physician's/QHP's work in the telephone/Internet/EHR interprofessional consultation (99452).

Interprofessional Consultation Reporting by an Attending/Primary Physician

The treating/requesting physician or other QHP may report code 99452 or prolonged service (99354–99357; 99358, 99359).

◉ Code 99452 may be reported when 16 to 30 minutes is spent by the requesting individual in a service day preparing for the referral and/or communicating with the consultant.

◉ Time spent in discussion with the consultant may also be reported with prolonged service codes if the total time of service exceeds 30 minutes beyond the typical time of the associated E/M service.

     ❖ Direct prolonged service codes 99354–99357 may be reported when the patient is present (on site) and accessible to the requesting physician in the office or other outpatient setting during the time of service that extends more than 30 minutes beyond the typical time of the associated E/M service.

❖ Prolonged services of more than 30 minutes in a day without the patient present are reported with codes **99358** and **99359**. For more information on prolonged services, see Chapter 7, Evaluation and Management Services in the Office and Outpatient Clinics, for prolonged services in an outpatient setting and Chapter 16, Noncritical Hospital Evaluation and Management Services, for prolonged services in an inpatient setting.

Interprofessional Consultation Reporting by a Consultant

Guidelines for the consultant reporting interprofessional telephone/Internet/EHR consultations include

- Telephone/Internet/EHR consultations of less than 5 minutes are not reported. For codes **99446–99449**, more than 50% of the time reported as interprofessional consultation must have been spent in medical consultative discussion rather than review of data (eg, medical records, test results). Both verbal and written reports are required for completion of the services represented by codes **99446–99449**.
- Code **99451** is reported based on the total time of review and interprofessional consultation. Only a written report is required for code **99451**.
- A single interprofessional consultation code is reported for the cumulative time spent in discussion and information review regardless of the number of contacts necessary to complete the service. Codes **99446–99451** are not reported more than once in a 7-day interval.
- Time spent in telephone or online consultation with the patient and/or family may be reported using codes **99441–99444** or **98966–98968**, and the time related to these services is not included in the time attributed to interprofessional consultation services.
- When the purpose of communication is to arrange a transfer of care or face-to-face patient encounter, interprofessional consultation codes are not reported.
- Interprofessional consultation services are not reported if the consultant has provided a face-to-face service to the patient within the past 14 days or when the consultation results in scheduling of a face-to-face service within the next 14 days or at the consultant's next available appointment date.
- Time spent by the consultant reviewing pertinent medical records, studies, or other data is included in the interprofessional consultation and not separately reported. Do not report prolonged E/M service before and/or after direct patient care (**99358**, **99359**) for any time within the service period if reporting **99446–99451**.
- As with all consultations, the request for advice or opinion should be documented in the patient record. For a new patient with no record, one will have to be created to document this service.

Examples

➤ **A 10-year-old boy with attention-deficit/hyperactivity disorder (ADHD) has become increasingly aggressive at home and school.** The child's pediatrician arranges a telephone consultation with a child and adolescent psychiatrist and forwards the child's history records prior to the telephone consultation. The pediatrician and psychiatrist spend a total of 16 minutes in discussion. On a second date, the pediatrician provides a face-to-face E/M service to the child to discuss recommendations based on the prior interprofessional consultation. A new care plan is developed for achieving better control of the child's predominantly hyperactive ADHD and is agreed to by the mother. The total face-to-face time for the pediatrician is approximately 25 minutes with 15 minutes spent in counseling and/or coordination of care.

	ICD-10-CM	CPT®	
First date of service (interprofessional consultation)	Both physicians report **F90.1** (ADHD, predominantly hyperactive type).	The consultant reports **99447** (11–20 minutes of medical discussion and review) for the service on the first date.	The pediatrician reports **99452** for the 16 minutes spent in interprofessional referral service.
Second date of service (pediatrician only)			The pediatrician reports **99214** (15 of 25 minutes [face-to-face] spent in counseling/coordination of care) for services on the second date.

Teaching Point: In this vignette, the patient and mother are not present for the interprofessional consultation. The primary care physician may report code 99452 for 16 to 30 minutes of interprofessional consultation. Had the pediatrician's time prior to the face-to-face visit exceeded 30 minutes, prolonged service before and/or after direct patient care codes 99358 and 99359 would be appropriately reported. Prolonged service before and/or after direct patient care requires that a related face-to-face encounter take place in proximity to the non–face-to-face prolonged service.

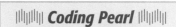

> **Coding Pearl**
>
> See codes for general behavioral health integration care management in Chapter 14, Mental and Behavioral Health Services, for a potential ongoing management option for the patient in the first example in this section.

> **A physician at a rural hospital admits a child with acute lymphoblastic leukemia who developed a *Streptococcus pneumoniae* infection.** The physician communicates with the child's hematologist, who is located several hours away, via a secure health information exchange for advice about treatment. The hematologist spends a total of 25 minutes reviewing hospital records and communicating with the attending physician. The attending physician's total time spent on the unit/floor providing and/or coordinating care for this patient is 70 minutes, with 40 minutes in preparation for and participation in the interprofessional consultation service and another 5 minutes counseling patient/caregivers following the consultation.

ICD-10-CM	CPT®	
Both physicians report A49.1 (streptococcal infection, unspecified site) and C91.00 (acute lymphoblastic leukemia not having achieved remission).	The consultant reports 99448 (21–30 minutes of medical consultative discussion and review).	The pediatrician reports 99223 (typical time 70 minutes) based on time spent in counseling and/or coordination of care.
The categories for leukemia have codes indicating whether the leukemia has achieved remission. Coders are instructed to ask the physician for status if documentation is unclear.		

Teaching Point: Interprofessional consultation services would not be reported if the consultant has provided a face-to-face service to the patient within the past 14 days or if the consultation results in scheduling of a face-to-face service within the next 14 days or at the consultant's next available appointment date.

> **A hospitalized 2-day-old develops poor feeding and tachypnea and is diagnosed with group B streptococcal septicemia.** The patient's primary care physician telephones an infectious disease specialist located several hours away for treatment advice. The physicians spend 8 minutes discussing the child's condition and treatment options. The infectious disease specialist reports this service with

ICD-10-CM	CPT®
P36.0 (sepsis of newborn due to streptococcus, group B)	The consultant reports 99446 (interprofessional consultation, 5–10 minutes) The pediatrician reports the appropriate E/M service, as the time of service does not support 99452 or prolonged service.

Teaching Point: The attending physician will include this work in the per diem charge for intensive or critical care services based on the type of care rendered.

Chapter 20: Digital Medicine Services: Technology-Enhanced Care Delivery

Part 5:
Coding Education Quiz/ Continuing Education Units (CEUs) for American Academy of Professional Coders

This publication has prior approval of the American Academy of Professional Coders (AAPC) for 4.0 continuing education units (CEUs). Granting of this approval in no way constitutes endorsement by the AAPC of the publication, content, or publication sponsor.

To earn your CEUs, complete the 40-question quiz online (www.aap.org/cfp). Click on "2019 Coding for Pediatrics Quiz." A passcode will be required; enter AAPCFP24.

You will only need the current *Coding for Pediatrics 2019* publication and *Current Procedural Terminology*® and *International Classification of Diseases, 10th Revision, Clinical Modification* manuals to answer the questions. A 70% score or better is required to earn the CEUs. You will be notified immediately whether or not you have passed. If you pass the test, you will receive a CEU certificate. If you do not receive a passing score, the test will be returned to you graded. However, it may be resubmitted for possible credit. NOTE: You may also take this quiz for a certificate of completion for your own records or to use for Category II Continuing Medical Education credits. Refer to the online site for more details.

This quiz will expire on October 1, 2019.

E-mail aapcodinghotline@aap.org if you have any questions.

4.0 Continuing Education Units

1. Which of the following conditions is not represented by modifier 59?
   A. Two or more physicians performed different and unrelated procedures.
   B. The procedure involved a different site or organ system.
   C. The procedure was a different procedure or surgery.
   D. The procedure required a separate incision or excision.
2. Which of the following is not an official code set for provision of supplies and services in a physician office?
   A. *Current Procedural Terminology (CPT®)*
   B. Healthcare Common Procedure Coding System (HCPCS)
   C. National Drug Code
   D. *International Classification of Diseases, 10th Revision, Procedure Coding System*
3. Typical Medically Unlikely Edit values for procedures done on finger and toe procedures are what?
   A. 10, based on performance of a single procedure on each digit
   B. 2, based on reporting of bilateral services
   C. 1, based on use of anatomic modifiers for procedures performed on multiple digits
   D. 1, but modifier 59 is always used to report additional procedures.
4. The *International Classification of Diseases, 10th Revision, Clinical Modification (ICD-10-CM)* tabular list includes instructions at which level?
   A. Block
   B. Category
   C. Code
   D. All of the above
5. *ICD-10-CM* codes assigned to support performance measurement of the "Weight Assessment and Counseling for Nutrition and Physical Activity for Children and Adolescents" measure include which of the following?
   A. Z71.3, dietary counseling and surveillance, and Z71.82, counseling for physical activity
   B. Z00.121, encounter for routine child health examination with abnormal findings
   C. 3008F, body mass index (BMI), documented
   D. Z68.51–Z68.54, BMI percentile, pediatric
6. When should physicians expect to receive requests for medical records related to the Healthcare Effectiveness Data and Information Set (HEDIS) quality measurement?
   A. Between July and October of each year
   B. When a payer identifies the physician's coding as higher than his or her peers
   C. Between January 1and May 15
   D. When physicians have not provided the appropriate care within the designated time frames
7. If services provided in a facility setting are reported *as if* provided in a physician's clinic, what may occur?
   A. The physician may be paid less than when reported as provided in a facility setting.
   B. The physician may be overpaid.
   C. The claim will always be denied due to disagreement between the place of service code and address listed on the claim.
   D. Nothing. The claim processes the same regardless of the location.
8. Fraud is what?
   A. Charging in excess for services or supplies
   B. Using only the 1995 guidelines for evaluation and management (E/M) code selection
   C. Waiving co-payments or deductibles for patients with financial hardship
   D. Requiring that a patient return for a procedure that could have been performed on the same day
9. Which of the following *is not* an element of the Office of Inspector General–recommended compliance program?
   A. Monitor all use of cut-and-paste functionality in the electronic health record.
   B. Implement written compliance and practice standards.
   C. Develop open lines of communication.
   D. Enforce disciplinary standards through well-publicized guidelines.

10. How many elements are included in an extended history of present illness (HPI)?
    A. 1 to 3 elements
    B. At least 10
    C. 4 or more
    D. 2 to 7

11. Documentation of a new patient office visit includes a chief complaint; 4 elements of HPI; 1 system reviewed; 1 element each of past, family, and social history (PFSH); a detailed examination; and low-complexity medical decision-making (MDM). Which code is appropriately reported for this service per the E/M documentation guidelines?
    A. **99201**
    B. **99203**
    C. **99202**
    D. **99204**

12. A complete PFSH for an established patient office visit requires which of the following?
    A. No PFSH is required for established patient visits.
    B. 1 specific item from each of the 3 history areas
    C. At least 2 items for each of the 3 history areas
    D. 1 specific item from 2 of the 3 history areas

13. Which of the following is supportive of a consultation rather than a transfer of care?
    A. Patient referred by pediatrician for E/M of dysphagia
    B. Patient referred by pediatrician for evaluation and advice on management of dysphagia
    C. Patient seen today for management of dysphagia
    D. Patient with dysphagia referred by family member

14. Which of the following supports reporting an E/M service based on time?
    A. 15 minutes spent in counseling and/or coordination of care
    B. Total face-to-face time is 40 minutes.
    C. 20 of 40 minutes was spent face-to-face providing counseling.
    D. 40 minutes was spent on the unit, with approximately 25 minutes spent counseling patient and parents on treatment options.

15. A physician provides an E/M service to a patient in a group home for children with complex medical conditions. What type of service is this?
    A. Home visit E/M service
    B. Initial nursing facility care
    C. Domiciliary, rest home, or custodial care service
    D. Subsequent nursing facility care

16. The diagnosis code for a minor problem or chronic condition requiring only insignificant E/M is reported with what codes when performed on the same date as a preventive medicine E/M service?
    A. **Z00.129**; insignificant problems are not abnormal findings.
    B. Do not report a code for conditions not requiring significant E/M.
    C. Assign a code for the problem but not the preventive service.
    D. **Z00.121** and a code for the problem

17. Which of the following screenings is not reported with code **96110**?
    A. Screen for Child Anxiety Related Disorders (SCARED)
    B. Modified Checklist for Autism in Toddlers (M-CHAT)
    C. Parents' Evaluation of Developmental Status (PEDS)
    D. Ages & Stages Questionnaires (ASQ)

18. Global periods are defined by which of the following?
    A. The clinical judgment of a physician or other qualified health care professional (QHP)
    B. *CPT®*
    C. Medicare Physician Fee Schedule
    D. HCPCS

19. Which of the following are considered inherent to an E/M service?
    A. Removal of an umbilical clamp
    B. Removal of impacted cerumen
    C. Removal of an earring requiring an incision
    D. Removal of an intranasal foreign body

20. True or false? The encounter form is not part of the medical record.
    A. True
    B. False

21. Which of the following codes is correct for reporting automated dipstick urinalysis with microscopy?
    A. 81003
    B. 81001
    C. 81002
    D. 81009

22. An adolescent patient presents for an intradermal tuberculosis test required by his employer. What code does the physician report for this encounter?
    A. 99211
    B. 36415
    C. 86580
    D. 86480

23. A physician documents 30 minutes spent developing a comprehensive care plan and coordinating a patient's care with other providers, parents, and teachers during a calendar month. The physician's nurse also documents 15 minutes spent providing parents with education and assistance in obtaining community resources for the same patient. Based on this information, what *CPT* code(s) should be reported for the physician's service?
    A. 99490, 99491
    B. 99491
    C. 99490
    D. 99487, 99489

24. A child is discharged from inpatient hospital care by a hospitalist to the care of her primary care pediatrician on the evening of Saturday, June 1. The pediatrician's office is closed on weekends. By what date must the pediatrician or her clinical staff make direct contact with the patient/caregiver to report transitional care management services?
    A. June 3
    B. June 2
    C. The date that the hospital lists as the discharge date
    D. June 4

25. Which of the following encounters *does not* describe a service that may be reported as incident to a physician's service as defined by Medicare?
    A. A medical assistant performs venipuncture as ordered by a nurse practitioner.
    B. A nurse administers a developmental screening instrument during a well-child visit.
    C. A nurse provides patient education on diabetes as directed by a physician's plan of care.
    D. A physician assistant provides an unplanned E/M service for an injury to a patient of a physician in the same group practice.

26. If the intent of the cause of an injury or other condition is unknown or unspecified, code the intent as
    A. Undetermined intent
    B. Sequela
    C. Accidental intent
    D. Suspected abuse, not ruled out

Part 5: Continuing Education Units (CEUs) for American Academy of Professional Coders

27. What determines the code(s) reported for developmental testing per *CPT*?
    A. The physician's total time of testing, interpretation, and report
    B. Whether the tests were administered by a physician, technician, or computer
    C. Only the physician's face-to-face time in testing the patient
    D. The patient's total time in the examination room

28. Codes in category Z05 (encounter for observation and evaluation of newborn for suspected diseases and conditions ruled out) may be reported for which of the following?
    A. A newborn affected by fetal growth restriction or slow intrauterine growth
    B. A newborn suspected of being affected by a localized maternal infection
    C. A symptomatic neonate is suspected of having an abnormal condition that, after examination and observation, is ruled out.
    D. A neonate without signs or symptoms is suspected of having an abnormal condition that, after examination and observation, is ruled out.

29. Code 99217 is reported when
    A. A patient is admitted to and discharged from observation on the same date.
    B. A patient is discharged from observation care on a date after the admission date.
    C. A physician other than the attending physician provides observation care.
    D. A patient is admitted to inpatient status on the same date the patient was admitted to observation.

30. Which of the following codes requires no PFSH?
    A. 99221
    B. 99234
    C. 99233
    D. 99218

31. An allied health care professional provides asthma control education and training to 4 patients using a standardized curriculum. The time of service is 50 minutes. What code(s) is appropriate for this service?
    A. 98960 × 2 units
    B. 98961
    C. 98960, 98961
    D. 98961 × 2 units

32. Attendance at delivery (when requested by the delivering physician or other QHP) and initial stabilization of newborn may be reported in conjunction with which of the following codes?
    A. 99027
    B. 0188T
    C. 99477
    D. 99465

33. Which type of code do many states require an emergency department (ED) physician to report that may not be required of physicians in other settings?
    A. *CPT*®
    B. External cause of injury codes
    C. Codes for discharge diagnoses
    D. Category II performance measurement codes

34. Which codes identify services provided in an urgent care clinic?
    A. 99201–99215 with place of service code 20
    B. 99281–99285 with place of service code 21
    C. The code is determined by the emergent nature of the presenting problem.
    D. 99281–99285 with place of service code 11

35. Which of the following is true when selecting a code for an ED E/M visit?
    A. The ED physician may report both an ED visit and initial observation care when provided on the same date.
    B. A new patient for an ED visit is one who has not received a face-to-face service by the ED physician or another ED physician in the same group practice in the past 3 years.
    C. ED physicians should always document time because prolonged service may be reported for ED visits lasting 1 hour or more.
    D. Time spent in counseling and/or coordination of care cannot be used as a key or controlling factor in the selection of an ED code.
36. Which of the following criteria is sufficient to support reporting critical care services?
    A. A newborn is preterm and requires intensive monitoring.
    B. A surgeon provided critical care after performing repair of a diaphragmatic hernia.
    C. A combination of organ failure, risk of imminent deterioration, and high-complexity MDM are required.
    D. The patient is admitted to an intensive or critical care unit.
37. Imaging is separately reported when provided in conjunction with which of the following procedures?
    A. 36570 or 36571
    B. 36568 or 36569
    C. 36572 or 36573
    D. 36584
38. Which of the following is reported with code 43752?
    A. A physician places a nasogastric tube without imaging guidance.
    B. A physician places a nasogastric tube with fluoroscopic guidance because clinical staff are unavailable to perform the placement.
    C. A physician uses fluoroscopy to place a nasogastric tube after attempts by nursing staff fail.
    D. A physician places a gastric tube and performs lavage for ingested poisons.
39. Telemedicine services include which of the following?
    A. Physician consultations provided via real-time audiovisual technology
    B. Physician E/M services conducted via telephone
    C. A physician service provided via e-mail
    D. A physician analyzes data collected and stored in a computer.
40. Code 99457 represents which type of service?
    A. Continuous glucose monitoring
    B. 20 minutes or more of time spent using the results of physiologic monitoring to manage a patient under a specific treatment plan
    C. A service performed only by physicians
    D. A service that requires no live interactive communication with the patient and/or caregivers

Part 5: Continuing Education Units (CEUs) for American Academy of Professional Coders

Appendixes

More coding resources, including online forms for the documents listed herein, can be accessed at www.aap.org/cfp. Use access code AAPCFP24.

I. Sample Assessment/Testing Tools

NOTE: These are provided as examples only; the American Academy of Pediatrics implies no endorsement or restriction of code use to these instruments. If you choose to use an instrument not listed below, be sure it is validated/standardized.

Instrument	Abbreviation	CPT® Code
Ages & Stages Questionnaires—3rd Edition	ASQ-3	96110
Ages & States Questionnaires: Social-Emotional, 2nd Edition	ASQ:SE-2	96127
Australian Scale for Asperger's Syndrome	ASAS	96127
Beck Anxiety Inventory	BAI	96127
Beck Depression Inventory	BDI	96127
Beck Youth Inventories—2nd Edition	BYI-2	96127
Beery-Buktenica Developmental Test of Visual-Motor Integration—6th Edition	Beery VMI	96112 and 96113
Behavior Assessment System for Children—2nd Edition	BASC-2	96127
Behavioral Rating Inventory of Executive Function	BRIEF	96127
Child Behavior Checklist	CBCL	96127
Children's Depression Inventory 2	CDI 2	96127
Clinical Evaluation of Language Fundamentals—5th Edition	CELF-5	96112 and 96113
Clinical Evaluation of Language Fundamentals—Preschool-2	CELF-Preschool-2	96112 and 96113
Columbia DISC Depression Scale		96127
Comprehensive Test of Nonverbal Intelligence—2nd Edition	CTONI-2	96112 and 96113
Conners Comprehensive Behavior Rating Scales	Conners CBRS	96127
Developmental Test of Visual Perception—3rd Edition	DTVP-3	96112 and 96113
Hamilton Anxiety Rating Scale	HAM-A	96127
Hamilton Rating Scale for Depression	HRSD	96127
Kaufman Brief Intelligence Test—2nd Edition	KBIT-2	96112 and 96113
Modified Checklist for Autism in Toddlers—Revised	M-CHAT-R	96110
Multidimensional Anxiety Scale for Children—2nd Edition	MASC 2	96127
NICHQ Vanderbilt Assessment Scales		96127
Parents' Evaluation of Developmental Status	PEDS	96110
Patient Health Questionnaire	PHQ-2 or PHQ-9	96127
Peabody Picture Vocabulary Test—4th Edition	PPVT-4	96112 and 96113
Pediatric Symptom Checklist	PSC or PSC-Y	96127
Screen for Child Anxiety Related Disorders	SCARED	96127
Test of Auditory Processing Skills—3rd Edition	TAPS-3	96112 and 96113
Test of Language Competence—Expanded Edition	TLC-Expanded	96112 and 96113
Test of Nonverbal Intelligence—4th Edition	TONI-4	96112 and 96113
Test of Problem Solving 3—Elementary Version	TOPS 3 Elementary	96112 and 96113
Test of Word Knowledge	TOWK	96112 and 96113
Woodcock-Johnson Test of Cognitive Abilities—4th Edition	WJ IV	96112 and 96113

Appendixes

II. Vaccine Products: *Commonly Administered Pediatric Vaccines*

This list was current as of July 1, 2018.

For updates, visit https://www.aap.org/en-us/Documents/coding_vaccine_coding_table.pdf.

CPT® Product Code	Separately report the administration with CPT® codes 90460–90461 or 90471–90474. See below.	Manufacturer	Brand	# of Vaccine Components
90702	Diphtheria and tetanus toxoids (**DT**), adsorbed when administered to <7 years, for IM use	SP	**Diphtheria and Tetanus Toxoids Adsorbed**	2
90700	Diphtheria, tetanus toxoids, and acellular pertussis vaccine (**DTaP**), when administered to <7 years, for IM use	SP GSK	**DAPTACEL INFANRIX**	3
90696	Diphtheria, tetanus toxoids, and acellular pertussis vaccine and inactivated poliovirus vaccine (**DTaP-IPV**), when administered to children 4–6 years of age, for IM use	GSK SP	**KINRIX Quadracel**	4
90697	Diphtheria, tetanus toxoids, acellular pertussis vaccine, inactivated poliovirus vaccine, Haemophilus influenza type b PRP-OMP conjugate vaccine, and hepatitis B vaccine (**DTaP-IPV-Hib-HepB**), for IM use	⚡	⚡	6
90723	Diphtheria, tetanus toxoids, acellular pertussis vaccine, Hepatitis B, and inactivated poliovirus vaccine (**DTaP-Hep B- IPV**), for IM use	GSK	**PEDIARIX**	5
90698	Diphtheria, tetanus toxoids, acellular pertussis vaccine, haemophilus influenza Type B, and inactivated poliovirus vaccine (**DTaP-IPV/Hib**), for IM use	SP	**Pentacel**	5
90633	Hepatitis A vaccine (**Hep A**), pediatric/adolescent dosage, 2 dose, for IM use	GSK Merck	**HAVRIX VAQTA**	1
90740	Hepatitis B vaccine (**Hep B**), dialysis or immuno-suppressed patient dosage, 3 dose, for IM use	Merck	**RECOMBIVAX HB**	1
90743	Hepatitis B vaccine (**Hep B**), adolescent, 2 dose, for IM use	Merck	**RECOMBIVAX HB**	1
90744	Hepatitis B vaccine (**Hep B**), pediatric/adolescent dosage, 3 dose, for IM use	Merck GSK	**RECOMBIVAX HB ENGERIX-B**	1
90746	Hepatitis B vaccine (**Hep B**), adult dosage, for IM use	Merck GSK	**RECOMBIVAX HB ENGERIX-B**	1
90747	Hepatitis B vaccine (**Hep B**), dialysis or immuno-suppressed patient dosage, 4 dose, for IM use	GSK	**ENGERIX-B**	1
90647	Hemophilus influenza B vaccine (**Hib**), PRP-OMP conjugate, 3 dose, for IM use	Merck	**PedvaxHIB**	1
90648	Hemophilus influenza B vaccine (**Hib**), PRP-T conjugate, 4 dose, for IM use	SP GSK	**ActHIB HIBERIX**	1

Appendixes

CPT® Product Code	Separately report the administration with CPT® codes 90460–90461 or 90471–90474. See below.	Manufacturer	Brand	# of Vaccine Components
90651	Human Papillomavirus vaccine types 6, 11, 16, 18, 31, 33, 45, 52, 58, nonavalent (**HPV**), 2 or 3 dose schedule, for IM use	Merck	**GARDASIL 9**	1
90630	**Influenza virus vaccine, quad (IIV4), split virus, preservative free, for intradermal use**	SP	**Fluzone Intradermal Quad**	1
90672	**Influenza virus vaccine, quad (LAIV), live, intranasal use**	MedImmune	**Flumist Quad**	1
90674	**Influenza virus vaccine, quad (ccIIV4), derived from cell cultures, subunit, preservative and antibiotic free, 0.5 mL dosage, IM**	Seqirus	**Flucelvax Quad**	1
90682	**Influenza virus vaccine, quad (RIV4), derived from recombinant DNA, HA protein only, preservative and antibiotic free, IM use**	SP	**Flublok Quad**	1
90685	**Influenza virus vaccine, quad (IIV4), split virus, preservative free, 0.25mL dose, for IM use**	SP	**Fluzone Quad**	1
90686	**Influenza virus vaccine, quad (IIV4), split virus, preservative free, 0.5mL dose, for IM use**	Seqirus SP GSK GSK	**Afluria Fluzone Quad FLUARIX Quad FLULAVAL**	1
90687	**Influenza virus vaccine, quad (IIV4), split virus, 0.25mL dose, for IM use**	SP	**Fluzone Quad**	1
90688	**Influenza virus vaccine, quad (IIV4), split virus, 0.5mL dose, for IM use**	Seqirus SP GSK	**Afluria Quad Fluzone Quad FLULAVAL**	1
90756	**Influenza virus vaccine, quad (ccIIV4), derived from cell cultures, subunit, antibiotic free, 0.5mL dose, for IM use**	Seqirus	**Flucelvax Quad**	1
90656	**Influenza virus vaccine, tri (IIV3), split virus, preservative free, 0.5mL dose, for IM use**	Seqirus	**Afluria**	1
90658	**Influenza virus vaccine, tri (IIV3), split virus, 0.5mL dose, for IM use**	Seqirus	**Afluria**	1
90673	**Influenza virus vaccine, tri (RIV3), derived from recombinant DNA, HA protein only, preservative and antibiotic free, IM use**	SP	**Flublok**	1
90707	Measles, mumps, and rubella virus vaccine (**MMR**), live, for subcutaneous use	Merck	**M-M-R II**	3
90710	Measles, mumps, rubella, and varicella vaccine (**MMRV**), live, for subcutaneous use	Merck	**ProQuad**	4
90620	**Meningococcal** recombinant protein and outer membrane vesicle vaccine, serogroup B (MenB-4C), 2 dose schedule, for IM use	GSK	**Bexsero**	1
90621	**Meningococcal** recombinant lipoprotein vaccine, serogroup B, 2 or 3 dose schedule, for IM use	Pfizer	**Trumenba**	1

Appendixes

CPT® Product Code	Separately report the administration with *CPT*® codes 90460–90461 or 90471–90474. See below.	Manufacturer	Brand	# of Vaccine Components
90734	**Meningococcal** conjugate vaccine, serogroups A, C, Y and W-135 quad (MenACWY or MCV4), for IM use	SP GSK	**Menactra** **Menveo**	1
90670	**Pneumococcal** conjugate vaccine, 13 valent (PCV13), for IM use	Pfizer	**PREVNAR 13**	1
90732	**Pneumococcal** polysaccharide vaccine, 23-valent (PPSV23), adult or immunosuppressed patient dosage, when administered to ≥2 years, for subcutaneous or IM use	Merck	**PNEUMOVAX 23**	1
90713	**Poliovirus** vaccine (**IPV**), inactivated, for subcutaneous or IM use	SP	**IPOL**	1
90680	**Rotavirus** vaccine, pentavalent (RV5), 3 dose schedule, live, for oral use	Merck	**RotaTeq**	1
90681	**Rotavirus** vaccine, human, attenuated (RV1), 2 dose schedule, live, for oral use	GSK	**ROTARIX**	1
90714	Tetanus and diphtheria toxoids (**Td**) adsorbed, preservative free, when administered to ≥7 years, for IM use	MBL SP	**Td (adult) adsorbed** **TENIVAC**	2
90715	Tetanus, diphtheria toxoids and acellular pertussis vaccine (**Tdap**), when administered to ≥7 years, for IM use	SP GSK	**ADACEL BOOSTRIX**	3
90716	**Varicella** virus vaccine (VAR), live, for subcutaneous use	Merck	**VARIVAX**	1
90749	**Unlisted vaccine or toxoid**	Please see *CPT* manual.		
Immunization Administration (IA) Codes				
IA Through Age 18 With Counseling				
90460	IA through 18 years of age via any route of administration, with counseling by physician or other qualified health care professional; first or only component of each vaccine or toxoid component administered (Do not report with 90471 or 90473)			
+90461	IA through 18 years of age via any route of administration, with counseling by physician or other qualified health care professional; each additional vaccine or toxoid component administered			
Immunization Administration				
90471	IA, one injected vaccine (*Do not report with* 90460 *or* 90473)			
+90472	IA, each additional injected vaccine			
90473	IA by intranasal/oral route; one vaccine (*Do not report with* 90460 *or* 90471)			
+90474	IA by intranasal/oral route; each additional vaccine			

III. Chronic Care Management Worksheet

Chronic Care Management Worksheet		
Reporting month/year	Patient	
DOB	MR#	Type of residence[a]
Chronic condition(s):		
Other medical conditions:		
Other needs (social, access to care):		
Physician/QHP	Date initial plan of care developed	
Date plan of care provided to patient/caregiver		

Clinical Staff Documentation: In the following table, include date, activity description, time spent, and location of any associated documentation (eg, plan of care, call notes). Activities may include

- Communication (with patient, family members, guardian/caregiver, surrogate decision-makers, or other professionals) about aspects of care
- Communication with home health agencies and other community services used by the patient
- Collection of health outcomes data and registry documentation
- Patient or family/caregiver education to support self-management, independent living, and activities of daily living
- Assessment of and support for treatment regimen adherence and medication management
- Identification of available community and health resources
- Facilitating access to care and services needed by the patient/family
- Management of care transitions not reported as part of transitional care management (99495, 99496)
- Ongoing review of patient status, including review of laboratory and other studies not reported as part of an E/M service
- Development and maintenance of a comprehensive care plan

Date	Activity (include reference to other documentation when indicated)	Time (start and stop)	Total Time	Clinical Staff Signature (legible/ credentials)
		Total Time	min	

____ 99487 first hour of clinical staff time with care plan establishment/substantial revision, per calendar month
____ 99489 each additional 30 minutes of clinical staff time per calendar month (Enter number of units.)
____ 99490 at least 20 minutes of clinical staff time per calendar month

Supervising physician/QHP signature _____

Date_____

Abbreviations: DOB, date of birth; E/M, evaluation and management; MR, medical record; QHP, qualified health care professional.

[a] Specify if patient lives in a private residence, group home, or other type of domiciliary. Do not report chronic care management services for patients residing in a facility that provides more than minimal medical care (eg, nursing facility).

Appendixes

IV. Care Plan Oversight Encounter Worksheet

Care Plan Oversight Encounter Worksheet

See www.aap.org/cfp for an online version of this worksheet (access code AAPCFP24).

Physician: _____ Patient Name: _____

Services Provided:
The letter that corresponds with each service provided should be placed in column #2.
A. Regular physician development and/or revision of care plans
B. Review of subsequent reports of patient status
C. Review of related laboratory or other studies
D. Communication (including telephone calls not separately reported with codes 99441–99443) with other health care professionals involved in patient's care
E. Integration of new information into the medical treatment plan and/or adjustment of medical therapy
F. Other (Attach additional explanatory materials on the services provided.)

Date of Service XX/XX/XXXX	Services Provided	Contact Name and Agency	Start Time	End Time	Total Minutes	Monthly Subtotal

Explanation for additional services provided:

Date:_____/_____
_____

Date:_____/_____
_____

Date:_____/_____
_____

Time Requirements per Calendar Month	Patient in Home, Domiciliary, or Rest Home (eg, assisted living facility)	Patient Under the Care of a Home Health Care Agency	Hospice Patient	Nursing Facility Patient
15–29 min	99339	99374	99377	99379
≥30 min	99340	99375	99378	99380
≥30 min Medicare code		G0181	G0182	

Monthly Total: _____ CPT® Code: _____

V. Global Per Diem Critical Care Codes: Direct Supervision and Reporting Guidelines

Global Per Diem Critical Care Codes: Direct Supervision and Reporting Guidelines

The delivery of neonatal and pediatric critical care has undergone significant changes in the last 2 decades, incorporating expanded technology and services and new patterns of delivery of care. Neonatal intensive care units (NICUs) have grown dramatically as improvements in perinatal care have led to markedly improved survival rates of the small preterm neonate. There has also been a growing national population with major socioeconomic shifts. These changes have led to a large increase in NICU beds. Simultaneous to these demographic and epidemiologic changes, serious Accreditation Council for Graduate Medical Education and Residency Review Committee limitations in resident and fellow work hours and, more specifically, to those hours allocated to clinical care in the NICU have reduced the number of house officers providing neonatal critical care. There has been a rapid expansion of other neonatal providers working as a team in partnership with an attending physician to meet expanding bedside patient care needs. These nonphysician providers (NPPs by Centers for Medicare & Medicaid Services nomenclature) are primarily neonatal nurse practitioners (NNPs). They have assumed a critical role in assisting the attending physician in caring for this expanding population of patients.

Neither NNPs nor residents or fellows are substitutes for the attending physician, who continues to remain fully in charge of these patients and directly supervises NNPs and residents or fellow physicians as well as other ancillary providers (eg, registered nurses, respiratory therapists, nutritionists, social workers, physical therapists, occupational therapists), who all play important contributory roles in the care of these critical patients. Unlike the supervision for residents or fellows enrolled in graduate medical education programs, the attending physician's supervision and documentation of care provided by NNPs is not covered by Physicians at Teaching Hospitals (PATH) guidelines. The attending physician is not "sharing services" with the NNP or resident or fellow. The attending physician (the physician responsible for the patient's care and reporting the service for that date) remains solely responsible for the supervision of the team and development of the patient's plan of care. In developing that plan, the attending physician will use the information acquired by and discussed with other members of the care team, including that of the resident or fellow and NNP.

When supervising residents or fellows, the attending physician will use this collective information as part of his or her own documentation of care. The attending physician must demonstrate in his or her own note that he or she has reviewed this information, performed his or her own focused examination of the patient, documented any additional findings or disagreements with the resident's or fellow's findings, and discussed the plan of care with the resident or fellow to meet PATH guideline requirements. These rules allow the attending physician to use the resident or fellow note as a major component of his or her own note and in determining the level of care the attending physician will report for that patient on that date.

Physicians at Teaching Hospitals guidelines do not apply to patients cared for by NNPs because NNPs are not enrolled in postgraduate education. This is true whether the NNP is employed by the hospital, medical group, or independent contractor. Centers for Medicare & Medicaid Services rules prohibit NPPs (in this case NNPs) and the reporting physician from reporting "shared or split services" when critical care services are provided. The reporting physician may certainly review and use the important information and observation of the NNPs, but the physician also provides his or her own evaluation along with documentation of the services he or she personally provided. Documentation expectations for the reporting physician include review of the notes and observations of other members of the care team; an independent-focused, medically appropriate bedside examination of the patient; and documentation that he or she has directed the plan of care for each patient whose services the physician reports. In many critically ill but stable patients, this requirement can be met by a single daily note. In situations in which the patient is very unstable and dramatic changes and major additional interventions are required to maintain stability, more extensive or frequent documentations are likely and may be entered by any qualified member of the care team.

In some states NNPs, through expanded state licenses, are permitted to independently report their services. If these NNPs are credentialed by the hospital and health plan to provide critical care services and procedures and possess their own National Provider Identifier (NPI), they may independently report the services they provide. In these states they can function as independent contractors or as employees of the hospital or a medical group, reporting their services under their own NPI. It is important to emphasize again that the

Appendixes

Global Per Diem Critical Care Codes: Direct Supervision and Reporting Guidelines

NNP and the physician do not report a shared critical care service. Critical care services are reported under the NNP or physician NPI, dependent on who was primarily providing the patient service and directing the care of the patient. Two providers may not report a global per diem critical care code (eg, **99468**, **99469**) on the same date of service. In most situations the physician is serving as responsible and supervising provider and the NNP (employed by the group or hospital) is acting as a member of the team of providers the physician supervises.

Physician Supervision

Current Procedural Terminology (*CPT*®) states that codes **99468–99476** (initial and subsequent inpatient neonatal and pediatric critical care, per day, for the evaluation and management of a critically ill neonate or child through 5 years of age) are used to report services provided by a physician directing the inpatient care of a critically ill neonate or young child. *Current Procedural Terminology* makes clear that the reporting provider is not required to maintain 24-hour, in-hospital physical presence. *Current Procedural Terminology* notes that the physician or other reporting provider must be physically present and at bedside at some time during the 24-hour period to examine the patient and review and direct the patient's care with the health care team. The physician must be readily available to the health care team if needed but does not have to provide 24-hour, in-house coverage. One provider reports the appropriate code only once per day, even though multiple providers may have interacted with the patient during the 24-hour global period (eg, on-call physician, NNP).

Medical Record Documentation

The medical record serves the dual purpose of communicating the medical status and progress of the patient and documenting the work of the reporting provider.

Based on the information presented previously, it is the suggestion of the American Academy of Pediatrics Committee on Coding and Nomenclature that the medical record documentation by the reporting physician or NPP supporting critical care codes should contain at a minimum

- Documentation of the critical status of the infant or child (This is not to be inferred.)
- Documentation of the *bedside* direction and supervision of all aspects of care
- Review of pertinent historical information and verification of significant physical findings through a medically indicated, focused patient examination
- Documentation of all services provided by members of the care team and discussion and direction of the ongoing therapy and plan of care for the patient
- Additional documentation of any major change in patient course requiring significant hands-on intervention by the reporting provider

The following are *not* required of the reporting physician or NPP:
- Twenty-four–hour presence in the facility or bedside
- Two or more documented notes a day
- Personally ordering all tests, medications, and therapies
- Performing all or any of the bundled procedures
- Documenting a daily comprehensive physical examination
- Documenting stable or unstable status so long as the infant or child meets critical care criteria

Each patient has a different level of illness(es), grouping of diagnoses, and medical and socioeconomic problems. The following are only examples of notes and should not be interpreted as requirements in every note for each patient:

A. The following note represents a sample attestation that could be appended to a resident or fellow's progress note:

"I have reviewed the resident's progress note and the baby has been seen and examined by me. He continues to be critically ill with respiratory failure requiring mechanical ventilation. I concur with the resident's evaluation and findings, though I did not appreciate abdominal tenderness on examination. I have discussed and agreed on a plan of care with the resident."

Global Per Diem Critical Care Codes: Direct Supervision and Reporting Guidelines

B. The following 2 paragraphs represent a single sample documentation that a reporting physician might write when care is delivered by an NNP and physician team. This note could be appended by the reporting physician to the NNP documentation or written as separate physician documentation.

"(Name) has been seen and examined by me on bedside rounds. The interval history, laboratory findings, and physical examination of the patient have been reviewed with members of the neonatal team. The notes have been reviewed. All aspects of care have been discussed, and I have agreed on an assessment and plan for the day with the care team.

"(Name) continues to be critically ill, requiring high-frequency jet ventilation. On examination, her breath sounds are coarse but equal, there is no heart murmur, and the abdomen is soft and non-tender. Her oxygen requirements have been at 100% for the past 12 hours. She remains on antibiotics for *Proteus* sepsis. At the recommendation of infectious disease, we have changed her antibiotic coverage to cefotaxime and gentamicin. Her blood pressure is acceptable today, but her urine output is only at 1 mL/kg/h. We are watching this closely and may need to restart dopamine. She remains NPO and is on total parenteral nutrition."

Approach to Documentation

This information deals largely with neonatal care. However, the same coding and documentation principles apply for critical care services provided to all children through the age of 5 years. The guidelines provided in this statement represent clarification of documentation recommendations for this unique code set. They are intended to create clarity going forward for physicians and other parties as they incorporate this new guidance into their documentation processes. Physicians should structure their documentation such that on review of a medical record representing a physician-rendered per-day neonatal or pediatric critical care service, one should be able to discern the reporting physician's unique documentation in support of the physician's role in that patient's care. It is especially important that an electronic health record used in documenting these services be configured to uniquely identify the author of each entry and allow for timely response to requests for documentation substantiating billed services. It is equally as important to log out of the record when your documentation is complete.

Appendixes

Sample Appeal Letter: Well/Sick Same Day

Date:

Insurance Carrier Claims Review Department and address *or*
Insurance Carrier Medical Director and address
Dear:

RE: Claim #:

I am writing regarding the aforementioned claim and <u>(Insurance Carrier Name)'s</u> practice of bundling preventive medicine service codes and office/outpatient service codes. *Current Procedural Terminology* (*CPT®*) guidelines indicate that in certain cases, it is appropriate to report a preventive medicine service code (99381–99397) in conjunction with an office/outpatient service code (99201–99215) on the same date of service.

According to American Medical Association *CPT* guidelines, "If an abnormality(ies) is encountered or a preexisting problem is addressed in the process of performing a preventive medicine evaluation and management service, and if the problem/abnormality(ies) is significant enough to require additional work to perform the key components of a problem-oriented service, then the appropriate office/outpatient code should also be reported. Modifier 25 should be added to the office/outpatient code to indicate that a significant, separately identifiable evaluation and management service was provided by the same physician on the same day as the preventive medicine service. The appropriate preventive medicine service is additionally reported." These statements clearly indicate that a "well" and a "sick" visit should be recognized as separate services when reported on the same day.

Unfortunately, many carriers are not familiar with the *CPT* guidelines that allow for the reporting of 2 visits on the same day of service by use of modifier 25. Further, there are no diagnosis (*International Classification of Diseases, 10th Revision, Clinical Modification* [*ICD-10-CM*]) requirements tied to the use of modifier 25. In fact, "The descriptor for modifier 25 was revised to clarify that since the E/M service may be prompted by the symptom or condition for which the procedure and/or service was provided, different diagnoses are not required to report the E/M services on the same date" (*CPT Assistant.* May 2000;10[5]). This basic tenet of *CPT* coding underscores the fact that it is *inherently incorrect for carriers to place restrictions on the number, type, or order of diagnoses associated with the reporting of 2 visits on the same day.*

There are also some carriers that, through failure to recognize all services provided during a single patient session, *potentially increase the number of visits necessary to address a patient's concerns.* If a patient is seen for a preventive medicine visit and the physician discovers that the patient has symptoms of otitis media during the examination, clinical protocol and common sense would dictate that the physician take care of the well-child examination and the treatment of the otitis media during that single patient visit. Unfortunately, the fact that some carriers fail to fairly pay the physician for providing both services will motivate providers to address only the acute problem and have the patient/parent return at a later date for the preventive medicine visit. This situation is frustrating for everyone involved, especially for the insureds.

While there is no legal mandate requiring private carriers to adhere to the aforementioned *CPT* guidelines, it is considered a good-faith gesture for them to do so, given that the guidelines are the current standard within organized medicine. Because providers are clearly instructed that an office/outpatient "sick" visit cannot be reported unless it represents a significant, separately identifiable service beyond the preventive medicine service, carriers should feel confident that the reporting of 2 visits on a single date of service *will not occur unless it is justified.*

Enclosed is a copy of the original claim that was submitted with a request that you process payment as indicated on the claim. I look forward to receiving your response.

If you have any questions, please feel free to contact me at _____

Sincerely,

VI. Coding for Pediatrics 2019 *Resource List*

Coding for Pediatrics 2019 (*www.aap.org/cfp [access code AAPCFP24]*)

ICD-10-CM Pediatric Office Superbill

"The Business Case for Pricing Vaccines"

"2019 RBRVS: What Is It and How Does It Affect Pediatrics?"

"Gainsharing and Shared Savings"

AAP Coding Hotline

FAQ: Immunization Administration

Coding at the AAP (*https://aap.org/coding*)

Coding Calculator (https://www.aap.org/en-us/professional-resources/practice-transformation/getting-paid/Coding-at-the-AAP/Pages/Coding-Calculator.aspx)

AAP Pediatric Coding Webinars (https://www.aap.org/webinars/coding)

Oral Health Coding Fact Sheet for Primary Care Physicians (https://www.aap.org/en-us/Documents/coding_factsheet_oral_health.pdf)

What is Included in Preventive Medicine Encounters Template Letter

AAP Pediatric Coding Newsletter™ (*http://coding.aap.org [subscription required]*)

ICD-10-CM Collection (https://coding.solutions.aap.org/icd10.aspx)

"Reporting the National Drug Code: A Refresher" (August 2014) (https://coding.solutions.aap.org/article.aspx?articleid=1906527)

"The Surgical Package and Related Services" (May 2018) (https://coding.solutions.aap.org/article.aspx?articleid=2679119)

"Revisiting Modifier 25: Still Confused After All These Years" (February 2016) (https://coding.solutions.aap.org/article.aspx?articleid=2483202)

"When Are Modifiers Necessary?" (November 2016) (https://coding.solutions.aap.org/article.aspx?articleid=2571212)

"Back to Basics: The National Correct Coding Initiative" (March 2015) (https://coding.solutions.aap.org/article.aspx?articleid=2169307)

"Place of Service: Not Always Office" (April 2015) (https://coding.solutions.aap.org/article.aspx?articleid=2199612)

"Denials to Dollars: Resubmissions and Appeals" (August 2016) (https://coding.solutions.aap.org/article.aspx?articleid=2536856)

"What Does Your EHR Documentation Say?" (March 2017) (https://coding.solutions.aap.org/article.aspx?articleid=2606145)

Time-based reporting of evaluation and management services (multiple articles) (March 2016) (https://coding.solutions.aap.org/issues.aspx#issueid=935013)

"Coding for Special Services In and Out of the Office" (May 2018) (https://coding.solutions.aap.org/article.aspx?articleid=2679118)

"History in the Preventive Service" (June 2015) (https://coding.solutions.aap.org/article.aspx?articleid=2297658)

"Sports and Camp Physicals" (June 2017) (https://coding.solutions.aap.org/article.aspx?articleid=2629481)

"Preparing for Preparticipation Physical Evaluations" (July 2018) (https://coding.solutions.aap.org/article.aspx?articleid=2685958)

"National Drug Code Unit Errors Prompt Refund Requests" (December 2017) (https://coding.solutions.aap.org/article.aspx?articleid=2664489)

Payer Appeal Letters for Claims Denial (https://coding.solutions.aap.org/ss/resources.aspx)

Appendixes

"Reporting Terminated Procedural Services" (November 2014) (https://coding.solutions.aap.org/article. aspx?articleid=1921435)

"You Code It! Removal of Sutures" (March 2018) (https://coding.solutions.aap.org/article.aspx?articleid=2673748)

"You Code It! Removal of Sutures (Answer)" (March 2018) (https://coding.solutions.aap.org/article. aspx?articleid=2673749)

"Professional Component Services: More Than Codes" (July 2014) (https://coding.solutions.aap.org/article. aspx?articleid=1906541)

Chronic care management (multiple articles) (April 2017) (https://coding.solutions.aap.org/issues. aspx#issueid=936144)

"Transitional Care Management: Revisiting the Basics" (July 2017) (https://coding.solutions.aap.org/article. aspx?articleid=2634452)

"Lactation Counseling: Payer Policies Drive Coding" (April 2018) (https://coding.solutions.aap.org/article. aspx?articleid=2676731)

"Newborn Resuscitation and the T-piece" (May 2015) (https://coding.solutions.aap.org/article. aspx?articleid=2276791)

"Observation Care Services: *CPT* or Medicare" (August 2014) (https://coding.solutions.aap.org/article. aspx?articleid=1906524)

"Concurrent Care: A Refresher" (May 2014) (https://coding.solutions.aap.org/article.aspx?articleid=1906512)

"Coding for Bedside Ultrasound: No Hocus POCUS" (November 2015) (https://coding.solutions.aap.org/article. aspx?articleid=2464173)

"Starting Over With Moderate Sedation" (October 2016) (https://coding.solutions.aap.org/article. aspx?articleid=2555995)

"Beyond Moderate Sedation: Coding for Anesthesia Services" (April 2014) (https://coding.solutions.aap.org/article. aspx?articleid=1906504)

"Documentation of Deep Sedation Services (Online Exclusive)" (May 2014) (https://coding.solutions.aap.org/ article.aspx?articleid=1906514)

AAP News

"PPAAC: Chapter pediatric councils work with payers on medical home programs" (www.aappublications.org/ news/2016/03/18/PPAAC031816)

AAP Policy Statements

"A New Era in Quality Measurement: The Development and Application of Quality Measures" (http://pediatrics. aappublications.org/content/139/1/e20163442)

"Application of the Resource-Based Relative Value Scale System to Pediatrics" (http://pediatrics.aappublications. org/content/133/6/1158)

"Patient- and Family-Centered Care Coordination: A Framework for Integrating Care for Children and Youth Across Multiple Systems" (http://pediatrics.aappublications.org/content/early/2014/04/22/peds.2014-0318)

AAP Practice Transformation: Getting Paid (https://www.aap.org/en-us/professional-resources/ practice-transformation/getting-paid/Pages/default.aspx)

Private Payer Advocacy: Letters to Carriers

Oops We've Overpaid You: How to Respond to Payer Audits

Value Based Payment

Accountable Care Organizations (ACOs) and Pediatricians: Evaluation and Engagement

AAP Webinar Series on Alternative Payment Models

AAP Pediatric Councils

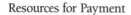

Resources for Payment

Hassle Factor Form Concerns with Payers (https://www.aap.org/en-us/professional-resources/practice-transformation/getting-paid/Pages/Hassle-Factor-Form-Concerns-with-Payers.aspx)

Managing the Practice: HIPAA Privacy and Security Compliance Manuals (https://www.aap.org/en-us/professional-resources/practice-transformation/managing-practice/Pages/HIPAA-Privacy-and-Security-Compliance-Manuals.aspx)

AAP Sections

State-specific information on coding for oral health services (https://www.aap.org/en-us/about-the-aap/Committees-Councils-Sections/Oral-Health/Map/Pages/State-Information-and-Resources-Map.aspx)

AMA *Current Procedural Terminology (CPT®)*

CPT (https://www.ama-assn.org/practice-management/cpt-current-procedural-terminology)

Category II codes (https://www.ama-assn.org/practice-management/cpt-category-ii-codes)

Category III codes (https://www.ama-assn.org/practice-management/cpt-category-iii-codes)

American Medical Association/Specialty Society Relative Value Scale Update Committee (RUC)

"Understanding the RUC Survey Instrument" (https://www.augs.org/assets/1/6/AMA_Understanding_the_RUC_Survey_Instrument.pdf)

Code Valuation and Payment RBRVS (https://www.aap.org/en-us/professional-resources/practice-transformation/getting-paid/Coding-at-the-AAP/Pages/Code-Valuation-and-PaymentRBRVS.aspx)

Care Coordination

Boston Children's Hospital Care Coordination Curriculum (www.childrenshospital.org/care-coordination-curriculum)

Centers for Medicare & Medicaid Services (CMS)

Multiple surgery indicators and adjustments—*Medicare Claims Processing Manual*, Chapter 12, Section 40.6 (www.cms.gov/Regulations-and-Guidance/Guidance/Manuals/Downloads/clm104c12.pdf)

Medicare Physician Fee Schedule (https://www.cms.gov/Medicare/Medicare-Fee-For-Service-Payment/PhysicianFeeSched/Index.html)

Place of Service Codes for Professional Claims (www.cms.gov/Medicare/Coding/place-of-service-codes/Place_of_Service_Code_Set.html)

Accountable Care Organizations (ACOs): General Information (https://innovation.cms.gov/initiatives/ACO/index.html)

Medicaid National Correct Coding Initiative (https://www.medicaid.gov/medicaid/program-integrity/ncci/index.html)

Program Integrity: Documentation Matters Toolkit (https://www.cms.gov/Medicare-Medicaid-Coordination/Fraud-Prevention/Medicaid-Integrity-Education/documentation-matters.html)

Incident-to services—*Medicare Claims Processing Manual*, Chapter 12, Section 30.6 (www.cms.gov/Regulations-and-Guidance/Guidance/Manuals/Downloads/clm104c12.pdf); *Medicare Benefit Policy Manual*, Chapter 15, Section 60 (http://cms.gov/manuals)

Claim Form and Billing Resources

Claim adjustment reason codes and remittance advice remark code descriptions—Washington Publishing Company (www.wpc-edi.com/reference)

Appendixes

Clinical Laboratory Improvement Amendments (CLIA)

CMS list of CLIA-waived procedures (by code) (www.cms.hhs.gov/CLIA)

CLIA - Clinical Laboratory Improvement Amendments—Currently Waived Analytes (www.accessdata.fda.gov/scripts/cdrh/cfdocs/cfClia/analyteswaived.cfm)

Health Insurance Portability and Accountability Act of 1996 (HIPAA)

Questions and Answers About HIPAA's Access Right (www.hhs.gov/hipaa/for-professionals/privacy/guidance/access/index.html#newlyreleasedfaqs)

Hypospadias Repair: Policy of the American Urological Association

"Pediatric Hypospadias Repair: A New Consensus Document on Coding" (https://www.auanet.org/Documents/practices-resources/coding-tips/Pediatric-Hypospadias-Repair.pdf)

International Classification of Diseases, 10th Revision, Clinical Modification (Centers for Disease Control and Prevention, National Center for Health Statistics)

ICD-10-CM code files (www.cdc.gov/nchs/icd/icd10cm.htm)

National Drug Codes

US Food and Drug Administration National Drug Code Directory (www.fda.gov/drugs/informationondrugs/ucm142438.htm)

Pediatrics (http://pediatrics.aappublications.org)

"Pediatric Accountable Care Organizations: Insight From Early Adopters" (February 2017) (http://pediatrics.aappublications.org/content/139/2/e20161840)

Preventive Services

AAP/Bright Futures "Recommendations for Preventive Pediatric Health Care" (insert) (www.aap.org/periodicityschedule)

Centers for Disease Control and Prevention Vaccines for Children Program (VFC) (www.cdc.gov/vaccines/programs/vfc/index.html)

Quality Measurement Information and Resources

US Department of Health and Human Services, Agency for Healthcare Research and Quality, National Quality Measures Clearinghouse (www.qualitymeasures.ahrq.gov)

CPT® Category II codes (https://www.ama-assn.org/practice-management/cpt-category-ii-codes)

PCPI (www.thepcpi.org)

Telemedicine

American Telemedicine Association State Policy Resource Center (https://www.americantelemed.org/policy-page/state-policy-resource-center)

Current listing of services covered under Medicare—*Medicare Claims Processing Manual*, Chapter 12 (https://www.cms.gov/Regulations-and-Guidance/Guidance/Manuals/downloads/clm104c12.pdf)

‖‖‖‖

Subject Index
Code Index

‖‖‖‖

Get hands-on, how-to help for your toughest coding and payment challenges with 2019 coding resources from the AAP!

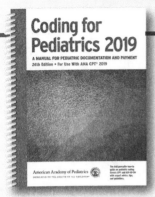

Coding for Pediatrics 2019
A Manual for Pediatric Documentation and Payment, 24th Edition

This year's completely updated 24th edition includes all changes in *CPT®* and *ICD-10-CM* codes for 2019 — complete with expert guidance for their application. The book's many clinical vignettes and examples, as well as the many coding pearls throughout, provide added guidance needed to ensure accuracy and payment.

Spiral-bound, 2018—590 pages
MA0875
Book ISBN 978-1-61002-203-3 · eBook ISBN 978-1-61002-204-0
Price: $134.95 *Member Price: $107.95*

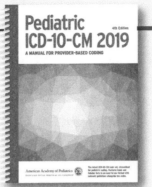

Pediatric ICD-10-CM 2019
A Manual for Provider-Based Coding, 4th Edition

Purpose-built to streamline the coding process, this important guide condenses the vast *ICD-10-CM* code set into a more manageable collection of only pediatric-centered guidelines and codes. Completely updated for 2019, including all new *ICD-10-CM* codes.

Spiral-bound, 2018—546 pages
MA0874
Book ISBN 978-1-61002-201-9 · eBook ISBN 978-1-61002-202-6
Price: $114.95 *Member Price: $91.95*

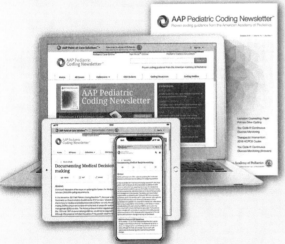

AAP Pediatric Coding Newsletter™

Streamline coding with a subscription to *AAP Pediatric Coding Newsletter*. Each issue is packed with time-saving how-to strategies to help your practice reduce errors, avoid over/under-coding, and get payment approved more quickly.

FOR INDIVIDUAL (SINGLE-USER)
ITEM#: SUB1005

Annual Subscription Price: $235
Member Price: $200

Subscribe for 2 years and save!
Price: $423 *Member Price: $360*

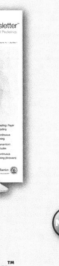

2019 Quick Reference Coding Tools for Pediatrics

NEW! **Quick Reference Guide to Coding Pediatric Preventive Services 2019**
MA0909
ISBN 978-1-61002-299-6
Price: $21.95 *Member Price: $16.95*

NEW! **Quick Reference Guide to Coding Pediatric Mental Health 2019**
MA0910
ISBN 978-1-61002-300-9
Price: $21.95 *Member Price: $16.95*

Pediatric Evaluation and Management Coding Card 2019
MA0877
ISBN 978-1-61002-207-1
Price: $21.95 *Member Price: $16.95*

Quick Reference Guide to Coding Pediatric Vaccines 2019
MA0876
ISBN 978-1-61002-205-7
Price: $21.95 *Member Price: $16.95*

Newborn Coding Decision Tool 2019
MA0878
ISBN 978-1-61002-209-5
Price: $21.95 Member Price: $16.95

Pediatric Office Superbill 2019
MA0879
ISBN 978-1-61002-211-8
Price: $21.95 *Member Price: $16.95*

Order at **shop.aap.org/books**, or call toll-free **888/227-1770** to order today!

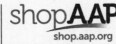 shop**AAP**
shop.aap.org

American Academy of Pediatrics
DEDICATED TO THE HEALTH OF ALL CHILDREN®

(continued)

19. Confirm initial screen was accomplished, verify results, and follow up, as appropriate. The Recommended Uniform Newborn Screening Panel (http://www.hrsa.gov/advisorycommittees/mchbadvisory/heritabledisorders/recommendedpanel/uniformscreeningpanel.pdf), as determined by The Secretary's Advisory Committee on Heritable Disorders in Newborns and Children, and state newborn screening laws/regulations (http://genes-r-us.uthscsa.edu/sites/genes-r-us/files/nbsdisorders.pdf) establish the criteria for and coverage of newborn screening procedures and programs.

20. Verify results as soon as possible, and follow up, as appropriate.

21. Confirm initial screening was accomplished, verify results, and follow up, as appropriate. See "Hyperbilirubinemia in the Newborn Infant ≥35 Weeks' Gestation: An Update With Clarifications" (http://pediatrics.aappublications.org/content/124/4/1193).

22. Screening for critical congenital heart disease using pulse oximetry should be performed in newborns, after 24 hours of age, before discharge from the hospital, per "Endorsement of Health and Human Services Recommendation for Pulse Oximetry Screening for Critical Congenital Heart Disease" (http://pediatrics.aappublications.org/content/129/1/190.full).

23. Schedules, per the AAP Committee on Infectious Diseases, are available at http://redbook.solutions.aap.org/SS/Immunization_Schedules.aspx. Every visit should be an opportunity to update and complete a child's immunizations.

24. See "Diagnosis and Prevention of Iron Deficiency and Iron-Deficiency Anemia in Infants and Young Children (0–3 Years of Age)" (http://pediatrics.aappublications.org/content/126/5/1040.full).

25. For children at risk of lead exposure, see "Low Level Lead Exposure Harms Children: A Renewed Call for Primary Prevention" (http://www.cdc.gov/nceh/lead/ACCLPP/Final_Document_030712.pdf).

26. Perform risk assessments or screenings as appropriate, based on universal screening requirements for patients with Medicaid or in high prevalence areas.

27. Tuberculosis testing per recommendations of the AAP Committee on Infectious Diseases, published in the current edition of the AAP *Red Book: Report of the Committee on Infectious Diseases*. Testing should be performed on recognition of high-risk factors.

28. See "Integrated Guidelines for Cardiovascular Health and Risk Reduction in Children and Adolescents" (https://www.nhlbi.nih.gov/health-topics/integrated-guidelines-for-cardiovascular-health-and-risk-reduction-in-children-and-adolescents).

29. Adolescents should be screened for sexually transmitted infections (STIs) per recommendations in the current edition of the AAP *Red Book: Report of the Committee on Infectious Diseases*.

30. Adolescents should be screened for HIV according to the USPSTF recommendations (http://www.uspreventiveservicestaskforce.org/uspstf/uspshivi.htm) once between the ages of 15 and 18, making every effort to preserve confidentiality of the adolescent. Those at increased risk of HIV infection, including those who are sexually active, participate in injection drug use, or are being tested for other STIs, should be tested for HIV and reassessed annually.

31. See USPSTF recommendations (http://www.uspreventiveservicestaskforce.org/uspstf/uspscerv.htm). Indications for pelvic examinations prior to age 21 are noted in "Gynecologic Examination for Adolescents in the Pediatric Office Setting" (http://pediatrics.aappublications.org/content/126/3/583.full).

32. Assess whether the child has a dental home. If no dental home is identified, perform a risk assessment (https://www.aap.org/RiskAssessmentTool) and refer to a dental home. Recommend brushing with fluoride toothpaste in the proper dosage for age. See "Maintaining and Improving the Oral Health of Young Children" (http://pediatrics.aappublications.org/content/134/6/1224).

33. Perform a risk assessment (https://www.aap.org/RiskAssessmentTool). See "Maintaining and Improving the Oral Health of Young Children" (http://pediatrics.aappublications.org/content/134/6/1224).

34. See USPSTF recommendations (http://www.uspreventiveservicestaskforce.org/uspstf/uspsdnch.htm). Once teeth are present, fluoride varnish may be applied to all children every 3–6 months in the primary care or dental office. Indications for fluoride use are noted in "Fluoride Use in Caries Prevention in the Primary Care Setting" (http://pediatrics.aappublications.org/content/134/3/626).

35. If primary water source is deficient in fluoride, consider oral fluoride supplementation. See "Fluoride Use in Caries Prevention in the Primary Care Setting" (http://pediatrics.aappublications.org/content/134/3/626).

Summary of Changes Made to the
Bright Futures/AAP Recommendations for Preventive Pediatric Health Care
(Periodicity Schedule)

This schedule reflects changes approved in February 2017 and published in April 2017.
For updates, visit www.aap.org/periodicityschedule.
For further information, see the *Bright Futures Guidelines*, 4th Edition, *Evidence and Rationale chapter* (https://brightfutures.aap.org/Bright%20Futures%20Documents/BF4_Evidence_Rationale.pdf).

CHANGES MADE IN FEBRUARY 2017

HEARING

- Timing and follow-up of the screening recommendations for hearing during the infancy visits have been delineated. Adolescent risk assessment has changed to screening once during each time period.

- Footnote 8 has been updated to read as follows: "Confirm initial screen was completed, verify results, and follow up, as appropriate. Newborns should be screened, per 'Year 2007 Position Statement: Principles and Guidelines for Early Hearing Detection and Intervention Programs' (http://pediatrics.aappublications.org/content/120/4/898.full)."

- Footnote 9 has been added to read as follows: "Verify results as soon as possible, and follow up, as appropriate."

- Footnote 10 has been added to read as follows: "Screen with audiometry including 6,000 and 8,000 Hz high frequencies once between 11 and 14 years, once between 15 and 17 years, and once between 18 and 21 years. See 'The Sensitivity of Adolescent Hearing Screens Significantly Improves by Adding High Frequencies' (http://www.jahonline.org/article/S1054-139X(16)00048-3/fulltext)."

PSYCHOSOCIAL/BEHAVIORAL ASSESSMENT

- Footnote 13 has been added to read as follows: "This assessment should be family centered and may include an assessment of child social-emotional health, caregiver depression, and social determinants of health. See 'Promoting Optimal Development: Screening for Behavioral and Emotional Problems' (http://pediatrics.aappublications.org/content/135/2/384) and 'Poverty and Child Health in the United States' (http://pediatrics.aappublications.org/content/137/4/e20160339)."

TOBACCO, ALCOHOL, OR DRUG USE ASSESSMENT

- The header was updated to be consistent with recommendations.

DEPRESSION SCREENING

- Adolescent depression screening begins routinely at 12 years of age (to be consistent with recommendations of the US Preventive Services Task Force [USPSTF]).

MATERNAL DEPRESSION SCREENING

- Screening for maternal depression at 1-, 2-, 4-, and 6-month visits has been added.

- Footnote 16 was added to read as follows: "Screening should occur per 'Incorporating Recognition and Management of Perinatal and Postpartum Depression Into Pediatric Practice' (http://pediatrics.aappublications.org/content/126/5/1032)."

NEWBORN BLOOD

- Timing and follow-up of the newborn blood screening recommendations have been delineated.

- Footnote 19 has been updated to read as follows: "Confirm initial screen was accomplished, verify results, and follow up, as appropriate. The Recommended Uniform Newborn Screening Panel (http://www.hrsa.gov/advisorycommittees/mchbadvisory/heritabledisorders/recommendedpanel/uniformscreeningpanel.pdf), as determined by The Secretary's Advisory Committee on Heritable Disorders in Newborns and Children, and state newborn screening laws/regulations (http://genes-r-us.uthscsa.edu/sites/genes-r-us/files/nbsdisorders.pdf) establish the criteria for and coverage of newborn screening procedures and programs."

- Footnote 20 has been added to read as follows: "Verify results as soon as possible, and follow up, as appropriate."

NEWBORN BILIRUBIN

- Screening for bilirubin concentration at the newborn visit has been added.

- Footnote 21 has been added to read as follows: "Confirm initial screening was accomplished, verify results, and follow up, as appropriate. See 'Hyperbilirubinemia in the Newborn Infant ≥35 Weeks' Gestation: An Update With Clarifications' (http://pediatrics.aappublications.org/content/124/4/1193)."

DYSLIPIDEMIA

- Screening for dyslipidemia has been updated to occur once between 9 and 11 years of age, and once between 17 and 21 years of age (to be consistent with guidelines of the National Heart, Lung, and Blood Institute).

SEXUALLY TRANSMITTED INFECTIONS

- Footnote 29 has been updated to read as follows: "Adolescents should be screened for sexually transmitted infections (STIs) per recommendations in the current edition of the AAP *Red Book: Report of the Committee on Infectious Diseases*."

HIV

- A subheading has been added for the HIV universal recommendation to avoid confusion with STIs selective screening recommendation.

- Screening for HIV has been updated to occur once between 15 and 18 years of age (to be consistent with recommendations of the USPSTF).

- Footnote 30 has been added to read as follows: "Adolescents should be screened for HIV according to the USPSTF recommendations (http://www.uspreventiveservicestaskforce.org/uspstf/uspshivi.htm) once between the ages of 15 and 18, making every effort to preserve confidentiality of the adolescent. Those at increased risk of HIV infection, including those who are sexually active, participate in injection drug use, or are being tested for other STIs, should be tested for HIV and reassessed annually."

ORAL HEALTH

- Assessing for a dental home has been updated to occur at the 12-month and 18-month through 6-year visits. A subheading has been added for fluoride supplementation, with a recommendation from the 6-month through 12-month and 18-month through 16-year visits.

- Footnote 32 has been updated to read as follows: "Assess whether the child has a dental home. If no dental home is identified, perform a risk assessment (https://www.aap.org/RiskAssessmentTool) and refer to a dental home. Recommend brushing with fluoride toothpaste in the proper dosage for age. See 'Maintaining and Improving the Oral Health of Young Children' (http://pediatrics.aappublications.org/content/134/6/1224)."

- Footnote 33 has been updated to read as follows: "Perform a risk assessment (https://www.aap.org/RiskAssessmentTool). See 'Maintaining and Improving the Oral Health of Young Children' (http://pediatrics.aappublications.org/content/134/6/1224)."

- Footnote 35 has been added to read as follows: "If primary water source is deficient in fluoride, consider oral fluoride supplementation. See 'Fluoride Use in Caries Prevention in the Primary Care Setting' (http://pediatrics.aappublications.org/content/134/3/626)."